Every Decker book is accompanied by a CD-ROM.

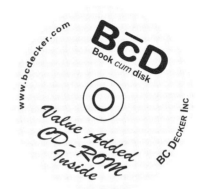

The disk appears in the front of each copy, in its own sealed jacket. Affixed to the front of the book will be a distinctive BcD sticker **"Book *cum* disk"**.

The disk contains the complete text and illustrations of the book, in fully searchable PDF files. The book and disk will be sold *only* as a package; neither will be available independently, and no prices will be available for the items individually.

BC Decker Inc is committed to providing high quality electronic publications that will compliment traditional information and learning methods.

We trust you will find the Book/CD Package invaluable and invite your comments and suggestions.

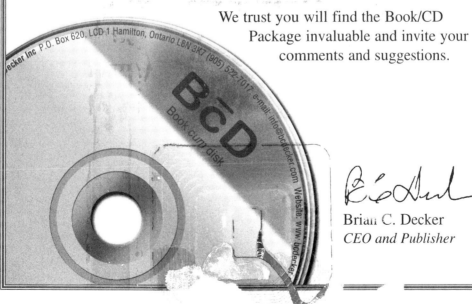

Brian C. Decker
CEO and Publisher

American Cancer Society
Atlas of
Clinical Oncology

Published

Blumgart, Fong, Jarnagin	*Hepatobiliary Cancer (2001)*
Cameron	*Pancreatic Cancer (2001)*
Char	*Tumors of the Eye and Ocular Adnexa (2001)*
Silverman	*Oral Cancer (1998)*
Sober, Haluska	*Skin Cancer (2001)*
Wiernik	*Adult Leukemias (2001)*
Willett	*Cancer of the Lower Gastrointestinal Tract (2001)*
Winchester, Winchester	*Breast Cancer (2000)*

Forthcoming

Carroll, Grossfeld, Reese	*Prostate Cancer (2001)*
Clark, Duh, Jahan, Perrier	*Endocrine Tumors (2002)*
Droller	*Urothelial Cancer (2002)*
Eifel, Levenback	*Cancer of the Female Lower Genital Tract (2001)*
Fuller	*Uterine and Endometrial Cancer (2003)*
Ginsberg	*Lung Cancer (2001)*
Grossbard	*Malignant Lymphomas (2001)*
Ozols	*Ovarian Cancer (2002)*
Pollock	*Soft Tissue Sarcomas (2001)*
Posner, Vokes, Weichselbaum	*Cancer of the Upper Gastrointestinal Tract (2001)*
Prados	*Brain Cancer (2001)*
Raghavan	*Germ Cell Tumors (2002)*
Shah	*Head and Neck Cancer (2001)*
Steele, Richie	*Kidney Tumors (2003)*
Volberding	*Cancer in the Immunocompromised Host (2003)*
Yasko	*Bone Tumors (2002)*

American Cancer Society

Atlas of

Clinical Oncology

Editors

GLENN D. STEELE JR, MD
Geisinger Health System

THEODORE L. PHILLIPS, MD
University of California

BRUCE A. CHABNER, MD
Harvard Medical School

Managing Editor

TED S. GANSLER, MD, MBA
Director of Health Content, American Cancer Society

American Cancer Society

Atlas of
Clinical Oncology

Adult Leukemias

Peter H. Wiernik, MD

Professor of Medicine and Radiation Oncology
New York Medical College
Valhalla, New York
Director, Comprehensive Cancer Center
Our Lady of Mercy Medical Center
Bronx, New York

2001
BC Decker Inc
Hamilton • London

BC Decker Inc
20 Hughson Street South
P.O. Box 620, L.C.D. 1
Hamilton, Ontario L8N 3K7
Tel: 905-522-7017; 1-800-568-7281
Fax: 905-522-7839
E-mail: info@bcdecker.com
Website: www.bcdecker.com

ISBN 1–55009–111-5
Printed in Canada

Cover figure submitted by Dr. Weirnik for Chapter 9, Extramedullary Manifestations of Adult Leukemia.

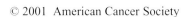

Sales and Distribution

United States
BC Decker Inc
P.O. Box 785
Lewiston, NY 14092-0785
Tel: 905-522-7017; 1-800-568-7281
Fax: 905-522-7839; 1-888-311-4987
E-mail: info@bcdecker.com
Website: www.bcdecker.com

Canada
BC Decker Inc
20 Hughson Street South
P.O. Box 620, L.C.D. 1
Hamilton, Ontario L8N 3K7
Tel: 905-522-7017; 1-800-568-7281
Fax: 905-522-7839
E-mail: info@bcdecker.com
Website: www.bcdecker.com

Foreign Rights
John Scott & Company
International Publishers' Agency
P.O. Box 878
Kimberton, PA 19442
Tel: 610-827-1640
Fax: 610-827-1671

U.K., Europe, Scandinavia, Middle East
Harcourt Publishers Limited
Customer Service Department
Foots Cray High Street
Sidcup, Kent
DA14 5HP, UK
Tel: 44 (0) 208 308 5760
Fax: 44 (0) 181 308 5702
E-mail: cservice@harcourt_brace.com

Australia, New Zealand
Harcourt Australia Pty. Limited
Customer Service Department
STM Division
Locked Bag 16
St. Peters, New South Wales, 2044
Australia
Tel: (02) 9517-8999
Fax: (02) 9517-2249
E-mail: stmp@harcourt.com.au
Website: www.harcourt.com.au

Japan
Igaku-Shoin Ltd.
Foreign Publications Department
3-24-17 Hongo
Bunkyo-ku,Tokyo, Japan 113-8719
Tel: 3 3817 5680
Fax: 3 3815 6776
E-mail: fd@igaku.shoin.co.jp

Singapore, Malaysia, Thailand, Philippines, Indonesia, Vietnam, Pacific Rim, Korea
Harcourt Asia Pte Limited
583 Orchard Road
#09/01, Forum
Singapore 238884
Tel: 65-737-3593
Fax: 65-753-2145

Notice: The authors and publisher have made every effort to ensure that the patient care recommended herein, including choice of drugs and drug dosages, is in accord with the accepted standard and practice at the time of publication. However, since research and regulation constantly change clinical standards, the reader is urged to check the product information sheet included in the package of each drug, which includes recommended doses, warnings, and contraindications. This is particularly important with new or infrequently used drugs.

Contributors

MIR YOUSUF ALI, MD
Northwestern University Medical School
Robert H. Lurie Comprehensive Cancer Center
Northwestern Memorial Hospital
Chicago, Illinois
Treatment of Adult Acute Leukemia

JANICE P. DUTCHER, MD
Professor of Medicine
New York Medical College
Our Lady of Mercy Cancer Center
Bronx, New York
Supportive Care

M. KATHRYN FOUCAR, MD
Professor, Department of Pathology
Health Sciences Center
University of New Mexico
Albuquerque, New Mexico
Morphology of Acute and Chronic Leukemia

MARSHALL HORWITZ, MD, PHD
Associate Professor
Department of Medicine
Division of Medical Genetics
University of Washington
Seattle, Washington
*Epidemiology and Genetics of Acute
 and Chronic Leukemia*

PIERRE LANEUVILLE, MD, FRCPC
Director, Division of Hematology
McGill University Health Centre
McGill University
Montreal, Quebec
*Moleceular Etiology and Pathogenesis
 of Leukemia*

HEATHER A. LEITCH, MD, PHD
Division of Medical Oncology
British Columbia Cancer Agency
University of British Columbia
Vancouver, British Columbia
*Molecular Etiology and Pathogenesis
 of Leukemia*

WILSON H. MILLER JR., MD, PHD
Lady Davis Institute
Jewish General Hospital
McGill University
Montreal, Quebec
*Molecular Etiology and Pathogenesis
 of Leukemia*

ELISABETH PAIETTA, PHD
Professor of Medicine
New York Medical College
Valhalla, New York
Our Lady of Mercy Cancer Center
Bronx, New York
Immunodiagnostics
Cytogenetics

PETER PAPENHAUSEN, PHD, FACMG
Fellow of the American College of
  Medical Genetics
National Director of Genetics
Laboratory Corporation of America in RTP,
  North Carolina
Research Triangle Park, North Carolina
Adjunct Associate Professor
Moffitt Cancer Center
Tampa, Florida
Cytogenetics

AARON P. RAPOPORT, MD
Assistant Professor
Greenebaum Cancer Center
University of Maryland School of Medicine
Baltimore, Maryland
Diagnosis

JACOB M. ROWE, MD
Professor
Technion Israel Institute of Technology
Rambam Medical Center
State of Israel, Ministry of Health
Haifa, Israel
Diagnosis

CLARENCE SARKODEE-ADOO, MD
Assistant Professor of Medicine
Greenebaum Cancer Center
University of Maryland School of Medicine
Baltimore, Maryland
Diagnosis

MARTIN S. TALLMAN, MD
Associate Professor of Medicine
Northwestern University Medical School
Robert H. Lurie Comprehensive Cancer Center
Northwestern Memorial Hospital
Chicago, Illinois
Treatment of Adult Acute Leukemia

PETER H. WIERNIK, MD
Professor of Medicine and Radiation Oncology
New York Medical College
Valhalla, New York
Director, Comprehensive Cancer Center
Our Lady of Mercy Medical Center
Bronx, New York
Extramedullary Leukemia
Complications of Treatment

Contents

Dedication

This book is dedicated to the more than 140 hematology and medical oncology fellows whom I have had the honor of mentoring over the past 30 years, especially those who have had successful careers in cancer treatment research: Joseph Aisner, James F. Bishop, Dean E. Brenner, Janice P. Dutcher, Mark R. Green, Rasim Gucalp, Michael J. O'Connell, Douglas D. Ross, John C. Ruckdeschel, Charles A. Schiffer, Joseph A. Sparano, David A. Van Echo, James C. Wade, Jan A. Walewski, and Howard J. Weinstein.

Preface

When I was a second-year medical student at the University of Virginia in 1962, the chairman of the Department of Medicine, the brilliant William Parson, presented a patient with acute myelocytic leukemia to us during one of his weekly professor rounds with students. The patient was a young man of 19 who was nervously smoking a cigarette as he sat up in bed to vomit blood, which was being lost at least as rapidly as it was being replaced. He was fully conscious and scared to death. He had been diagnosed about a week before we visited him, and in the hall Dr. Parson told us he would probably die of sepsis and hemorrhage within a few days and that there was nothing that could be done. I decided at that moment to spend the next 40 or 50 years learning all I could about the leukemias and to try my best to play some role in improving the outcome for future patients with those and other neoplasms.

I was fortunate to grow up in an era when the scientific method was beginning to be applied to cancer treatment research in an increasingly rigorous fashion. The great minds of those early days of cancer treatment research, especially Emil J. Freireich, James F. Holland, and Emil Frei III, were convinced early on that major understanding of the nature of leukemia and effective treatment for it would evolve during our lifetimes if the scientific method that they embraced prevailed in our clinics and our laboratories. They were right.

The great effort and expense expended over the last several decades studying the leukemias, which are relatively uncommon, not only rewarded us with a much better understanding of the nature of those diseases and more effective treatments for them, it also taught us lessons that, when applied to the study of the more common cancers, rewarded us even more.[1] Some of those lessons are: 1) medicine can cure cancer; 2) combinations of drugs with different mechanisms of action and different toxicities are usually more effective cancer treatments than single agents; 3) treatment of minimal residual disease enhances the cure rate; 4) the complete natural history of a given neoplasm is not fully appreciated until there is an effective treatment that prolongs survival for that neoplasm; 5) supportive care improvements allow patients to survive long enough to receive adequate cancer treatment to which they are more likely to respond; 6) adverse prognostic factors diminish in importance after effective cancer therapy is developed; and 7) one can learn to cure neoplasms of unknown etiology by prospective clinical trials.

This small book summarizes advances in leukemia biology and treatment primarily for those physicians who have recently embarked on a mission to tackle the remaining obstacles to cure and for those who wish to apply the most successful treatments currently available.

I wish to thank the publisher, Mr. Brian C. Decker, for the opportunity to edit this book, and Christina Philips, Production Editor at BC Decker, Inc, who through gentle persuasion and expert advice and assistance is responsible for the completion of this effort within a reasonable period of time.

Peter H. Wiernik, MD
June, 2001

REFERENCE

Wiernik PH. Lessons learned about treatment of the more common neoplasms from the study of acute leukemia. Cancer J Sci Am 1996;2:356-359.

Epidemiology and Genetics of Acute and Chronic Leukemia

MARSHALL HORWITZ, MD, PhD

The state of knowledge of the ultimate origins of leukemia has reached a paradox. The molecular genetic mechanisms in the leukemic cell are now reasonably well defined and adhere to a paradigm in which somatic mutation disrupts the function of key genes involved in the regulation of cellular growth, the maintenance of the differentiated hematopoietic cellular phenotype, or the fidelity of the genome. Reasonably uniform access to medical care in industrialized nations and public health surveillance data provide for accurate forecasts of the numbers, types, and demographic distribution of leukemia in any given year. Thus, it can be said with high reliability that about 31,000 Americans will develop leukemia within the next 12 months.[1] We cannot name who these unfortunate individuals will be or identify what it is, if anything, that links the actions of their daily lives to the molecular pathogenesis of the disease. But it is not for want of trying; as of this writing, a Web-based PubMed search of the literature for "leukemia epidemiology" lists more than 11,000 publications. Thus, a nearly endless roster of potential agents has been scrutinized over the years for possible associations with leukemia. To make a long story short, there are only four unambiguously known causes of leukemia: ionizing radiation, benzene, chemotherapy, and some rare inherited syndromes (and even the literature on benzene may be subject to some indecision). Since most leukemic patients have neither of these factors in their history, further epidemiologic investigation seems warranted. Yet, the jury is still out on whether a multitude of other exposures, ranging from such unlikely culprits as maternal hot dog consumption to electromagnetic fields, are significant factors in conferring leukemia risk. The tentative conclusion can only be that if there are unidentified risk factors, they must be either so exceptionally rare so as to avoid detection for so long or they must be so common that they have escaped suspicion in spite of their ubiquity. This chapter will examine both tenants of this supposition and contrast it with the null hypothesis that the origins of leukemia result from failure of intrinsically error-prone mechanisms of the cell that are out of reach of the abuses and good intentions of our lifestyle.

INCIDENCE

The reported frequency of leukemia increased in the first half of the twentieth century, began slowing in its rate of acceleration in the 1940s, and has stabilized for the last 30 or so years.[2] Improved diagnostic technology presumably accounts for this secular trend. There has been recent controversy as to whether childhood leukemia has become more common. Data from the National Cancer Institute SEER program, which tracks cancer in 14 percent of the United States population, however, have found relatively stable rates of leukemia and other pediatric cancers since the 1980s, while allowing for diagnostic improvements and reporting changes.[3]

There are approximately 31,500 total cases of leukemia in the United States per year (Figure 1–1). The male to female ratio is 1.28:1. Acute myelogenous leukemia (AML) comprises 32 percent of the

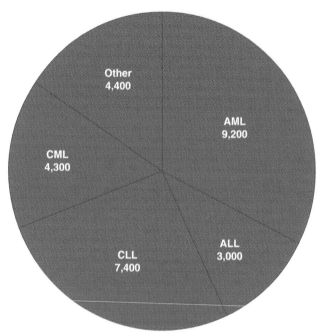

Figure 1–1. Incidence of leukemia in the United States projected for 2001 (from Parker et al.[1]). Numbers of cases indicated are for both sexes, of all ages.

total, followed by chronic lymphocytic leukemia (CLL) at 26 percent of the total, chronic myelocytic leukemia (CML) with 15 percent, and acute lymphoblastic leukemia (ALL) encompassing 11 percent; the remainder is unclassified.

Acute lymphoblastic leukemia is the predominant form of leukemia among children, occurring at an approximate 3:1 ratio in comparison to AML among the Caucasian population of most Western nations.[4] The peak incidence occurs between the ages of 2 and 5 years[5] but then begins to exponentially increase in frequency beginning from the mid to late adult years.

The incidence of AML remains generally constant through childhood and the early adult years and then begins to exponentially increase in frequency from about the age of 30 years. Myelodysplastic syndrome (MDS) appears to linearly increase in frequency from about the age of 50 years, before which it is uncommon. About 30 percent of patients with MDS progress to AML, varying from 8 percent for the refractory anemia (RA) subtype to 60 percent for the RA with excess blasts in transformation (RAEB-t) form.[6]

Chronic myelocytic leukemia occurs mainly among middle-aged adults, although juvenile forms

can be a feature of the neurofibromatosis I tumor suppressor gene syndrome (see below).

Chronic lymphocytic leukemia tends to be a disease of older men and, overall, is about twice as common among men.

ENVIRONMENTAL FACTORS

Clusters

The repeated observation of "clustering" of cases of leukemia and lymphoma within a geographic region, school, household, or place of employment has prompted the investigation of potential causative environmental and infectious agents. Perhaps the best known of these was a cluster of mostly childhood ALL in Woburn, Massachusetts, thought by some residents to be associated with local toxic waste dumps,[7] which resulted in a legal case and was the subject of a book[7] and later a movie starring John Travolta. With a few notable exceptions, the results of most such investigations have proven inconclusive.

Among the most imaginative methods to examine potential clusters of leukemia is a study[8] based on the "small-world" observation that two strangers in a chance encounter can often identify a common "friend of a friend" that links them socially through a circle of acquaintances (used as the basis for the party game "Six Degrees of Kevin Bacon"). For example, almost any two Americans can be linked by an average of no more than five to seven intermediaries.[9] Employing this seldom-used technique, social networks of 13,409 residents, including 42 patients with leukemia and lymphoma, of Orleans County, New York, between 1967 and 1972, were elaborated. The study found no significant difference for direct acquaintanceship between patients with leukemia or lymphoma compared to the background population; however, the authors found that leukemia or lymphoma patients could be linked, on average, through a smaller number of acquaintances than the population at large and that this remained significant even when controlling for socioeconomic status (although there was no independent control for either race or apparent exclusion of medical personnel from the acquaintance network).

Blood-borne Factors

Leukemic blood and bone marrow have at times been deliberately transfused into healthy subjects in an attempt to transfer leukemia.[10–13] Such bizarre experiments remain irreproducible in the presently enlightened era of ethical safeguards on human experimentation. Nevertheless, multiple attempts to transmit leukemia all failed, even with follow-up periods for as long as several years. Surveillance studies of blood transfusion recipients from donors later found to be leukemic have also failed to show leukemia transmission.[14,15] Presumably, immunologic barriers would account for a host versus leukemia response that would prevent transmission of leukemia between two histoincompatible individuals. These studies would also seem to speak for a relative scarcity, or at least establish a long period of latency, of infectious factors capable of causing leukemia, for blood-borne viruses should also have been transmitted through such experimentation.

Human T-Cell Leukemia Viruses 1 and 2

An exception to viral etiologies of leukemia is human T-cell leukemia virus 1 (HTLV-1). Human T-cell leukemia virus 1[16] is endemic to southwest Japan, the Caribbean basin, parts of Central Africa, and other parts of the world. Chronic HTLV-1 infection is associated with a form of adult T-cell leukemia/lymphoma (ATL). Human T-cell leukemia virus 1 also appears to be responsible for a neurodegenerative disorder, tropical spastic paraparesis. Breast-feeding is a likely means of vertical transmission of the virus. Other routes of infection are through sexual activity and exchange of blood products.

About 2 to 5 percent of HTLV-1 infected individuals will develop ATL, with a latency period thought to be between 20 and 30 years duration. Human T-cell leukemia virus 1 causes four different types of hematopoietic malignancy. About 60 percent of patients develop acute ATL, clinically characterized by a short prodrome, rapid course with poor prognosis (median survival of 6 months), lymphocytosis, and skin and pulmonary involvement. About 20 percent of HTLV-1–associated ATL is of the lymphomatous type, in which lymphadenopathy is a more prominent feature than the circulating proliferation of lymphocytes. Chronic and smoldering forms of ATL are less common. All of these subtypes represent monoclonal proliferations of CD4+ T cells arising from clonal proviral integration events and clonal T-cell receptor gene rearrangements.

Human T-cell leukemia virus 2 was first isolated from a patient with a rare T-cell variant of the—usually B cell in origin—hairy cell leukemia. However, conclusive evidence that HTLV-2 is a consistent cause of hematopoietic neoplasia remains elusive.

CHEMICAL CARCINOGENS

Benzene

Benzene is the only nontherapeutic chemical agent for which there is persuasive evidence that it is a cause of leukemia.[17,18] Its exposure is a well-recognized cause of aplastic anemia. The association with leukemiagenesis is strongest for AML, but there is correlation with MDS and ALL. The evidence draws on numerous anecdotal reports, first observed in the Italian rotogravure and shoe industries in the 1920s and 1930s, as well as systematic occupational surveys. The latency period between exposure and development of leukemia has ranged from 2 to 20 or more years. Corroborating evidence comes from animal studies, many of which demonstrate (not always reproducibly) leukemia, lymphoma, and solid tumors on benzene exposure.

Tobacco

Cigarette smoking has been consistently associated with a small (about 30 to 50%) but not definitive elevation in risk for AML in a number of studies.[18]

Ionizing Radiation

Exposure to ionizing radiation can cause leukemia.[19] The earliest evidence linking leukemia to ionizing radiation comes from occupational exposures, including among radiologists and radium dial painters in the early parts of the twentieth century. The strongest evidence linking radiation to leukemia is found in survivors of the atomic bombings of Hiroshima and Nagasaki in 1945. All forms of leukemia except for CLL are elevated in this population. The effects of exposure began to show up as early as 1.5 years following the blasts, reached a peak at 6 to 7 years following exposure, and returned to baseline levels by around 1970. The minimum exposure associated with leukemia is in the order of 20 to 50 cGy. It is difficult to determine with certainty whether levels of exposure lower than this in the Japanese survivor population are also associated with leukemia or what may be the potential shape of the dose-response curve in this group.

A variety of medical exposures to ionizing radiation have proven to elevate leukemia risk. Among the most carefully documented are studies of individuals receiving radiation treatment for ankylosing spondylitis from 1935 through 1954[20] in the United Kingdom. The exposures ranged between 100 and 3,000 cGy. Leukemia incidence, mostly acute, began to increase within 2 years of exposure, reached a peak (of a greater than 10-fold relative risk) at 3 to 5 years following exposure, and returned to baseline values after 18 years. Individuals exposed to external beam radiation used in the treatment of Hodgkin's and non-Hodgkin's lymphoma and breast cancer also demonstrate an increased risk of leukemia, although the contributions from concomitant chemotherapy are often difficult to differentiate.[19]

TREATMENT-RELATED LEUKEMIA

About 6 percent of AML and 2.3 percent of ALL appear secondary to treatment of a prior malignancy with cytotoxic chemotherapy or therapeutic irradiation.[6,21] Treatment-related leukemia is a significant complication of Hodgkin's and non-Hodgkin's lymphoma, myeloma, breast cancer, ovarian cancer, testicular carcinoma, and polycythemia. The features of AML differ depending on the type of chemotherapy agent employed (alkylating agent versus topoisomerase II inhibitor). Acute myelogenous leukemia occurring in individuals exposed to alkylating agents is similar to AML arising in patients with antecedent MDS in that both demonstrate a preleukemic phase, trilineage dysplasia, frequent cytogenetic abnormality of chromosomes 5 and 7, and a poor prognosis. In contrast, in individuals exposed to topoisomerase inhibitors, the AML is

usually not preceded by a preleukemic phase, and there are frequent balanced translocations involving chromosome 11q23 and often a broad distribution of cytogenetic abnormalities within a single patient.

The relative risk for developing secondary AML following treatment can be estimated from a recent large study registering 3,865 Italian patients with acute leukemia from the mid 1990s.[21] Two hundred patients were identified in which leukemia was the second malignancy. The patients were divided as to whether their first malignancy was treated with chemotherapy and/or radiation therapy (about two-thirds of the population) versus surgery without either chemotherapy or radiation therapy (about one-third of the population). The inference of this study is that chemotherapy and/or radiation therapy doubles the risk for treatment-related leukemia, but, surprisingly, there is a significant elevation in risk for AML and ALL among individuals with a prior malignancy who were not exposed to these therapies. An unusual elevation in the frequency of M3 AML was also reported in this study. One interpretation of these results is that there is an increased predisposition to leukemia among all cancer patients, presumably as a result of an environmental or genetic effect.

MATERNAL FACTORS

Maternal-Fetal Transmission

At least four potential cases of maternal to fetal prenatal transmission of leukemia have been reported, including CML, AML, and ALL.[22–25] In neither of the families were other individuals affected with leukemia. Clonal markers were not examined in any study. Potential etiologies for this phenomenon would include inheritance, transplacental metastasis of leukemia, or coincidence. There are another five instances of maternal leukemia cells metastatic to the placenta but without fetal transmission.[26] Maternal transmission of leukemia remains a rare event, given that over 400 occurrences of leukemia during pregnancy have been documented.[27] Additionally, long-term follow-up of 17 children between the ages of 4 to 22 years born to mothers with acute leukemia treated with chemotherapy during pregnancy documented normal growth and development; none had leukemia or hematologic abnormality peripherally or on bone marrow examination.[28] Undoubtedly, even greater numbers of women of child-bearing age have had incipient leukemia during pregnancy or developed leukemia without transmitting it to their children. Once again, this observation would seem to point away from the presence of infectious agents and environmental factors that might be common to both mother and fetus.

Advanced Maternal Age

Some older studies have associated advanced maternal age with an approximately 50 percent increased risk for leukemia development in childhood.[29,30] Advanced maternal age is associated with risk for Down syndrome, itself having a higher incidence of leukemia, but the risk remained even after correction for cases of Down syndrome. As the childhood leukemia cases have also been linked to a higher incidence of minor congenital malformations,[31] it is possible that such studies point to occult cytogenetic effects that could predispose to leukemia. More recent studies, however, have failed to confirm an association between maternal age and childhood leukemia.[32,33]

Birth Order

An inverse association between birth order and risk for childhood leukemia has been documented.[34,35] This observation has been taken as evidence for a hypothesis that delayed exposure to infection may increase the risk for leukemia, particularly ALL. An alternative explanation is that lower birth orders can only be achieved in couples with high fecundity and that lower fecundity may be associated with occult cytogenetic factors.

Breast-feeding

A recent case-control study found that breast-feeding was associated with a reduced risk for leukemia,[36] although the findings were of borderline statistical significance. A protective effect against Hodgkin's disease and lymphoma has been suggested from prior smaller studies. Such findings, if proven reliable, could indicate that the immune-modulating effects of breast-feeding could somehow relate to leukemia vulnerability. A study from the same group and along the same lines addressed potential effects of vaccination and childhood leukemia[37] and found no association, although a trend linking the *Haemophilus influenzae* type B (Hib) vaccine and pediatric ALL was suggested.

ETHNIC AND GEOGRAPHIC DIFFERENCES

A variety of data have been used to develop evidence that the risk for leukemia varies across racial and geographic boundaries.

Hispanics

An excess of M3 AML (acute promyelocytic leukemia) occurs among some Latino populations. In the Los Angeles area in the 1980s and 1990s, M3 was 2.9 to 5.8 times more common among patients identified as Hispanic compared to non-Hispanic individuals.[38] A higher proportion of M3 AML was noted for Madrid.[39] These observations are difficult to interpret in light of the cultural and ethnic heterogeneity between European and American Hispanic populations.[40] An elevated rate of secondary AML was found among children of Mexican ancestry who were treated for ALL.[40]

Asians

CLL appears to be rare in Japan, China, and Korea and among Japanese and Chinese Americans.[41,42] To differentiate between genetic and environmental factors, a study of Japanese immigrants to the United States stratified occurrence by generation and found no significant difference among those born in Japan compared to those born and raised in America,[43] in contrast to atherosclerotic vascular disease and breast cancer, which tends to normalize with adoption of Western lifestyles.

African Americans

A reduced frequency of ALL among African Americans has been noted. In the 1950s, the differences were reasonably attributed to under-reporting and reduced access to care.[44] Nevertheless, the differences have persisted at about a two-fold level at least through the late 1980s[45] and are greatest for early childhood ALL.[4] Acute leukemia is particularly less common among elderly African Americans compared to Caucasians.[46] As multiple myeloma is approximately two-fold more common among African Americans[47] and occurs among the same-aged population, it is unlikely that the rate differences are an artifact of diagnosis and reporting. The disparity in childhood ALL between Caucasians and African Americans has normalized somewhat in recent years, and some have argued that this speaks for an environmental factor that may equate with socioeconomic status.[48] Two such environmental factors that have been entertained include diagnostic x-rays and a delayed exposure to early childhood infections.

Jews

A number of studies have found a higher frequency (generally on the order of two-fold) of CLL, AML, and CML (generally in that order) among Jews of European ancestry (Ashkenazi) compared with those of Asian or Latin origin (Sephardic), in both the United States and Israel.[44,49,50] However, not all studies have appreciated differences in leukemia frequency between Jews and gentiles.[51,52] An anecdotal series suggested a high rate of treatment-related AML among Ashkenazi Jews with multiple myeloma.[53]

FAMILIAL CLUSTERING

Consanguinity

A higher than expected frequency of an illness among an inbred population often suggests autosomal-recessive inheritance or the presence of a major gene conferring risk for a complex disorder. Consanguinity has been addressed in two American and one Japanese communities. Among Hutterite children with ALL, an excess of parental consanguinity was observed.[54] In a Syrian Jewish community of New York that practiced consanguineous marital arrangements, a 30-fold excess of pediatric ALL was present.[55] In a study of 20 Japanese families in which there were two or more cases of all different types of leukemia, 10 (50%) of these families were consanguineous compared with a finding of consanguinity of 4.5 percent among the parents of 200 sporadic individuals with leukemia[56] and a much lower rate of consanguinity among the general Japanese population. Furthermore, the mean age of onset of leukemia was at a younger age among individuals in the consanguineous families. These studies among isolated populations suggest that there may be low-penetrance genes acting in a dosage-dependent manner to confer leukemia risks.

Twins

A time-honored approach to deciphering the causative role of genetic and environmental factors in the occurrence of a disease is to compare monozygous and dizygous twins. Given the rarity of leukemia, it was predicted in the 1960s that if leukemia were an independent event in monozygotic twins, then just a single concordant pair should appear in the United States over the next 200 or so years.[57] However, at least about 50 case reports of concordant monozygotic twins have become apparent since that time. The concordance rate for identical twins indicates that congenital factors confer leukemia risk.

In fact, the concordance rate for monozygous twins approaches 100 percent if one member of the pair develops leukemia prior to 12 months of age[58] but declines with advancing age.[59] The explanation for this phenomenon is now clear and points to somatic rather than constitutional genetic factors as being causative. Most of the reported pairs of monozygous twins with leukemia have identical cytogenetic and clonal markers.[60] These observations are compatible with a hypothesis[61] that leukemia results from somatic mutations beginning in utero in one twin. The leukemic cells most likely metastasize across the common placental circulation and are not rejected by the immunologically identical second twin. In fact, one recent study[61A] found that TEL-AML1 fusions in a pair of twins concordant for development of ALL at ages 2 and 5 years could be identified using reverse transcriptase-mediated polymerase chain reaction in routinely obtained neonatal blood spots, thereby proving that the translocation was present at birth and must have occurred congenitally. Moreover, this study found that the TEL-AML1 chromosomal translocation could be detected in these Guthrie blood spots in six of nine nontwin childern with ALL, the oldest of whom was 5 years. The interesting implication from this otherwise rare phenomenon is that it probably arises congenitally in most instances, emphasizing that maternal factors and exposures cannot easily be dismissed when evaluating the epidemiologic literature.

Proband Effects

So-called proband studies identify an individual with a particular illness and then determine if other members of the families face an elevated risk. Such studies can point to the presence of complex genetic factors whose influence might fall short of that expected for a single gene disorder.

Overall, there appears to be an elevated risk for any sort of hematopoietic malignancy among family members. There was a 3.62-fold relative risk for any type of hematopoietic malignancy among first- and second-degree relatives observed in a large Israeli population in the late 1980s.[62] The majority of malignancies found in relatives were of a different type than those occurring in the proband. The authors interpreted this as evidence of an inherited defect in the pluripotent hematopoietic stem cell.

Comprehensive studies of proband effects have been performed in Utah, where state cancer registries are linked to Mormon Church genealogic records.[63,64] Using data from 125,000 cancer patients from 1952 to 1966, the relative risk for the same type of malignancy among first-degree relatives of probands with leukemia was 5.69 for lymphocytic types and 2.97 for myeloid types.

Strong proband effects have also been observed in CLL. A relative risk of 6.57 among first-degree relatives of index patients with CLL was observed in a study of Baltimore patients with CLL diagnosed between 1969 and 1982.[65] A similar effect was found in a study of Serbian patients with CLL in the 1990s,[66] in which there was found to be no significant increase in risk for other types of cancer. It should be cautioned that proband effects cannot be easily isolated from environmental factors. In fact, one small study of patients with CLL observed sig-

nificant spousal concordance,[67] although of less magnitude than observed in first-degree relatives in other series.

Families Inheriting Leukemia through a Single Gene

A remarkably successful approach used to identify genes causing cancer (tumors suppressor and DNA repair genes in particular) is to identify the subset of families who inherit common forms of malignancy. This strategy has resulted in great advances in the understanding of cancers of the colon, breast, thyroid, skin, and other organs. Although rare, a number of families are known in which leukemia appears to be transmitted as a result of a highly penetrant single gene in Mendelian fashion. These families, in general, lack identifying features of established syndromes of which a risk for hematopoietic malignancy may be a component feature.

Such families could be under-reported. In the Utah cancer registry,[63] the relative risk for first-degree relatives of probands with breast and colorectal carcinoma was 1.83 and 2.67, respectively. This is lower than the risk observed for leukemia in this same population. Since now sizable minorities of all cases of breast and colorectal cancer are attributed to Mendelian inheritance, it is possible that single genes conferring risks for malignancy may be as common, or even more common, as a phenomenon for leukemia. Supportive evidence comes from surveys of leukemia incidence that are confined to a limited geographic distribution. For example, careful ascertainment of the families of probands with leukemia and lymphoma diagnosed in sparsely populated central Nebraska between 1958 and 1963 identifed 39 families from a total of 151 probands (25.8%) in which Mendelian transmission was suspected.[68]

In many of the reported families, the particular type of hematopoietic malignancy is constant among the different affected family members.

At least 14 families[60] have been reported with the probable autosomal-recessive inheritance of childhood-onset myelodysplasia. In these families, somatic loss of chromosome 7 (monosomy 7) is nearly invariant. Genetic studies have all but eliminated the possibility, however, that the responsible gene maps to chromosome 7.[69] In one sibship comprised of two affected brothers,[70] both had a constitutional inversion at chromosome 1p22-q23, potentially implicating a locus in this region.

A relatively large number of families are known to demonstrate autosomal-dominant transmission of AML and myelodysplasia.[60] Some of these families are exceptionally large; one Australian pedigree identified at least 17 individuals who have developed AML across five generations. In some of these families,[71] affected individuals have developed a variety of different subtypes of AML and myelodysplasia, indicating that the defective gene likely acts early in the course of differentiation of the hematopoietic stem cell. One of these families demonstrated weak evidence for linkage to chromosome 16q.[72] A subset of AML families, however, has been identified in which affected individuals specifically develop M6 erythroleukemia or its characteristic myelodysplastic precursor, "erythremic myelosis."[73,74]

An exceptional syndrome of AML in association with an aspirin-like platelet granule defect is known.[75] These families clinically present with a bleeding diathesis, mild to moderate thrombocytopenia, and morphologic and functional defects in platelet granules (Figure 1–2). Many of the affected individuals develop hematopoietic malignancy, AML being the most common, but also including lymphoid leukemia, lymphoma, and sarcoma. The gene was mapped to chromosome 21q using a genome-wide screen for linkage, and mutations were subsequently identified in *CBFA2* (AML1). The mutations are predicted to result in haploinsufficiency. It is too early to tell whether a "second hit" is required, as is the case with tumor suppressor gene mechanisms. *CBFA2* is among the most common site of acquired chromosome translocation in sporadic cases of leukemia.

Interestingly, heterozygous mutations of *CBFA2* were also detected at a high frequency among sporadic Japanese patients with AML and ALL.[76] This study did not differentiate between somatic and constitutional mutation. Therefore, it is possible that some heterozygous mutations of *CBFA2* could represent high-frequency, low-penetrance alleles for a gene conferring leukemia risk. Future studies of this gene should be enlightening.

A number of other families transmitting what would appear to be a single gene capable of causing each type of leukemia are known. (For an extensive review, see Horwitz.[60]) At least 17 families with apparent autosomal-dominant CLL have been reported. The affected individuals in these families tend to mirror the demographics of sporadic occurrence of CLL in that the majority of patients tend to be male, with the age of onset in the mid to late adult years. In still other families with multiple cases of CLL, the pattern of inheritance could also be consistent with autosomal-recessive inheritance.

At least eight families are described with the autosomal-dominant inheritance of ALL.

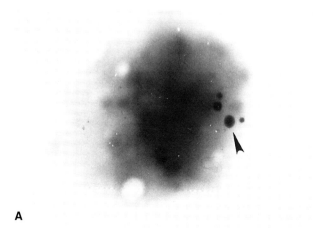
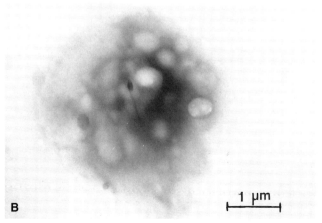

Figure 1–2. Characteristic dense platelet granule defects from a family with *CBFA2* mutations causing familial AML. Transmission electron micrographs of platelet whole mounts from a normal control (*A*) and affected member of a family (*B*). Calcium imparts an electron-dense property to human platelet dense granules, allowing them to be viewed directly by electron microscopy with no additional staining (*arrowhead*). Normal individuals have four to eight dense granules per platelets. The affected individual has no evident dense granules in this platelet. (Photographs courtesy of Dr. Sara Israels, Manitoba Institute of Cell Biology, University of Manitoba.)

Hairy cell leukemia is an uncommon chronic lymphoproliferative disorder of B cells. Somewhat surprisingly, at least eight families segregating hairy cell leukemia have been reported. In general, in most families in which there are multiple affected individuals, the leukemias tend to be all, or mostly, of the same type. Nevertheless, a few families have been reported in which different members developed different types of leukemia, crossing boundaries between myeloid and lymphoid cell types and acute versus chronic onset.[77] Some of this clinical heterogeneity, at least among the older reports, is probably the result of the less well-refined diagnostic capabilities of that era.

Nearly all autosomal-dominant leukemia families, with the possible exception of the families with the platelet granule defect now attributed to heterozygous mutation of *CBFA2*, demonstrate "anticipation."[78] Anticipation describes a declining age of onset or worsening severity of disease with each subsequent generation. In hereditary neurodegenerative illness, such as Huntington's disease and myotonic dystrophy, anticipation molecularly results from unstable trinucleotide repeat sequences. At present, there is no molecular explanation for anticipation in leukemia. Efforts to identify unstable repetitive sequences prone to dynamic mutation have proven unsuccessful. The possibility of a statistical bias in ascertainment cannot be totally dismissed, although there are few, if any, cases in such families in which a child develops leukemia at a later age than a parent.

CONSTITUTIONAL CHROMOSOMAL ABNORMALITIES PREDISPOSING TO LEUKEMIA

Down Syndrome

Trisomy 21 Down syndrome (Figure 1–3) results in a 10- to 18-fold elevated risk for leukemia,[79] in addition to mental retardation, cardiac and gastrointestinal malformations, and other developmental anomalies. A high frequency of individuals with Down syndrome develops a usually transient myeloproliferative syndrome during the neonatal period.[80] In early childhood, before approximately 3 years of age, the most common leukemia type is M7 AML.[81] With advancing age, ALL comprises a predominating proportion of cases.[82] Some individuals with Down syndrome are chromosomally mosaic for both a trisomy 21 population of cells and cells with a normal karyotype; in these individuals, the leukemoid reactions of infancy and the leukemia always demonstrate a tri-

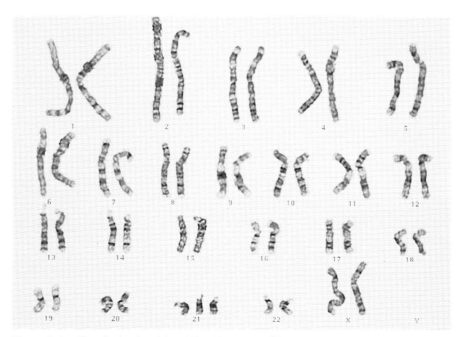

Figure 1–3. Constitutional peripheral blood karyotype of Down syndrome demonstrating trisomy 21. (Photograph courtesy of Wayne Guest and Dr. Christine Disteche, University of Washington.)

somy 21 karyotype.[83] Therefore, it is probable that excessive dosage of a gene on chromosome 21 is responsible for leukemia risk in Down syndrome.

It has been proposed that the risk for leukemia in Down syndrome results from a gene dosage effect attributed to an allelic variant common in the population.[84] One of the parents would be heterozygous for this allelic variant, and the trisomic individual would inherit two copies of this allele of the risk gene as a result of the nondisjunction duplicating chromosome 21. Presumably, this allele would be common in the general population to account for the high frequency of leukemia among the Down syndrome population yet be of such low penetrance that autosomal-recessive inheritance of leukemia would not be appreciated. Down syndrome usually results from maternal nondisjunction in meiosis I, which is well known to be associated with advanced maternal age. Taking advantage of an observation that the transient leukemia of infancy may be more commonly seen in Down syndrome individuals atypically resulting from meiosis II nondisjunction events, attempts have been made to map the regions of limited uniparental disomy in which such a gene would reside.[85] The proposed gene remains unidentified at present, but its predicted location overlaps with *CBFA2*, responsible for inherited AML in association with platelet granule defects. Therefore, *CBFA2* remains a candidate for the leukemia risk elevating gene of Down syndrome. Of course, it is also possible that the leukemia risk in Down syndrome cannot be attributed to a single gene but rather is the effect of contiguous genes on chromosome 21.

Trisomy 8 Mosaicism

Trisomy 8 mosaicism is a rare constitutional abnormality resulting in mental retardation and multiple developmental defects. (Complete trisomy 8 does not appear to result in a viable birth, so trisomy 8 exists only in the mosaic state.) Acute and chronic leukemia, aplastic anemia, and myelodysplasia have been reported at high frequency in individuals with trisomy 8.[86] As with Down syndrome, the leukemic population of cells invariably derives from the trisomic population of cells. Since trisomy 8 is among the most common cytogenetic abnormalities

observed in leukemia and myelodysplasia, there is presumably a gene or group of genes residing on this chromosome that confers leukemia risk in a dosage-dependent manner.

Other Chromosomal Abnormalities

At various times, a variety of other constitutional chromosomal abnormalities have been identified in case reports of individuals with leukemia or hematologic malignancy. These include Klinefelter's syndrome (XXY) and other sex chromosome abnormalities, Robertsonian translocations (resulting from fusion of the long arms of acrocentric chromosomes), the Christchurch chromosome (loss of the short arm of acrocentric chromosomes, first observed in New Zealand), paracentric inversion of the long arm of chromosome 7, and numerous "private" abnormalities that appear to segregate in a family in association with hematopoietic malignancy. For the most part, there is insufficient evidence at present to conclude that these abnormalities are causative of the hematopoietic malignancy in which they have been observed. In the specific case of Klinefelter's syndrome, some case series have failed to reproducibly find an increased risk of leukemia.[87] Additionally, in one Klinefelter mosaic who developed leukemia,[88] cytogenetic analysis of the blasts demonstrated both XY and XXY cells, suggesting that, in contrast to Down syndrome and trisomy 8, the signal events leading to malignancy preceded the emergence of this cytogenetic abnormality. Nevertheless, Klinefelter's syndrome is probably associated with an increased frequency of male breast cancer and germ cell tumors of the mediastinum.[89]

GENETIC SYNDROMES THAT INCLUDE LEUKEMIA AS A COMPONENT

DNA Repair Disorders

Bloom Syndrome

The clinical features of Bloom syndrome (Figure 1–4) consist of autosomal-recessive inheritance, growth retardation, a characteristic facial appearance, photosensitive telangiectatic erythema, café-

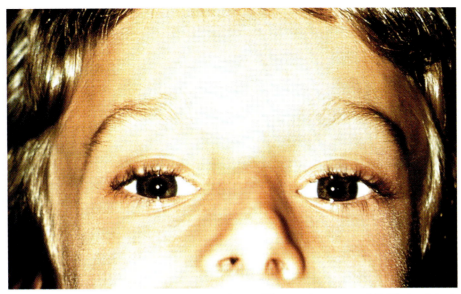

Figure 1–4. Bloom syndrome. Note facial erythema. (Photograph courtesy of Dr. Virgina Sybert, University of Washington. Reprinted with permission from Sybert VP. Genetic skin disorders. New York: Oxford University Press; 1997.)

au-lait skin pigmentation, and immunodeficiency with recurrent infections.[90] Approximately one-quarter of patients develop ALL, AML, lymphoma, or other malignancy. Cells from individuals with Bloom syndrome demonstrate an increased frequency of sister chromatid exchanges (Figure 1–5). The locus is on chromosome 15q26.1 and encodes a DNA helicase.[91] The helicase is in the RecQ family (named after the conserved *Escherichia coli* protein); other human diseases resulting from mutations in RecQ-like helicases include Werner's syndrome, with features of premature aging, and the osteogenic sarcoma-predisposing Rothmund-Thomson syndrome. There are founder mutations in the Ashkenazi Jewish population that account for a relatively high frequency of Bloom syndrome in this population.[92] In fact, the observation of these mutations among North and Central American non-Jewish patients of Spanish ancestry with Bloom syndrome has been taken as evidence of the presence of a Jewish population among early Spanish colonialists.[93]

Ataxia Telangiectasia

Ataxia telangiectasia (Figure 1–6) is an autosomal-recessive disorder comprised of progressive cerebellar ataxia, telangiectatic skin lesions, and recurrent sinopulmonary infections consequent to the

effects of both neurologic depression and mild immunodeficiency.[94] About 15 percent of patients develop malignancy, typically by age 15 years. The malignancies are usually of lymphoid origin and include Hodgkin's and non-Hodgkin's lymphoma and T-cell ALL. The locus resides on chromosome 11q22-q23 and encodes ataxia telangiectasia mutated (ATM), a phosphatidyliniositol kinase related to yeast proteins involved in meiotic recombination and cell-cycle regulation. Cells from patients with ataxia telangiectasia display a phenotype in which they fail to heed the G1-S cell-cycle checkpoint following DNA damage.[95] This likely

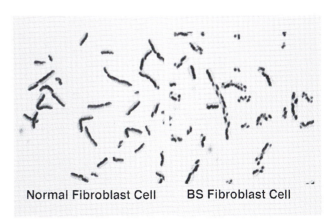

Normal Fibroblast Cell   BS Fibroblast Cell

Figure 1–5. Bloom syndrome, demonstrating increased frequency of sister chromatid exchange with BrdU labeling. (Photograph courtesy of Dr. Nathan Ellis, Memorial Sloan-Kettering Cancer Center.)

predisposes cells to accumulate somatic mutation without appropriate DNA repair. Spontaneous chromosome breaks are therefore a frequent feature of ataxia telangiectasia.

An enduring controversy is whether heterozygous carriers of ataxia telangiectasia are at an increased risk for breast cancer. Some studies have failed to detect an association, whereas others have.[96]

There are some less common ataxia telangiectasia-like disorders that share similar clinical features but result from mutations in different genes. Nijmegen chromosomal breakage syndrome (also known as Berlin breakage syndrome) is clinically differentiated from ataxia telangiectasia by microcephaly and a "bird-like" facies. The gene[97] resides on chromosome 8q21 and encodes p95, a component of the MRE11/RAD50 double-strand break repair complex. A second disorder with clinical and cellular phenotypic features inseparable from ataxia telangiectasia also maps to the long arm of chromosome 11 but at cytogenetic band 11q21, and results from mutations in the gene encoding MRE11.[98] It is estimated that about 6 percent of ataxia telangiectasia cases are attributable to this second locus.

Fanconi's Anemia

Fanconi's anemia (Figure 1–7) is a genetically heterogeneous autosomal-recessive disorder whose clinical features include pancytopenia and a variety of congenital abnormalities such as short stature and skeletal dysplasia with hypoplastic thumbs, mental and sexual retardation, skin pigmentary changes, and renal malformations.[99] Cells from individuals with Fanconi's anemia demonstrate a high frequency of chromosomal breaks following treatment with mitomycin C or diepoxybutane. Patients with Fanconi's anemia display a 15,000-fold increase in relative risk for MDS and AML. About half of patients develop myelodysplasia or AML by age 40.[100] At least eight different cellular complementation groups have been defined.[101] The genes responsible for complementation group C residing on chromosome 9q22.3,[102] complementation group A residing on chromosome 16q24.3,[103,104] and complementation group F[105] on 11p15 have all been identified. The locus for complementation group F has been mapped to chromosome 6p22-p21,[106] but the gene has not yet been identified. The protein products of these genes are heterogeneous, and the biochemical pathways through which they interact have yet to be fully defined.

Tumor Suppressor Gene Syndromes

Li-Fraumeni Syndrome

Li-Fraumeni syndrome results from inherited mutations of the *p53* tumor suppressor gene residing on

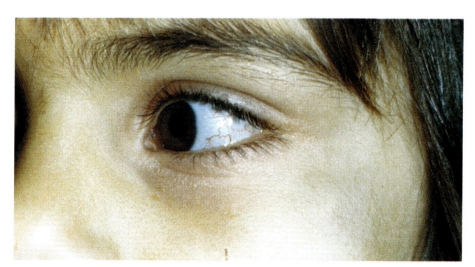

Figure 1–6. Ataxia telangiectasia. The telangiectasia is particularly prominent across the slcerae. (Photograph courtesy of Dr. Virgina Sybert, University of Washington. Reprinted with permission from Sybert VP. Genetic skin disorders. New York: Oxford University Press; 1997.

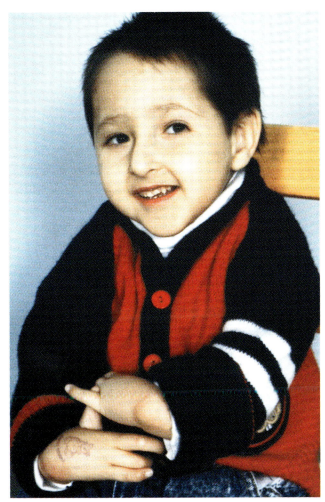

Figure 1–7. Fanconi's anemia. Note the defect of the radial ray and microcephaly. (Photograph courtesy of Dr. Roberta Pagon, University of Washington.)

chromosome 17p13.1. Leukemia and lymphoma occur in Li-Fraumeni syndrome but are less common features than sarcomas, brain tumors, melanoma, and breast cancer in this disorder.[107] Germline mutations in *p53* have been excluded as a potential etiology of autosomal-dominant AML and ALL.[108]

Neurofibromatosis I

Neurofibromatosis I (Figure 1–8) is a common (1/3,000) autosomal-dominant disorder comprised of café-au-lait skin lesions, intertrigineous freckling, and neurofibromas. It is caused by mutations in the GAP family neurofibromin tumor suppressor gene on chromosome 17q11.2, which result in defective down-regulation of the *p21* ras proto-oncogene.[109] Neurofibromatosis I predisposes to the development

of tumors of the central and peripheral nervous system including gliomas, schwannomas, neurofibrosarcomas, and skeletal muscle rhabdomyosarcomas. Neurofibromatosis I is also associated with a risk for hematopoietic malignancy, particularly juvenile CML, usually in conjunction with monosomy 7.[110] There may also be an elevated risk for non-Hodgkin's lymphoma, ALL, and myelodysplasia. Curiously, juvenile CML in neurofibromatosis I has mostly been observed with maternal inheritance,[111] although the gene is not known to demonstrate parental imprinting at a molecular level.

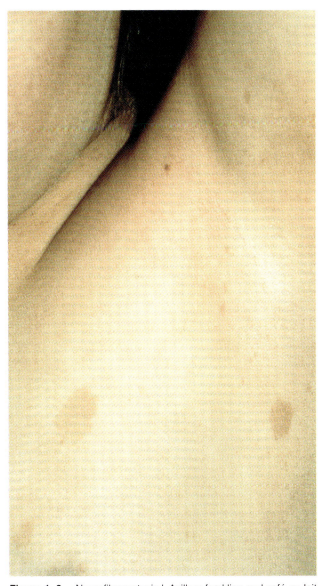

Figure 1–8. Neurofibromatosis I. Axillary freckling and café-au-lait spots are visible. (Photograph courtesy of Dr. Virgina Sybert, University of Washington. Reprinted with permission from Sybert VP. Genetic skin disorders. New York: Oxford University Press, 1997.

Congenital Cytopenias

Blackfan-Diamond Anemia

Blackfan-Diamond anemia consists of congenital hypoplastic anemia with growth retardation and a characteristic facial appearance.[112] There is an increased risk for AML. It is thought to be transmitted by both autosomal-dominant and autosomal-recessive inheritance. Heterozygous mutations in apparent autosomal-dominant cases have been found in the RPS19 encoding the S19 ribosomal protein.[113]

Severe Congenital Neutropenia and Cyclic Hematopoiesis

Severe congenital neutropenia refers to congenital onset of low numbers of circulating neutrophils (typically fewer than 500 μL^{-1}). There is typically arrest of differentiation evident on bone marrow histopathology.[114] The disorder was first reported by Kostmann in the 1950s in Norbotten County in Sweden where it results from autosomal-recessive inheritance among individuals who appear to be related through descent from a common founder. The eponym Kostmann's syndrome has thus come to describe severe congenital neutropenia, but the term is confusing because the majority of cases outside of Sweden appear to be sporadic or, in a few cases, result from autosomal-dominant inheritance. Neutrophils are the major blood phagocyte, and neutropenia predisposes to opportunistic infections. Many of the individuals who survive infectious complications, at least 10 to 20 percent, ultimately develop myelodysplasia or AML.[115] Treatment with recombinant granulocyte colony-stimulating factor (G-CSF) increases circulating neutrophils to levels sufficient to reduce the frequency of infection but may increase the risk of leukemic transformation.[116]

The etiology of the disorder is further confused by the report in the mid-1990s that mutations of the gene encoding the G-CSF receptor are the cause of severe congenital neutropenia in a minority of the non-Swedish patients.[117] In fact, mutations in the gene encoding the G-CSF receptor are now believed to arise somatically in a minority of patients, usually in association with progression to leukemia.[118]

Our laboratory recently found that mutations in the gene ELA2, encoding the neutrophil granule serine protease neutrophil elastase, are the cause of the majority of cases of severe congenital neutropenia. We began these studies through the positional cloning of the gene responsible for a different illness, cyclic hematopoiesis. Cyclic hematopoiesis is an autosomal-dominant illness of humans in which there is a 21-day oscillatory production of neutrophils and monocytes. It is genetically homogeneous and results from mutations in the gene encoding neutrophil elastase,[119] which resides on chromosome 19pter. On a candidate gene basis, we found that about 70 percent of sporadic and small multigenerational families with severe congenital neutropenia result from mutations in the gene encoding neutrophil elastase (unpublished). The sporadic cases are then the result of new mutations, most of which appear to occur as a consequence of deamination of methylcytosine at CpG sequences.

Schwachman Syndrome

Schwachman syndrome (also known as Schwachman-Diamond and Schwachman-Bodian pancreatic lipomatosis) is an autosomal-recessive syndrome of pancreatic insufficiency with congenital pancreatic lipomatosis and moderate dwarfism. Bone marrow pathology resembles that of Fanconi's anemia with early-onset pancytopenia and a similar distribution of hematopoietic malignancy,[120] as well as pediatric myelodysplasia.[121] The relative risk for developing leukemia has been estimated at 27 times that of the general population. Our laboratory excluded mutations in the gene encoding neutrophil elastase as the cause of the Schwachman syndrome (unpublished). The chromosomal locus presently remains unassigned.

CONCLUSION

Only a few strong environmental and genetic factors appear definitely associated with leukemia risk. Since most individuals developing leukemia are neither exposed to these carcinogens nor have a family history of hematopoietic malignancy, it seems reasonable to conclude that the majority of leukemia is most likely the result of ubiquitous environmental and genetic factors that each confer incremental liability to a background risk resulting from spontaneous cellular events. That environmental and genetic factors are capable of interacting to potentiate leukemia risk is vividly demonstrated in studies of secondary AML among individuals with previous malignancy. The coming years will likely see rapid advancement in defining at least the genetic factors. With the recent identification of *CBFA2* mutations in a subset of exceptionally rare familial AML, it now becomes important to readdress other data on the frequency of *CBFA2* mutations and question whether mutations in this gene might not be constitutional, rather than acquired, as has been the prior assumption. Resolution of whether ataxia telangiectasia heterozygote carriers are predisposed to cancer will also likely point toward the probability of similarly acting genetic factors. It is possible that leukemia risk in Down syndrome is the result of common, but low-penetrance, alleles of a gene in the general population. The continued accumulation of a series of rare families inheriting different types of leukemia as single gene traits will further elucidate early genetic events in leukemia and, no doubt, provide additional candidate genes.

REFERENCES

1. Greenlee RT, Hill-Harman MB, Murray T, et al. Cancer statistics, 2001. CA Cancer J Clin 2001;51:15–36.
2. Wingo PA, Ries LA, Giovino GA, et al. Annual report to the nation on the status of cancer, 1973–1996, with a special section on lung cancer and tobacco smoking. J Natl Cancer Inst 1999;91:675–90.
3. Linet MS, Ries LA, Smith MA, et al. Cancer surveillance series: recent trends in childhood cancer incidence and mortality in the United States. J Natl Cancer Inst 1999;91:1051–8.
4. Linet MS, Devesa SS. Descriptive epidemiology of childhood leukaemia. Br J Cancer 1991;63:424–9.
5. Court Brown WM, Doll R. Leukaemia in childhood and young adult life. BMJ 1961;1:981–994.
6. Leone G, Mele L, Pulsoni A, et al. The incidence of secondary leukemias. Haematologica 1999;84:937–45.
7. Durant JL, Chen J, Hemond HF, Thilly WG. Elevated incidence of childhood leukemia in Woburn, Massachusetts: NIEHS Superfund Basic Research Program searches for causes. Environ Health Perspect 1995;103(Suppl 6):93–8.
8. Greenwald P, Rose JL, Daitch PB. Acquaintance networks among leukemia and lymphoma patients. Am J Epidemiol 1979;110:162–77.
9. Travers J, Milgram S. An experimental study of the small world problem. Sociometry 1969;32:425–43.
10. Schupfer F. Studi sulle leucemie e sulle pseudoleucemie. Nota il: l'influenza che sulla leucemia esercitano le mallattie infettive intercorrenti ed il suo valore terapeutico. Policlinico (Med) 1905;12:145.
11. Thiersch JB. Attempted transmission of human leukemia in man. J Lab Clin Med 1945;30:866–74.
12. Bierman HR, Byron RL, Kelley KH, et al. Studies on cross circulation in man. I. Methods and clinical changes. Blood 1951;6:487–503.
13. Ianman JT, Bierman HR, Byron RL. Transfusion of leukemic leukocytes in man—hematologic and physiologic changes. Blood 1950;5:1099–113.
14. Gramen K. Accident-transfusion of leukaemic blood. Acta Clin Scand 1928;64:369–73.
15. Greenwald P, Woodard E, Nasca PC, et al. Morbidity and mortality among recipients of blood from preleukemic and prelymphomatous donors. Cancer 1976;38:324–8.
16. Franchini G. Molecular mechanisms of human T-cell leukemia/lymphotropic virus type I infection. Blood 1995;86:3619–39.
17. Snyder R, Kalf GF. A perspective on benzene leukemogenesis. Crit Rev Toxicol 1994;24:177–209.
18. Savitz DA, Andrews KW. Review of epidemiologic evidence on benzene and lymphatic and hematopoietic cancers. Am J Ind Med 1997;31:287–95.
19. Heath CW. Epidemiology and hereditary aspects of acute leukemia. In: Wiernik PH, Canellos GP, Dutcher JP, Kyle RA, editors. Neoplastic diseases of the blood. New York: Churchill Livingstone; 1996.
20. Smith PG, Doll R. Mortality among patients with ankylosing spondylitis after a single treatment course with x rays. BMJ 1982;284:449–60.
21. Pagano L, Pulsoni A, Tosti ME, et al. Acute lymphoblastic leukaemia occurring as second malignancy: report of the GIMEMA archive of adult acute leukaemia. Gruppo Italiano Malattie Ematologiche Maligne dell'Adulto. Br J Haematol 1999;106:1037–40.
22. Olah E, Stenszky V, Kiss A, et al. Familial leukemia: Ph1 positive acute lymphoid leukemia of a mother and her infant. Blut 1981;43:265–72.
23. Cramblett HG, Friedman JL, Najjar S. Leukemia in an infant born of a mother with leukemia. N Engl J Med 1958;259:727–9.
24. Osada S, Horibe K, Oiwa K, et al. A case of infantile acute monocytic leukemia caused by vertical transmission of the mother's leukemic cells. Cancer 1990;65:1146–9.

25. Jannini P. Leucemia familiar (cronica y aguda) en dos generaciones sucesivas. Sangre 1967;12:331–2.

26. Dildy GA, Moise KJ, Carpenter RJ, et al. Maternal malignancy metastatic to the products of conceptions: a review. Obstet Gynecol Surv 1989;91:1059–69.

27. Antonelli NM, Dotters DJ, Katz VL, Kuller JA. Cancer in pregnancy: a review of the literature. Part II. Obstet Gynecol Surv 1996;51:135–42.

28. Aviles A, Niz J. Long-term follow-up of children born to mothers with acute leukemia during pregnancy. Med Pediatr Oncol 1988;16:3–6.

29. MacMahon B, Newill VA. Birth characteristics of children dying of malignant neoplasms. J Natl Cancer Inst 1962;28:231–44.

30. Stark CR, Mantel N. Effects of maternal age and birth order on the risk of mongolism and leukemia. J Natl Cancer Inst 1966;37:687–698.

31. Mehes K, Kajtar P, Sandor G, et al. Excess of mild errors of morphogenesis in childhood lymphoblastic leukemia. Am J Med Genet 1998;75:22–7.

32. Shaw G, Lavey R, Jackson R, Austin D. Association of childhood leukemia with maternal age, birth order, and paternal occupation. A case-control study. Am J Epidemiol 1984;119:788–95.

33. Zack M, Adami HO, Ericson A. Maternal and perinatal risk factors for childhood leukemia. Cancer Res 1991;51:3696–701.

34. Petridou E, Trichopoulos D, Kalapothaki V, et al. The risk profile of childhood leukaemia in Greece: a nationwide case-control study. Br J Cancer 1997;76:1241–7.

35. Westergaard T, Andersen PK, Pedersen JB, et al. Birth characteristics, sibling patterns, and acute leukemia risk in childhood: a population-based cohort study. J Natl Cancer Inst 1997;89:939–47.

36. Shu XO, Linet MS, Steinbuch M, et al. Breast-feeding and risk of childhood acute leukemia. J Natl Cancer Inst 1999;91:1765–72.

37. Groves FD, Gridley G, Wacholder S, et al. Infant vaccinations and risk of childhood acute lymphoblastic leukaemia in the USA. Br J Cancer 1999;81:175–8.

38. Douer D, Preston-Martin S, Chang E, et al. High frequency of acute promyelocytic leukemia among Latinos with acute myeloid leukemia. Blood 1996; 87:308–13.

39. Tomas JF, Fernandez-Ranada JM. About the increased frequency of acute promyelocytic leukemia among Latinos: the experience from a center in Spain. Blood 1996;88:2357–8.

40. Villalona-Calero MA. Secondary acute myelogenous leukemia in children with Latin-American ancestry [letter; comment]. J Clin Oncol 1993;11:2286.

41. Shimkin MB, Loveland DB. A note on the mortality from lymphatic leukemia in Oriental populations of the United States. Blood 1961;17:763–6.

42. Lee M, Lee JO, Seo HZ. Clinical and statistical observations on malignant tumors. Korean J Hematol 1967;2:23–6.

43. Haenszel W, Kurihara M. Studies of Japanese migrants. I. Mortality from cancer and other diseases among Japanese in the United States. J Natl Cancer Inst 1968;40:43–68.

44. MacMahon B, Koller KF. Ethnic differences in the incidence of leukemia. Blood 1957;12:1–10.

45. Hernandez JA, Land K, McKenna RW. Leukemias, myeloma, and other lymphoreticular neoplasm. Cancer 1995;75:381–94.

46. McPhedran P, Heath CW Jr, Garcia JS. Racial variations in leukemia incidence among the elderly. J Natl Cancer Inst 1970;45:25–8.

47. Bergsagel D. The incidence and epidemiology of plasma cell neoplasms. Stem Cells 1995;13(Suppl 2):1–9.

48. McWhirter WR. The relationship of incidence of childhood lymphoblastic leukaemia to social class. Br J Cancer 1982;46:640–5.

49. Bartal A, Bentwich Z, Manny N, Izak G. Ethnical and clinical aspects of chronic lymphocytic leukemia in Israel: a survey on 288 patients. Acta Haematol 1978;60:161–71.

50. Haenszel W. Cancer mortality among U.S. Jews. Isr J Med Sci 1971;7:1437–50.

51. King H, Diamond E, Bailar JC. Cancer mortality and religious preference—a suggested method in research. Milbank Mem Fund Q 1965;43:349–358.

52. Cuneo JM. Leukemia incidence and ethnicity in Nassau County, New York. Am J Public Health 1976; 66:1094–5.

53. Mittelman M, Lewinski UH, Weiss H, et al. Secondary myelodysplastic syndrome in multiple myeloma—a study of nine patients with an attempt to detect myeloma patients at risk. Haematologia 1994;26: 67–74.

54. Martin AO, Dunn JK, Genetics of neoplasia in a human isolate. In: Gelboin HV, editor. Genetic and environmental factors in experimental and human cancer. Tokyo: Japan Scientific Society; 1980. p. 291–302.

55. Feldman JG, Lee SL, Seligman B. Occurrence of acute leukemia in females in a genetically isolated population. Cancer 1976;38:2548–50.

56. Kurita S, Kamei Y, Ota K. Genetic studies on familial leukemia. Cancer 1974;34:1098–101.

57. Pearson HA, Grello FW, Cone TE. Leukemia in identical twins. N Engl J Med 1963;268:1151–6.

58. Degos L. Depidemiologie de la leucemie aigue humaine. Le risque de leucemie aigue. Rev Prat 1973;23:91–4.

59. Buckley JD, Buckley CM, Breslow NE, et al. Concordance for childhood cancer in twins. Med Pediatr Oncol 1996;26:223–9.

60. Horwitz M. The genetic basis of common diseases. In: King RA, Rotter JI, Motuslky AG, editors. New York: Oxford University Press; in press.

61. Clarkson BD, Boyse EA. Possible explanation of the high concordance for acute leukaemia in monozygous twins. Lancet 1971;1:669–701.

61A. Wiemels JL, Cazzaniga G, Daniotti M, et al. Prenatal origin of acute lymphoblastic leukemia in children. Lancet 1999;354:1499–1503.

62. Shpilberg O, Modan M, Modan B, et al. Familial aggregation of haematological neoplasms: a controlled study. Br J Haematol 1994;87:75–80.

63. Goldgar DE, Easton DF, Cannon-Albright LA, Skolnick MH. Systematic population-based assessment of cancer risk in first-degree relatives of cancer probands. J Natl Cancer Inst 1994;86:1600–8.

64. Cannon-Albright L, Thoma A, Goldgar DE, et al. Familiarity of cancer in Utah. Cancer Res 1994;54:2378–85.

65. Linet MS, Van Natta ML, Brookmeyer R, et al. Familial cancer history and chronic lymphocytic leukemia. Am J Epidemiol 1989;130:655–64.

66. Radovanovic Z, Markovic-Denic L, Jankovic S. Cancer mortality of family members of patients with chronic lymphocytic leukemia. Eur J Epidemiol 1994;10:211–3.

67. Cuttner J. Increased incidence of hematologic malignancies in first-degree relatives of patients with chronic lymphocytic leukemia. Cancer Invest 1992;10:103–9.

68. Rigby PG, Pratt PT, Rosenlof RC, Lemon HM. Genetic relationships in familial leukemia and lymphoma. Arch Intern Med 1968;121:67–71.

69. Shannon KM, Turhan AG, Chang SSY, et al. Familial bone marrow monosomy 7. Evidence that the predisposing locus is not on the long arm of chromosome 7. J Clin Invest 1989;84:984–9.

70. Paul B, Reid MM, Davison EV, et al. Familial myelodysplasia: progressive disease associated with emergence of monosomy 7. Br J Haematol 1987;65:321–3.

71. Horwitz M, Sabath DE, Smithson WA, Radich J. A family inheriting different subtypes of acute myelogenous leukemia. Am J Hematol 1996;52:295–304.

72. Horwitz M, Benson KF, Li F-Q, et al. Genetic heterogeneity in familial acute myelogenous leukemia: evidence for a second locus at chromosome 16q21-23.2. Am J Hum Genet 1997;61:873–81.

73. Lee EJ, Schiffer CA, Misawa S, Testa JR. Clinical and cytogenetic features of familial erythroleukaemia. Br J Haematol 1987;65:313–20.

74. Horwitz M. The genetics of familial leukemia. Leukemia 1997;11:1347–59

75. Song WJ, Sullivan MG, Legare RD, et al. Haploinsufficiency of CBFA2 causes familial thrombocytopenia with propensity to develop acute myelogenous leukaemia. Nat Genet 1999;23:166–75.

76. Osato M, Asou N, Abdalla E, et al. Biallelic and heterozygous point mutations in the runt domain of the AML1/PEBP2alphaB gene associated with myeloblastic leukemias. Blood 1999;93:1817–24.

77. Weiner L. A family with high incidence of leukemia and unique Ph' chromosome findings. Blood 1965;26:871–9.

78. Horwitz M, Goode EL, Jarvik GP. Anticipation in familial leukemia. Am J Hum Genet 1996;59:990–8.

79. Evans DIK, Steward JK. Down's syndrome and leukaemia. Lancet 1972;2:1322.

80. Seibel NL, Sommer A, Miser J. Transient neonatal leukemoid reactions in mosaic trisomy 21. J Pediatr 1984;104:251.

81. Epstein CJ. Down syndrome (trisomy 21). In: Scriver CR, Beaudet AL, Sly WS, Valle D, editors. The metabolic and molecular bases of inherited disease. Vol. I. New York: McGraw-Hill; 1995. p. 749–94.

82. Stiller CA, Kinnier Wilson LM. Down syndrome and leukaemia. Lancet 1981;2:1343.

83. Rowley JD. Down syndrome and acute leukaemia: increased risk may be due to trisomy 21. Lancet 1981;2:1020–2.

84. Iselius L, Jacobs P, Morton N. Leukaemia and transient leukaemia in Down syndrome. Hum Genet 1990;85:477–85.

85. Niikawa N, Deng H-X, Abe K, et al. Possible mapping of the gene for transient myeloproliferative syndrome at 21q11.2. Hum Genet 1991;87:561–6.

86. Zollino M, Genuardi M, Bajer J, et al. Constitutional trisomy 8 and myelodysplasia: report of a case and review of the literature. Leuk Res 1995;9:773–6.

87. Horsman DE, Tapio Pantzar J, Dill FJ, Kalousek DK. Klinefelter's syndrome and acute leukaemia. Cancer Genet Cytogenet 1987;26:275–6.

88. Shaw MP, Eden OB, Grace E, Ellis PM. Acute lymphoblastic leukemia and Klinefelter's syndrome. Pediatr Hematol Oncol 1992;9:81–5.

89. Robinson A, de la Chapelle A. Sex chromosome abnormalities. In: Rimoin DL, Connor JM, Pyeritz RE, editors. Emery and Rimoin's principles and practice of medical genetics. 3rd ed. Vol. 1. New York: Churchill Livingstone; 1997. p. 985.

90. German J. Bloom's syndrome: incidence, age of onset, and types of leukemia in the Bloom's Syndrome Registry. In: Bartsocas CS, Loukopoulos D, editors. Genetics of hematological disorders. Washington, DC: Hemisphere; 1992. p. 241–58.

91. Ellis NA, Groden J, Ye T-Z, et al. The Bloom's syndrome gene product is homologous to RecQ helicases. Cell 1995;83:655–666.

92. Li L, Eng C, Desnick RJ, et al. Carrier frequency of the Bloom syndrome blmAsh mutation in the Ashkenazi Jewish population. Mol Genet Metab 1998;64:286–90.

93. Ellis NA, Ciocci S, Proytcheva M, et al. The Ashkenazic Jewish Bloom syndrome mutation blmAsh is present in non-Jewish Americans of Spanish ancestry. Am J Hum Genet 1998;63:1685–93.

94. Taylor AMR, Metcalfe JA, Thick J, Mak Y-F. Leukemia and lymphoma in ataxia telangiectasia. Blood 1996;87:423–38.

95. Hartwell L. Defects in a cell cycle checkpoint may be responsible for the genomic instability of cancer cells. Cell 1992;71:543–6.

96. Bebb DG, Yu Z, Chen J, et al. Absence of mutations in the ATM gene in forty-seven cases of sporadic breast cancer. Br J Cancer 1999;80:1979–81.

97. Carney JP, Maser RS, Olivares H, et al. The hMre11/hRad50 protein complex and Nijmegen breakage syndrome: linkage of double-strand break repair to the cellular DNA damage response. Cell 1998;93:477–86.

98. Stewart GS, Maser RS, Stankovic T, et al. The DNA double-strand break repair gene hMRE11 is mutated in individuals with an ataxia-telangiectasia-like disorder. Cell 1999;99:577–87.

99. Auerbach AD. Fanconi anemia. In: Cohen PR, Kurzrock R, editors. Dermatologic clinics. Vol. 13. Philadelphia: WB Saunders; 1995. p. 41–9.

100. Butturini A, Gale RP, Verlander PC, et al. Hematologic abnormalities in Fanconi anemia: an international Fanconi anemia registry study. Blood 1994;84:1650–5.

101. Joenje H, Oostra AB, Wijker M, et al. Evidence for at least eight Fanconi anemia genes. Am J Hum Genet 1997;61:940–4.

102. Strathdee CV, Gavish H, Shannon WR, Buchwald M. Cloning of cDNAs for Fanconi's anaemia by functional complementation. Nature 1992;356:763–7.

103. Lo Ten Foe JR, Rooimans MA, Bosnoyan-Collins L, et al. Expression cloning of a cDNA for the major Fanconi anaemia gene, FAA. Nat Genet 1996;14:320–3.

104. Positional cloning of the Fanconi anaemia group A gene. The Fanconi Anaemia/Breast Cancer Consortium. Nat Genet 1996;14:324–8.

105. de Winter JP, Rooimans MA, van Der Weel L, et al. The Fanconi anaemia gene FANCF encodes a novel protein with homology to ROM. Nat Genet 2000;24:15–6.

106. Waisfisz Q, Saar K, Morgan NV, et al. The Fanconi anemia group E gene, FANCE, maps to chromosome 6p. Am J Hum Genet 1999;64:1400–5.

107. Malkin D. Germline p53 mutations and heritable cancer. Annu Rev Genet 1994;28:443–65.

108. Felix CA, D'Amico D, Mitsudomi T, et al. Absence of hereditary p53 mutations in 10 familial leukemia pedigrees. J Clin Invest 1992;90:653–8.

109. Gutmann DH, Collins FS. von Recklinghausen neurofibromatosis. In: Scriber CR, Beaudet AL, Sly WS, Valle D, editors. The metabolic and molecular bases of inherited disease. Vol. I. New York: McGraw-Hill; 1995. p. 677–96.

110. Stiller CA, Chessels JM, Fitchett M. Neurofibromatosis and childhood leukaemia/lymphoma: a population-based UKCCSG study. Br J Cancer 1994;70:969–72.

111. Shannon KM, Watterson J, Johnson P, et al. Monosomy 7 myeloproliferative disease in children with neurofibromatosis, type 1: epidemiology and molecular analysis. Blood 1992;79:1311–8.

112. Halperin DS, Freedman MH. Diamond-Blackfan anemia: etiology, pathophysiology, and treatment. Am J Pediatr Hematol Oncol 1989;11:380–94.

113. Draptchinskaia N, Gustavsson P, Andersson B, et al. The gene encoding ribosomal protein S19 is mutated in Diamond-Blackfan anaemia. Nat Genet 1999;21:169–75.

114. Kostmann R. Infantile genetic agranulocytosis: a review with presentation of ten new cases. Acta Paediatr Scand 1975;64:362–8.

115. Welte K, Dale D. Pathophysiology and treatment of severe chronic neutropenia. Ann Hematol 1996;72:158–65.

116. Bonilla MA, Dale D, Zeidler C, et al. Long-term safety of treatment with recombinant human granulocyte colony-stimulating factor (r-metHuG-CSF) in patients with severe congenital neutropenias. Br J Haematol 1994;88:723–30.

117. Dong F, Brynes RK, Tidow N, et al. Mutations in the gene for the granulocyte colony-stimulating-factor receptor in patients with acute myeloid leukemia preceded by severe congenital neutropenia. N Engl J Med 1995;333:487–93.

118. Tidow N, Pilz C, Teichmann B, et al. Clinical relevance of point mutations in the cytoplasmic domain of the granulocyte colony-stimulating factor receptor gene in patients with severe congenital neutropenia. Blood 1997;89:2369–75.

119. Horwitz M, Benson KF, Person RE, et al. Mutations in ELA2, encoding neutrophil elastase, define a 21-day biological clock in cyclic haematopoiesis. Nat Genet 1999;23:433–6.

120. Woods WG, Roloff JS, Lukens JN, Krivit W. The occurrence of leukemia in patients with the Schwachman syndrome. J Pediatr 1981;99:425–8.

121. Passmore SJ, Hann IM, Stiller CA, et al. Pediatric myelodysplasia: a study of 68 children and a new prognostic scoring system. Blood 1995;85:1742–50.

2

Molecular Etiology and Pathogenesis of Leukemia

HEATHER A. LEITCH, MD, PhD
PIERRE LANEUVILLE, MD
WILSON H. MILLER JR, MD, PhD

Leukemia is an uncontrolled or malignant outgrowth of hematopoietic cells arrested at an incompletely differentiated stage of development. The term *leukemia* was coined by Virchow in the mid 1800s[1] and translated literally means "white blood," an appearance conferred by overabundance of cells of the leukemic clone (Figure 2–1). In the late twentieth century, it became increasingly common to detect leukemia on the basis of abnormalities found on routine blood work, early in the evolution of the disease, and before a high peripheral blood white count was manifest. Certain leukemias, such as hairy cell leukemia (HCL) or leukemia secondary to myelodysplasia or prior chemotherapy, may present with low peripheral white cell counts. Thus, despite linguistic origins, leukemic blood is not inevitably white.

In chronic leukemia, a relatively mature phenotype is typical of leukemic cells, whereas in acute leukemia, an overabundance of immature blood-forming cells or blasts predominates. Our understanding of leukemia has evolved enormously over the past several decades. Initial descriptions were based on morphology, in conjunction with attempts to elucidate predisposing factors on a population level. Recent advances in cell and molecular biology have led to an increasingly sophisticated appreciation of the intercellular, intracellular, and molecular mechanisms of blood cell communication and growth regulation. This insight has largely been gained by investigation of the mechanisms that regulate altered cellular behavior. This chapter will describe the contribution of predisposing host and environmental factors to the development of leukemia. An underlying predisposition to genetic

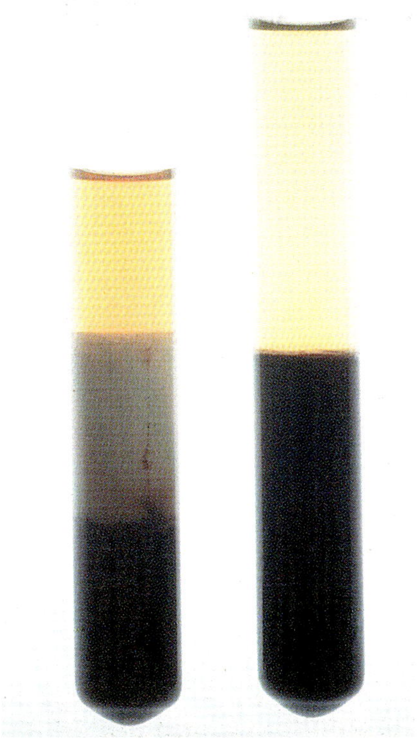

Figure 2–1. Buffy coat preparation of peripheral blood from a leukemic patient (left) and a normal control (*right*) showing a dramatic expansion of the white blood cell compartment due to the presence of leukemic cells.

changes that may lead to a leukemic phenotype is reviewed, as are steps at which cellular growth control may become dysregulated. Classic environmental factors linked to leukemogenesis and our current understanding of selected leukemia syndromes are discussed in the context of genomic instability.

CLASSIFICATION OF LEUKEMIA

In the early part of the twentieth century, leukemia was classified on the basis of descriptive cellular morphology by light microscopy. Classification was further refined by histochemical techniques, which exploited the reaction of cellular components of leukemic blasts with special stains. The French-American-British classification is based on these techniques and is still widely used today.[2,3] Leukemia is divided into acute versus chronic and lymphoid versus myeloid. Lymphoid and myeloid leukemias are further subdivided by the predominant lineage and stage of differentiation of leukemic blasts.

With further technical advances, antibodies specific for certain proteins or cell markers were used to identify cell types by immunohistochemistry or to sort cells by the fluorescence activated cell sorter. Changes are recognized on the chromosomal and molecular level by classic cytogenetic banding techniques and by the more recently established tools of fluorescent in situ hybridization (FISH) and polymerase chain reaction (PCR). Both cell surface and molecular markers are taken into account in the proposed World Health Organization (WHO) classification of leukemia.[4] The WHO classification recognizes several molecular categories of acute myelogenous leukemia (AML) and acute lymphocytic leukemia (ALL) as distinct disease entities. In addition, secondary AML (s-AML) arising from myelodysplastic syndrome (MDS) or previous chemotherapy or radiation therapy (t-AML) is placed into a separate category. Evolving systems of classification reflect an improved understanding of the molecular pathophysiology of leukemia, which links pathways of hematopoietic development to the origin of specific leukemias. Individual leukemic syndromes are defined by the stage in hematopoietic development where their malignant clone may originate.

HEMATOPOIESIS

Our understanding of the etiology of leukemia relies heavily on the study of normal hematopoiesis. Hematopoiesis is the development of blood cells from blood-forming cells in the bone marrow. This process involves an exquisitely regulated balance between self-renewal and terminal differentiation. Mature cells become senescent and must be removed and replaced on a continual basis, a process that takes place on a massive scale; about 10^{11} are produced hourly,[5] or 1 trillion cells daily. Replacement of hematopoietic cells is achieved via differentiation of primitive pluripotent stem cells through a series of cell divisions.

Stem cells constitute 0.1 percent of the nucleated cells of the bone marrow, and the majority of these are quiescent. The cells, once stimulated to cycle, undergo asymmetric division to form an early progenitor cell and another stem cell. Progenitor cells undergo further cell divisions, becoming progressively more differentiated and more restricted in their capacity for self-renewal. Differentiation and lineage commitment occur under the influence of a complex array of signals from the extracellular environment, including signals provided by important cytokines, such as stem cell factor, interleukin-3 (IL-3), granulocyte-macrophage colony-stimulating factor (GM-CSF), and granulocyte colony-stimulating factor (G-CSF). Binding of cytokines to cell surface receptors results in the initiation of a cascade of signal transduction events within the cell. A series of negative regulators and amplification circuits provide additional control over the process of hematopoiesis.[6–8] Whether a cell will remain quiescent or proliferate and terminally differentiate depends on its lineage of differentiation, its activation state, and the balance of signals acting on it. The processes of proliferation and differentiation are normally tightly coupled, and normal hematopoiesis reflects a balance between cell survival and division, differentiation, and death. In leukemia, this balance is disrupted, leading to partial uncoupling of these processes and dysregulation of hematopoiesis. Accumulation of leukemic cells disrupts production of nonclonal hematopoietic cells, which are displaced in the bone marrow by the leukemic clone. Other complications secondary to the presence of the leukemic cells themselves may occur, giving rise to the clinical picture that accompanies leukemic presentation.

DEVELOPMENT OF TECHNIQUES TO UNDERSTAND HEMATOPOIESIS

Much of our understanding of hematopoiesis was gained via in vitro hematopoietic assays, including colony assays and long-term marrow cultures, and led to the development of current terminology. Clonogenic assays demonstrating hematopoietic progenitor cells were first studied in the mouse.[9] Lethally irradiated mice were rescued with bone marrow from syngeneic donors, resulting in hematopoietic reconstitution and formation of hematopoietic colonies in the spleen. The observation that a limiting number of cells resulted in colonies containing cells of all hematopoietic lineages was the first demonstration of the pluripotent stem cell, an observation that has been confirmed using retrovirally marked stem cells.[10]

Culture of hematopoietic cells in vitro in agar or methylcellulose allows assessment of factors influencing colony formation. Characteristics of progenitor cells are inferred from that of their progeny. The colony-forming unit (CFU) is a cell capable of giving rise in vitro to a colony of cells of a certain pheno-

type. Similarly, colony-stimulating factors (CSFs) were originally defined by the lineage of cells observed in colonies formed in vitro in their presence (Figure 2–2). With purification and cloning techniques, these factors were identified as proteins or glycoproteins with the function of cytokines; they are secreted by cells, act on cell surface receptors, and activate the receptors or associated cytoplasmic signaling molecules. These, in turn, transmit signals to the cell nucleus, ultimately leading to alteration of cellular growth and differentiation.

Colony assays were used to define the lineage commitment of progenitor cells. However, these assays produced clones of cells with limited survival in vitro, an indication that culture conditions did not closely approximate conditions of hematopoiesis in vivo. Strategies to obtain long-term in vitro growth of marrow cells led to a more physiologic assay system and allowed an increased understanding of the role of bone marrow stroma in supporting hematopoietic cell growth and differentiation. The long-term marrow culture, developed by Dexter and colleagues, involves incubation of marrow cells under appropriate conditions in liquid culture and results in formation of an adherent layer of stromal cells, consisting of fibroblasts, adipocytes, endothelial cells, and macrophages.[11]

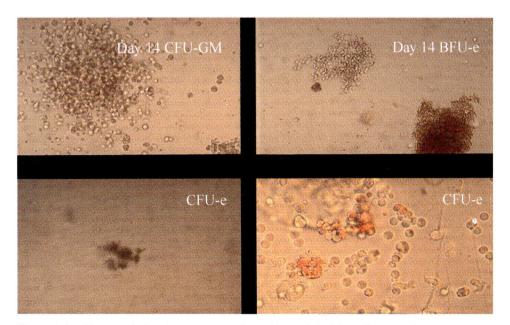

Figure 2–2. Hematopoietic colony assays performed in methylcellulose. The top left panel depicts a granulocyte-macrophage colony-forming unit (CFU-GM). Erythroid burst-forming units (BFU-e) and erythroid colony-forming units (CFU-e) are shown in the top right and lower panels, respectively.

These are in intimate contact with primitive hematopoietic cells and provide a microenvironment, thought to be similar to that of the bone marrow, which supports the survival and maturation of hematopoietic cells (Figure 2–3).[12] Direct contact with stromal cells is required for maintenance of hematopoiesis; if physically separated from the stroma, the hematopoietic cells die.[5] As the cells mature, they are released into the supernatant in vitro, presumably in a similar manner to their release from the bone marrow into the circulation in vivo. Using Dexter cultures in combination with cell-sorting techniques, the physical characteristics of early progenitor cells, including the long-term culture-initiating cell, were defined.[13]

ADVANCES IN THE MOLECULAR BIOLOGY OF LEUKEMIA

Understanding the crucial steps of hematopoiesis has led directly to our current classification schema for leukemia. Primary leukemic cells, as well as a multitude of cell lines derived from both murine and human leukemia, can be studied by these techniques. Leukemic and normal hematopoietic cells can be identified by the array of proteins and glycoproteins expressed on the cell surface. Cluster designation (CD) antigens are cell surface markers of variable structure and function identified using antibodies. To date, over 100 CD antigens have been named. Important CD antigens in leukemia include CD34, a stem cell marker; CD33, an early myeloid marker expressed on virtually all AML; CD20 and CD3, markers for B and T cells, respectively; and CD45, a lymphocyte activation marker. Cell surface markers have recently been exploited for therapeutic purposes using murine monoclonal or humanized antibodies to CD33 or other markers, alone or conjugated to chemotherapeutic agents or radionuclides.[14,15]

With the advent of molecular biology, it became possible to identify specific genetic changes associated with hematologic malignancies. The first recurring chromosomal abnormality associated with a human malignancy, the Philadelphia chromosome (Ph) of chronic myelogenous leukemia (CML), was identified in CML metaphases and was a landmark observation.[16] By cytogenetic techniques, it became clear that Ph results from juxtaposition of the long arm of chromosome 9 with chromosome 22, t(9;22) (Figure 2–4). With refinement in molecular tech-

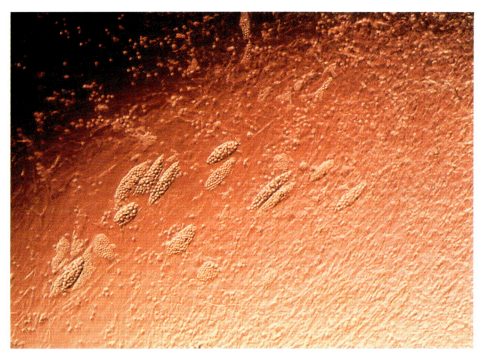

Figure 2–3.   Long-term marrow culture of normal bone marrow cells. An adherent layer of stromal cells is seen, which supports the survival and differentiation of "cobblestone areas" of hematopoietic precursors.

niques, the cellular genes involved in this translocation, bcr and abl, have been characterized. The normal functions provided by these gene products have been clarified, as have several ways in which these functions are disrupted by t(9;22)(q34;q11). Although far from completely understood, the functions of bcr and abl, and the resulting bcr-abl chimeric protein, were the first to be defined in human leukemia and remain among the most thoroughly studied. Chronic myelogenous leukemia is the first human malignancy in which a treatment was specifically designed to target the function of the fusion protein. An inhibitor of the tyrosine kinase activity of bcr-abl is currently in clinical trials.[17] This form of treatment, if effective, has the potential to revolutionize the treatment of human cancer.

Another novel strategy targeting a fusion product of the translocation t(15;17)(q21;q11) has already led to a major improvement in survival in AML-M3. The t(15;17) results in disruption of the retinoic acid receptor (RAR) (Figure 2–5), making cells expressing the disrupted receptor refractory to the differentiation-inducing effects of physiologic levels of retinoic acid (RA).[18,19] Pharmacologic levels of all-*trans* RA (ATRA), in contrast, lead to remission induction by differentiation of cells of the leukemic clone.[20] By combining ATRA with induction and consolidation chemotherapy, AML-M3 now has one of the more favorable outcomes of the acute leukemias. Although its use preceded and, indeed, led to the elucidation of the molecular disruption conferred by t(15;17), this is the first example of correlation of a genetic defect with a targeted and specific treatment.

The presence of t(9;22) or other characteristic translocations can be detected by several techniques, in addition to cytogenetics, which include FISH and PCR. Fluorescent in situ hybridization is a technique in which molecular probes for specific nucleotide sequences are conjugated to fluorochromes and hybridized to metaphase or interphase chromosomes; the abnormality is detected by direct visualization (Figure 2–6). Spectral karyotyping or multicolor FISH uses multiple fluorochrome-labeled chromosome-specific probes simultaneously. Abnormalities are detected through sophisticated computer programming. These techniques have allowed identification of previously unrecognized genetic changes.[21]

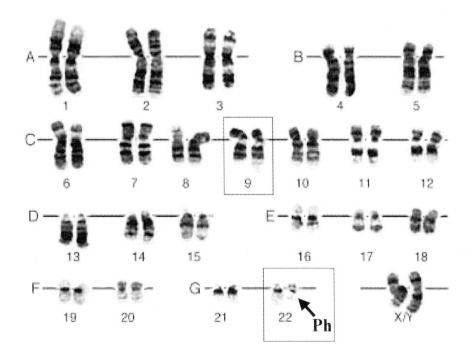

Figure 2–4. The Philadelphia chromosome (Ph) is the cytogenetic hallmark of chronic myelogenous leukemia and is a translocation created by the reciprocal exchange of the long arms of chromosomes 9 and 22.

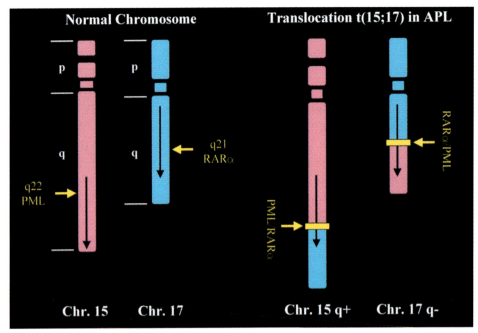

Figure 2–5.   The t(15;17) translocation is characteristic of APL and creates a fusion of the PML gene from chromosome 15 and the RAR-α gene from chromosome 17.

By PCR, nucleotide sequences of interest are amplified by many logs using primers of specific sequence in conjunction with repeated cycles of nucleotide extension. This exponential amplification gives PCR an extraordinary sensitivity and specificity for detecting genetic fusions, which is useful both in diagnosis and in monitoring for minimal residual disease following treatment.

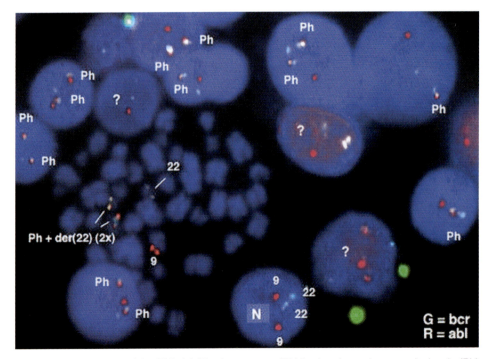

Figure 2–6.   Detection of the Philadelphia chromosome (Ph) in chronic myelogenous leukemia (Ph) by fluorescent in situ hybridization (FISH) of *BCR* (*green*) and *ABL* (*red*) specific probes. The presence of Ph is revealed by the superimposition of red and green fluorescence signals (*arrow*).

Additional new techniques hold promise for increasing the sophistication of our understanding of molecular changes in leukemia. Chromosome painting uses fluorochome-conjugated chromosome-specific probes to detect translocation or duplication of DNA sequences. By this technique, a previously unrecognized translocation, the t(12;21) of childhood ALL, was defined. This is important, as the t(12;21) was subsequently recognized to be one of the most common molecular changes in childhood leukemia and to be associated with a particularly good prognosis.[22]

Thus, the identification of chromosomal markers has defined subgroups of patients whose prognosis differs substantially. Molecular markers indicating good prognosis are the t(8;21) of AML-M2, the t(15;17) of AML-M3, the inv(16) of AML-M4, and the t(12;21) of childhood ALL. Poor prognosis occurs in AML harboring alterations in chromosomes 11q23 or 7, deletion of 5, or presence of Ph. Thus, in addition to defining pathophysiology and prognosis, recognition of molecular changes in leukemia is important in tailoring therapy.

MURINE MODELS CAN ISOLATE THE ROLE OF INDIVIDUAL GENES

Murine models are convenient systems for in vivo manipulation of a gene product. The first murine systems used involved reconstitution of lethally irradiated mice with hematopoietic cells containing the gene of interest.[23] In transgenic animals, a mutation is introduced by microinjection of a genetically engineered transgene into a fertilized egg (Figure 2–7). This is introduced on a vector carrying a specific promoter in addition to the coding sequences of interest. The vector incorporates randomly into the genome and can be expressed in all cell types, including germ cells, or more selectively, depending on the chosen promoter. By breeding, mouse lines with incorporated transgene can be identified and selected.

With knock-in mice, abnormal gene products expressed in human malignancy, such as chimeric proteins, may be introduced in the germline, which is useful in generating animal models of human disease. This technique directs the transgene to the appropriate promoter via homologous recombina-

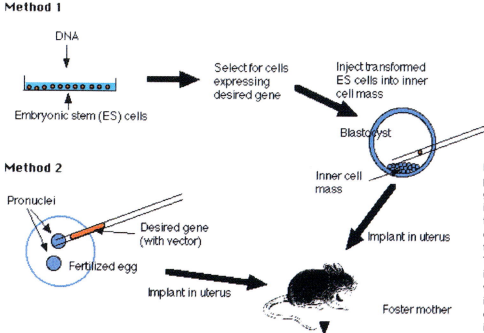

Figure 2–7. There are two principal methods for generating transgenic mice bearing a foreign gene of interest. In the first approach, totipotent embryonic stem cells are transduced in vitro with a DNA vector containing the foreign gene of interest. Transfected cells are then introduced into a blastocyst by microinjection, where they become incorporated into the inner cell mass. These cells differentiate following implantation into the uterus of a surrogate mother to appear in various tissues of the adult animal. In the second method, the DNA vector is injected directly into a fertilized ovum, which is then implanted in a surrogate mother.

tion. Since the vector containing the transgene contains no promoter sequences, the gene will only be expressed if incorporated into the genome. Homologous recombination is unlikely to occur near unrelated promoters; thus, the transgene is expressed in a tissue-specific manner and subjected to normal cellular controls. Gene function may also be revealed by deletion or inactivation of a gene of interest. This strategy is employed in knock-out mice, which are created in a manner similar to knock-in mice. These animal models not only allow definition of gene function but are convenient model systems for exploring new therapies.

ANALYSIS OF THE MULTISTEP NATURE OF LEUKEMOGENESIS: USE OF GENE ARRAY TECHNOLOGY

The above discussion focuses on identification of single genetic changes in specific leukemia syndromes. Both clinical and genetic observations, however, suggest that development of a fully malignant phenotype involves accumulation of several mutations. Analysis of blood samples taken years before clinical presentation of leukemia occasionally shows the presence of characteristic molecular defects.[24,25] Familial susceptibility to leukemia is occasionally reported. Inherited mutations in germline tumor suppressor genes occur, but additional mutations in other genes are necessary before a leukemic phenotype is manifest. This progression has been reproduced experimentally in animal models with inactivated tumor suppressor genes. Finally, progression of several malignancies, including CML, is associated with a number of additional cytogenetic changes.[26,27] However, each characteristic change occurs in only a minority of cases, and, to date, none have been pathognomonic. This suggests the involvement of multiple pathways of cell regulation in leukemogenesis and that changes in one of several overlapping pathways of signal transduction may lead to a similar phenotype.

With the introduction of microarrays using DNA chip technology, the ability to detect changes in patterns of gene expression is unprecedented.[28–31] The expression of multiple genes may be analyzed simultaneously by transcriptional profiling. Oligonucleotide arrays of specified sequence or products of cDNA inserts are used as probes and fixed to a solid support. Labeled cellular messenger ribonucleic acid (mRNA) is hybridized to probes on a solid support, and the relative abundance of each message, or its relative expression, is measured by detection of label. Software programming helps to identify patterns of gene expression present in a particular sample.[30] By this method, the ability to distinguish between AML and ALL with high sensitivity and specificity was demonstrated, illustrating potential application to diagnosis. In addition, two predominant types of gene expression were identified in a subtype of non-Hodgkin's lymphoma (NHL, diffuse large B-cell lymphoma), which corresponded to separate stages of B-cell development as putative cells of origin. One of the NHL groups had a significantly better overall survival than the other.[32] Thus, a subgroup of patients was identified in whom worse outcome could be expected and who might benefit from altered therapeutic strategies.

GENOMIC INSTABILITY: ETIOLOGY OF GENETIC CHANGE LEADING TO LEUKEMIA

In the past two decades, much effort has focused on the description and characterization of abnormal molecules predisposing to leukemia, without a clear mechanism by which these alterations are produced in the first place. In this section, data implicating an underlying phenomenon of genomic instability are reviewed. The involvement of illegitimate V(D)J recombination is discussed, as are defects in DNA repair. Finally, specific sequences with increased susceptibility to DNA breaks are described.

Whereas some leukemia subtypes are associated with recurring chromosomal abnormalities, only acute promyelocytic leukemia (APL) and CML have a change that is specific to almost all cases. In others, a multitude of abnormalities are associated with a minority of cases. The recent demonstration that some chromosomal translocations found in leukemia occur in the blood-forming cells of normal healthy individuals is consistent with the view that leukemogenesis is a multistep process.[33,34] Recent work has investigated the mechanisms by which leukemia cells might become predisposed to the accumulation of mutations.

On a chromosomal level, changes associated with leukemia development and/or prognosis include hyperdiploidy[35] and loss of heterozygosity.[36] In MDS, multiple chromosomal abnormalities not detectable by standard cytogenetics were revealed by FISH.[37]

In CML, the role of genomic instability was initially raised by the observation of additional cytogenetic changes preceding blast crisis in one-third to one half of cases. These observations have been supported in several experimental systems. An increase in sensitivity to ionizing radiation has been noted in cells expressing P210 bcr-abl.[38] Cell lines carrying a vector expressing P210 bcr-abl were unstable, with evolution to abrogation of growth factor dependence, increased cell proliferation, and the appearance of new chromosomal abnormalities.[39] Evolution of clonal immunoglobulin (Ig) rearrangements occurring with clinical progression was also observed.[40]

The issue of whether bcr-abl is the result of genomic instability or itself contributes to instability was addressed directly by inducing expression of P190 bcr-abl. Mutation frequency was measured in P190 bcr-abl transgenic mice, which develop leukemia by day 100 (Figure 2–8). Point

mutations were increased five-fold in the preleukemic phase, suggesting that genomic instability is induced by expression of bcr-abl before leukemic transformation.[41]

More recently, large deletions adjacent to the translocation breakpoints were seen in a subgroup of patients with CML. The deletions spanned several megabases, suggesting that loss of one or several genes might occur. Whether the deletions preceded or were a result of the translocation was unclear, but the presence of the deletions did correlate with poor survival.[42] Deletions around breakpoints in other leukemias involving translocations also occur. The t(4;11) of ALL involves deletions, duplications, and insertions around participating breakpoints, indicating a defect in DNA repair.[43] Chromosomal deletions have also been noted in leukemias involving t(8;21), inv(16), and 11q23.[44–46] These observations suggest that alteration of secondary target genes accompanying translocation of the leukemia-specific fusion might be a common mechanism of mutation in leukemogenesis.

ILLEGITIMATE V(D)J RECOMBINATION

The V(D)J recombinase system coordinates the formation of Ig and T-cell receptor (TCR) chains during B- and T-cell maturation by juxtaposition of nonad-

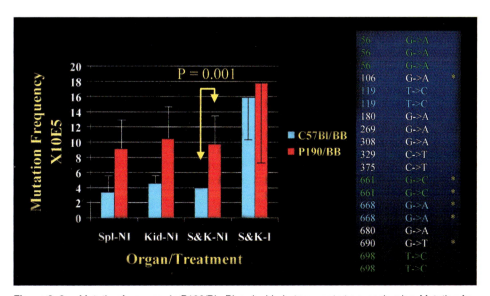

Figure 2–8. Mutation frequency in P190/Big Blue double heterozygote transgenic mice. Mutation frequency was measured in various tissues from control and P190 transgenic mice. In spleen (spl), kidney (Kid), and spleen plus kidney (S&K), the number of mutations (*right*) was higher in P190 mice than in controls, implicating bcr-abl in the induction of a mutator phenotype.[41]

jacent DNA sequences, resulting in antigen receptors with sufficient diversity to respond to environmental stimuli. Rarely, recombination via V(D)J
recombinase may occur to an inappropriate location
and may result in gene activation and/or transformation of lymphoid or even myeloid cells. Many examples of leukemia involving illegitimate V(D)J
recombination exist in the literature. There are
reports of myeloid leukemias in which Ig or TCR
gene rearrangements occur. In AML, the presence of
Ig heavy-chain (IgH) rearrangement resulted in significantly worse survival of 29 percent at 25 months,
compared with 88 percent for patients with germline
IgH.[47] Oligoclonal rearrangements of IgH and TCR
loci have been noted in lymphoid malignancies, as
have cross-lineage rearrangements of either TCR in
B-cell leukemias or Ig genes in T-cell leukemia.[48,49]
Aberrant rearrangements of IgH switch regions were
found in CLL and clustered to a particular region
suggestive of a recombinational hot spot.[50] Illegitimate V(D)J recombination in a human lymphoid
leukemia cell line was precipitated by etoposide, a
chemotherapeutic agent implicated in t-AML, linking a known leukemogenic exposure to a particular
mechanism of aberrant DNA recombination.[51] The
presence of breakpoint sequences consistent with
V(D)J recombination occurred in conjunction with
site-specific deletions of the *HPRT* gene, suggesting
alterations in a DNA repair gene by illegitimate
V(D)J recombination. Several instances of disruption of nuclear factors or tumor suppressors by
V(D)J recombination have been described.[52,53]

MICROSATELLITE INSTABILITY, DNA MISMATCH REPAIR

The genes that mediate repair of DNA in the cell have
been increasingly implicated as tumor suppressors in
that defects in their function are associated with a
growing variety of malignancies. One measure of
genomic instability is microsatellite instability (MSI),
which detects defects in DNA mismatch repair
(MMR). Microsatellites are short, repeated DNA
sequences that exist throughout the genome.
Microsatellite instability has been detected in several
lymphoid and myeloid malignancies, as well as major
nonhematopoietic cancers.[54] It is associated with a

higher proportion of relapsed AML than AML in
remission or at presentation, suggesting an association with leukemia progression.[55] Loss of genes medi-
ating MMR has been associated with MSI in
leukemia and lymphoma cell lines, as well as patient
samples, linking MSI to MMR.[56,57] Secondary
leukemias, which have a wide variety of chromosomal abnormalities, have been reported to frequently
show abnormal expression of the MMR gene *MSH2*.[58]

SPECIFIC DNA SEQUENCES AND STRUCTURE

Although it is important to clarify the mechanisms
by which DNA mutation and translocation occur and
alter expression of key genes, chemical and enzymatic modifications to the DNA of a cell may be
equally important in the development of leukemia.
Several DNA structural features have been implicated as targets in leukemogenesis, including methylation, telomeres, and *alu* sequences.

DNA methylation frequently occurs at limited
genomic regions called CpG islands, which contain
a high density of CpG dinucleotides, and is detected
by a PCR technique specific for methylated
sequences (Figure 2–9), Southern blotting using
methylation-specific restriction enzymes, or
immunofluorescence.[59] Most CpG islands occur in
the promoter region or 5' end of genes, implicating
methylation in transcriptional control (Figure 2–10).
DNA methylation is inversely correlated with DNA
transcriptional activity, with hypermethylation in
transcriptionally inactive regions, and treatment
with demethylating agents results in induction of
gene expression. Methylation-mediated transcriptional control may occur by several mechanisms.
Methylation of a promoter may directly block the
binding of nuclear proteins required for transcription, as observed in the erythropoietin gene.[60]
Methyl-CpG binding proteins (MeCPs and MDBP)
repress transcription by binding to regions of methylated DNA[61] and/or by recruitment of histone
deacetylase (HDAC). This, in turn, induces a transcriptionally inactive state of chromatin by removing
acetyl groups from histones bound to regulatory
sequences of DNA.[62,63] Thus, the location and density of DNA methylation influence the transcrip-

tional regulation of genes either directly or by influencing the binding of regulatory proteins to DNA.

Several observations have led to the suggestion that abnormal patterns of methylation may be important in leukemia. Methylation status was associated with particular subtypes of leukemia.[64-66] DNA methylation may alter the expression of several classes of genes involved in cellular growth control and has been implicated in the transcriptional silencing of tumor suppressor genes,[67-69] including *p53* and *RB*.[70] Hypomethylation in human leukemia also occurs in genes whose products are important in cell-cycle control.[65] Altered methylation of promoters of MMR genes was demonstrated in t-AML and associated with abnormal expression of these genes in AML,[58] implicating differential methylation with control of DNA repair.[71]

Aberrant methylation of DNA at certain regions of the genome may also destabilize their structure, predisposing to recombination or mutation.[72] Progression of CML is marked by changes in methylation pattern.[73] Abnormal methylation patterns were rare in chronic phase but found in a majority of cases in accelerated phase, blast crisis, and acute leukemia.[74] Furthermore, changes in methylation status correlated to response to treatment.[75-77] Indeed, methylation levels may play a role in the substantial biologic and clinical differences between the chronic leukemia mediated by the p210 form of bcr-abl and the acute leukemia of p190 bcr-abl.[78] In other leukemias, the promoter of the multidrug resistance (MDR) gene appears to be hypomethylated in leukemia, providing a possible basis for its overexpression and resistance to cytotoxic agents.[79] Thus, methylation changes may reflect transcriptional control of genes involved in cell-cycle control, DNA repair, and drug resistance and in some cases are correlated with outcome.

A body of work addresses the role of telomere length and telomerase activity in hematologic malignancies. Telomeres are the physical ends of eukaryotic chromosomes and are composed of hexameric DNA nucleotide repeats. These struc-

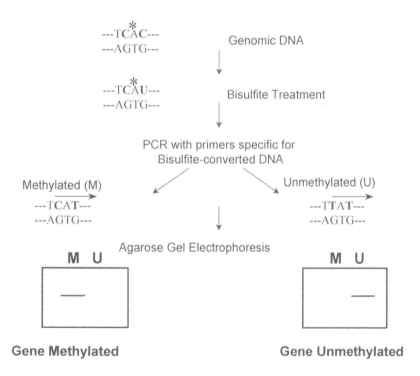

Figure 2–9. Polymerase chain reaction (PCR)-based detection for the methylation status of genomic DNA. This assay entails initial modification of genomic DNA by sodium bisulfite, converting all unmethylated (C), but not methylated (C*), cytosines to uracil. Subsequent PCR amplification is performed with primers designed to distinguish methylated (M) and unmethylated (U) in a specific promoter of the gene of interest. Amplified bands will be visualized at M or U when PCR products are electrophoresed on agarose gel, as shown.

tures preserve chromosomal integrity, providing protection against degradation and recombination and ensuring the complete replication of genes. Telomere erosion occurs with cell division, a process that might be important in regulation of cell senescence. This is partially compensated by the activity of telomerase, a ribonucleoprotein enzyme that adds DNA to the ends of chromosomes (Figure

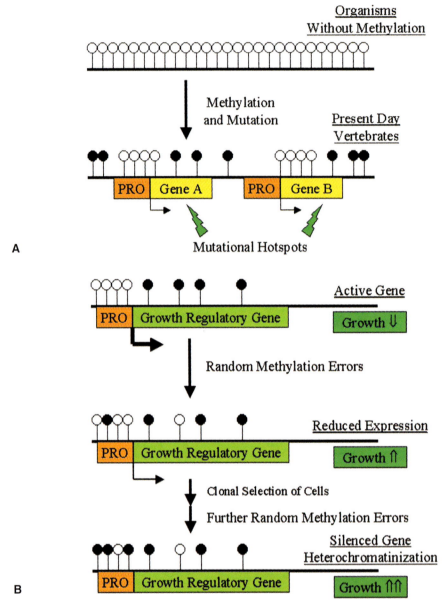

Figure 2–10.   *A*, Evolution of CpG islands. Organisms without cytosine methylation show no suppression in the frequency of occurrence of the CpG methylation site, as indicated in the upper part of the figure. Cytosine methylation (*filled circles*) in vertebrates and other organisms has led to an approximately 80 percent suppression in the frequency of occurrence of the CpG site (*lower part of figure*). The remaining CpG sites are either clustered in 0.5- to 2-kb regions called CpG islands or are dispersed, in which case they are mostly methylated. These sites are often mutational hotspots and contribute very significantly to the generation of polymorphisms, germline mutations, and cancer-causing mutations in the *p53* and other genes. *B*, Model for the progressive inactivation of tumor suppressor genes by abnormal methylation of CpG islands. Several tumor suppressor genes contain CpG islands, which, in common with other autosomal genes, are not normally methylated. Random methylation errors of these CpG sites leads to reduced gene expression, resulting in the clonal selection of cells with these heritable epigenetic defects. Further methylation can result in the eventual paralysis of the gene by heterochromatinization, giving rise to further selection of cells with methylation defects. Tumor cells often contain reduced methylation of the dispersed CpG sites, resulting in a decreased overall level of methylation at the same time as focal hypermethylation of CpG islands is observed.[69]

2–11). The lifespan of normal human fibroblasts and epithelial cells can be extended in vitro by increased expression of telomerase,[80] and the activity of telomerase is highest in cells with high growth requirements, such as stem cells and activated lymphocytes, and in most malignant cells.

High telomerase activity has been demonstrated in hematologic malignancies in numerous studies,[81–84] with activity returning to baseline after successful treatment.[85,86] Although it is unclear whether increased activity of telomerase is a primary defect or is secondary to high cell division requirements in hematologic malignancies, analysis of telomere length and telomerase activity may give prognostic information. Several studies have looked for correlations between telomerase activity and prognosis.[84,87–89] In one recent study, telomere length was significantly shorter in individuals with advanced CML, as compared with those in chronic phase. In this study, patients in chronic phase who went on to develop blast crisis within 2 years had significantly shorter telomere length than those who remained in chronic phase.[89] Telomerase may be specifically inhibited, presenting a potential target for the development of novel treatments of hematologic malignancies.[90]

MOLECULAR BASIS OF HEMATOPOIETIC DYSREGULATION, ALTERATION OF SIGNAL TRANSDUCTION

Previous sections discussed mechanisms by which the integrity of cellular DNA and its function can be disrupted. This section will focus on specific genes that illustrate the diverse signaling pathways in hematopoietic cells that can be dysregulated in malignancy.

Specific genes whose abnormal function mediate malignant cell growth have been called oncogenes. Oncogenes were first recognized in association with retroviruses, which essentially pirated cellular genes involved in growth control. In many cases, the activity of such viral oncogenes (v-onc) was up-regulated via mutation. Once reintegrated into the eukaryotic

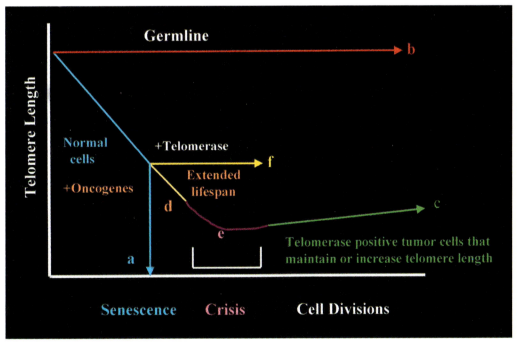

Figure 2–11. The correlation between telomere maintenance and telomerase activity served as a foundation for the telomere hypothesis, first proposed by Calvin Harley in 1991. Maintenance of telomere length generally correlates with the presence of telomerase activity in the germline (*b*) and tumor cells (*c*) but not in most somatic cells (*a*). Absence of telomerase in most normal cells leads to telomere shortening and replicative senescence in culture in vitro (*a*). Alterations in key cellular pathways by the introduction of oncogenes in normal cells lead to an extension of lifespan of the cells in culture (*d*). At a point termed crisis, most of the cells die (*e*). Cells that survive crisis generally have reactivated telomerase (*c*). In certain normal cell types, including hematopoietic progenitors, the expression of telomerase is sufficient for telomere maintenance and extension of lifespan and is one step in tumorigenesis.

genome, the oncogenic potential of these genes became clear. The cellular homologues of these genes are referred to as cellular oncogenes (c-onc) or proto-oncogenes. These genes mediate a variety of cellular functions, from interactions with the extracellular environment and among cells to transcription in the nucleus.

Hematopoietic signaling and thus control of differentiation and proliferation can be disrupted at these levels. Extracellular, cytoplasmic, and nuclear proteins altered by mutation may mediate abnormal hematopoiesis. Up-regulation of signals leading to cell proliferation, or disruption of signals resulting in differentiation, quiescence, or cell death, may result in clonal outgrowth. Alterations of dozens of signaling molecules have been described in leukemia. This section will examine how alterations in signaling from the extracellular environment, at the cell surface, within the cytoplasm, and within the nucleus contribute to leukemogenesis. Factors involved in cell-cycle progression, nuclear transcription factors, and tumor suppressor genes are discussed. Although not an exhaustive review of such mechanisms, this section is meant to illustrate the levels at which cellular growth regulation may become disrupted and result in leukemia.

EXTRACELLULAR SIGNALING

Adhesion molecules mediate interaction of hematopoietic cells with the extracellular matrix and with stromal and other cells. Although the precise signals that govern the adhesion, transport, and release of hematopoietic cells are not clear, several molecules are involved in adhesion. These include components of the extracellular matrix[91–95] and three families of cell surface adhesion molecules, the integrins, selectins, and endothelial cell adhesion molecules, or intercellular adhesion molecules.[8,96,97]

Defects in adhesive interactions of hematopoietic cells were first described in CML[98,99] and result in "marrowization of the peripheral blood," in which the circulation of immature progenitor cells, which are normally undetectable, is universal.[100] Release of immature cells into the peripheral blood in CML may make them less susceptible to down-regulatory signals provided by the bone marrow microenviron-

ment. Normalization of defects in cellular adhesion in CML cells has been correlated with a restored sensitivity to apoptosis.[101]

Adhesion defects may also contribute to the ability of leukemic cells to evade detection by the immune system. For example, CLL cells lack expression of accessory molecules required for T-cell binding and activation, such as CD154, the ligand for CD40. The forced expression of CD154 by CLL cells stimulates a cytotoxic lymphocyte (CTL) response against CLL.[102]

Angiogenesis, or the formation of new blood vessels, is an essential feature linking the growth of solid tumors to their environment. Increased angiogenesis has more recently been demonstrated in hematologic malignancies. Using immunohistochemical staining of tissue sections for vascular endothelial growth factor or von Willebrand factor, a higher number of vessels per millimeter in leukemic bone marrow was demonstrated compared to normal[103,104] (Figure 2–12). Based on these and related data, antiangiogenic agents are in clinical trials in myeloma, leukemia, and preleukemic syndromes.[105–107]

ALTERATION OF CYTOPLASMIC SIGNALING PATHWAYS

Alterations in both positive and negative regulatory cytokines have been described in leukemia. Cytokines secreted by AML blasts and CML cells can induce a variety of effects including autocrine growth,[108,109] induction of expression of receptors for other cytokines,[110] and suppression of growth of nonclonogenic cells.[111–113] These mechanisms may contribute to the progressive dominance of the leukemic clone over normal hematopoietic cells, a phenomenon that may be reversed by appropriate growth conditions in vitro. Stromal cell layers may contribute to altered cytokine expression in leukemogenesis; for example, stromal expression of G-CSF is lost in CML blast crisis.[114,115]

Cytokines typically bind to receptors that traverse the cell membrane and regulate signal transduction by intrinsic tyrosine kinase activity within their cytoplasmic domains. Other receptors, such as Ras, bind to and activate cytoplasmic signaling molecules. P21 Ras is a cytoplasmic signaling protein frequently implicated in hematopoietic and non-hematopoietic malignancies. Ras is a monomeric guanosine diphosphate (GDP) binding protein activated by signals received from receptors with intrinsic tyrosine kinase activity. Similar to the related G protein family of signal transducers, Ras has intrinsic guanosine triphosphate (GTP)ase activity, which is up-regulated by G protein activating proteins (GAPs). Activation of Ras has pleiotropic effects that may result in proliferation, transformation, immune modulation, or differentiation.[116,117] The downstream and even upstream regulators of Ras are complex and only beginning to be understood.

Abnormalities in the Ras gene have prognostic implications in leukemias, as well as solid tumors. In AML, mutations of *ras* were associated with a reduced chance of complete remission after induction chemotherapy.[118,119] Evidence for a causal role of *ras* mutations in leukemia has come from animal models. Lethally irradiated mice were reconstituted with bone marrow cells carrying activated N-ras in a retroviral vector. A majority of these mice developed syndromes that resembled CML, AML, or MDS, implicating *ras* mutation in leukemogenesis.[120] Ras activity has also been shown to be required for

BCR-ABL-mediated inhibition of apoptosis,[121,122] for BCR-ABL-mediated cellular transformation,[123] and for proliferation of CML cells.[124]

Other well-characterized nonreceptor signaling molecules are involved in leukemia. The bcr-abl fusion of CML results in up-regulated abl tyrosine kinase activity, which, in turn, activates several signal transduction pathways via phosphorylation of tyrosine residues (Figure 2–13). *JAK*, or Janus kinase, is a family of tyrosine kinases that bind the cytoplasmic portion of cell surface receptors and phosphorylate them, creating docking sites for other proteins.[125] Fusions between *TEL* and *JAK2*, which lead to constitutive activation of JAK, occur in B-cell precursor ALL and in chronic myelomonocytic leukemia (CMML).[126,127]

Activation of signaling in leukemia has been linked to altered transcription in the nucleus. STAT comprises a family of transcription factors that exist in latent form in the cell cytoplasm and are substrates for JAK. Requirement for activation of STAT by JAK is abrogated in CML, as bcr-abl directly phosphorylates STAT, resulting in translocation of STAT to the nucleus and activation of its nuclear functions.[128,129] In in vitro cell culture, a constitu-

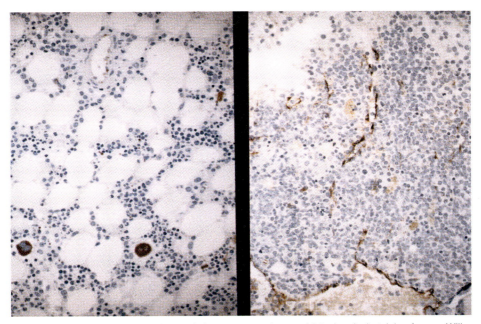

Figure 2–12. Angiogenesis in leukemic bone marrow. Immunohistochemical staining for von Willebrand factor, which stains endothelial cells, megakaryocytes, and platelets, is depicted. The slide on the left is normal marrow, which is negative but for megakaryocytes. An increased number of vessels is seen in AML marrow (*right*). (Photographs courtesy of Dr. Aly Karsan, Division of Laboratory Medicine, University of British Columbia, Vancouver, Canada.)

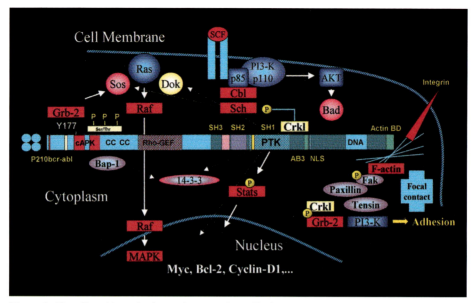

Figure 2–13.   Signal transduction pathways activated by bcr-abl. A complex array of pathways is activated by bcr-abl, leading to nuclear effects and alteration of cellular metabolism and growth control. Some of the key effects include the functional activation of the ras pathway (involving proteins grb-2, sos, crkl, dok), the activation of growth factor signal transduction pathways (SCF), inhibition of apoptosis, and altered cellular adhesion (by interaction with membrane-associated focal adhesion complexes).

tively active mutant of *STAT5* induces growth factor independence.[129] Although no evidence directly links increased activity of STAT to leukemogenesis, its direct activation by bcr-abl in conjunction with the known leukemogenic effects of bcr-abl indicates that STAT is likely an important protein in cellular growth control and dysregulation.

NUCLEAR FACTORS

Nuclear transcription factors and associated molecules are the final common pathway driving gene expression and thus cellular behavior and lineage commitment.[130] Nuclear proto-oncogenes, many of which are transcription factors, mediate increased cell survival and proliferation. The juxtaposition of strong regulatory sequences near the promoter of a proto-oncogene can result in its overexpression, leading to the oncogenic phenotype and increased proliferation. The classic example of this process is the t(8;14) of Burkitt's leukemia, a translocation that brings the IgH enhancer element in proximity to the coding sequence of the proto-oncogene *c-myc*. This results in up-regulation of the expression of *c-myc*, transcription of genes regulated by *c-myc*, and increased cell division.[131]

Chromosomal translocations involving transcription factors can have several other consequences, including creation of chimeric proteins with new or altered function. For example, DNA binding specificity may be altered by replacement of one DNA binding domain with another. This occurs in the t(1;19) of pre–B-cell ALL, in which *PBX* is fused to *E2A*. The carboxy terminal HLH domain of E2A is replaced with the homeobox (*HOX)* domain of *PBX;* thus, the chimeric product interacts with genes regulated by *PBX*. Activity of a transcription factor can also be altered by fusion to an unrelated protein in a way that changes the binding characteristics to key protein partners, as illustrated by the PML/RAR and other fusions seen in APL syndromes.[132]

TUMOR SUPPRESSOR GENES

Tumor suppressor genes are genes whose loss of function, often by deletion or point mutation, is associated with the malignant phenotype. Classic tumor suppressor genes include *Rb* of retinoblastoma and *p53*. Inheritance of one mutation in the germline, as seen in families with a defective allele, results in an increased rate of tumors in these individuals. A "second hit," in which the second allele is inactivated by somatic mutation, dramatically increases the incidence of tumor formation. For example, germline mutation of *p53*, a tumor suppressor gene mutated in many solid tumors and hematologic malignancies, is associated with Li-Fraumeni syndrome, a congenital syndrome with anomalies that include cancer predisposition. Genomic instability may be a common cause of somatic *p53* inactivation since *p53* mutations have been associated with mutagenic drugs in t-AML and with MSI.[133,134]

p53 was originally characterized in virally infected cells. Binding of viral proteins to *p53* sequestered it and led to inactivation of its tumor suppressor function and cellular outgrowth. *p53* normally functions in the cell as a regulator of progression through the cell cycle. With genotoxic damage, p53 mediates delay in cell-cycle progression, allowing time for DNA repair.[8,135,136] Should too much DNA damage be present for efficient repair to take place, p53 may induce mediators of programmed cell death. p53 binds to the promoter of the human mismatch repair gene *hMSH2*[137] and to proteins involved in nucleotide excision repair[138]; thus, its effect on DNA repair may be indirect. However, it also has intrinsic 3'-5' exonuclease activity, suggesting a direct role in DNA repair in addition.[139–141]

Although the regulation of *p53* is not fully understood, it exists in the cell in an inactive form that is inefficient at DNA binding. Its expression and DNA binding activity are up-regulated in response to genotoxic stress such as exposure to ionizing radiation or chemicals and from double-stranded DNA breaks such as those occurring during V(D)J recombination.[142–145]

In cells that have lost p53 or other surveillance mechanisms, genotoxic damage can lead to persistent changes that may further progress toward a malignant phenotype (Figure 2–14). A number of observations have linked alterations in *p53* with leukemia. Germline *p53* mutation was associated with MLL segmental jumping translocation, the dispersal of multiple copies of the *MLL* gene throughout the genome, in t-AML.[146] Alterations in *p53* were associated with ALL in relapse and coincided with acquisition of complex cytogenetic abnormalities.[147] The *ATM* gene of ataxia telangiectasia (AT), a congenital syndrome of chromosomal instability, appears to function upstream of p53 in signaling DNA damage due to ionizing radiation, and normal *ATM* function is required for cell-cycle arrest.[148] Most recently, the *PML* gene, a tumor suppressor rearranged in APL, has been shown to induce cellular senescence in a p53-dependent man-

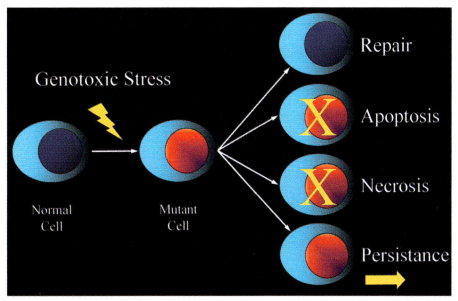

Figure 2–14. Disposition of cells with acquired DNA damage. Three mechanisms ensure that DNA damage is not passed on to the next generation of cells. Damaged cells may die by necrosis or apoptosis or may be stalled in a nonreplicative phase of the cell cycle in order to undergo DNA repair. Should these mechanisms fail, the cell may accumulate mutations that, under appropriate circumstances, result in leukemic transformation.

ner.[149] Thus, mutation of p53 is associated both with congenital syndromes predisposing to leukemogenesis and with gene mutation and cytogenetic abnormalities known to confer a poor prognosis.

CELL-CYCLE-SPECIFIC PROTEINS

For cell division to occur, DNA must be accurately replicated and distributed to daughter cells. Checkpoints in the cell cycle allow delay of cell division should genotoxic damage occur, thus allowing time for DNA repair. These checkpoints are at the G1/S (growth phase 1/DNA synthesis) transition, in the S phase itself, and at the G2/M (growth phase 2/mitosis) transition. A series of cyclins and cyclin-dependent kinases (CDKs) control progression through each phase of the cell cycle and transition between phases (Figure 2–15).[8,150] An important control point is the G1/S transition, which is regulated by p53 via differential phosphorylation of Rb. In its dephosphorylated state, Rb binds to several transcription factors, sequestering them. Phosphorylation of Rb releases these transcription factors, allowing DNA synthesis to occur.

Abnormalities in cell-cycle progression occur with alterations in p53, Rb, cyclins, or the associated

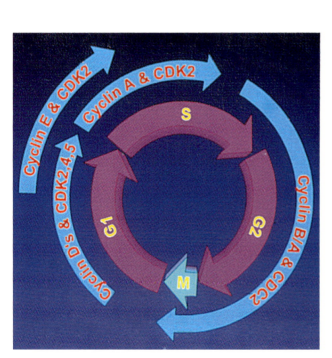

Figure 2–15. Schematic diagram correlating the phases of the cell cycle with the expression of specific cyclins. Also shown are the kinases that modify the activity of the indicated cyclins.

CDKs. Cyclin D1, also known as PRAD-1, CCND1, and Bcl-1, mediates progression through G1 and transition from G1 to S phase. The expression of cyclin D1 is up-regulated in several lymphoproliferative disorders, including mantle cell lymphoma (MCL), in which the t(11;14)(q13;132) juxtaposes regulatory elements of the IgH locus with coding sequences for cyclin D1.[151] Dysregulation of cell-cycle-specific proteins occurs in HCL, with overexpression of cyclin D1. Unlike MCL, no detectable rearrangements or amplifications are defined in HCL, and the mechanism of gene activation in HCL is currently unknown.[152,153] Other abnormalities in cell-cycle-specific proteins include inactivating point mutations in the CDK inhibitor *p16*, which is common in ALL.

ETIOLOGY OF LEUKEMIA

Role of Host Factors

The growing encyclopedia of molecular abnormalities associated with leukemia begins to explain how cells escape the complex growth regulatory systems that control the life cycle of normal cells. Equally important is to understand why these changes occur in some individuals but not most. Risk factors for leukemia involve the genetic makeup of the host, particularly with regard to the function of the immune system, as well as the environment.

An intact immune system is important in protecting against tumorigenesis, a process referred to as "tumor surveillance." An increased incidence of leukemia is seen in some syndromes of congenital immunodeficiency. Although an increase in hematologic malignancies occurs in the setting of acquired immunodeficiency such as infection with the human immunodeficiency virus (HIV), this mainly takes the form of NHL. Non-Hodgkin's lymphoma in HIV and with iatrogenic immunosuppression will be discussed briefly in this section to illustrate themes that may be important in the maintenance of immunity against all hematologic malignancies.

Non-Hodgkin's lymphoma is increased 100- to 150-fold in HIV compared to age-matched individuals. Non-Hodgkin's lymphoma in this setting tends to be clinically aggressive. Pathophysiology may involve chronic antigen stimulation from HIV itself, from

Epstein-Barr virus (EBV), or from concomitant opportunistic infections (OIs). This may lead to cytokine dysregulation, which, in conjunction with decreased immune surveillance, may predispose to clonal outgrowth and further transforming events.[154,155] In keeping with this hypothesis, a polyclonal activation of B cells is commonly seen in HIV, accompanied by a polyclonal or oligoclonal increase in Igs.[156]

In terms of phenotype and clinical presentation, HIV-NHL is reminiscent of malignancies that occur in the setting of iatrogenic immunosuppression. A similar excess of NHL is seen with immunosuppression following organ transplantation. Approximately 2 percent of transplant recipients develop post-transplant lymphoproliferative disorder (PTLD), compared to an incidence of NHL between 0.1 and 9 per 100,000 in the general population, an increase of 20- to 120-fold. The incidence of PTLD varies according to type and intensity of immunosuppression.[157–159] An association with EBV is supported by several lines of evidence, including epidemiologic data, measurement of neutralizing antibodies, CTL activity, and viral load.[158,160–165] Like NHL in HIV, lesions range from polymorphic and polyclonal to monomorphic and monoclonal.[166,167] In some cases, several clones can be detected in different lesions. It could be argued that immunosuppression in conjunction with EBV primary infection or reactivation in PTLD or OI in HIV leads to the establishment of one or several clones. Further transforming events may then occur and lead to clonal outgrowth and truly malignant behavior.

The importance of the immune system in keeping abnormal cell growth in check is further suggested by the recent unexpected observation of abnormal fusion transcripts in normal healthy individuals. Using sensitive PCR techniques, the bcr-abl fusion characteristic of CML was detected in a significant proportion of healthy adults (12 of 16 and 22 of 73) and in non-CML hematopoietic cell lines, and included transcripts for both P190 and P210.[168,169] As CML is a rare disorder, it is unlikely that the majority of adults harboring a bcr-abl rearrangement will go on to develop CML. Other fusion sequences associated with hematologic malignancies demonstrated in normal healthy persons include the t(14;18) of follicular lymphoma. No data have yet linked the observation of this translocation in the healthy to subsequent development of lymphoma. In addition, transcripts consistent with partial duplication of MLL or fusion transcripts involving MLL have been found in normals.[170–172] Cells expressing fusion oncoproteins may be unable to overcome the normal cellular regulatory controls without infrequent additional mutations. Alternatively, expression of transcript in a cell at a critical stage of differentiation may be required for transformation.

For example, an intact immune system in an individual with a human leukocyte antigen (HLA) haplotype capable of presenting bcr-abl fusion sequences from chimeric proteins as antigen would make clonal expansion and transformation unlikely. Consistent with this assumption is the observation that a proportion of patients who remain Ph or bcr-abl positive following hematopoietic stem cell transplantation lose positivity over time. Conversely, re-emergence of a Ph clone following the attainment of Ph negativity after bone marrow transplantation (BMT) is predictive of relapse and is an indication for donor lymphocyte infusion, which induces a graft versus leukemia immune response, often leading to renewed cytogenetic remission. Similarly, the reappearance of t(15;17) in APL by cytogenetic analysis or PCR is associated with subsequent relapse and is an indication for therapy.[173,174]

In contrast, in AML-M2, the detection of t(8;21) following therapy does not predict relapse and does not indicate further therapy.[175] Thus, in this case, other factors must be important in determining leukemic outgrowth. Factors that predispose to the subsequent development of a hematologic malignancy are likely to include host immunity overall and specific immunity to the abnormal cells and proteins, which may be influenced by HLA type.

Recent evidence has implicated HLA both in susceptibility to the development of CML and in treatment outcome, phenomena that may be related to immunity or to other factors. The European Bone Marrow Transplant Group conducted a case-control study and meta-analysis to clarify this issue. Using 1,899 patients and over 500,000 bone marrow donors as controls, a protective effect against the development of CML of 27 percent was found for HLA-B8, 10 percent for HLA-A3, and 49 percent for the combination of HLA-B8 and -A3. A 29 percent risk reduction for HLA-B8 was confirmed. In another study, a decreased incidence of HLA-DRw6 antigen was observed in patients with CML.[176] The protective effect of HLA type may be mediated by the ability to present bcr-abl fusion peptides as antigen on the cell surface, inducing a protective immune response.[177] Indeed, a correlation between HLA-DR type and the ability to obtain CD4+ and CTL responses to bcr-abl peptides has been observed.[178]

In CML, HLA may also correlate with response to treatment. Of 239 patients with CML treated with interferon-α, patients with HLA-B27 had a better response rate; 10 of 14 (71%) had a major cytogenetic response, and 57 percent had a complete cytogenetic response, compared with 59 percent and 30 percent, respectively, overall. In addition, there was a trend for better survival in patients with HLA-B27, whereas those with HLA-A2, -B7, and -B18 had a trend for shorter survival.[179]

Chronic lymphocytic leukemia has been reported in families, and in at least some cases, disturbances in immune function such as immunodeficiency and autoimmunity were prevalent, further linking leukemogenesis to immune defects.[180,181] A number of reports have noted an association between the HLA-C locus alleles and the occurrence of acute leukemia. Although the mechanism of increased frequency of leukemia is difficult to explain, it has been suggested that HLA-C may determine susceptibility to natural killer cell-mediated cytolysis.[181,182] Thus, a multitude of examples link global or specific defects in immunity, some of which may be mediated by HLA haplotype, to a predisposition to hematologic malignancies.

Etiology of Leukemia on a Population Level

Epidemiologic data indicate that some congenital syndromes influence predisposition to leukemia. Both epidemiologic data and the occurrence of case clustering have led to the view that acquired and environmental factors such as physical agents, toxins, occupational exposures, and possibly infectious agents are involved in leukemogenesis. However, with the exception of ionizing radiation, which is associated with the occurrence of myeloid leukemia, data are often contradictory, and firm conclusions are scanty. Leukemia is a rare disorder, with an inci-

dence of 9 to 10 cases per 100,000 persons per year in the United States; thus, it is difficult to link an increase in risk to a particular exposure.

The association of genetic syndromes with leukemia is firmly established. Genetic syndromes in which an increased incidence of leukemia occurs include syndromes of immune deficiency and of chromosomal instability by mechanisms discussed above. Leukemia is increased in Down syndrome, which includes defects of cell-cycle control and T-cell immunity.[181] Heritable immunodeficiency states associated with leukemia include severe combined immunodeficiency, X-linked hypogammaglobulinemia, common variable immunodeficiency, and Wiskott-Aldrich syndrome.[183,184] Other inherited disorders of chromosome breakage and abnormal DNA repair that predispose to leukemogenesis include ataxia telangiectasia (AT), Bloom syndrome, and Li-Fraumeni syndrome. Two congenital syndromes present interesting models of leukemogenesis: AT and Fanconi's anemia (FA).

Ataxia telangiectasia is a rare, autosomal-recessive, progressive neurologic disorder characterized by increased risk of cancer. Heterozygotes develop a variety of solid tumors and hematopoietic malignancies.[185] The homozygous state is characterized by radiosensitivity and genomic instability; 40 percent of affected persons develop lymphoid malignancies, including T-ALL, T-lymphoma, and T-CLL.[184] T-cell lymphoproliferations occur at four to five times the frequency of B-cell malignancies and are characterized by nonrandom inversions and translocations involving the Ig and TCR loci.[186–190] This finding has led to the suggestion that an underlying defect in AT may be an increase in V(D)J-mediated rearrangements. However, a defect in cell-cycle checkpoint control also occurs, with inappropriate decrease in cell-cycle arrest in response to genomic damage induced by ionizing radiation.[191] This leads to an inappropriate increase in *p53*-mediated apoptosis in response to nonlethal damage. Other defects may include an inability to activate systems of DNA repair.[192]

The gene mutated in AT, *ATM*, has been identified and is located at chromosome 11q22-23.[193] The role of the protein is not fully understood, but it may be involved in cell-cycle progression. Inactivation of *ATM* is seen in 20 to 40 percent of sporadic

CLL.[194,195] Mutations in this setting are missense and in-frame deletions.[196,197] The loss of function mutations observed in this gene suggests that it may normally function as a tumor suppressor.

Fanconi's anemia is an autosomal-recessive disorder characterized by developmental defects, bone marrow failure, and AML. Diagnosis is confirmed by an increased hypersensitivity to DNA cross-linking agents such as diepoxybutane and mitomycin C in vitro. Analysis by the International Fanconi Anemia Registry reveals that by age 40, 98 percent of patients will develop hematologic abnormalities, 52 percent will develop MDS or AML, and 81 percent will die of hematologic causes.[198] Indeed, the incidence of AML is increased 15,000-fold compared to the general population.[198] Acute myelogenous leukemia in FA involves deletions characteristic of those that occur secondary to exposure to alkylating agents, such as abnormalities of chromosomes 5 and 7.[199,200]

The gene responsible for FA, *FAC*, has a structure suggestive of a transcriptional repressor and is homologous to *PZLF*, a gene involved in a variant translocation in APL.[201] The major underlying defect appears to be a disturbance in cell-cycle progression. In contradistinction to AT, G2 arrest is increased in FA, except when evolved to MDS or AML.[202] However, other mechanisms that may be important in FA are illustrated by the demonstration of site-specific deletions at the site of a consensus heptamer sequence similar to that found at Ig and TCR genes. This suggests that V(D)J-mediated recombination may be involved in the development of hematologic abnormalities in FA.

Multigeneic Hereditary Predisposition

A bimodal distribution of the incidence of leukemia with age suggests different etiologies for childhood and adult leukemias. A prenatal origin to childhood leukemia has been suggested by the results of twin concordance studies, in which an increased incidence of leukemia is seen in each twin. However, in this setting, the relative influence of genetics and shared uterine environment are difficult to define.[181] In adult leukemia, no twin concordance has been demonstrated, suggesting that acquired factors are more likely to be important in this group. However, racial clustering has been noted in some forms of leukemia, including an increased incidence of APL in Hispanics, where the proportion of APL was 37.5 percent, versus 6.5 percent in non-Hispanics.[203] This observation remained significant after adjusting for the younger age of Hispanic patients. Similarly, in Los Angeles, a higher proportion of AML-M2 (52%) was noted in Orientals.[204] Chronic myelogenous leukemia occurs more frequently in African Americans than Caucasians, and both CML and CLL are twice as common in Jews.[180] It is not clear, as in twin studies, whether these associations are secondary to a genetic predisposition or a common acquired factor, such as an environmental exposure. For example, ethnic Asians show an increased incidence of CLL in North America compared to the Orient, which is not altered by immigration, suggesting environmental factors.[180,183,205]

Environmental Factors: Link to Infections

In children, a link between socioeconomic status and the incidence of leukemia is noted in some studies.[206] This has led to speculation that exposure to infectious agents might be important in leukemogenesis[207-209] and that changes in the pattern of childhood infection might lead to alterations in the immune system that predisposes to the development of leukemia.[210] Consistent with this hypothesis is the observed link between inflammatory conditions such as vasculitis and inflammatory bowel disease and leukemia.[211] The roles of EBV in African Burkitt's lymphoma and the retrovirus human T-cell lymphocyte virus-1 (HTLV-I) in adult T-cell lymphocytic leukemia (ATL) are well documented.

Adult T-cell lymphocytic leukemia is endemic in the Orient and the Caribbean, with small foci in the Middle East. Human T-cell lymphocyte virus-1 infection results in transformation of peripheral CD4 cells and can present in a variety of ways. The acute form presents aggressively, with high leukocyte counts, hepatosplenomegaly, hypercalcemia, and lytic bony lesions, and has poor survival. Less common are the lymphomatous, chronic, and smoldering forms.[212] Infection with HTLV-I may predispose to genomic instability; MSI was demonstrated in a large proportion of patients with ATL and in higher numbers than other hematologic malignancies.[213] However, with these exceptions, no studies to date have convincingly demonstrated a link between infectious agents and leukemia.

Ionizing Radiation

Although most environmental factors predisposing to leukemia remain unidentified, a convincingly documented leukemogenic exposure is ionizing radiation. This has been linked to the development of myeloid leukemia, particularly CML.[180,214] The data implicating ionizing radiation have existed for several decades and arose largely from follow-up of survivors of the nuclear bombings at Hiroshima and Nagasaki (Figure 2–16).[215] These data demonstrate a positive correlation between radiation dose and leukemia incidence, with a dramatic link between leukemia risk and distance from the epicenter of the nuclear blast. The incidence and timing of leukemia are also related to the relative emissions of nuclear particle types and linear energy transfer.[216] A correlation between nuclear tests in the United States and waves of myeloid leukemia and ALL in children and adolescents was noted, as was the occurrence of multiple cytogenetic abnormalities in a group of Japanese fishermen exposed to fallout from the nuclear testing at Bikini. Ionizing radiation results in the generation of free radicals, which can induce double-stranded DNA breaks, reciprocal translocations, and sister chromatid exchange.[217] Leukemia-associated transcripts following exposure of cell lines to ionizing radiation have been demonstrated.[218,219]

In addition to the data from nuclear misadventures, some studies of occupational exposure to ionizing radiation have confirmed an association with increased risk of leukemia,[220] particularly in medical personnel exposed to radiation prior to the era of uniform shielding and monitoring.[180,182] Finally, there is evidence that patients exposed to ionizing radiation for therapeutic purposes have an increased risk of leukemia, particularly ΛML.[180,182,183] Patients who received total body irradiation as conditioning for hematopoietic stem cell transplantation are at increased risk for the development of a variety of secondary malignancies, including leukemia. In contrast, results of studies of nonionizing radiation, such as from electromagnetic fields, are contradictory.[182]

Occupational Risks

An association between other occupations and the incidence of leukemia has been demonstrated in some studies. For example, CLL was noted in rubber industry workers exposed to solvents and in tailors, furniture workers, and printers.[180] The occupations of electrician and welder were associated with leukemia.[221] Brewery workers and auto mechanics were associated with CML. Aside from ionizing radiation, the most persuasive evidence links environmental exposure to benzene and its metabolites with leukemia risk.[222–224] Although some groups have failed to demonstrate such a relationship,[225] the discrepancy in results may reflect extent of exposure. Most affected patients in case series had a history of intense exposure for prolonged periods.[180] Workers exposed to 15 to 150 parts per million (ppm) had a five- to six-fold increased risk for AML

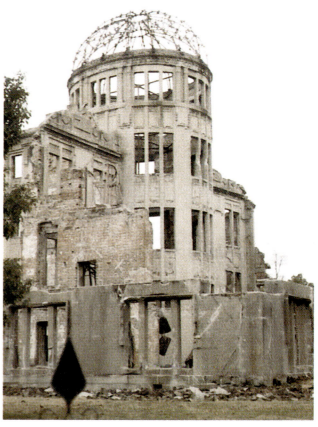

Figure 2–16.   The war memorial at Hiroshima, Japan. This building was at the epicenter of the nuclear blast and was the only structure left standing within a wide radius, as energy from the explosion traveled circumferentially.

and CML, whereas those exposed to less than 1 ppm were at no discernible increased risk.

Potential mechanisms for these associations have been explored in animal models in vitro. Exposure of mice to benzene resulted in spindle fiber disruption and the occurrence of chromosomal translocations characteristic of MDS and acute leukemia.[226] Hydroquinone, a benzene metabolite, alters the differentiation of leukemic cell lines in vitro; it blocks the differentiation of HL-60 cells to monocytes,[227] while facilitating differentiation of the same cell line to neutrophils.[228] Data on other chemicals and environmental toxins such as pesticides and herbicides are contradictory.[180]

Some information links the effects of tobacco smoking to the development of leukemia.[180] Time to blast crisis in CML is shorter in smokers, and a two- to three-fold increased risk of AML is seen in persons with a 20 pack-year smoking history.[229] Bad prognosis cytogenetics such as –7, 7q-, and +8 occur more frequently in smokers. Although these effects may be related to benzene inhalation, the presence of multiple carcinogens in tobacco smoke confounds analysis. A small number of studies show an increased risk of childhood leukemia with marijuana use during pregnancy.[182] This effect is confounded by the possibility of other lifestyle issues that might put the fetus at risk.

Leukemia Associated with Previous Chemotherapy

There is a large and persuasive body of evidence implicating previous exposure to chemotherapeutic agents to the development of t-AML, which accounts for 10 to 20 percent of all AML cases and occurs in 5 to 15 percent of patients previously treated with chemotherapy. These agents include the topoisomerase II inhibitors or epidophyllotoxins, such as etoposide, and alkylating agents such as cyclophosphamide or chlorambucil. It was noted that patients treated with chlorambucil for the myeloproliferative syndrome polycythemia vera were at significant risk of death due to leukemia (20%), compared with patients who received phlebotomy alone, of whom 7 percent died of leukemia.[230] Defined syndromes result; leukemia secondary to alkylating agents usu-

ally presents at an interval of approximately 5 years following exposure and is characterized by cytopenias, dysplasia, and abnormalities of chromosomes 5 and 7, all poor prognostic features.[231,232] Survival is in the order of several months. In contrast, patients with leukemia following exposure to topoisomerase II inhibitors have an interval to leukemia of approximately 2 years and often have rearrangements involving chromosome 11q23, the locus for MLL.[233] Although these leukemias respond favorably to induction chemotherapy, survival is short. Acute myelogenous leukemia secondary to chemotherapy has many features in common with AML that occurs in the elderly, including the particular chromosomal abnormalities involved, poor response to therapy, and short survival.[234] Patients with t-AML may benefit from intensive therapeutic regimens, including high-dose cytarabine or BMT.[235,236] However, the probability of survival even following BMT is a mere 8 percent in patients with the subtype of MDS refractory anemia with excess blasts in transformation or AML.[237]

The magnitude of risk for t-AML can be estimated from cohort studies of patients previously treated with the implicated agents. In most series, the majority of patients with t-AML had prior breast cancer, Hodgkin's disease, or NHL.[238] The relative risk of patients receiving chlorambucil for the treatment of NHL was estimated at 6.5 (confidence interval 1.6–26) after receiving a cumulative dose of at least 1,300 mg. In contrast, regimens containing cyclophosphamide were associated with a relative risk of 1.8 (0.7–4.9) at a cumulative dose less than 20,000 mg. On this basis, it was concluded that an excess of four leukemias over a period of 10 years would be seen in a group of 10,000 patients receiving chemotherapy, including cyclophosphamide for NHL.[239]

Through a monitoring program at the National Cancer Institute, the 6-year cumulative risk of AML following treatment with etoposide was 0.7 to 3.3 percent, for which no dose response was seen,[240] and was mainly related to the pretransplant chemotherapy regimen.[241,242] Patients receiving etoposide for stem cell mobilization prior to autologous stem cell transplantation for NHL were at a 12.3-fold risk for the development of t-AML,[243] and patients receiving BEAM for NHL (carmustine, etoposide, cytosine-arabinoside, and melphalan) had a relative risk of 357 (43–1,290) for t-AML.[242]

In summary, leukemia risk from environmental exposure involves the disruption of mostly unidentified and likely multiple cellular genes and signaling pathways. Inherited abnormalities may contribute to effects of mutations acquired through the action of mostly unidentified physical or chemical agents. Congenital syndromes and environmental factors implicated in leukemogenesis share with sporadic leukemia a predisposition to or acquisition of genomic instability and/or the accumulation of multiple genetic changes leading to cellular transformation.

LEUKEMIA SYNDROMES

Philadelphia Chromosome-Positive Leukemias

Chronic myelogenous leukemia is a chronic leukemia characterized by the overabundance of structurally normal neutrophils and neutrophil precursors in the peripheral blood. The chronic phase of CML may be asymptomatic and lasts a median of 3 years. Although variable in timing, CML inevitably progresses through an accelerated phase and blast crisis to acute leukemia (Figure 2–17). The acute transformation of CML may be either myeloid or lymphoid in type. Both analysis of X-chromosome-linked polymorphism and cellular distribution of the Ph chromosome in CML have indicated that the underlying defect in this leukemia is harbored in the pluripotent stem cell.

The t(9;22) of CML, which results in the Ph chromosome, is one of the best characterized transloca-tions in human leukemia. Like many translocations, the t(9;22) causes an in-frame fusion between the coding sequences of two loci, resulting in a bcr-abl fusion transcript and protein. Although much remains to be understood about the specific events directed by the normal gene products bcr and abl, a large body of evidence documents signal transduction pathways disrupted in CML. Chronic myelogenous leukemia was one of the first human malignancies in which function of the genes and gene products involved in recurring chromosomal abnormalities was dissected (Figures 2–18 and 2–19). It is an excellent example of the ways in which the techniques of molecular biology can be harnessed for diagnostic purposes and to design new and specific therapies that target genetic changes. Recent strategies have targeted both the molecular translocation in CML using antisense oligonucleotides to *bcr-abl* and the function of the fusion protein using specific inhibitors of its signal transduction activity, in an attempt to reverse the leukemic phenotype. These strategies may be complemented by attempts to elicit specific immunity to the fusion region of the bcr-abl polypeptide.[178]

The t(9;22) results in several forms of BCR-ABL, which are associated with distinct leukemic syndromes (see Figure 2–18). The form associated with CML results from breaks in the 5.8 kilobase major breakpoint cluster region (M-bcr) and results in fusion between the exons b2 or b3 of bcr and a2 of abl. This fuses the regulatory regions and N-terminal 13 to 14 exons of bcr to the 10 C-terminal exons of abl, resulting in a protein of 210 kilodaltons (kDa), or P210. P190, which is associated with acute leukemia, results from translocation between the minor bcr (m-bcr) and

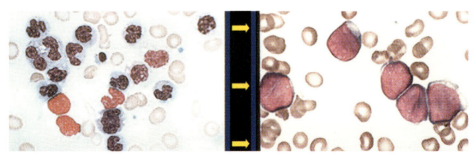

Figure 2–17.   Evolution of CML and genomic instability. Evolution from chronic phase, characterized by overabundance of mature neutrophils and their precursors (*left*), to blast crisis and acute leukemia (*right*), is accompanied by the acquisition of secondary cytogenetic abnormalities in clinical specimens, cell lines, and transgenic murine models. Other abnormalities accompanying leukemic progression include altered gene methylation inhibition of apoptosis and cell-cycle abnormalities.

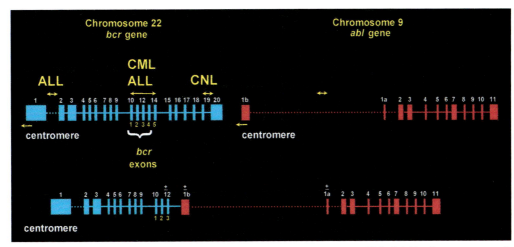

Figure 2–18. Gene structure of *c-bcr*, *c-abl*, and *bcr-abl*. Translocations in Philadelphia chromosome-positive leukemias occur in the major breakpoint cluster region (M-bcr) in CML and ALL. This is between exons 10 to 14 of the *bcr* gene; all translocations fuse portions of *bcr* to the first or second exon of *abl*. This fusion yields the protein P210. The m-bcr, between exons 1 and 2 of *bcr*, occurs in ALL, and the fusion results in a shorter protein, P190. In chronic neutrophilic leukemia (CNL), the μ-bcr between *bcr* exons 19 and 20 yields the fusion protein P230.

abl and fuses the first exons of bcr to the same exons of abl. Finally, a P230 form of bcr-abl has been described, in which fusion at the micro-bcr connects 19 bcr exons to 10 exons of abl. This form is associated with chronic neutrophilic leukemia, a leukemia associated with a more indolent course than CML.

About 25 percent of adults and 5 percent of children with acute ALL carry Ph. Half of these patients express P210 bcr-abl, whereas the remaining patients express the shorter P190 bcr-abl protein. P190 has stronger transforming activity than P210 in experimental models[244] and in the clinical setting,[245] which may be a result of relatively increased tyrosine kinase activity or loss of as yet undefined regulatory domains. Although no function for the reciprocal translocation product abl-bcr has been defined,

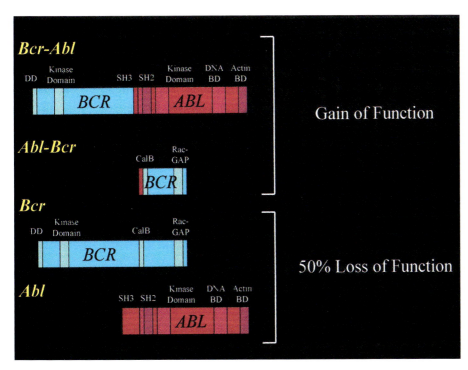

Figure 2–19. Gene products in Philadelphia chromosome-positive leukemias. A reciprocal translocation has the potential to create two novel genes from the breakpoints of the two derivative chromosomes and necessarily destroys one of the two normal copies of each loci involved. The t(9;22) translocation associated with CML and ALL results in the expression of both *bcr-abl* and *abl-bcr* gene products (ie, gain of function). Although the expression of *bcr-abl* has been shown to be essential for leukemogenesis, the expression of *abl-bcr* does not seem to play a role, given that it is not expressed in all patients and that the natural history of *abl-bcr*-positive patients is similar to that of *abl-bcr*-negative individuals. The effect of losing one normal copy of the bcr and abl alleles is unclear (ie, loss of function). Mice bearing only a single copy of the *bcr* gene appear to be normal. In contrast, heterozygous *abl* knock-out mice are cancer prone when exposed to genotoxic stress, suggesting that loss of *abl* function could facilitate cellular transformation by the *bcr-abl* gene product.

abl-bcr, bcr-abl, and the untranslocated abl and bcr alleles are all coexpressed in CFU-GM from patients with CML.[246] abl-bcr is also detected in a majority of patients with CML.[247]

Several lines of evidence, including in vitro and in vivo models, indicate that bcr-abl is important in cellular transformation. Introduction of P210 bcr-abl into hematopoietic cell lines results in growth factor independence and tumorigenicity.[248] Reconstitution of mice with bone marrow cells infected with a retroviral vector carrying P210 bcr-abl resulted in hematologic malignancy, including a CML-like syndrome and lymphoid malignancies.[19,249] These tumors were inconsistently transplantable, an indication that bcr-abl confers a proliferative advantage but that complete cellular transformation involves additional genetic changes. The observation that t(9;22) occurs in normal individuals[168] supports the concept that bcr-abl is necessary but not sufficient for leukemic transformation.

abl is a protein tyrosine kinase that is distributed in both the cytoplasm and the nucleus in normal cells and is involved in inhibition of progression through the cell cycle. Fusion with bcr relocates abl to the cytoplasm, in proximity to the cytoskeleton, suggesting that loss of down-regulatory functions of abl in the nucleus might be important in addition to gain of constitutive tyrosine kinase activity in the cytoplasm.

The activation of c-abl is triggered by genotoxic stress and results in growth arrest in the G1 phase of the cell cycle, a mechanism mediated by p53.[250–252] abl may also directly down-regulate CDK2 and cause growth arrest and is capable of inducing caspases and apoptosis (Figure 2–20).[253] These observations suggest that abl usually functions as a negative regulator of cell growth, a concept supported by the observation that overexpression of dominant negative abl disrupts cell-cycle control and enhances transformation by several oncogenes.[251]

Less is known about the contribution of bcr to transformation in CML. However, bcr has both serine/threonine kinase activity and is a GAP for the Ras-related protein Rac. It has a structural domain important in binding an abl src homology domain called SH2, which is important in regulation of signal transduction in bcr-abl-positive cells. bcr retains several domains important in binding to other pro-

teins, presumably substrates for phosphorylation, and domains that enable bcr-abl fusion protein to form heterodimers, which is thought to be important for its activity.

Further cytogenetic abnormalities that accompany CML progression are characteristic, but none occur in a majority. The most common change is duplication of Ph. Mutations of p53 have been documented in up to one-quarter of patients in accelerated phase.[254] In a transgenic mouse model, it was demonstrated that loss of a p53 allele induces blastic transformation in hematopoietic cells expressing P210 bcr-abl and that this was accompanied by loss of the normal p53 allele.[255] Recently, a mouse strain transgenic for P210 bcr-abl and heterozygous for p53 was created. In these mice, loss of the wild-type p53 allele occurred frequently, suggesting that it was a nonrandom change. This was accompanied by acceleration in mutation rate and accelerated transition to blast crisis. Thus, this model provides a useful system for further study of the interaction between bcr-abl and p53 in leukemogenesis[255] and should allow further elucidation of the role of p53 in CML.

Inhibition of the tyrosine kinase activity of bcr-abl has been made possible by the development of specific tyrosine kinase inhibitors. In experimental models, the 2-phenylaminopyrimidine derivative STI 571 (signal transduction inhibitor, formerly known as CGP 57148) preferentially inhibits formation of colonies by bcr-abl-positive primary cells and cell lines as well as reversing the effects of bcr-abl in murine models.[256–259] Normal adhesion of CML cells to the extracellular matrix is restored in the presence of STI 571, and apoptosis is induced.[260–262] STI 571 has little cross-reactivity for other tyrosine kinases and is active as an oral formulation, making it convenient for potential clinical use. STI 571 is currently in clinical trials in patients with CML.[17,257]

Leukemia Syndromes Associated with Abnormal Transcriptional Activation and Repression

Recently, a considerable amount of research effort into leukemogenesis has been aimed at investigating the mechanism by which activators and repressors of transcription interact to influence cellular pheno-

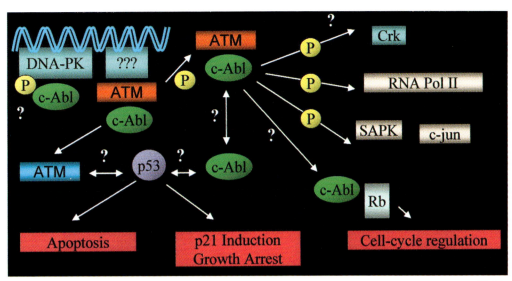

Figure 2–20.   Role of c-abl in DNA repair. Abl is involved in DNA repair indirectly through interaction with Rb, thus influencing cell-cycle regulation. In addition, it phosphorylates a number of substrates involved in cellular metabolism, including RNA polymerase II (RNA pol II). Through putative interactions with p53 and ATM (protein mutated in ataxia telangiectasia), it may also influence apoptosis and DNA metabolism.

type. Several recurring chromosomal translocations in human leukemia result in alterations of transcriptional regulators, including the t(15;17) of APL and the core binding factor mutations t(12;21) of ALL, t(8;21) of AML-M2, and inv(16) of AML-M4.

Chromatin is packaged into nucleosomes consisting of 146 base pairs of double-stranded DNA wrapped around a core of eight histone molecules (Figure 2–21). Internucleosomal regions consist of stretches of up to 100 base pairs of DNA. The structure of nucleosomes is stabilized by hydrogen bonds and electrostatic interactions, which, in turn, are influenced by primary DNA sequence, features of secondary structure, and possibly modifications such as methylation. For transcription to occur, DNA must dissociate from the nucleosome structure and other chromatin-associated proteins to be accessible to transcription factors, which occurs in part by acetylation of histones.[63] Histone acetyl transferases (HAT) move the acetyl moiety from acetyl coenzyme A to the internal lysine residue in the amino terminal tail of histones. Acetylation results in altered electrostatic interactions and steric hindrance and destabilizes the histone-DNA complex, relieving nucleosomal repression and allowing access of the transcriptional machinery to the DNA template.[263] Histone acetylation is tightly controlled in the cell by the balance between HAT activity and HDAC.

Acute Promyelocytic Leukemia

Alterations in histone acetylation play a key role in transcriptional regulation of APL. Acute promyelocytic leukemia is a syndrome characterized by accumulation of leukemic promyeloblasts in the bone marrow. It represents about 10 percent of AML, with a median age at presentation in the early 30s. Although generally responsive to classic therapy, APL is associated with an excess of bleeding at presentation due to hyperfibrinolysis and disseminated intravascular coagulation, a result of the characteristics of the leukemic cells. The characteristic recurring chromosomal translocation of APL is the t(15;17), which fuses the gene *PML* (promyelocytic leukemia) to the *RAR-α*. This, in turn, results in a fusion transcript and protein (Figure 2–22).

A dynamic process of histone acetylation and deacetylation is involved in the regulation of RA responsive genes (Figure 2–23). Retinoic acid receptor-α in the absence of ligand forms a heterodimer with the nuclear protein RXR and binds to a sequence in the promoter region of RA responsive genes, repressing transcription. Other proteins involved in transcriptional repression complexes include nuclear receptor co-repressor molecules, such as N-CoR, and silencing mediator of retinoid and thyroid receptors (SMRT). Co-repressors recruit

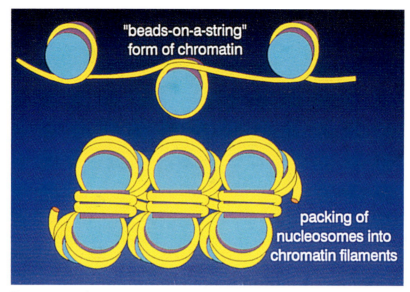

Figure 2–21. Structure of chromatin. Double-stranded DNA is wrapped around a core complex of histone proteins to form a nucleosome. This occurs every 160 base pairs and in interphase chromosomes confers a "beads-on-a-string" appearance. Histone binding is released from DNA regulatory regions by acetylation, allowing access of transcription factors.

HDAC activity, both directly and via intermediary proteins such as Sin3. Binding of the ligand RA induces a conformational change in RAR-α, resulting in release of co-repressors and thus HDAC. Retinoic acid receptor-α is then free to bind a complex that enhances transcriptional activation including several proteins with HAT activity.[18] Factors that may participate in this complex include P/CAF, members of the SRC1 family of 160-kDa proteins, p300, and cyclic AMP response element binding protein (CBP).

In APL, the fusion protein PML-RAR-α has an enhanced interaction with the transcriptional co-repressor complex, resulting in repression of transcription at physiologic levels of RA. SMRT/N-CoR and thus HDAC is not released from PML-RAR-α until pharmacologic concentrations of RA are achieved. Thus, only at pharmacologic concentrations of RA does transcription of RA responsive genes result and differentiation of PML blasts occur (Figure 2–24).

Acute promyelocytic leukemia is an intriguing model of transcriptional regulation in human leukemia for several reasons. Retinoic acid is now regularly used as first-line therapy for APL in conjunction with chemotherapy. Thus, APL is the first human malignancy in which the disruption of a nuclear transcription factor leads to a differentiation blockade and malignant growth that can be overcome by a treatment directed to the dysregulated

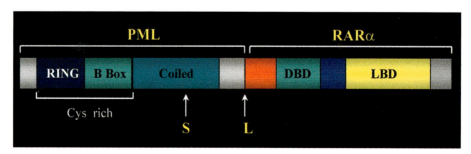

Figure 2–22. Structure of PML-RAR-α. The N-terminal portions of PML from chromosome 15q22 are fused to the C-terminal portions of RAR-α from 17q21. This results in a fusion protein with altered ability to release transcriptional repression in the presence of the ligand RA.

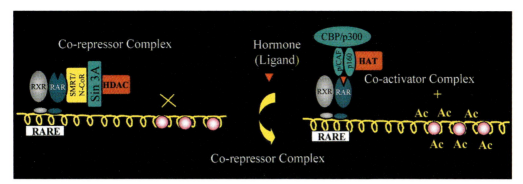

Figure 2–23. Transcriptional co-repression and co-activation. In normal cells, the co-repressor complex, consisting of SMRT, N-CoR, Sin3A, and HDAC, is recruited to the vicinity of the RAR-α/RXR heterodimer and mediates the low state of acetylation of repressed chromatin. Binding of ligand causes release of the co-repressor and recruitment of a co-activator complex, which may include CBP, p300, p/CAF, and P160. These induce histone acetylation (Ac), which is associated with an activated state of chromatin.

receptor. Further, it is the first in which co-regulatory factors downstream of the molecular disruption were described and were themselves targeted as a potentially useful treatment. In one case of RA-resistant APL, an inhibitor of HDAC was used to overcome the block to retinoid-induced transcription and the APL phenotype.[264]

The lack of response to RA-induced differentiation in the variant t(11;17)(q23;q12) of APL is explained by the fusion of PZLF to RAR-α. Unlike PML, PZLF itself has the capacity to bind SMRT and N-CoR directly.[132] Thus, pharmacologic concentrations of RA are unable to release co-repressors from PZLF-RAR, resulting in maintenance of deacetylated chromatin in the vicinity of the RA-responsive element and transcriptional repression. Consistent with this mechanism, repression can be partially overcome by direct inhibition of HDAC.

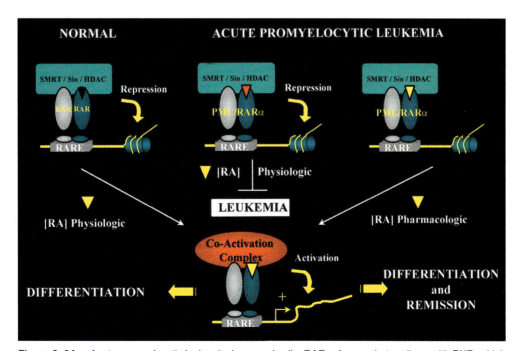

Figure 2–24. Acute promyelocytic leukemia. In normal cells, RAR-α forms a heterodimer with RXR, which binds the co-repressor complex SMRT, Sin, and HDAC. This results in transcriptional repression. Physiologic levels of RA release the co-repressor, and a co-activator complex is recruited, resulting in transcription. In APL, the fusion of PML to RAR-α does not allow release of the co-repressor at physiologic levels of RA. At pharmacologic levels of RA, however, the co-repressor is released, co-activators are recruited, and transcription occurs, resulting in cellular differentiation and remission induction.

The importance of histone acetylation in leukemogenesis is underscored by the observation of translocations directly involving histone acetylases. For example, t(8;16)(p11;p13) fuses the co-activator of transcription and histone acetylation, CBP, to MOZ (monocytic leukemia zinc finger gene) in AML-M4 and -M5.[265] Of note, in addition to their HAT activity, CBP and p300 acetylate nonhistone nuclear proteins, including p53, which strongly increases binding of p53 to DNA. Thus, protein acetylation by histone acetylases may provide indirect mechanisms of transcriptional control in addition to its direct effects on chromatin.[266]

Core Binding Factor Leukemias

Other acute leukemia subtypes alter transcription factors whose regulation involves histone acetylation, suggesting similar mechanisms of leukemogenesis and possibly similar approaches to the development of novel therapies. Core binding factor (CBF) is a nuclear transcription factor involved in the transcription of several genes encoding for cytokines and enzymes important in hematopoietic cells; these include IL-3, GM-CSF, M-CSF, neutrophil elastase, and myeloperoxidase. Core binding factor is a heterodimer composed of an alpha subunit, CBF-α, also known as CBFA1 or AML1, and a beta subunit, CBF-β. Three recurring translocations in human leukemia target either *AML1* or *CBF*-β. The t(12;21)(p13;q22) resulting in the *TEL-AML1* fusion is associated with ALL, the t(8;21)(q22;q22) resulting in the *AML1-ETO* fusion is associated with AML-M2 (Figure 2–25), and the inv(16) resulting in the *CBF-β-MYH1* fusion is associated with AML-M4 with eosinophilia (*AML-M4eo*) (Figure 2–26). Core binding factor is disrupted in addition by the t(3;21), resulting in the *AML1-EVI1* fusion of MDS. The targeting of CBF in at least three subtypes of leukemia and leukemias of both myeloid and lymphoid lineage suggests that alterations in CBF transcriptional regulation affect a convergent pathway leading to the leukemic phenotype. It is interesting to note that the three leukemias in which alterations of either subunit of CBF have been described all have a good prognosis.

AML1, through heterodimerization with CBF-β, acts as an activator of transcription. To date, *AML1* is the most frequently documented gene targeted in chromosomal translocations in human leukemia. Gene knock-out experiments reveal that AML1 is essential for hematopoiesis and that loss of *AML1* results in embryonic lethality.[267] Conversely, knock-in experiments using *AML1* fusion genes demonstrate for the most part a dominant negative effect on AML1 responsive genes.

AML1 is involved in a substantial minority of childhood ALL. Due to a similar banding pattern by cytogenetic techniques of the juxtaposed regions, t(12;21) was not recognized until the advent of chromosomal painting. Using this technique, the presence of material from chromosome 12 was demonstrated on chromosome 21. By molecular analysis, t(12;21) was shown to be the most common abnormality in childhood ALL, occurring in as many as 25 percent of cases. Clinical correlations suggest that it is a leukemia with a very good prognosis, so it is possible that less intensive therapeutic regimens will be developed for this group of patients.[22,268]

The t(12;21) translocation results in an in-frame fusion of the transcription factor TEL (*ETV6*) to AML-1, resulting in a chimeric protein. Thus, the promoter sequences and N-terminal portion of *TEL* are joined to nearly the entire coding sequence of *AML1*. Results of cell transcription assays suggest that TEL-AML1 may function by dominant inhibition of AML1 function.[269,270] The function of TEL is not well understood; however, the normal *TEL* allele is frequently deleted in cells harboring *TEL-AML1*. This suggests a tumor suppressor function, the loss of which might be important in leukemic progression.[164] Other fusions involving *TEL* include the *TEL-PDGF* receptor chimera formed in chronic myelomonocytic leukemia.[271]

Acute myelogenous leukemia-M2 is also known as acute myeloblastic leukemia with differentiation and is a common subtype of AML, accounting for about 15 percent of AML overall. Approximately 30 percent of AML-M2 harbor the translocation t(8;21)(q22;q22), which results in an in-frame fusion of the *AML1* gene from chromosome 21 to the *ETO* gene from chromosome 8 (see Figure 2–25). This results in the chimeric transcript and protein product AML1-ETO (eight twenty one). AML1-ETO forms a complex that in general

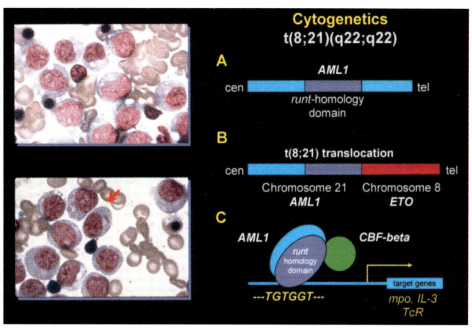

Figure 2–25. AML-M2 involving alteration of CBF. A subset of AML-M2 is associated with fusion between AML1 (CBF-α) of chromosome 21 and ETO of chromosome 8. This occurs by translocation t(8;21)(q22;q22) and gives rise to AML cells, as shown.

represses the transcription of AML1 responsive genes, an effect that may be mediated by more efficient recruitment of CBF-β by AML1-ETO than by AML1.[272] Gene knock-in experiments indicate that AML1-ETO is a dominant negative inhibitor of AML1 function.[273,274] Repression is mediated through the C-terminal zinc finger domains of ETO, which interacts with N-CoR and thus recruits Sin3 and HDAC to the vicinity of the gene promoter.

Acute myelomonocytic leukemia-M4 is another subtype of AML involving alteration in CBF. Although AML-M4 has an intermediate to poor prognosis, a subtype of patients with AML-M4eo do well. Acute myelomonocytic leukemia-M4eo is associated with the inv(16)(p13;q22), which results in an in-frame fusion of *CBF*-β to the smooth muscle myosin heavy-chain gene *MYH1*, resulting in a fusion protein (see Figure 2–26). Although the function of *CBF*-β-*MYH1* is less well understood than either *TEL-AML1* or *AML1-ETO*, the breakpoint in *CBF*-β is conserved and results in incorporation of domains necessary for interaction with AML1. In contrast, breakpoints are variable within the *MYH1*, but all fusion transcripts incorporate an oligomerization domain, suggesting that this domain and

probably protein-protein interactions are important in the function of the fusion protein.

To summarize, the transcription factor CBF is a heterodimer of AML1 and CBF-β and is disrupted by the t(12;21) of childhood ALL, the t(8;21) of AML-M2, and the inv(16) of AML-M4eo. At least two of these translocations, *TEL-AML1* and *AML1-ETO*, result in a fusion protein that acts as a dominant negative inhibitor of AML1. Although many of the genes controlled by CBF remain to be defined, one of the genes under its regulation is the MDR involved in cellular resistance to chemotherapeutic agents, disruption of which could at least partially account for the better prognosis associated with these leukemias. Current research strategies aim to clarify the mechanisms of activation and repression of transcription associated with these fusion products. It has been demonstrated that AML1-ETO recruits the same repressor complex as PML-RAR-α and that inhibition of histone deacetylation results in displacement of this repressor. Thus, manipulation of histone acetylation and deacetylation may well have a role in future therapy of leukemias involving alterations in CBF in addition to APL.

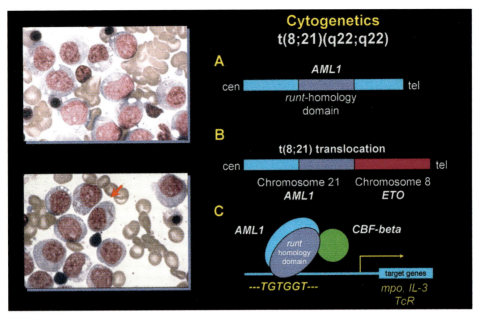

Figure 2–26. AML-M4eo involving alteration of CBF. A subset of AML-M4 is associated with fusion between CBF-β from chromosome 16q and the *MYH11* myosin heavy-chain gene from chromosome 10p. This occurs by inversion of a portion of chromosome 16, inv(16)(p13;q22) or translocation t(16;16)(p13;q22). AML-M4 blasts are shown along with atypical eosinophils (*arrows*), whose large basophilic inclusions are characteristic of M4.

Chromosomal Aberrations Involving 11q23

Abnormalities involving the mixed-lineage leukemia (*MLL*) locus on chromosome 11q23 occur in 5 to 10 percent of primary AML and are seen frequently in t-AML following exposure to topoisomerase II inhibitors. Up to 85 percent of t-AML may show changes involving 11q23, and abnormalities of this locus are associated with several AML subtypes (Figure 2–27). Alterations of *MLL* also involve the t(4;11) of pediatric ALL—hence, one of its other names, *ALL1* (*MLL* is also known as *HRX* or *HTRX*). Abnormalities include a multitude of translocations, with over 40 fusion sites identified and 20 fusion partners cloned. Another frequently recurring abnormality of *MLL* is a partial tandem duplication spanning exons 2 through 6 or 8, which appears to occur as a result of homologous recombination between *Alu* elements.[275,276] In primary AML, 11 percent of patients with normal cytogenetics by standard banding techniques had rearrangements of *MLL*, in most cases, the partial tandem duplication, detected by more sensitive methods. This finding is important since up to 40 percent of patients with adult AML may present with normal cytogenetics.[277] Thus, this abnormality could exist in a significant number of patients with AML and have prognostic implications; patients had a significantly worse complete remission duration compared to those without *MLL* abnormalities. Other changes affecting 11q23 include trisomy 11, which results in duplication of *MLL* in primary AML, the first example of such amplification as a result of recurrent trisomy in human cancer. Deletions involving 11q23 may involve *MLL* and/or other genes.[278]

Inhibitors of topoisomerase II stabilize homodimeric intermediates of DNA replication. It has been suggested that monomeric subunits of topoisomerase II inhibitors bound to DNA might exchange binding partners in some circumstances, leading to chromosomal translocation.[279] Breakpoints in t-AML occur in the 3' half of the MLL bcr, which contains several topoisomerase II consensus sites. In contrast, in de novo leukemias involving 11q23, breakpoints occur in the 5' region of the bcr.[280] This provides a potential molecular basis for the differences in cellular behavior observed in secondary versus de novo leukemias.

The *MLL* gene encodes a 430-kDa protein, with features suggestive of a function in transcriptional regulation.[281,282] *MLL* contains an N-terminal methyltransferase domain that is preserved in translocated fusion products. Although the significance of this finding is not clear, it is tempting to speculate that disruptions in regulatory mechanisms by translocations involving 11q23 may be related to alterations in DNA methylation. Other features of MLL include a C-terminal SET domain, a region involved in binding of the nuclear proteins SWI and SWF. This is predicted to alter chromatin structure in an adenosine triphosphate (ATP)-dependent manner, resulting in release of DNA from the nucleosome core structure and facilitating gene expression. The SET domain is lost in most abnormalities involving 11q23, suggesting that the ability to dissociate certain DNA elements from nucleosome structure may be lost or compromised in many translocations involving 11q23. Partial tandem duplications of *MLL* result in duplication of AT hooks, involved in DNA binding and of DNA methyltransferase domains.

Translocations involving *MLL* fuse the N-terminal domains of *MLL* to C-terminal portions of the partner protein, with expression of the resulting fusion protein under control of the *MLL* promoter. The reciprocal fusion gene resulting from the translocation is usually deleted, out of frame, or not expressed. The fusion partners, although not well characterized, appear to encode proteins with structural features suggestive of involvement in transcriptional regulation. For example, both *CBP* and *p300* are partner genes to *MLL* in translocations involved in human leukemia; t(11;16)(q23;p13.3) fuses *MLL* to *CBP* in t-AML and CMML,[283] and t(11;22) fuses *MLL* to *p300* in AML.[284,285]

Finally, abnormalities of 11q23 appear to fall into two categories. Patients with AML and balanced translocations involving 11q23 typically had involvement of the *MLL* gene, had a history of exposure to topoisomerase II, were more frequently of M4 and M5 subtype, expressed HLA-DR, and had shorter disease-free survival. Conversely, patients with unbalanced translocations of 11q23, which frequently do not fall within MLL, had more splenomegaly, lower white blood cell count, and a lower probability of entering CR.[286]

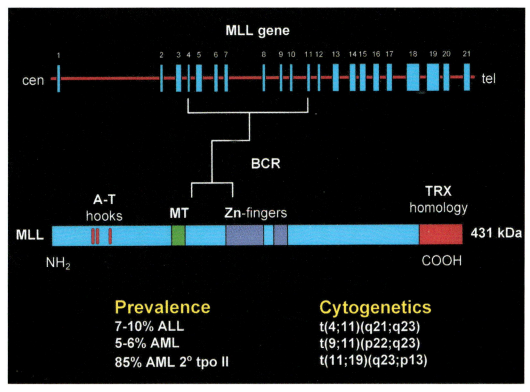

Figure 2–27. Acute myelogenous leukemia-associated 11q23 translocations. Translocations involving the MLL of 11q23 occur in about 10 percent of sporadic AML and up to 85 percent of AML occurring secondary to treatment with epidophyllotoxins. The *MLL* gene has features of a transcription factor, including AT hooks involved in DNA binding and zinc fingers involved in protein-protein interactions.

Chronic Lymphocytic Leukemia: A Model of Decreased Apoptosis

Accidental cell death occurs by necrosis, a process by which intracellular contents are released into the extracellular environment and stimulate an inflammatory response. In contrast, apoptosis, or programmed cell death, is a process by which cells implode in an orderly fashion, by an active process that requires RNA transcription and protein synthesis.[287] It involves the activation of proteolytic enzymes and degradation of cellular contents. Degraded cellular material is packaged into membranous particles, which are released and engulfed by phagocytes. It is triggered intrinsically; for example, neutrophils at the end of their lifespan spontaneously undergo apoptosis, or by external stimuli such as cytokine withdrawal or exposure to either chemotherapeutic agents or ionizing radiation. A decrease in the ability to undergo apoptosis results in prolonged cellular lifespan and is thought to be important in hematologic and other malignancies.

Stimuli that cause DNA damage can result in a number of events. Necrosis may be precipitated, cellular transformation may occur, or DNA repair or apoptosis may result. The latter two effects are both mediated by p53. Following DNA damage, p53 stimulates pathways that induce growth arrest in the G1 phase of the cell cycle. This allows time for repair to take place and ensures that DNA damage is not passed on by cell division. However, p53 may also induce proapoptotic mediators, such as BAX. Induction of apoptosis involves the expression of IL-1β converting enzyme proteases, also known as caspases, critical effector molecules of apoptosis. Other proapoptotic signals include binding of the cell surface protein Fas, or CD95, to ligand or antibody. This induces caspases through an intracytoplasmic "death domain" called FADD (Fas associated protein with a death domain). This pathway may also be stimulated by tumor necrosis factor (TNF) via the TNF receptor and the associated TRADD (TNF receptor associated death domain protein). Finally, the insertion of perforins into the target cell membrane by CTL results in release of degradative enzymes called granzymes into the target cell, activation of caspases, degradation of cellular contents, and cell death.[8,94]

A prototype malignancy for the study of apoptosis is follicular lymphoma, which harbors the t(14;18). This translocation results in up-regulated expression of BCL-2, a mitochondrial protein with antiapoptotic activity and the first cellular proto-oncogene recognized to be important in regulation of programmed cell death.[288] Chronic lymphocytic leukemia is a leukemia in which resistance to apoptosis is important. Apoptosis and the expression of BCL-2 are dysregulated in CLL by an unknown mechanism as no translocation involving the *bcl-2* locus occurs in this malignancy.

Although no rearrangements of *bcl-2* have been demonstrated in CLL, up to 85 percent of cases express high levels of this antiapoptotic protein. Resistance to apoptosis in CLL might also be mediated by pathways involving Fas. Cell surface expression of Fas is low in CLL, but enforced up-regulation of Fas does not result in apoptosis of CLL cells. B-CLL cells modulate their microenvironment by the production of cytokines, and T cells in the vicinity in turn produce antiapoptotic cytokines such as IL-4 and IFN-γ. Thus, several pathways of resistance to apoptosis may be important in CLL.

SUMMARY AND FUTURE DIRECTIONS

Our understanding of leukemia susceptibility, etiology, and pathogenesis has evolved over several decades with refinement in technology. Initial epidemiologic observations on a population level in conjunction with crude measures of cellular characteristics by morphology give way to characterization of abnormal genes and proteins associated with tumorigenesis in general and to recurrent abnormalities associated with specific leukemic syndromes. Understanding of the mechanisms by which these proteins influence transcriptional control and thus cellular growth control continues to evolve. In some instances, these insights have led to promising new therapeutic strategies targeting specific functions altered in specific leukemic phenotypes. Further refinements will likely address both the role of genetics in immunity and the underlying mechanisms that lead to a phenotype predisposing to genetic mistakes. This may be greatly aided by analysis of transcriptional profiling, allowing insight into altered expression of dozens of genes simultaneously, or altered signaling cascades. Other future directions will involve analysis of the contribution of post-transcriptional modifications such as translational and post-translation modification and protein interactions that may be important in cellular behavior.

REFERENCES

1. Henderson ES. History of leukemia. In: Henderson ES, Lister TA, Greaves MF, editors. Leukemia. Philadelphia: WB Saunders; 1996. p. 1–7.
2. Bennett JM, Catovsky D, Daniel MT, et al. Proposed revised criteria for the classification of acute myeloid leukemia. A report of the French-American-British Cooperative Group. Ann Intern Med 1985;103:620–5.
3. Catovsky D, Matutes E. The classification of acute leukaemia. Leukemia 1992;6(Suppl 2):1–6.
4. Harris NL, Jaffe ES, Diebold J, et al. World Health Organization classification of neoplastic diseases of the hematopoietic and lymphoid tissues: report of the Clinical Advisory Committee meeting-Airlie House, Virginia, November 1997. J Clin Oncol 1999;17:3835–49.
5. Allen TD, Dexter TM, Simmons PJ. Marrow biology and stem cells. In: Dexter TM, Garland JM, Testa NG, editors. Colony-stimulating factors, Immunology Series. New York: Marcel Dekker, Inc.; 1990. p. 1–38.
6. Metcalf D. Haemopoietic growth factors 1. Lancet 1989;15:825–7.
7. Witte ON. Steel locus defines new multipotent growth factor. Cell 1990;63:5–6 [published erratum appears in Cell 1990;63:1112].
8. Israels LG, Israels ED. Mechanisms in hematology. Winnipeg, MB: The University of Manitoba University Press; 1996.
9. Till JE, McCulloch EA. A direct measurement of the radiation sensitivity of normal mouse bone marrow cells. Radiat Res 1961;14:215–22.
10. Dexter TM, Spooncer E. Growth and differentiation in the hemopoietic system. Annu Rev Cell Biol 1987;3:423–41.
11. Dexter TM, Allen TD, Lajtha LG. Conditions controlling the proliferation of haemopoietic stem cells in vitro. J Cell Physiol 1977;91:335–44.
12. Metcalf D. Control of granulocytes and macrophages: molecular, cellular, and clinical aspects. Science 1991;254:529–33.
13. Szilvassy SJ, Lansdorp PM, Humphries RK, et al. Isolation in a single step of a highly enriched murine hematopoietic stem cell population with competitive long-term repopulating ability. Blood 1989;74:930–9.
14. Sievers EL, Appelbaum FR, Spielberger RT, et al. Selective ablation of acute myeloid leukemia using antibody-targeted chemotherapy: a phase I study of an anti-CD33 calicheamicin immunoconjugate. Blood 1999;93:3678–84.
15. Matthews DC, Appelbaum FR, Eary JF, et al. Radiolabeled anti-CD45 monoclonal antibodies target lymphohematopoietic tissue in the macaque. Blood 1991;78:1864–74.
16. Nowell PC, Hungerford DA. A minute chromosome in human chronic granulocytic leukemia. Science 1960;132:1497–502.
17. Druker BJ, Lydon NB. Lessons learned from the development of an abl tyrosine kinase inhibitor for chronic myelogenous leukemia. J Clin Invest 2000; 105:3–7.
18. Kakizuka A, Miller WH Jr, Umesono K, et al. Chromosomal translocation t(15;17) in human acute promyelocytic leukemia fuses RAR alpha with a novel putative transcription factor, PML. Cell 1991;66:663–74.
19. de The H, Lavau C, Marchio A, et al. The PML-RAR alpha fusion mRNA generated by the t(15;17) translocation in acute promyelocytic leukemia encodes a functionally altered RAR. Cell 1991;66: 675–84.
20. Warrell RP Jr, de The H, Wang ZY, Degos L. Acute promyelocytic leukemia. N Engl J Med 1993;329: 177–89.
21. Rowley JD. The role of chromosome translocations in leukemogenesis. Semin Hematol 1999;36(Suppl 7): 59–72.
22. McLean TW, Ringold S, Neuberg D, et al. TEL/AML-1 dimerizes and is associated with a favorable outcome in childhood acute lymphoblastic leukemia. Blood 1996;88:4252–8.
23. Daley GQ, Van Etten RA, Baltimore D. Induction of chronic myelogenous leukemia in mice by the P210bcr/abl gene of the Philadelphia chromosome. Science 1990;247:824–30.
24. Wiemels JL, Ford AM, Van Wering ER, et al. Protracted and variable latency of acute lymphoblastic leukemia after TEL-AML1 gene fusion in utero. Blood 1999;94:1057–62.
25. Wiemels JL, Cazzaniga G, Daniotti M, et al. Prenatal origin of acute lymphoblastic leukaemia in children. Lancet 1999;354:1499–503.
26. Faderl S, Talpaz M, Estrov Z, et al. The biology of chronic myeloid leukemia. N Engl J Med 1999; 341:164–72.
27. Hagemeijer A. Chromosome abnormalities in CML. Baillieres Clin Haematol 1987;1:963–81.
28. Pallisgaard N, Hokland P, Riishoj DC, et al. Multiplex reverse transcription-polymerase chain reaction for simultaneous screening of 29 translocations and chromosomal aberrations in acute leukemia. Blood 1998;92:574–88.
29. De Risi J, Penland L, Brown PO, et al. Use of a cDNA microarray to analyse gene expression patterns in human cancer. Nat Genet 1996;14:457–60.

30. Golub TR, Slonim DK, Tamayo P, et al. Molecular classification of cancer: class discovery and class prediction by gene expression monitoring. Science 1999;286:531–7.

31. Kurian KM, Watson CJ, Wyllie AH. DNA chip technology [editorial]. J Pathol 1999;187:267–71.

32. Alizadeh AA, Eisen MB, Davis RE, et al. Distinct types of diffuse large B-cell lymphoma identified by gene expression profiling. Nature 2000;403:503–11.

33. Witte ON. Mechanisms of leukemogenesis. In: Stamatoyannopoulos G, editor. The molecular basis of blood diseases. Philadelphia: WB Saunders; 1994.

34. Hunter T. Cooperation between oncogenes. Cell 1991;64:249–70.

35. Block AW, Sait SN, Kakati S, et al. Massive hyperdiploidy and near-tetraploidy in acute myeloid leukemia [abstract]. Blood 1999;94(Suppl 1):200b.

36. Sweetser DA, Chen C-S, Flowers DA, et al. Loss of heterozygosity occurs in childhood de novo acute myeloid leukemia and is associated with an elevated white blood cell count [abstract]. Blood 1999; 94(Suppl 1):494a.

37. Kearns WG, Liu J, Aridgides L, et al. Genomic instability in bone marrow failure syndromes: high frequency of aneuploidy by fluorescence in situ hybridization and identification of a spindle checkpoint gene mutation [abstract]. Blood 1999;94(Suppl 1):674a.

38. Santucci MA, Anklesaria P, Laneuville P, et al. Expression of p210 bcr/abl increases hematopoietic progenitor cell radiosensitivity. Int J Radiat Oncol Biol Phys 1993;26:831–6.

39. Laneuville P, Sun G, Timm M, Vekemans M. Clonal evolution in a myeloid cell line transformed to interleukin-3 independent growth by retroviral transduction and expression of p210bcr/abl. Blood 1992;80: 1788–97.

40. Laneuville P, Sullivan AK. Clonal succession and deletion of bcr/abl sequences in chronic myelogenous leukemia with recurrent lymphoid blast crisis. Leukemia 1991;5:752–6.

41. Salloukh HF, Laneuville P. Increase in mutant frequencies in mice expressing the bcr-abl activated tyrosine kinase. Leukemia 2000;14:1401–4.

42. Sinclair PB, Nacheva EP, Leversha M, et al. Large deletions at the t(9; 22) breakpoint are common and may identify a poor-prognosis subgroup of patients with chronic myeloid leukemia. Blood 2000;95:738–43.

43. Gillert E, Leis T, Repp R, et al. A DNA damage repair mechanism is involved in the origin of chromosomal translocations t(4;11) in primary leukemic cells. Oncogene 1999;18:4663–71.

44. Shimizu K, Miyoshi H, Kozu T, et al. Consistent disruption of the AML1 gene occurs within a single intron in the t(8;21) chromosomal translocation. Cancer Res 1992;52:6945–8.

45. Marlton P, Claxton DF, Liu P, et al. Molecular characterization of 16p deletions associated with inversion 16 defines the critical fusion for leukemogenesis. Blood 1995;85:772–9.

46. Corral J, Forster A, Thompson S, et al. Acute leukemias of different lineages have similar MLL gene fusions encoding related chimeric proteins resulting from chromosomal translocation. Proc Natl Acad Sci U S A 1993;90:8538–42.

47. Kyoda K, Nakamura S, Matano S, et al. Prognostic significance of immunoglobulin heavy chain gene rearrangement in patients with acute myelogenous leukemia. Leukemia 1997;11:803–6.

48. Szczepanski T, Beishuizen A, Pongers-Willemse MJ, et al. Cross-lineage T cell receptor gene rearrangements occur in more than ninety percent of childhood precursor-B acute lymphoblastic leukemias: alternative PCR targets for detection of minimal residual disease. Leukemia 1999;13:196–205.

49. Stolz F, Panzer S, Fischer S, Panzer-Grumayer ER. Oligoclonal immunoglobulin heavy-chain and T-cell receptor delta rearrangements persist in a recurrent acute lymphoblastic leukemia with one immunoglobulin kappa rearrangement as a clonal marker. Mod Pathol 1999;12:819–26.

50. Crossen PE, Morrison MJ. Aberrant rearrangements of the immunoglobulin heavy chain switch region in chronic B-cell leukemia. Leuk Lymphoma 1998;31: 559–65.

51. Chen CL, Fuscoe JC, Liu Q, Relling MV. Etoposide causes illegitimate V(D)J recombination in human lymphoid leukemic cells. Blood 1996;88:2210–8.

52. Hatano M, Roberts CW, Minden M, et al. Deregulation of a homeobox gene, HOX11, by the t(10;14) in T cell leukemia. Science 1991;253:79–82.

53. Cayuela JM, Gardie B, Sigaux F. Disruption of the multiple tumor suppressor gene MTS1/p16(INK4a)/ CDKN2 by illegitimate V(D)J recombinase activity in T-cell acute lymphoblastic leukemias. Blood 1997;90:3720–6.

54. Kodera T, Kohno T, Takakura S, et al. Microsatellite instability in lymphoid leukemia and lymphoma cell lines but not in myeloid leukemia cell lines. Genes Chromosomes Cancer 1999;26:267–9.

55. Tasaka T, Lee S, Spira S, et al. Microsatellite instability during the progression of acute myelocytic leukaemia. Br J Haematol 1997;98:219–21.

56. Hangaishi A, Ogawa S, Mitani K, et al. Mutations and loss of expression of a mismatch repair gene, hMLH1, in leukemia and lymphoma cell lines. Blood 1997;89:1740–7.

57. Indraccolo S, Minuzzo S, Nicoletti L, et al. Mutator phenotype in human hematopoietic neoplasms and its association with deletions disabling DNA repair genes and bcl-2 rearrangements. Blood 1999;94: 2424–32.

58. Zhu YM, Das-Gupta EP, Russell NH. Microsatellite instability and p53 mutations are associated with abnormal expression of the MSH2 gene in adult acute leukemia. Blood 1999;94:733–40.

59. Bensaada M, Kiefer H, Tachdjian G, et al. Altered patterns of DNA methylation on chromosomes from leukemia cell lines: identification of 5-methylcytosines by indirect immunodetection. Cancer Genet Cytogenet 1998;103:101–9.

60. Yin H, Blanchard KL. DNA methylation represses the expression of the human erythropoietin gene by two different mechanisms. Blood 2000;95:111–9.

61. Meehan RR, Lewis JD, McKay S, et al. Identification of a mammalian protein that binds specifically to DNA containing methylated CpGs. Cell 1989;58:499–507.

62. Jones PL, Veenstra GJ, Wade PA, et al. Methylated DNA and MeCP2 recruit histone deacetylase to repress transcription. Nat Genet 1998;19:187–91.

63. Redner RL, Wang J, Liu JM. Chromatin remodeling and leukemia: new therapeutic paradigms. Blood 1999;94:417–28.

64. Aggerholm A, Guldberg P, Hokland M, Hokland P. Extensive intra- and interindividual heterogeneity of p15INK4B methylation in acute myeloid leukemia. Cancer Res 1999;59:436–41.

65. Guo SX, Taki T, Ohnishi H, et al. Hypermethylation of p16 and p15 genes and RB protein expression in acute leukemia. Leuk Res 2000;24:39–46.

66. Nakamura M, Sugita K, Inukai T, et al. p16/MTS1/INK4A gene is frequently inactivated by hypermethylation in childhood acute lymphoblastic leukemia with 11q23 translocation. Leukemia 1999;13:884–90.

67. Meehan R, Lewis J, Cross S, et al. Transcriptional repression by methylation of CpG. J Cell Sci Suppl 1992;16:9–14.

68. Taylor SM, Jones PA. Multiple new phenotypes induced in 10T1/2 and 3T3 cells treated with 5-azacytidine. Cell 1979;17:771–9.

69. Jones PA. DNA methylation errors and cancer. Cancer Res 1996;56:2463–7.

70. Guinn BA, Mills KI. p53 mutations, methylation and genomic instability in the progression of chronic myeloid leukaemia. Leuk Lymphoma 1997;26:211–26.

71. Krichevsky S, Siegfried Z, Asimakopoulos FA, et al. Methylation of the promoter regions of DNA repair and genotoxic stress response genes in therapy-related but not primary leukemia [abstract]. Blood 1999;94(Suppl 1):594a.

72. Litz CE, Etzell J. Aberrant DNA methylation of genomic regions translocated in myeloid malignancies. Leuk Lymphoma 1998;30:1–9.

73. Nelkin BD, Przepiorka D, Burke PJ, et al. Abnormal methylation of the calcitonin gene marks progression of chronic myelogenous leukemia. Blood 1991;77:2431–4.

74. Baylin SB, Fearon ER, Vogelstein B, et al. Hypermethylation of the 5' region of the calcitonin gene is a property of human lymphoid and acute myeloid malignancies. Blood 1987;70:412–7.

75. Issa JP, Kantarjian H, Mohan A, et al. Methylation of the abl1 promoter in chronic myelogenous leukemia: lack of prognostic significance. Blood 1999;93:2075–80.

76. Asimakopoulos FA, Shteper PJ, Krichevsky S, et al. abl1 methylation is a distinct molecular event associated with clonal evolution of chronic myeloid leukemia. Blood 1999;94:2452–60.

77. Ben Yehuda D, Krichevsky S, Rachmilewitz EA, et al. Molecular follow-up of disease progression and interferon therapy in chronic myelocytic leukemia. Blood 1997;90:4918–23.

78. Siegfried Z, Shteper PJ, Asimakopoulos FA, et al. Methylation of abl1 in acute lymphatic leukemia (ALL) [abstract]. Blood 1999;94(Suppl 1):595a.

79. Nakayama M, Wada M, Harada T, et al. Hypomethylation status of CpG sites at the promoter region and overexpression of the human MDR1 gene in acute myeloid leukemias. Blood 1998;92:4296–307.

80. Bodnar AG, Ouellette M, Frolkis M, et al. Extension of life-span by introduction of telomerase into normal human cells. Science 1998;279:349–52.

81. Engelhardt M, Mackenzie K, Drullinsky P, et al. Telomerase activity and telomere length in acute and chronic leukemia, pre- and post-ex vivo culture. Cancer Res 2000;60:610–7.

82. Uchida N, Otsuka T, Arima F, et al. Correlation of telomerase activity with development and progression of adult T-cell leukemia. Leuk Res 1999;23:311–6.

83. Xu D, Gruber A, Peterson C, Pisa P. Telomerase activity and the expression of telomerase components in acute myelogenous leukaemia. Br J Haematol 1998;102:1367–75.

84. Ohyashiki JH, Ohyashiki K, Iwama H, et al. Clinical implications of telomerase activity levels in acute leukemia. Clin Cancer Res 1997;3:619–25.

85. Engelhardt M, Ozkaynak MF, Drullinsky P, et al. Telomerase activity and telomere length in pediatric patients with malignancies undergoing chemotherapy. Leukemia 1998;12:13–24.

86. Zhang W, Piatyszek MA, Kobayashi T, et al. Telomerase activity in human acute myelogenous leukemia: inhibition of telomerase activity by differentiation-inducing agents. Clin Cancer Res 1996;2:799–803.

87. Bechter OE, Eisterer W, Pall G, et al. Telomere length and telomerase activity predict survival in patients with B cell chronic lymphocytic leukemia. Cancer Res 1998;58:4918–22.

88. Boultwood J, Peniket A, Watkins F, et al. Telomere length shortening in chronic myelogenous leukemia is associated with reduced time to accelerated phase. Blood 2000;96:358–61.

89. Brummendorf TH, Holyoake TL, Rufer N, et al. Prognostic implications of differences in telomere length between normal and malignant cells from patients with chronic myeloid leukemia measured by flow cytometry. Blood 2000;95:1883–90.

90. Jin J, Hauberg M, Heidorn K, et al. Inhibition of telomerase by homoharringtonine induces apoptosis in a human Burkitt lymphoma cell line [abstract]. Blood 1999;94(Suppl 1):88a.

91. Gordon MY, Riley GP, Clarke D. Heparan sulfate is necessary for adhesive interactions between human early hemopoietic progenitor cells and the extracellular matrix of the marrow microenvironment. Leukemia 1988;2:804–9.

92. Aruffo A, Stamenkovic I, Melnick M, et al. CD44 is the principal cell surface receptor for hyaluronate. Cell 1990;61:1303–13.

93. Campbell AD, Long MW, Wicha MS. Haemonectin, a bone marrow adhesion protein specific for cells of granulocyte lineage. Nature 1987;329:744–6.

94. Allen PD, Bustin SA, Newland AC. The role of apoptosis (programmed cell death) in haemopoiesis and the immune system. Blood Rev 1993;7:63–73.

95. Williams DA, Rios M, Stephens C, Patel VP. Fibronectin and VLA-4 in haematopoietic stem cell-microenvironment interactions. Nature 1991;352:438–41.

96. Schwartz MA, Schaller MD, Ginsberg MH. Integrins: emerging paradigms of signal transduction. Annu Rev Cell Dev Biol 1995;11:549–99.

97. Arkin S, Naprstek B, Guarini L, et al. Expression of intercellular adhesion molecule-1 (CD54) on hematopoietic progenitors. Blood 1991;77:948–53.

98. Gordon MY, Dowding CR, Riley GP, et al. Altered adhesive interactions with marrow stroma of haematopoietic progenitor cells in chronic myeloid leukaemia. Nature 1987;328:342–4.

99. Takahashi M, Keating A, Singer JW. A functional defect in irradiated adherent layers from chronic myelogenous leukemia long-term marrow cultures. Exp Hematol 1985;13:926–31.

100. Banavali S, Silvestri F, Hulette B, et al. Expression of hematopoietic progenitor cell associated antigen CD34 in chronic myeloid leukemia. Leuk Res 1991;15:603–8.

101. Upadhyaya G, Guba SC, Sih SA, et al. Interferon-alpha restores the deficient expression of the cytoadhesion molecule lymphocyte function antigen-3 by chronic myelogenous leukemia progenitor cells. J Clin Invest 1991;88:2131–6.

102. Kato K, Cantwell MJ, Sharma S, Kipps TJ. Gene transfer of CD40-ligand induces autologous immune recognition of chronic lymphocytic leukemia B cells. J Clin Invest 1998;101:1133–41.

103. Hussong JW, Rodgers GM, Shami PJ. Evidence of increased angiogenesis in patients with acute myeloid leukemia. Blood 2000;95:309–13.

104. Perez-Atayde AR, Sallan SE, Tedrow U, et al. Spectrum of tumor angiogenesis in the bone marrow of children with acute lymphoblastic leukemia. Am J Pathol 1997;150:815–21.

105. Singhal S, Mehta J, Desikan R, et al. Antitumor activity of thalidomide in refractory multiple myeloma. N Engl J Med 1999;341:1565–71.

106. Thomas DA, Aguayo A, Estey E, et al. Thalidomide as anti-angiogenesis therapy in refractory or relapsed leukemias [abstract]. Blood 1999;94(Suppl 1):507a.

107. Raza A, Lisak L, Andrews C, et al. Thalidomide produces transfusion independence in patients with long-standing refractory anemias and myelodysplastic syndromes (MDS) [abstract]. Blood 1999;94(Suppl 1):661a.

108. Young DC, Griffin JD. Autocrine secretion of GM-CSF in acute myeloblastic leukemia. Blood 1986;68:1178–81.

109. Falcinelli F, Onorato M, Falzetti F, et al. Activation of the granulocyte-monocyte colony stimulating factor gene in acute myeloid leukaemia cells is not related to gene rearrangement. Leuk Res 1991;15:957–61.

110. Kobari L, Weil D, Lemoine FM, et al. Secretion of tumor necrosis factor-alpha by fresh human acute nonlymphoblastic leukemic cells: role in the disappearance of normal CFU-GM progenitors. Exp Hematol 1990;18:1187–92.

111. Backx B, Broeders L, Bot FJ, Lowenberg B. Positive and negative effects of tumor necrosis factor on colony growth from highly purified normal marrow progenitors. Leukemia 1991;5:66–70.

112. Elbaz O, Budel LM, Hoogerbrugge H, et al. Tumor necrosis factor downregulates granulocyte-colony-stimulating factor receptor expression on human acute myeloid leukemia cells and granulocytes. J Clin Invest 1991;87:838–41.

113. Leitch HA, Levy JG. Reversal of CAMAL-mediated alterations of normal and leukemic in vitro myelopoiesis using inhibitors of proteolytic activity. Leukemia 1994;8:605–11.

114. Otsuka T, Eaves CJ, Humphries RK, et al. Lack of evidence for abnormal autocrine or paracrine mechanisms underlying the uncontrolled proliferation of primitive chronic myeloid leukemia progenitor cells. Leukemia 1991;5:861–8.

115. Klein H, Becher R, Lubbert M, et al. Synthesis of granulocyte colony-stimulating factor and its requirement for terminal divisions in chronic myelogenous leukemia. J Exp Med 1990;171:1785–90.

116. Weijzen S, Velders MP, Kast WM. Modulation of the immune response and tumor growth by activated Ras. Leukemia 1999;13:502–13.

117. Satoh T, Kaziro Y. Ras in signal transduction. Semin Cancer Biol 1992;3:169–77.

118. Kiyoi H, Naoe T, Nakano Y, et al. Prognostic implica-

tion of FLT3 and N-RAS gene mutations in acute myeloid leukemia. Blood 1999;93:3074–80.

119. Misawa S, Horiike S, Kaneko H, et al. Significance of chromosomal alterations and mutations of the N-RAS and TP53 genes in relation to leukemogenesis of acute myeloid leukemia. Leuk Res 1998;22:631–7.

120. MacKenzie KL, Dolnikov A, Millington M, et al. Mutant N-ras induces myeloproliferative disorders and apoptosis in bone marrow repopulated mice. Blood 1999;93:2043–56.

121. Cortez D, Stoica G, Pierce JH, Pendergast AM. The bcr-abl tyrosine kinase inhibits apoptosis by activating a Ras-dependent signaling pathway. Oncogene 1996;13:2589–94.

122. Sanchez-Garcia I, Martin-Zanca D. Regulation of Bcl-2 gene expression by bcr-abl is mediated by Ras. J Mol Biol 1997;267:225–8.

123. Sawyers CL, McLaughlin J, Witte ON. Genetic requirement for Ras in the transformation of fibroblasts and hematopoietic cells by the Bcr-Abl oncogene. J Exp Med 1995;181:307–13.

124. Skorski T, Kanakaraj P, Ku DH, et al. Negative regulation of p120GAP GTPase promoting activity by p210bcr/abl: implication for RAS-dependent Philadelphia chromosome positive cell growth. J Exp Med 1994;179:1855–65.

125. Ward AC, Touw I, Yoshimura A. The Jak-Stat pathway in normal and perturbed hematopoiesis. Blood 2000;95:19–29.

126. Schwaller J, Frantsve J, Aster J, et al. Transformation of hematopoietic cell lines to growth-factor independence and induction of a fatal myelo- and lymphoproliferative disease in mice by retrovirally transduced TEL/JAK2 fusion genes. EMBO J 1998;17:5321–33.

127. Ho JM, Beattie BK, Squire JA, et al. Fusion of the ets transcription factor TEL to Jak2 results in constitutive Jak-Stat signaling. Blood 1999;93:4354–64.

128. Nieborowska-Skorska M, Wasik MA, Slupianek A, et al. Signal transducer and activator of transcription (STAT)5 activation by bcr/abl is dependent on intact Src homology (SH)3 and SH2 domains of bcr/abl and is required for leukemogenesis. J Exp Med 1999;189:1229–42.

129. de Groot RP, Raaijmakers JA, Lammers JW, et al. STAT5 activation by bcr-Abl contributes to transformation of K562 leukemia cells. Blood 1999;94:1108–12.

130. Tenen DG, Hromas R, Licht JD, Zhang DE. Transcription factors, normal myeloid development, and leukemia. Blood 1997;90:489–519.

131. Lyons SF, Liebowitz DN. The roles of human viruses in the pathogenesis of lymphoma. Semin Oncol 1998;25:461–75.

132. Melnick A, Licht JD. Deconstructing a disease: RAR-alpha, its fusion partners, and their roles in the pathogenesis of acute promyelocytic leukemia. Blood 1999;93:3167–215.

133. Horiike S, Misawa S, Kaneko H, et al. Distinct genetic involvement of the TP53 gene in therapy-related leukemia and myelodysplasia with chromosomal losses of Nos 5 and/or 7 and its possible relationship to replication error phenotype. Leukemia 1999;13:1235–42.

134. Ben Yehuda D, Krichevsky S, Caspi O, et al. Microsatellite instability and p53 mutations in therapy-related leukemia suggest mutator phenotype. Blood 1996;88:4296–303.

135. Levine AJ. p53, the cellular gatekeeper for growth and division. Cell 1997;88:323–31.

136. Schwartz D, Almog N, Peled A, et al. Role of wild type p53 in the G2 phase: regulation of the gamma-irradiation-induced delay and DNA repair. Oncogene 1997;15:2597–607.

137. Scherer SJ, Welter C, Zang KD, Dooley S. Specific in vitro binding of p53 to the promoter region of the human mismatch repair gene hMSH2. Biochem Biophys Res Commun 1996;221:722–8.

138. Smith ML, Chen IT, Zhan Q, et al. Involvement of the p53 tumor suppressor in repair of u.v.-type DNA damage. Oncogene 1995;10:1053–9.

139. Offer H, Wolkowicz R, Matas D, et al. Direct involvement of p53 in the base excision repair pathway of the DNA repair machinery. FEBS Lett 1999;450:197–204.

140. Kohli M, Jorgensen TJ. Lack of dependence on p53 for DNA double strand break repair of episomal vectors in human lymphoblasts. Biochem Biophys Res Commun 1999;264:702–8.

141. Mallya SM, Sikpi MO. Evidence of the involvement of p53 in gamma-radiation-induced DNA repair in human lymphoblasts. Int J Radiat Biol 1998;74:231–8.

142. Guidos CJ, Williams CJ, Grandal I, et al. V(D)J recombination activates a p53-dependent DNA damage checkpoint in scid lymphocyte precursors. Genes Dev 1996;10:2038–54.

143. Lakin ND, Jackson SP. Regulation of p53 in response to DNA damage. Oncogene 1999;18:7644–55.

144. Milner J. Structures and functions of the tumor suppressor p53. Pathol Biol (Paris) 1997;45:797–803.

145. Okorokov AL, Milner J. Proteolytic cleavage of p53: a model for the activation of p53 in response to DNA damage. Oncol Res 1997;9:267–73.

146. Felix CA, Megonigal MD, Chervinsky DS, et al. Association of germline p53 mutation with MLL segmental jumping translocation in treatment-related leukemia. Blood 1998;91:4451–6.

147. Tang W, Willers H, Powell SN. p53 directly enhances rejoining of DNA double-strand breaks with cohesive ends in gamma-irradiated mouse fibroblasts. Cancer Res 1999;59:2562–5.

148. Artuso M, Esteve A, Bresil H, et al. The role of the ataxia telangiectasia gene in the p53, WAF1/

CIP1(p21)- and GADD45-mediated response to DNA damage produced by ionising radiation. Oncogene 1995;11:1427–35.

149. Pearson M, Carbone R, Sebastiani C, et al. PML regulates p53 acetylation and premature senescence induced by oncogenic Ras. Nature 2000;406:207–10.

150. Downward J. Cell cycle: routine role for Ras. Curr Biol 1997;7:R258–60.

151. Yatabe Y, Suzuki R, Tobinai K, et al. Significance of cyclin D1 overexpression for the diagnosis of mantle cell lymphoma: a clinicopathologic comparison of cyclin D1-positive MCL and cyclin D1-negative MCL-like B-cell lymphoma. Blood 2000;95:2253–61.

152. de Boer CJ, Kluin-Nelemans JC, Dreef E, et al. Involvement of the CCND1 gene in hairy cell leukemia. Ann Oncol 1996;7:251–6.

153. Bosch F, Campo E, Jares P, et al. Increased expression of the PRAD-1/CCND1 gene in hairy cell leukaemia. Br J Haematol 1995;91:1025–30.

154. Aboulafia D. Epidemiology and pathogenesis of AIDS-related lymphomas. Oncology (Huntingt) 1998;12:1068–81.

155. Straus DJ. Human immunodeficiency virus-associated lymphomas. Med Clin North Am 1997;81:495–510.

156. Vandermolen LA, Fehir KM, Rice L. Multiple myeloma in a homosexual man with chronic lymphadenopathy. Arch Intern Med 1985;145:745–6.

157. Penn I. The changing pattern of posttransplant malignancies. Transplant Proc 1991;23:1101–3.

158. Swinnen LJ. Treatment of organ transplant-related lymphoma. Hematol Oncol Clin North Am 1997;11:963–73.

159. Ambinder RF. Human lymphotropic viruses associated with lymphoid malignancy: Epstein-Barr and HTLV-1. Hematol Oncol Clin North Am 1990;4:821–33.

160. Riddler SA, Breinig MC, McKnight JL. Increased levels of circulating Epstein-Barr virus (EBV)-infected lymphocytes and decreased EBV nuclear antigen antibody responses are associated with the development of posttransplant lymphoproliferative disease in solid-organ transplant recipients. Blood 1994;84:972–84.

161. Zutter MM, Martin PJ, Sale GE, et al. Epstein-Barr virus lymphoproliferation after bone marrow transplantation. Blood 1988;72:520–9.

162. Lucas KG, Small TN, Heller G, et al. The development of cellular immunity to Epstein-Barr virus after allogeneic bone marrow transplantation. Blood 1996;87:2594–603.

163. Swinnen LJ, Gulley ML, Hamilton E, Schichman SA. EBV DNA quantification in serum is highly correlated with the development and regression of posttransplant lymphoproliferative disorder (PTLD) in solid organ transplant recipients [abstract]. Blood 1998;92(Suppl 1):314a.

164. Raynaud S, Cave H, Baens M, et al. The 12;21 translocation involving TEL and deletion of the other TEL allele: two frequently associated alterations found in childhood acute lymphoblastic leukemia. Blood 1996;87:2891–9.

165. Green M, Cacciarelli TV, Mazariegos GV, et al. Serial measurement of Epstein-Barr viral load in peripheral blood in pediatric liver transplant recipients during treatment for posttransplant lymphoproliferative disease. Transplantation 1998;66:1641–4.

166. Harris NL, Ferry JA, Swerdlow SH. Posttransplant lymphoproliferative disorders: summary of Society for Hematopathology Workshop. Semin Diagn Pathol 1997;14:8–14.

167. Knowles DM, Cesarman E, Chadburn A, et al. Correlative morphologic and molecular genetic analysis demonstrates three distinct categories of posttransplantation lymphoproliferative disorders. Blood 1995;85:552–65.

168. Bose S, Deininger M, Gora-Tybor J, et al. The presence of typical and atypical bcr-abl fusion genes in leukocytes of normal individuals: biologic significance and implications for the assessment of minimal residual disease. Blood 1998;92:3362–7.

169. Biernaux C, Loos M, Sels A, et al. Detection of major bcr-abl gene expression at a very low level in blood cells of some healthy individuals. Blood 1995;86:3118–22.

170. Marcucci G, Strout MP, Bloomfield CD, Caligiuri MA. Detection of unique ALL1 (MLL) fusion transcripts in normal human bone marrow and blood: distinct origin of normal versus leukemic ALL1 fusion transcripts. Cancer Res 1998;58:790–3.

171. Caldas C, So CW, MacGregor A, et al. Exon scrambling of MLL transcripts occur commonly and mimic partial genomic duplication of the gene. Gene 1998;208:167–76.

172. Uckun FM, Herman-Hatten K, Crotty ML, et al. Clinical significance of MLL-AF4 fusion transcript expression in the absence of a cytogenetically detectable t(4; 11)(q21; q23) chromosomal translocation. Blood 1998;92:810–21.

173. Miller WH Jr, Levine K, DeBlasio A, et al. Detection of minimal residual disease in acute promyelocytic leukemia by a reverse transcription polymerase chain reaction assay for the PML/RAR-alpha fusion mRNA. Blood 1993;82:1689–94.

174. Lo CF, Diverio D, Avvisati G, et al. Therapy of molecular relapse in acute promyelocytic leukemia. Blood 1999;94:2225–9.

175. Jurlander J, Caligiuri MA, Ruutu T, et al. Persistence of the AML1/ETO fusion transcript in patients treated with allogeneic bone marrow transplantation for t(8; 21) leukemia. Blood 1996;88:2183–91.

176. Caruso C, Lo CP, Botindari C, Modica MA. HLA anti-

gens in Sicilian patients affected by chronic myelogenous leukaemia. J Immunogenet 1987;14:295–9.

177. Posthuma EF, Falkenburg JH, Apperley JF, et al. HLA-B8 and HLA-A3 coexpressed with HLA-B8 are associated with a reduced risk of the development of chronic myeloid leukemia. The Chronic Leukemia Working Party of the EBMT. Blood 1999;93:3863–5.

178. Mannering SI, McKenzie JL, Fearnley DB, Hart DN. HLA-DR1-restricted bcr-abl (b3a2)-specific CD4+ T lymphocytes respond to dendritic cells pulsed with b3a2 peptide and antigen-presenting cells exposed to b3a2 containing cell lysates. Blood 1997;90:290–7.

179. Cortes J, Fayad L, Kantarjian H, et al. Association of HLA phenotype and response to interferon-alpha in patients with chronic myelogenous leukemia. Leukemia 1998;12:455–62.

180. Lin AY, Li FP. Etiology and epidemiology of chronic leukemias. In: Wiernik P, Canellos GP, Kyle RA, Schiffer CA, editors. Neoplastic diseases of the blood. New York: Churchill Livingstone; 1996. p. 9–20.

181. Taylor GM, Birch JM. The hereditary basis of human leukemia. In: Henderson ES, Lister TA, Greaves MF, editors. Leukemia. Philadelphia: WB Saunders; 1996. p. 210–245.

182. Sullivan AK. Classification, pathogenesis, and etiology of neoplastic diseases of the hematopoietic system. In: Lee GR, Bithell TC, Foerster J, et al., editors. Wintrobe's clinical hematology. Malvern, PA: Lea & Febiger; 1993. p. 1725–91.

183. Insel RA, Quaidoo EA. Disorders of lymphocyte function. In: Hoffman R, Benz EJ Jr, Shahil SJ, et al., editors. Hematology: basic principles and practice. Philadelphia: Churchill Livingstone; 2000. p. 762–82.

184. Taylor AM, Metcalfe JA, Thick J, Mak YF. Leukemia and lymphoma in ataxia telangiectasia. Blood 1996;87:423–38.

185. Peterson RD, Funkhouser JD, Tuck-Muller CM, Gatti RA. Cancer susceptibility in ataxia-telangiectasia. Leukemia 1992;6(Suppl 1):8–13.

186. Brito-Babapulle V, Catovsky D. Inversions and tandem translocations involving chromosome 14q11 and 14q32 in T-prolymphocytic leukemia and T-cell leukemias in patients with ataxia telangiectasia. Cancer Genet Cytogenet 1991;55:1–9.

187. Stern MH. Ataxia telangiectasia: a model for T-cell leukemogenesis. Nouv Rev Fr Hematol 1993;35:29–31.

188. Thick J, Sherrington PD, Fisch P, et al. Molecular analysis of a new translocation, t(X;14)(q28;q11), in premalignancy and in leukaemia associated with ataxia telangiectasia. Genes Chromosomes Cancer 1992;5:321–5.

189. Uppenkamp M, Dresen IG, Becher R, et al. Molecular analysis of an ataxia telangiectasia T-cell clone with a chromosomal translocation t(14;18)—evidence for a breakpoint in the T-cell receptor delta-chain gene. Leuk Res 1992;16:681–91.

190. Russo G, Isobe M, Gatti R, et al. Molecular analysis of a t(14;14) translocation in leukemic T-cells of an ataxia telangiectasia patient. Proc Natl Acad Sci U S A 1989;86:602–6.

191. Beamish H, Williams R, Chen P, Lavin MF. Defect in multiple cell cycle checkpoints in ataxia-telangiectasia postirradiation. J Biol Chem 1996;271: 20486–93.

192. Meyn MS. Ataxia-telangiectasia and cellular responses to DNA damage. Cancer Res 1995;55:5991–6001.

193. Hecht F, Hecht BK. Chromosome changes connect immunodeficiency and cancer in ataxia-telangiectasia. Am J Pediatr Hematol Oncol 1987;9:185–8.

194. Haidar MA, Kantarjian H, Manshouri T, et al. ATM gene deletion in patients with adult acute lymphoblastic leukemia. Cancer 2000;88:1057–62.

195. Stankovic T, Weber P, Stewart G, et al. Inactivation of ataxia telangiectasia mutated gene in B-cell chronic lymphocytic leukaemia. Lancet 1999;353:26–9.

196. Stankovic T, Kidd AM, Sutcliffe A, et al. ATM mutations and phenotypes in ataxia-telangiectasia families in the British Isles: expression of mutant ATM and the risk of leukemia, lymphoma, and breast cancer. Am J Hum Genet 1998;62:334–45.

197. Dar ME, Winters TA, Jorgensen TJ. Identification of defective illegitimate recombinational repair of oxidatively-induced DNA double-strand breaks in ataxia-telangiectasia cells. Mutat Res 1997;384:169–79.

198. Butturini A, Gale RP, Verlander PC, et al. Hematologic abnormalities in Fanconi anemia: an International Fanconi Anemia Registry study. Blood 1994; 84:1650–5.

199. Lensch MW, Rathbun RK, Olson SB, et al. Selective pressure as an essential force in molecular evolution of myeloid leukemic clones: a view from the window of Fanconi anemia. Leukemia 1999;13:1784–9.

200. Maarek O, Jonveaux P, Le Coniat M, et al. Fanconi anemia and bone marrow clonal chromosome abnormalities. Leukemia 1996;10:1700–4.

201. Hoatlin ME, Zhi Y, Ball H, et al. A novel BTB/POZ transcriptional repressor protein interacts with the Fanconi anemia group C protein and PLZF. Blood 1999;94:3737–47.

202. Berger R, Le Coniat M, Gendron MC. Fanconi anemia. Chromosome breakage and cell cycle studies. Cancer Genet Cytogenet 1993;69:13–6.

203. Douer D, Preston-Martin S, Chang E, et al. High frequency of acute promyelocytic leukemia among Latinos with acute myeloid leukemia. Blood 1996;87:308–13.

204. Keung YK, Chen SC, Groshen S, et al. Acute myeloid leukemia subtypes and response to treatment among ethnic minorities in a large US urban hospital. Acta Haematol 1994;92:18–22.

205. Montserrat E, Bosch F, Rozman C. B-cell chronic lymphocytic leukemia: recent progress in biology, diagnosis, and therapy. Ann Oncol 1997;8(Suppl 1): 93–101.
206. Swensen AR, Ross JA, Severson RK, et al. The age peak in childhood acute lymphoblastic leukemia: exploring the potential relationship with socioeconomic status. Cancer 1997;79:2045–51.
207. Smith M. Considerations on a possible viral etiology for B-precursor acute lymphoblastic leukemia of childhood. J Immunother 1997;20:89–100.
208. Labat ML. Possible retroviral origin of prion disease: could prion disease be reconsidered as a preleukemia syndrome? Biomed Pharmacother 1999;53:47–53.
209. Lehtinen T, Lehtinen M. Common and emerging infectious causes of hematological malignancies in the young. APMIS 1998;106:585–97.
210. Greaves M. Molecular genetics, natural history and the demise of childhood leukaemia. Eur J Cancer 1999;35:1941–53.
211. Caspi O, Polliack A, Klar R, Ben Yehuda D. The association of inflammatory bowel disease and leukemia—coincidence or not? Leuk Lymphoma 1995;17:255–62.
212. Kikuchi M, Mitsui T, Takeshita M, et al. Virus associated adult T-cell leukemia (ATL) in Japan: clinical, histological and immunological studies. Hematol Oncol 1986;4:67–81.
213. Hatta Y, Yamada Y, Tomonaga M, et al. Microsatellite instability in adult T-cell leukaemia. Br J Haematol 1998;101:341–4.
214. Jablon S, Kato H. Childhood cancer in relation to prenatal exposure to atomic-bomb radiation. Lancet 1970;2:1000–3.
215. Gale RP, Butturini A. Perspective: Chernobyl and leukemia. Leukemia 1991;5:441–2.
216. Kato H. Cancer mortality. In: Shigematsu I, Dagan A, editors. Cancer in atomic bomb survivors. Tokyo: Japan Scientific Societies Press.1986. p. 53–74.
217. Holmberg M. Is the primary event in radiation-induced chronic myelogenous leukemia the induction of the t(9;22) translocation? Leuk Res 1992;16:333–6.
218. Spencer A, Granter N. Leukemia patient-derived lymphoblastoid cell lines exhibit increased induction of leukemia-associated transcripts following high-dose irradiation. Exp Hematol 1999;27:1397–401.
219. Ito T, Seyama T, Mizuno T, et al. Induction of bcr-abl fusion genes by in vitro X-irradiation. Jpn J Cancer Res 1993;84:105–9.
220. Flodin U, Fredriksson M, Persson B, et al. Background radiation, electrical work, and some other exposures associated with acute myeloid leukemia in a case-referent study. Arch Environ Health 1986;41:77–84.
221. Stern FB, Waxweiler RA, Beaumont JJ, et al. A case-control study of leukemia at a naval nuclear shipyard. Am J Epidemiol 1986;123:980–92.
222. Smith MT, Zhang L, Wang Y, et al. Increased translocations and aneusomy in chromosomes 8 and 21 among workers exposed to benzene. Cancer Res 1998;58:2176–81.
223. Lewis SJ, Bell GM, Cordingley N, et al. Retrospective estimation of exposure to benzene in a leukaemia case-control study of petroleum marketing and distribution workers in the United Kingdom. Occup Environ Med 1997;54:167–75.
224. Rinsky RA, Smith AB, Hornung R, et al. Benzene and leukemia. An epidemiologic risk assessment. N Engl J Med 1987;316:1044–50.
225. Westley-Wise VJ, Stewart BW, Kreis I, et al. Investigation of a cluster of leukaemia in the Illawarra region of New South Wales, 1989–1996. Med J Aust 1999; 171:178–83.
226. Rithidech K, Dunn JJ, Bond VP, et al. Characterization of genetic instability in radiation- and benzene-induced murine acute leukemia. Mutat Res 1999; 428:33–9.
227. Oliveira NL, Kalf GF. Induced differentiation of HL-60 promyelocytic leukemia cells to monocyte/ macrophages is inhibited by hydroquinone, a hematotoxic metabolite of benzene. Blood 1992;79:627–33.
228. Kalf GF, O'Connor A. The effects of benzene and hydroquinone on myeloid differentiation of HL-60 promyelocytic leukemia cells. Leuk Lymphoma 1993;11:331–8.
229. Herr R, Ferguson J, Myers N, et al. Cigarette smoking, blast crisis, and survival in chronic myeloid leukemia. Am J Hematol 1990;34:1–4.
230. Berk PD, Goldberg JD, Donovan PB, et al. Therapeutic recommendations in polycythemia vera based on Polycythemia Vera Study Group protocols. Semin Hematol 1986;23:132–43.
231. Greenberg P, Cox C, Le Beau MM, et al. International scoring system for evaluating prognosis in myelodysplastic syndromes. Blood 1997;89:2079–88 [published erratum appears in Blood 1998;91:1100].
232. Rowley JD, Alimena G, Garson OM, et al. A collaborative study of the relationship of the morphological type of acute nonlymphocytic leukemia with patient age and karyotype. Blood 1982;59:1013–22.
233. Thirman MJ, Larson RA. Therapy-related myeloid leukemia. Hematol Oncol Clin North Am 1996; 10:293–320.
234. Taylor PR, Reid MM, Stark AN, et al. De novo acute myeloid leukaemia in patients over 55-years-old: a population-based study of incidence, treatment and outcome. Northern Region Haematology Group. Leukemia 1995;9:231–7.
235. Preisler HD, Raza A, Barcos M, et al. High-dose cytosine arabinoside as the initial treatment of poor-risk patients with acute nonlymphocytic leukemia: a Leukemia Intergroup Study. J Clin Oncol 1987; 5:75–82.

236. De Witte T, Zwaan F, Hermans J, et al. Allogeneic bone marrow transplantation for secondary leukaemia and myelodysplastic syndrome: a survey by the Leukaemia Working Party of the European Bone Marrow Transplantation Group (EBMTG). Br J Haematol 1990;74:151–5.

237. Witherspoon RP, Deeg HJ. Allogeneic bone marrow transplantation for secondary leukemia or myelodysplasia. Haematologica 1999;84:1085–7.

238. Leone G, Mele L, Pulsoni A, et al. The incidence of secondary leukemias. Haematologica 1999;84:937–45.

239. Travis LB, Curtis RE, Stovall M, et al. Risk of leukemia following treatment for non-Hodgkin's lymphoma. J Natl Cancer Inst 1994;86:1450–7.

240. Smith MA, Rubinstein L, Anderson JR, et al. Secondary leukemia or myelodysplastic syndrome after treatment with epipodophyllotoxins. J Clin Oncol 1999;17:569–77.

241. Sobecks RM, Le Beau MM, Anastasi J, Williams SF. Myelodysplasia and acute leukemia following high-dose chemotherapy and autologous bone marrow or peripheral blood stem cell transplantation. Bone Marrow Transplant 1999;23:1161–5.

242. Pedersen-Bjergaard J, Pedersen M, Myhre J, Geisler C. High risk of therapy-related leukemia after BEAM chemotherapy and autologous stem cell transplantation for previously treated lymphomas is mainly related to primary chemotherapy and not to the BEAM-transplantation procedure. Leukemia 1997;11:1654–60.

243. Krishnan A, Bhatia S, Slovak ML, et al. Predictors of therapy-related leukemia and myelodysplasia following autologous transplantation for lymphoma: an assessment of risk factors. Blood 2000;95:1588–93.

244. Kelliher M, Knott A, McLaughlin J, et al. Differences in oncogenic potency but not target cell specificity distinguish the two forms of the bcr/abl oncogene. Mol Cell Biol 1991;11:4710–6.

245. Radich J, Gehly G, Lee A, et al. Detection of bcr-abl transcripts in Philadelphia chromosome-positive acute lymphoblastic leukemia after marrow transplantation. Blood 1997;89:2602–9.

246. Diamond J, Goldman JM, Melo JV. bcr-abl, abl-bcr, bcr, and abl genes are all expressed in individual granulocyte-macrophage colony-forming unit colonies derived from blood of patients with chronic myeloid leukemia. Blood 1995;85:2171–5.

247. Melo JV, Gordon DE, Cross NC, Goldman JM. The abl-bcr fusion gene is expressed in chronic myeloid leukemia. Blood 1993;81:158–65.

248. Hariharan IK, Adams JM, Cory S. bcr-abl oncogene renders myeloid cell line factor independent: potential autocrine mechanism in chronic myeloid leukemia. Oncogene Res 1988;3:387–99.

249. Elefanty AG, Hariharan IK, Cory S. bcr-abl, the hallmark of chronic myeloid leukaemia in man, induces multiple haemopoietic neoplasms in mice. EMBO J 1990;9:1069–78.

250. Yuan ZM, Huang Y, Whang Y, et al. Role for c-Abl tyrosine kinase in growth arrest response to DNA damage. Nature 1996;382:272–4.

251. Sawyers CL, McLaughlin J, Goga A, et al. The nuclear tyrosine kinase c-Abl negatively regulates cell growth. Cell 1994;77:121–31.

252. Daniel R, Cai Y, Wong PM, Chung SW. Deregulation of c-abl mediated cell growth after retroviral transfer and expression of antisense sequences. Oncogene 1995;10:1607–14.

253. Dan S, Naito M, Seimiya H, et al. Activation of c-Abl tyrosine kinase requires caspase activation and is not involved in JNK/SAPK activation during apoptosis of human monocytic leukemia U937 cells. Oncogene 1999;18:1277–83.

254. Kelman Z, Prokocimer M, Peller S, et al. Rearrangements in the p53 gene in Philadelphia chromosome positive chronic myelogenous leukemia. Blood 1989;74:2318–24.

255. Honda H, Ushijima T, Wakazono K, et al. Acquired loss of p53 induces blastic transformation in p210(bcr/abl)-expressing hematopoietic cells: a transgenic study for blast crisis of human CML. Blood 2000;95:1144–50.

256. Carlo-Stella C, Regazzi E, Sammarelli G, et al. Effects of the tyrosine kinase inhibitor AG957 and an anti-Fas receptor antibody on CD34(+) chronic myelogenous leukemia progenitor cells. Blood 1999;93:3973–82.

257. Carroll M, Ohno-Jones S, Tamura S, et al. CGP 57148, a tyrosine kinase inhibitor, inhibits the growth of cells expressing bcr-abl, TEL-abl, and TEL-PDGFR fusion proteins. Blood 1997;90:4947–52.

258. Deininger MW, Goldman JM, Lydon N, Melo JV. The tyrosine kinase inhibitor CGP57148B selectively inhibits the growth of bcr-abl-positive cells. Blood 1997;90:3691–8.

259. le Coutre P, Mologni L, Cleris L, et al. In vivo eradication of human bcr/abl-positive leukemia cells with an abl kinase inhibitor. J Natl Cancer Inst 1999;91:163–8.

260. Verfaillie CM. Biology of chronic myelogenous leukemia. Hematol Oncol Clin North Am 1998;12:1–29.

261. Deininger M, Goldman JM, Melo JV. The induction of apoptosis in CML cells exposed to the tyrosine kinase inhibitor CGP57418B is associated with altered gene transcription. Blood 1997;90:83a (ab).

262. Gambacorti-Passerini C, le Coutre P, Mologni L, et al. Inhibition of the abl kinase activity blocks the proliferation of bcr/abl+ leukemic cells and induces apoptosis. Blood Cells Mol Dis 1997;23:380–94.

263. Imhof A, Wolffe AP. Transcription: gene control by targeted histone acetylation. Curr Biol 1998;8:R422–4.

264. Warrell RP Jr. Retinoid resistance [letter]. Lancet 1993;341:126.

265. Borrow J, Stanton VP Jr, Andresen JM, et al. The translocation t(8;16)(p11;p13) of acute myeloid leukaemia fuses a putative acetyltransferase to the CREB-binding protein. Nat Genet 1996;14:33–41.

266. Blobel GA. CREB-binding protein and p300: molecular integrators of hematopoietic transcription. Blood 2000;95:745–55.

267. Okuda T, van Deursen J, Hiebert SW, et al. AML1, the target of multiple chromosomal translocations in human leukemia, is essential for normal fetal liver hematopoiesis. Cell 1996;84:321–30.

268. Shurtleff SA, Meyers S, Hiebert SW, et al. Heterogeneity in CBF beta/MYH11 fusion messages encoded by the inv(16)(p13q22) and the t(16;16)(p13;q22) in acute myelogenous leukemia. Blood 1995;85:3695–703.

269. Hiebert SW, Sun W, Davis JN, et al. The t(12;21) translocation converts AML-1B from an activator to a repressor of transcription. Mol Cell Biol 1996;16:1349–55.

270. Meyers S, Lenny N, Sun W, Hiebert SW. AML-2 is a potential target for transcriptional regulation by the t(8;21) and t(12;21) fusion proteins in acute leukemia. Oncogene 1996;13:303–12.

271. Golub TR, Barker GF, Bohlander SK, et al. Fusion of the TEL gene on 12p13 to the AML1 gene on 21q22 in acute lymphoblastic leukemia. Proc Natl Acad Sci U S A 1995;92:4917–21.

272. Tanaka T, Tanaka K, Ogawa S, et al. An acute myeloid leukemia gene, AML1, regulates hemopoietic myeloid cell differentiation and transcriptional activation antagonistically by two alternative spliced forms. EMBO J 1995;14:341–50.

273. Yergeau DA, Hetherington CJ, Wang Q, et al. Embryonic lethality and impairment of haematopoiesis in mice heterozygous for an AML1-ETO fusion gene. Nat Genet 1997;15:303–6.

274. Okuda T, Cai Z, Yang S, et al. Expression of a knocked-in AML1-ETO leukemia gene inhibits the establishment of normal definitive hematopoiesis and directly generates dysplastic hematopoietic progenitors. Blood 1998;91:3134–43.

275. Strout MP, Marcucci G, Bloomfield CD, Caligiuri MA. The partial tandem duplication of ALL1 (MLL) is consistently generated by Alu-mediated homologous recombination in acute myeloid leukemia. Proc Natl Acad Sci U S A 1998;95:2390–5.

276. So CW, Ma ZG, Price CM, et al. MLL self fusion mediated by Alu repeat homologous recombination and prognosis of AML-M4/M5 subtypes. Cancer Res 1997;57:117–22.

277. Mrozek K, Heinonen K, dela Chapelle A, Bloomfield CD. Clinical significance of cytogenetics in acute myeloid leukemia. Semin Oncol 1997;24:17–31.

278. Harbott J, Mancini M, Verellen-Dumoulin C, et al. Hematological malignancies with a deletion of 11q23: cytogenetic and clinical aspects. European 11q23 Workshop participants. Leukemia 1998;12:823–7.

279. Zhou RH, Wang P, Zou Y, et al. A precise interchromosomal reciprocal exchange between hot spots for cleavable complex formation by topoisomerase II in amsacrine-treated Chinese hamster ovary cells. Cancer Res 1997;57:4699–702.

280. Broeker PL, Super HG, Thirman MJ, et al. Distribution of 11q23 breakpoints within the MLL breakpoint cluster region in de novo acute leukemia and in treatment-related acute myeloid leukemia: correlation with scaffold attachment regions and topoisomerase II consensus binding sites. Blood 1996;87:1912–22.

281. Hunger SP, Tkachuk DC, Amylon MD, et al. HRX involvement in de novo and secondary leukemias with diverse chromosome 11q23 abnormalities. Blood 1993;81:3197–203.

282. Cimino G, Rapanotti MC, Sprovieri T, Elia L. ALL1 gene alterations in acute leukemia: biological and clinical aspects. Haematologica 1998;83:350–7.

283. Satake N, Ishida Y, Otoh Y, et al. Novel MLL-CBP fusion transcript in therapy-related chronic myelomonocytic leukemia with a t(11;16)(q23;p13) chromosome translocation. Genes Chromosomes Cancer 1997;20:60–3.

284. Rowley JD, Reshmi S, Sobulo O, et al. All patients with the T(11;16)(q23; p13.3) that involves MLL and CBP have treatment-related hematologic disorders. Blood 1997;90:535–41.

285. Ida K, Kitabayashi I, Taki T, et al. Adenoviral E1A-associated protein p300 is involved in acute myeloid leukemia with t(11;22)(q23;q13). Blood 1997;90:4699–704.

286. Archimbaud E, Charrin C, Magaud JP, et al. Clinical and biological characteristics of adult de novo and secondary acute myeloid leukemia with balanced 11q23 chromosomal anomaly or MLL gene rearrangement compared to cases with unbalanced 11q23 anomaly: confirmation of the existence of different entities with 11q23 breakpoint. Leukemia 1998;12:25–33.

287. Williams GT. Programmed cell death: apoptosis and oncogenesis. Cell 1991;65:1097–8.

288. Strasser A, Whittingham S, Vaux DL, et al. Enforced BCL2 expression in B-lymphoid cells prolongs antibody responses and elicits autoimmune disease. Proc Natl Acad Sci U S A 1991;88:8661–5.

3

Diagnosis

CLARENCE SARKODEE-ADOO, MD
AARON P. RAPOPORT, MD
JACOB M. ROWE, MD

Leukemias, including acute myeloid (AML) or lymphoblastic (ALL), chronic lymphocytic (CLL), and chronic myelogenous leukemia (CML), are diagnosed in approximately 31,500 individuals per year in the United States.[1] Despite significant progress in understanding the biologic basis for many of these diseases, preventive and therapeutic measures remain limited in effectiveness, and the majority of patients eventually die of their disease. In the year 2001, 21,500 deaths in the United States are projected to be attributable to leukemia.[1] Although chemotherapy remains the major modality for the treatment of leukemia, additional therapeutic opportunities are being developed that exploit important biologic differences between neoplastic and normal cells. The physician involved in caring for patients with leukemia needs to be familiar with the traditional tests in use for these diseases, as well as newer diagnostic methods based on the cellular, immunologic, and molecular biology of leukemia. As before, clinicians also need to be competent in the clinical assessment of adults with leukemia to recognize specific problems that may require immediate attention and treatment. This chapter focuses on the clinical diagnosis of specific problems in adults with leukemia and the appropriate selection, use, and interpretation of diagnostic tests. Subsequent chapters will describe some of the more technical aspects underlying the performance of these diagnostic tests.

CLINICAL EVALUATION OF ADULTS WITH LEUKEMIA

A history of exposure to radiation or chemical toxins is important to elicit in patients with leukemia since this may provide clues to the etiology of the disease and possibly point to the diagnosis of a specific type of leukemic process. An increased incidence of AML follows exposure to ionizing radiation and possibly cigarette smoking. Other reports implicate exposure to pesticides, fungicides, and industrial chemicals, although with the exception of exposure to benzene, the epidemiologic literature is often contradictory and inconclusive. Previous treatment with chemotherapeutic drugs, particularly alkylating agents and topoisomerase II inhibitors, is also associated with an increased risk of developing acute leukemia. Acute myeloid leukemia may arise by transformation from other clonal disorders of hemopoiesis, including the myeloproliferative and myelodysplastic syndromes. Secondary CML (after radiation or chemotherapy), ALL (after myeloproliferative disorders), and myelodysplastic syndrome (MDS) (after toxic exposure or chemotherapy) have also been reported. With the exception of rare cases of erythroleukemia, adult-onset acute leukemia does not seem to be familial.[2,3] Rare cases of familial CLL and myeloproliferative disorders are also reported in the literature.[4,5]

Leukemias of all types disrupt normal hemopoiesis, although the degree and manner in which specific blood cell lineages are affected vary from disease to disease. Anemia is the most common clinical feature of leukemia. In many patients with CLL and CML, the anemia is slow in onset and therefore often associated with mild and nonspecific symptoms. In CLL, anemia due to marrow compromise must be differentiated from direct antiglobulin test-positive (DAT+) autoimmune hemolysis since the treatment approach may differ. In other leukemias, both acute and chronic, anemia is the result of dysplastic erythropoiesis or suppression of normal erythroid progenitors; most patients are DAT negative and have no biochemical evidence for hemolysis.

In addition to anemia, disordered hemopoiesis in acute leukemia is characterized by maturational arrests and functional defects in the other formed elements of blood, including neutrophils and platelets. It is important to recognize that defective function is not limited to blasts or other morphologically abnormal cells. Neutrophils that are deficient in myeloperoxidase (MPO), elastase, hexose monophosphate shunt enzymes, or the ability to reduce nitroblue tetrazolium have been described in patients with AML and ALL and may be the basis of functional defects in such processes as neutrophil adherence, chemotaxis, phagocytosis, and bactericidal activity. In one study, defective neutrophil function was found to confer shortened survival duration in acute leukemia patients. Currently, however, studies of neutrophil function are not commonly used for the determination of infection risk in patients with acute leukemia. On the other hand, the absolute neutrophil count (ANC; neutrophils plus bands) is easily obtained by automated blood counters and microscopy. The likelihood and severity of infections are inversely correlated with the ANC; thus, fever in acute leukemic patients with neutropenia (ANC < 1,500/μL) should be treated as evidence for potentially life-threatening bacterial infections. Clinical examination should focus on frequent sites of infection, including the throat, lungs, skin, and perirectal areas (Figure 3–1). Table 3–1 lists some of the symptoms and physical signs frequently encountered in patients with leukemia.

The majority of individuals with acute leukemia are thrombocytopenic at the time of initial diagnosis. Commonly, petechial rashes or purpura are observed on the lower limbs, and blisters may be evident in the

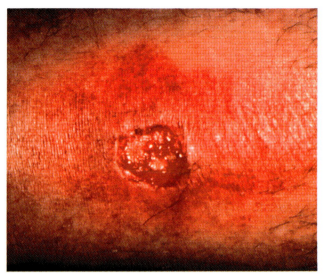

Figure 3–1. Ecthyma gangrenosum: necrotic skin ulcer due to *Pseudomonas aeruginosa* infection in a patient with neutropenia from acute leukemia.

buccal mucosa. Ophthalmoscopy may demonstrate retinal hemorrhages or, occasionally, leukemic infiltrates (Figure 3–2). Frank bleeding is observed less commonly, except when there is evidence of disseminated intravascular coagulation (DIC). Bleeding may be occult, and such symptoms as headache, back pain, or muscle swelling at sites of trauma should be investigated thoroughly. The platelet count should be verified by examination of the peripheral blood smear since platelet-sized fragments of circulating leukocytes (Figure 3–3) can be mistakenly enumerated as platelets by automated counters. Splenic

Table 3–1. CLINICAL AND LABORATORY FEATURES OF LEUKEMIA	
Clinical Features	**Laboratory Features**
Bruising, purpura, bleeding	Thrombocytopenia, DIC
Fever, infections	Neutropenia, abnormal neutrophils
Fatigue, angina, claudication, dyspnea	Anemia; occasionally autoimmune (CLL)
Skin lesions, gum swelling	Leukemic infiltration
Confusion, seizures, cranial nerve deficits	Brain involvement (radiographic studies) or leukemic meningitis (spinal fluid examination)
Early satiety, weight loss	Splenomegaly
Confusion, somnolence, dyspnea, angina	Leukostasis

DIC = disseminated intravascular coagulation; CLL = chronic lymphocytic leukemia.

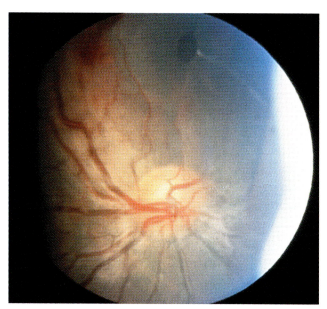

Figure 3–2. Retinal hemorrhage: a frequent finding in patients with severe thombocytopenia and anemia from acute leukemia.

sequestration may contribute to thrombocytopenia. Thrombocytopenia is usually more profound in acute than chronic leukemia at the time of diagnosis. Although patients with CML and other myeloprolif-erative disorders may present with thrombocytosis, bleeding complications may still develop due to defects in platelet function such as the acquired von

Willebrand's disease. Laboratory evidence of DIC is occasionally found at presentation in individuals with any form of AML and is commonly observed in those with acute promyelocytic leukemia (APL). Occasionally, the full clinical syndrome of DIC, with bleeding and concurrent microvascular thrombosis, may be present. In individuals with polycythemia or a very large buffy coat due to extreme leukocytosis, the prothrombin or partial thromboplastin time may be spuriously prolonged because of the presence of insufficient plasma in the blood volumes processed with fixed amounts of test reagent.

Skin infiltration by leukemia (leukemia cutis) is more commonly observed in the monocytic forms of AML. Typically, these lesions are raised, palpable, nonpigmented, and painless plaques (Figure 3–4) or nodules (chloroma; Figure 3–5). In individuals with AML, the presence of leukemia cutis implies a poorer prognosis, and in CML, it is suggestive of blast transformation; thus, punch biopsies of the skin are often needed to evaluate suspicious lesions. Other sites of extramedullary involvement are the gums in AML, especially monocytic subtypes, and the gums, spleen, and lymph nodes in ALL. Large mediastinal masses are frequently found in patients with T-cell ALL and less often in B-cell ALL of

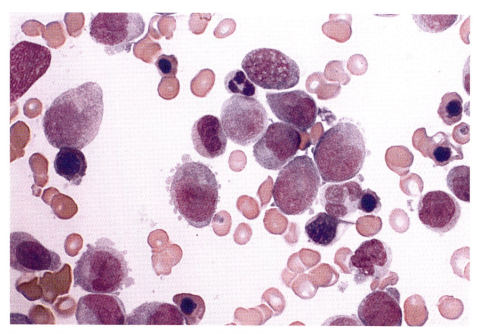

Figure 3–3. Bone marrow from a patient with AML, Wright-Giemsa stain. Note the cytoplasmic projections on the blasts in the center of the field. Leukocyte cytoplasmic fragments may be spuriously enumerated as platelets.

defines a more advanced stage in either the Rai or Binet staging systems. However, massively enlarged spleens (below the umbilicus) are more commonly seen in patients with CML, causing symptoms such as fatigue, early satiety, and weight loss. In studies of CML patients treated with chemotherapy, interferon, or bone marrow transplantation, the presence of moderate to massive splenomegaly has been found to confer inferior survival rates.

An unusual but potentially lethal manifestation of leukemia is the development of leukostasis due to extremely high numbers of circulating blasts (AML) or blasts and promyelocytes (CML).[6] Symptoms of leukostasis include impairments in the level of consciousness, dyspnea, priapism, and cardiac dysfunction. Leukostasis occurs at lower white cell counts in AML (especially monocytic subtypes) than ALL due to the larger size and lower pliability of myeloblasts and monoblasts than lymphoblasts. Because the sluggish microvascular blood flow is related to the total cytocrit (red cells and leukocytes; Figure 3–6), packed cell transfusions should be avoided if possible until the white cell count has been lowered by chemotherapy or leukapheresis. A high cytocrit may also be associated with spurious hypoglycemia or hypoxia due to consumption of glucose or oxygen in the sample submitted for laboratory testing.

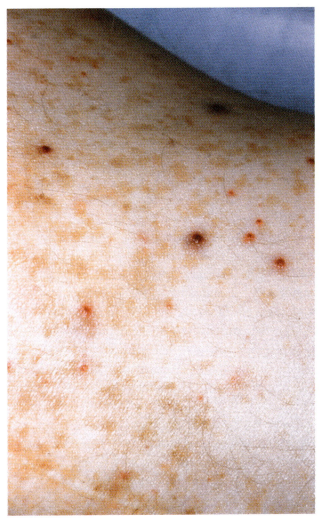

Figure 3–4. Leukemia cutis: widespread cutaneous involvement with acute leukemia. This is more commonly seen in monocytic subtypes of AML and T-cell subtypes of ALL.

mature B phenotype. Central nervous system involvement by ALL may manifest as cranial nerve deficits. Acute lymphoblastic leukemia is more commonly associated with meningeal involvement at the time of presentation than AML. Meningeal involvement may be asymptomatic and require magnetic resonance imaging or lumbar puncture (generally deferred until after the initiation of treatment) to demonstrate its presence. Rarely, localized infiltrates of myeloid blasts (granulocytic sarcoma) or chloroma may develop in a variety of other sites (breast, tonsil, gut, heart, bone) months or even years before widespread overt marrow involvement.

In the chronic leukemias (CLL, CML), splenomegaly is a common finding at the time of diagnosis. In patients with CLL, the presence of splenomegaly

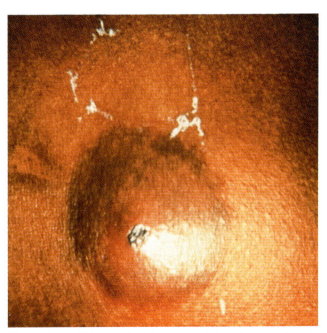

Figure 3–5. Chloroma (skin): extramedullary deposit of acute leukemic blasts.

BLOOD AND MARROW MORPHOLOGY IN THE DIAGNOSIS OF LEUKEMIA

Automated Blood Cell Counters

Automated blood cell counters have largely replaced manual methods for the routine measurement of hemoglobin concentration and red cell indices as well as platelet and leukocyte counts. The widespread use of these devices in Western countries has led to an increase in the number of individuals with leukemia (particularly CML and CLL) who are diagnosed while asymptomatic or during evaluation for other diseases. It is possible that this contributes to the trend toward increasing duration of chronic-phase CML observed in recent studies of that disease.

Modern counters generally use automated colorimetric methods for the measurement of hemoglobin concentration, in combination with cytometric methods for determination of red cell indices and cell counts. In addition, white blood cells may be separated into three- or five-part differentials based on cell size and nuclear and cytoplasmic characteristics (Figure 3–7). As with all laboratory procedures, stringent quality assurance procedures are necessary to ensure that automated counters perform within the required limits of accuracy and that reported limits of normalcy are valid. In addition, it is important to be constantly aware of the limits of measurement outside of which automated counters are not accurate. Modern devices can be set to "flag" laboratory values outside these limits, thus triggering an evaluation using a different method, such as manual cell counts. A useful practice in many laboratories is the manual review of peripheral slides selected randomly by various criteria. The alternative practice of reviewing peripheral smears for all patients with no previous evaluation on file is difficult to maintain in laboratories serving large populations.

Numeric abnormalities are the most frequently encountered triggers leading to evaluations that subsequently disclose a diagnosis of leukemia in adults. Leukocytosis is characteristic of CML, CLL, and the majority of acute leukemias. However, a significant number of patients with acute leukemia present with leukopenia. Abnormalities of the white cell differential or the presence of circulating blasts may be flagged by sensitive automated counters. The automated leukocyte count must be corrected for the presence of nucleated red blood cells if these are present in large number. Thrombocytopenia is a common feature of acute leukemia, MDS, or CLL. Occasionally, automated counters may underestimate the degree of thrombocytopenia in individuals with acute leukemia because of the enumeration of small leukocyte fragments as platelets (see Figure 3–3). Thrombocytosis as a presenting feature is quite common in CML and the myeloproliferative disorders. Thrombocytosis is also a feature of the 5q- syndrome, an uncommon form of MDS usually found in young women. In evaluating patients with abnormal automated blood counts, it is important to bear in mind that with the exception of splenic sequestration and Evans's syndrome of autoimmune hemolytic anemia and thrombocytope-

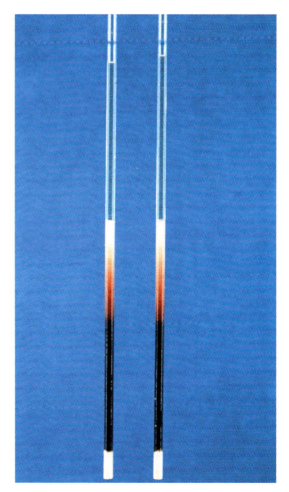

Figure 3–6. Hyperleukocytosis: capillary tube showing contributions of the "white cell-crit" (26%) and the "red cell-crit" (33%) to the total "cytocrit" (59%) in a patient with extreme leukocytosis. Since the symptoms of leukostasis correlate with the cytocrit, caution must be exercised in transfusing patients with anemia and extreme leukocytosis until the white cell number is lowered.

nia, most cases of bicytopenia or pancytopenia are due to an abnormality of the bone marrow, with MDS and leukemia being important diagnostic considerations. Thus, bone marrow aspiration and/or biopsy are usually indicated for the evaluation of bi- or pancytopenia.

Microscopic Evaluation of Blood and Marrow

The cornerstone of leukemia diagnosis is the examination of well-prepared blood and marrow slides by experienced personnel. Most laboratories now routinely perform Romanowsky-type stains, reserving other stains for special indications. Commonly employed stains are listed in Table 3–2. The relative value of blood or marrow as the source of specimens varies with the different leukemias. It is extremely important for the morphologist to be aware of the patient's history and physical findings at the time that samples were obtained. Pernicious anemia, a diagnosis of human immunodeficiency virus (HIV) infection, acute viral illness, and recent treatment with erythroid or myeloid growth factors are all common clinical features that profoundly affect the interpretation of blood and marrow morphology.

Familiarity with the morphologic features of normal marrow is an essential premise to the interpretation of diagnostic blood and marrow specimens in

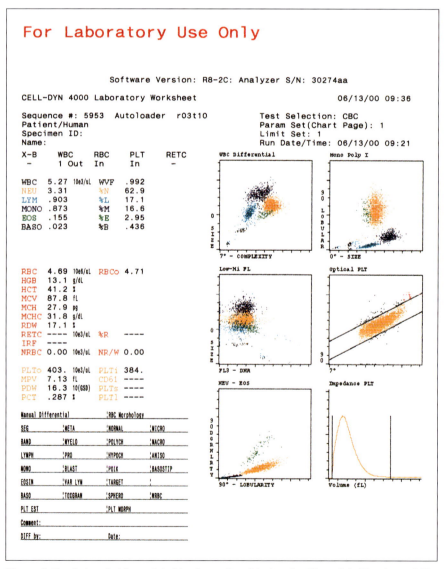

Figure 3–7. Automated "complete blood count" and leukocyte differential. (Courtesy of Ms. Nila deGrano, Hematology Laboratory, Greenbaum Cancer Center.)

Table 3–2. COMMONLY EMPLOYED STAINS IN LEUKEMIA DIAGNOSIS

Stain	Comments
Sudan black B	Myelomonocytic cells
Myeloperoxidase	Myelomonocytic cells
Chloroacetate esterase	Granulocytic blasts and cells
Alpha naphthylbutyrate esterase	Monocytic cells
Periodic acid–Schiff	Lymphoblasts, erythroblasts—block positivity; myeloblasts—speckled pattern
Terminal deoxynucleotidyl transferase	Most lymphoblasts; also some myeloblasts
Tartrate-resistant acid phosphatase	Hairy cell leukemia
Leukocyte alkaline phosphatase	Score is low in chronic myelogenous leukemia
Prussian blue	Iron stain—ring sideroblasts

patients with leukemia. Megakaryocytes are large, multinucleated cells with finely granular cytoplasm. At least three to five should normally be seen in each low power field. Blasts (Figure 3–8) are large cells with a high nuclear:cytoplasmic ratio. Their nuclear chromatin is loose and uniform, and one or more distinct nucleoli are usually found. Cytoplasmic granules are not normally found in blasts. Erythroblasts possess large round nuclei with open chromatin and a distinc-

tively dark blue cytoplasmic appearance in Wright-Giemsa preparations. Lymphoblasts cannot be reliably distinguished from myeloblasts morphologically. In patients lacking Auer rods or other overt signs of leukemia, normal blasts can also not be distinguished from leukemic blasts. The classification of blasts into types I, II, and III, based mainly on the nuclear:cytoplasmic ratio and number of cytoplasmic granules, is of some historic interest. In the United States, most morphologists do not include type III blasts in the differential counts for leukemia diagnosis.

Promyelocytes are usually the largest identifiable myeloid cell in the marrow. These cells have a large, fairly immature nucleus without nucleoli, surrounded by small to moderate amounts of cytoplasm containing primary or azurophilic granules. The presence of a well-developed paranuclear halo indicates further maturation; this is accompanied by progressive loss of the primary granules and their replacement with secondary neutrophilic, eosinophilic, or basophilic granules. Auer rods are linear crystals of dysplastic azurophilic granules, found only in the blasts of patients with AML (Figure 3–9). Normal myelocytes, metamyelocytes, and bands are defined primarily by the degree of nuclear indentation concurrent with cytoplasmic granulation. Segmentation and type of granules are used to identify neutrophils,

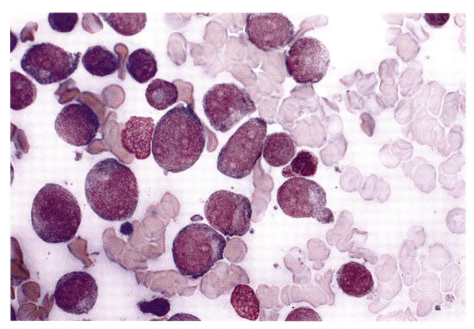

Figure 3–8. Bone marrow aspirate from a patient with acute myeloid leukemia; Wright-Giemsa stain. Note the presence of nucleoli in some of the blasts.

eosinophils, and basophils (Figure 3–10). Monocytes are large cells often with clefted nuclei and pale blue cytoplasm. Normal and abnormal lymphocytes are described below.

Morphologic Findings in Acute Myeloid Leukmia

Traditionally, acute leukemia was diagnosed based on the presence of more than 30 percent blasts (the denominator being all nucleated cells) in the bone marrow. It is worth emphasizing that in Romanowsky-type stains, the only reliable evidence of myeloid lineage in acute leukemia is the presence of Auer rods. Cytochemical stains (Table 3–3) are useful in differentiating most cases of AML from ALL and in further subclassifying AML (Tables 3–3 and 3–4) The differentiation of AML from ALL is based on the presence of positive staining ($\geq$ 3% of blasts) by Sudan black B (SBB) or MPO in most cases of AML (Figure 3–11). Because of a significant amount of overlap, terminal deoxynucleotide transferase (TdT) and periodic acid–Schiff (PAS) stains are not reliable for the separation of AML from ALL. Blasts of granulocytic lineage are identified by positive specific esterase (SE) staining, whereas, conversely, monoblasts react positively to nonspecific esterase (NSE) stains. Using the

percentage of residual maturing myeloid cells (promyelocytes, myelocytes, metamyelocytes, and granulocytes) as an indicator of maturation, a French, American, and British (FAB) cooperative group divided acute myeloblastic leukemia into two groups, M1 (without maturation) and M2 (with maturation)[7,8] (see Table 3–4). Extramedullary leukemia is more common in cases classified as M2. Some cases of M2, which exhibit blasts with heavier granulation and numerous Auer rods, likely represent a distinct entity since cytogenetic studies reveal the presence of t(8;21). The presence of t(8;21) has been associated with lower relapse rates than usually found with AML in general, even after adjusting for its relatively higher frequency in young adults.[9] Together, M1 and M2 account for 50 percent of adult AML.

Acute promyelocytic (or progranular) leukemia, which has been recognized as a distinct entity since 1957, was termed M3 by the FAB group. This form of leukemia derives its name from the appearance of blasts with very heavy granulation, reminiscent of promyelocytes. The granules have been found to be the source of procoagulant substances responsible for the development of DIC in many patients with this disease. Numerous Auer rods are usually found in the blasts in APL (Figure 3–12), and a careful search often reveals medium- to large-sized cells

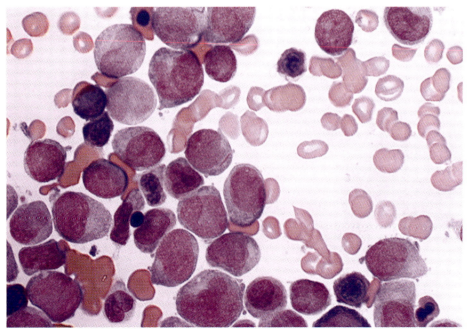

Figure 3–9.   Bone marrow aspirate from a patient with acute myeloid leukemia; Wright-Giemsa stain.

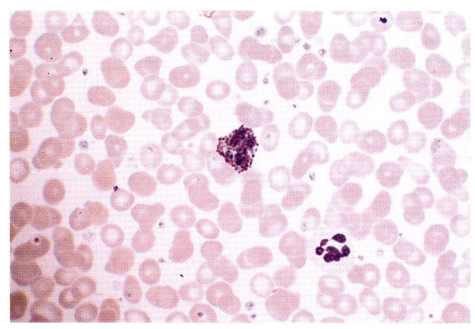

Figure 3–10. Peripheral blood smear; hematoxylin and eosin stain. Basophil and neutrophil.

containing bundles of Auer rods (faggot cells). Several blasts also exhibit bilobed nuclei; this appears to be a more consistent morphologic feature of APL since it is also found in the microgranular variants that lack heavy granulation (Figure 3–13). Although initially described as a distinct disease on the basis of clinical and morphologic features, more recently, cytogenetic studies in almost all cases have been found to show t(15;17) or one of its variants. This translocation, which juxtaposes the promyelocytic leukemia gene (*PML*) on chromosome 15 with the retinoic acid receptor-alpha gene (*RARA*) on chromosome 17, can also be demonstrated on the molecular level by polymerase chain reaction (PCR) or reverse transcriptase (RT)-PCR for the transcript. Cases that morphologically resemble classic APL but that lack cytogenetic or molecular evidence of this genetic abnormality often exhibit clinical characteristics quite unlike APL. Therapy targeted to the *PML/RARA* gene product (all-*trans* retinoic acid [ATRA]) has helped to transform APL into the most prognostically favorable subtype of AML, with survival rates in excess of 80 to 90 percent.[10]

Monocytic forms of AML (Figure 3–14) represent 30 to 35 percent of cases. Monoblasts are typically large cells with folded nuclei, surrounded by variable amounts of cytoplasm containing granules that stain positively for NSE and negatively for SE.

Table 3–3. CORRELATION OF HISTOCHEMICAL CHARACTERISTICS AND IMMUNOPHENOTYPE OF ACUTE LEUKEMIA CELLS		
FAB	**Cytochemical Stains**	**Markers**
M0	MPO–, SBB–, SE–, NSE–	CD13, CD33, CD34, TdT±, HLA-DR, icMPO
M1	MPO+, SBB+, SE+, NSE–	CD13, CD33, HLA-DR, icMPO
M2	MPO+, SBB+, SE+, NSE–	CD13, CD33, HLA-DR, icMPO
M3	MPO+, SBB+, SE+, NSE–	CD13, CD33, icMPO
M4	MPO+, SBB+, SE+, NSE+	CD13, CD33, HLA-DR, icMPO, CD14
M5	MPO±, SBB+, SE–, NSE+	CD13, CD33, HLA-DR, icMPO, CD14
M6	MPO+, SBB+, PAS+	CD13±, CD33±, icMPO, glycophorin
M7	MPO–, SBB±, PAS+	CD33, CD41, CD61, icMPO
ALL, L1/L2	MPO–, SBB–, PAS+	CD19, CD10±, sIg–
ALL, L3	MPO–, SBB–, PAS+	CD19, sIg+, κ or λ light chain
T-ALL	MPO–, SBB–, PAS+	CD3±, icCD3+

MPO = myeloperoxidase; SBB = Sudan black B; SE = specific esterase; NSE = nonspecific esterase; PAS = periodic acid–Schiff; ic = intracellular.

Table 3–4. SUBCLASSIFICATION OF ACUTE MYELOID LEUKEMIA				
	%*	Morphology	Common Cytogenetics	Prognosis
M0	< 5	MPO/SBB negative; myeloid by EM or immunologic methods		Poor
M1, acute myelogenous leukemia without maturation	~50	< 10% maturation	t(9;22), inv(3)	Mixed
M2, acute myelogenous leukemia with maturation		> 10% maturation	t(8;21)	Good with t(8;21)
M3, acute promyelocytic leukemia	~10	Abnormal promyelocytes counted as blasts; nuclear clefting; prominent granules, Auer rods	t(15;17)	Good
		Microgranular variant; without prominent granules, Auer rods	t(11:17), t(5;17)	
M4, acute myelomonocytic leukemia	~30	Monoblasts + promonocytes 20–80%		
		M4Eo, acute myelomonocytic leukemia with eosinophilia; abnormal eosinophil precursors present	inv 16	Good
M5, acute monocytic leukemia M5a M5b		Monoblasts + promonocytes > 80%	t(11)(q23) del(11)(q23)	Poor?
M6, acute erythrocytic leukemia	~2	Erythroid precursors > 50% nucleated cells; blasts > 30% nonerythroid cells	-5, 5q-, -7, 7q-	Poor
M7, acute megakaryoblastic leukemia	< 5	Immunologic confirmation of megakaryocytic lineage	t(1;22) (infants)	Poor

Except otherwise stated, blast counts refer to percentage of nonerythroid cells.
*Incidence rates reported in large North American series; may differ in other parts of the world.

In the FAB system, monocytic leukemias were divided into AML M4 (acute myelomonocytic leukemia), in which granulocytic blasts represent more than 20 percent of bone marrow, and M5 (acute monocytic leukemia), in which granulocytic blasts number fewer than 20 percent of bone marrow (the

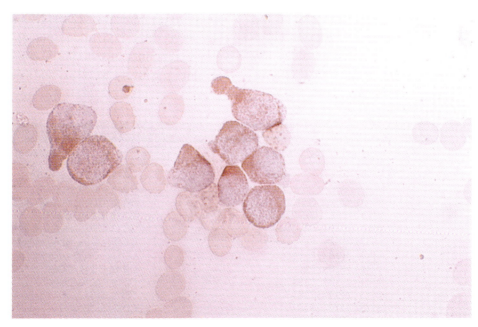

Figure 3–11.   Bone marrow aspirate from a patient with APL. Myeloperoxidase stain.

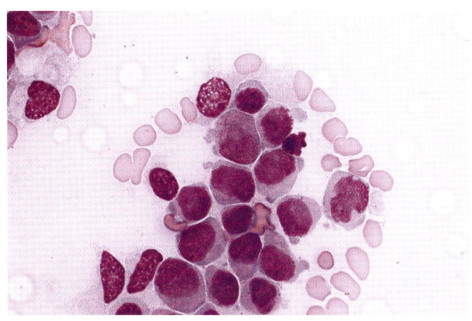

Figure 3–12. Bone marrow aspirate from same patient as Figure 3–9; Wright-Giemsa stain. Note the presence of an Auer rod.

difference being made up of monoblasts and promonocytes). The technique of double esterase staining, by which granulocytic and monocytic blasts can be demonstrated on the same slide with SE and NSE, facilitates the distinction of M4 from M5 leukemia. Auer rods are typically not found in M5. Two subtypes of M5 are described: in M5a, the majority of nonerythroid cells are monoblasts, whereas in M5b, promonocytes and monocytes make up a significant percentage. Chronic myelomonocytic leukemia (CMML), a clinically less acute disease in which circulating monocytes number more than 1,000/μL, was classified with the MDSs. Monocytic forms of AML can be difficult to differentiate from CMML. It is also important to note that SBB and MPO stains are occasionally negative in acute mono-

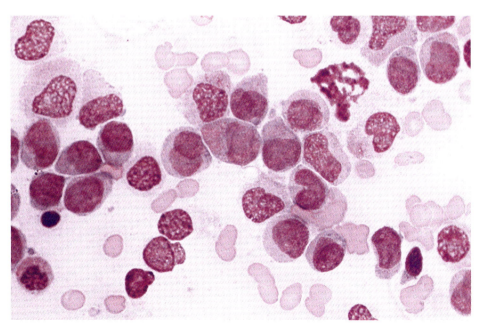

Figure 3–13. Bone marrow aspirate from patient with APL; Wright-Giemsa stain. Note nuclear clefting.

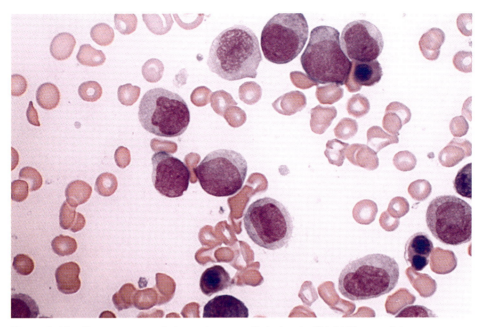

Figure 3–14.   Bone marrow aspirate, acute monocytic leukemia; Wright-Giemsa stain.

cytic leukemias. This, coupled with the rarity of Auer rods in monocytic leukemias in general, leads to occasional confusion with ALL. A distinct subtype of acute monocytic leukemia (with eosinophilia) is recognized, in which the marrow is interspersed with a variable number of abnormal monolobate eosinophilic precursors exhibiting very coarse, dark granules (Figure 3–15). Nonspecific esterase stains, which are normally positive in monoblasts, are usually unimpressive by light microscopy in this subtype of monoblastic leukemia, although electron microscopic studies have confirmed the presence of monocytic granules in the majority of cases evaluated.[11] Cytogenetic studies reveal abnormalities of chromosome 16, typically inversions at p13q22. Patients with this abnormality also generally fare better than those with other subtypes of AML.[12]

Acute erythroleukemia is the least common type of AML recognized distinctly by morphologic criteria (2 to 3%) (Figure 3–16). In this disease, erythroid precursors account for 50 percent or more of marrow nucleated cells. To distinguish acute erythrolcukemia from MDSs and chronic erythremic proliferations, some authors propose that more than 30 percent of the nonerythroid cells should be blasts.[8,13] Erythroblasts stain positively with the PAS technique, typically in a speckled pattern, although not distinctly enough to differentiate them from lymphoblasts, which typically stain in a block pattern. It has been suggested that the ratio of pronormoblasts to myeloblasts in the marrow of patients with erythroleukemia correlates with cytogenetic abnormalities and prognostic outcomes.[14] Care must also be taken to distinguish erythroleukemia from megaloblastic anemia, in which the bone marrow shares features of hypercellularity, erythroid hyperplasia, and nuclear-cytoplasmic asynchrony. The bone marrow in individuals with anemia due to parvovirus B19 infection may also have large, abnormal proerythroblasts reminiscent of erythroleukemia. During the recovery phase of parvovirus-induced anemia, erythroid hyperplasia may be seen, further confusing the picture.

Although classification systems based on morphology have received widespread attention, they have also been the subject of much critical debate (Table 3–5). Early studies demonstrated lack of consistency between various observers, particularly relating to the distinction between FAB M1 and M2, M2 and M4, and M4 and M5. Moreover, with few exceptions, it appeared that clinical features and treatment outcomes could not be reliably predicted by morphologic studies alone.[15,16] Morphologic studies also failed to recognize certain distinct forms of AML, such as acute megakaryocytic leukemia (Figure 3–17), acute basophilic leukemia, acute eosinophilic leukemia, and the more undifferentiated forms of

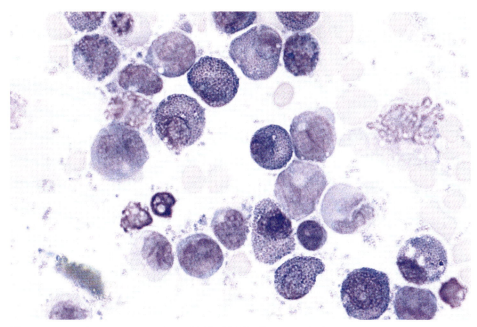

Figure 3–15. Bone marrow aspirate, M4Eo; Wright-Giemsa stain. Note abnormal eosinophils.

AML. Minimally differentiated AML and megakaryocytic leukemia are particularly problematic because the blasts are SBB and MPO negative at the light microscopic level, and their myeloid nature can only be demonstrated by electron microscopy or flow cytometry for myeloid markers.[17] To address some of these concerns, the National Cancer Institute sponsored a workshop in 1988, which proposed criteria for acute megakaryoblastic leukemia and the distinction of ALL from M0 (see below). More recently, it has been argued that other important morphologic criteria that were not included in the FAB descriptions but that are now known to be associated with distinct clinical features and treatment outcomes should be considered in the subclassification of AML. For example, individuals with AML in whom there are clear mor-

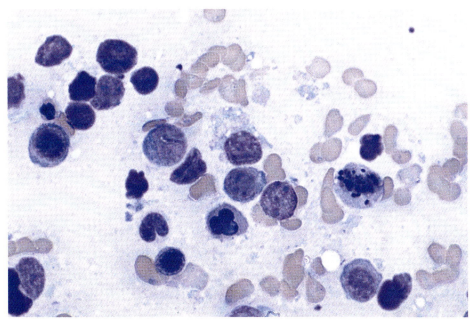

Figure 3–16. Bone marrow aspirate from patient with acute erythroleukemia; Wright-Giemsa stain. Note abnormal erythroid cells.

Table 3–5. COMMON LIMITATIONS OF PURELY MORPHOLOGIC CLASSIFICATION SYSTEMS

Failure to incorporate biologic characteristics of disease into diagnostic decisions
Dependence on observer judgment; lack of reproducibility
Frequent dependence on arbitrarily established categories
Lack of prognostic informativeness
Failure to identify modern therapeutic targets

phologic signs of multilineage dysplasia appear more likely to have disease that is resistant to chemotherapy. It is possible that the presence of multilineage dysplasia reflects leukemic derivation from a more primitive cell type, with likely preservation of biologic mechanisms that protect the malignant cell from xenobiotic injuries such as chemotherapy.

In general, the prognostic information provided by morphologic studies in AML is extremely limited, with cytogenetic and molecular studies (discussed below) providing much more biologically relevant data. This is not surprising since many of the widely used morphologic criteria are based on arbitrarily selected distinctions rather than true biologic correlates. In addition, clinical features such as a history of exposure to chemotherapy or antecedent MDS strongly influence the response to therapy and will likely be incorporated into future classification schemes.

Morphologic Findings in the Myelodysplastic Syndromes

Historically, blood and bone marrow morphology has been widely used for the diagnosis and classification of MDS, as it has been for AML (Table 3–6). The hallmark of MDS is the presence of peripheral blood cytopenias in the setting of bone marrow hypercellularity and dysplasia. This represents a form of ineffective erythropoiesis. Anemia is almost universal, with thrombocytopenia and/or neutropenia being found in about one half to two-thirds of all patients. Erythrocytes are usually slightly macrocytic, although they may be microcytic in individuals with sideroblastic anemia. Abnormally shaped erythrocytes and nucleated forms are commonly found. The reticulocyte count is usually decreased or insufficiently increased for the degree of anemia present. Leukopenia is found in about one-third of cases; monocyte counts in excess of 1,000/μL occur in CMML. Neutrophil dysplasia may be manifested as hypogranulation and abnormal segmentation patterns such as the pseudo Pelger-Huët (bilobed) anomaly. Immature myeloid cells including blasts may be found in smears made from peripheral blood. Thrombocytopenia is seen in up to two-thirds of patients. The platelets are quite frequently abnor-

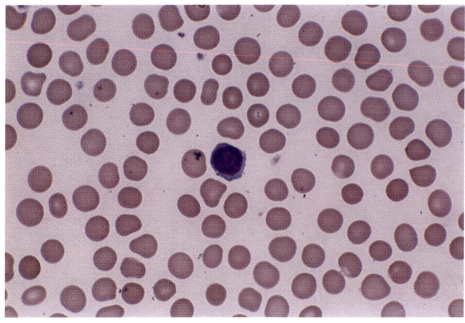

Figure 3–17. Blast from a patient with acute megakaryocytic leukemia. Peripheral blood; Wright-Giemsa stain. Note absence of any distinctive features.

Table 3–6. MORPHOLOGIC (FAB) CLASSIFICATION OF MDS

Relative Incidence	Features	Prognosis* Median Survival (mo)	% Leukemic Progression
Refractory anemia with ringed sideroblasts (20%)	> 15% ringed sideroblasts < 5% blasts	50	8
Refractory anemia (30%)	< 15% ringed sideroblasts < 5% blasts	50	12
Refractory anemia with excess blasts (20%)	5–20% blasts	11	44
Refractory anemia with excess blasts in transformation (15%)	20–30% blasts or presence of Auer rods	5	60
Chronic myelomonocytic leukemia (15%)	< 20% blasts, increased monocytes	11	14

*Data reported from MIC Cooperative Group Study of 1,081 cases.

mal in showing hypogranulation or abnormal size.

Bone marrow hypercellularity is characteristic of MDS, although a hypocellular variant has been described.[18,19] Nuclear-cytoplasmic asynchrony, resembling megaloblastoid changes, may be evident in erythrocyte or myeloid precursors. Iron stains frequently demonstrate increased iron stores. Erythroid precursor cells with perinuclear iron deposits (ring sideroblasts) may also be found. Leukocyte dysplasia and increased blast counts are common. Megakaryocytes may be decreased in number and often demonstrate dysplastic features such as hypolobulation and small size (micromegakaryocytes). In contrast to AML, cytochemical stains are usually not of value in the classification of MDS.

Myelodysplastic syndromes are usually classified on the basis of the foregoing features as refractory anemia, refractory anemia with ringed sideroblasts, refractory anemia with excess blasts (RAEB), or refractory anemia with excess blasts in transformation (RAEB-t).[20] A fifth group, CMML, shares many similarities with myeloproliferative disorders, such as leukocytosis and a lower incidence of thrombocytopenia as the presenting feature. Although these groups have been associated with different rates of transformation to AML and varying survival rates, cytogenetic studies have been found to provide even more important prognostic information, as in AML.[21] In particular, the arbitrarily selected percentages of bone marrow blasts that were used to separate RAEB, RAEB-t, and AML have come into question because of clinical studies showing similar outcomes in RAEB-t treated with intensive induction regimes as have been traditionally associated with AML. Several authors, as well as a clinical

advisory group convened to review World Health Organization (WHO) proposals for the classification of hematopoietic cell malignancies, have recommended the use of a blast percentage of 20 percent, instead of 30 percent, to separate AML from MDS.[21] However, biologically, the influence of blast counts on clinical outcomes is likely to fall along a continuum rather than a strict threshold number. In this disease, as in AML, cytogenetic and clinical features contribute significantly to prognosis.

Morphologic Findings in Acute Lymphoblastic Leukemia

Morphologically, ALL is differentiated from AML by the absence of Auer rods and MPO or SBB staining, although rare cases of SBB-positive ALL have been reported.[22] Periodic acid–Schiff stains typically demonstrate "block" positivity in ALL blasts, but this is not distinctive enough to be of much diagnostic use. Based on nuclear:cytoplasmic ratio, nucleolar characteristics, regularity of nuclear membrane outline, and blast cell size, three subtypes of ALL have been described: L1, L2, and L3.[23] The most distinctive form, mature B-cell ALL (the leukemic counterpart of Burkitt's lymphoma), represents only about 5 percent of ALL in adults. The blasts in this form of ALL are large, with large, uniform, round to oval nuclei. Nuclear chromatin is finely stippled, and nucleoli are usually single and distinct. The cytoplasm is intensely blue and often vacuolated (Figure 3–18).

The interobserver concordance rates between L1 and L2 (Figure 3–19), the other subtypes of ALL, are less than with L3. Moreover, treatment recommendations are similar for adult L1 and L2; thus, practically, the distinction between L1 and L2 is of little consequence. In contrast, L3, which is more reliably diagnosed morphologically, is usually associated with a distinctive mature B-cell phenotype. Cytogenetic studies frequently reveal t(8;14). L3 is usually an aggressive disease, with a higher propensity for central nervous system or meningeal involvement than other subtypes of ALL. Because of higher relapse rates, overall survival rates are lower than observed in other forms of ALL. Recently, however, brief duration, aggressive chemotherapy programs have been associated with improved treatment results compared to historical series. This association of specific morphologic, immunophenotypic, and cytogenetic features with a clinical entity provides yet another example of a biologically distinct leukemic disease. Indeed, even in other subtypes of ALL, cytogenetic and molecular studies are more important prognostic indicators than morphologic features.

Morphologic Findings in the Chronic Myeloproliferative Disorders

The myeloproliferative disorders CML, essential thrombocythemia, polycythemia rubra vera, and myelofibrosis with myeloid metaplasia (MMM) are a group of diseases in which clonal stem cell aberrations result in abnormal blood cell proliferation. Morphologically, the bone marrow differs from AML in showing orderly maturation and lower blast counts.[24] The distinction from MDS is based on the lack of severe multilineage dysplasia or profound peripheral blood cytopenias. In CML, the automated blood count demonstrates leukocytosis; the differential count shows absolute neutrophilia, but there is also an increase in the number of neutrophil precursors. A low leukocyte alkaline phosphatase score differentiates CML from benign leukemoid reactions. Chronic myeloid leukemia must also be distinguished from the more rare chronic neutrophilic leukemia, a similar disease in which the leukocyte differential shows mainly mature neutrophils.[25] Pronounced thrombocytosis, basophilia, and/or eosinophilia suggest a poorer prognosis in CML. Anemia is usually mild or moderate, and the platelet count is often normal or elevated. Bone marrow examination shows increased myeloid:erythroid ratio, with orderly myeloid maturation. Signs of dysplasia are subtle, often limited to the presence of micromegakaryocytes (very small, hypolobulated megakaryocytes). Special stains are generally not helpful in the evaluation of MPD, with the exception of reticulin or Masson's trichrome for

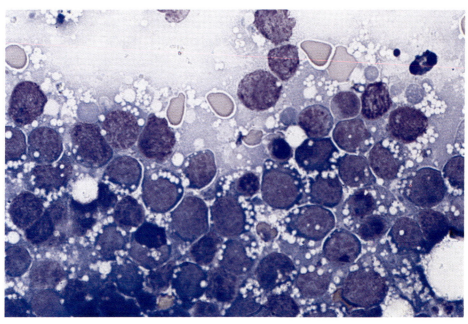

Figure 3–18. Bone marrow aspirate, L3; Wright-Giemsa stain. Note intensely basophilic cytoplasm with vacuolation.

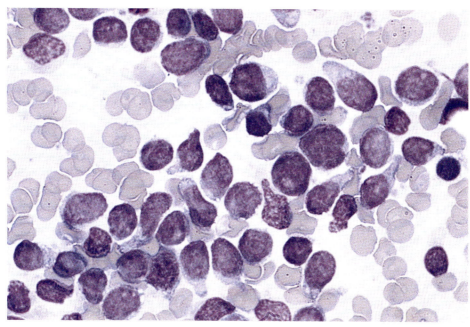

Figure 3–19. Bone marrow aspirate, ALL L1/L2; Wright-Giemsa stain.

demonstrating myelofibrosis in advanced stages. Other signs of transformation to MMM are the development of an erythroleukoblastic picture with nucleated red blood cells, leukocyte precursors, and sometimes megakaryocyte fragments found circulating in the peripheral blood. Teardrop cells and other abnormal erythrocytes may also be found (Figure 3–20). The majority of individuals with CML are diagnosed in the chronic phase. Progression to blast crisis is marked by an increase in bone marrow or circulating blasts or the development of leukemic skin or soft tissue infiltration.

Morphology of Chronic Lymphoproliferative Disorders

In those lymphoproliferative disorders presenting in a leukemic form, such as CLL, the diagnostic sample is most frequently blood or bone marrow; these are generally easier to obtain than lymph nodes or splenic tissue. Leukemic cells may be found circulating in the blood in the absence of marrow involvement, especially in the leukemia of large granular lymphocytes or the leukemic phase of lymphomas such as mantle cell lymphoma. In such diseases, bone marrow involvement signifies advanced disease. In CLL, some but not all studies have shown that the pattern of marrow involvement influences the prognosis, with diffuse infiltration being worse than a nodular pattern.[26,27] It is crucial to review bone marrow biopsies and aspirates since some lymphocytic disorders do not aspirate well, and the degree of involvement would otherwise be underestimated. For cytologic detail, however, well-stained peripheral blood or marrow aspirates are superior to biopsies (Figure 3–21).

Many different lymphoid cells can be recognized morphologically. Lymphoblasts have been described in the ALL section. Mature-looking lymphocytes are slightly larger than erythrocytes and possess a large round or slightly indented nucleus with dense chromatin and no nucleoli. The cytoplasm is pale bluish on Wright-Giemsa staining (Figure 3–22). Atypical lymphocytes are usually larger, and the cytoplasm is often irregular or molded around abutting cells. Prolymphocytes are found in some cases of CLL, although if they number more than 60 percent, a diagnosis of prolymphocytic leukemia should be rendered. Prolymphocytes generally have a smaller nuclear:cytoplasmic ratio than mature lymphocytes, and in addition, one or two indistinct nucleoli may be apparent. Large granular lymphocytes differ in the presence of a few coarse azurophilic granules. The lymphocytes of hairy cell leukemia (HCL) have a mature-looking nucleus; the cytoplasm bears fine

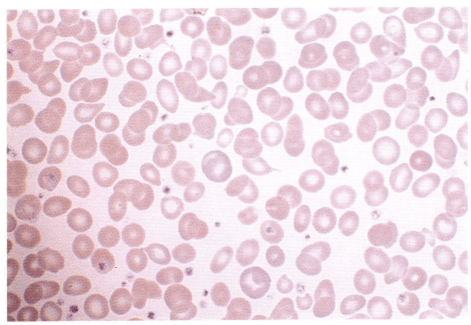

Figure 3–20. Peripheral smear from patient with myelofibrosis with myeloid metaplasia. Note dimorphic red cell morphology with tear drop-shaped red cells.

projections in well-prepared specimens. The tartrate-resistant acid phosphatase stain is positive in peripheral blood specimens in most patients with HCL and quite specific. It is important to regard as positive only those specimens that show some lymphocytes with very heavy staining (> 40 granules or granules obscuring the nucleus) in order not to overdiagnose HCL. The cytoplasmic projections of splenic lymphoma with villous lymphocytes are wider than those of HCL and generally more polarized to one side of the cell. Sézary cells are relatively large lymphocytes with cerebriform, usually clefted nuclei, and scanty

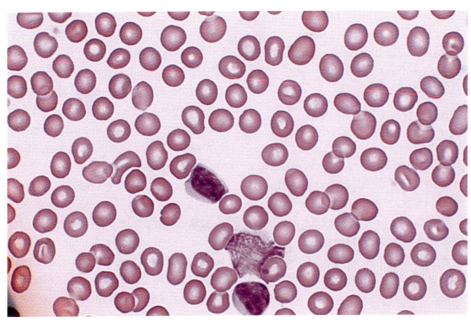

Figure 3–21. Peripheral blood from patient with CLL; hematoxylin and eosin stain. Note presence of a smudge cell. Smudge cells, which are the artefactual result of leukocyte damage during slide preparation, are a common finding in CLL but are not pathognomonic.

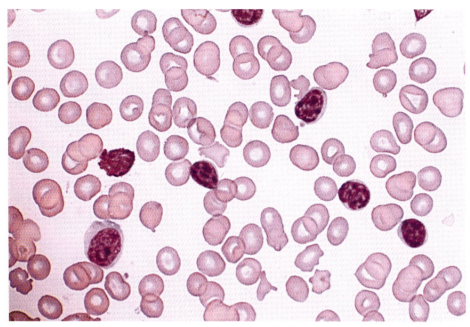

Figure 3–22. Peripheral blood from patient with CLL; hematoxylin and eosin stain. Note lymphocytosis, with mature-appearing lymphocytes.

cytoplasm, usually found circulating in patients with mycosis fungoides. In patients with adult T-cell leukemia/lymphoma associated with human T-cell leukemia virus-1 infection, lymphocytosis is composed of cells ranging from small, mature-looking lymphocytes to bizarre, hyperlobulated forms.

Mature plasma cells classically have an eccentric nucleus with alternating areas of dark and light chromatin and no nucleoli. The cytoplasm is a darker blue than that of lymphocytes, and a lighter blue perinuclear "halo" is usually present. Immature plasma cells have larger nuclei with more open chromatin. Plasmablasts exhibit an even more immature-looking nucleus, with fine, open chromatin and distinct nucleoli, and the nucleus is usually centrally placed. Plasma cells of all types are found in the blood and marrow of patients with plasma cell leukemia. Lymphoplasmacytic cells are lymphocytes with mature-looking, eccentrically placed nuclei and moderate to large amounts of pale blue cytoplasm. They are found in the bone marrow of patients with Waldenström's macroglobulinemia. "Hand mirror" cells are mononuclear cells with a small amount of cytoplasm limited to a single, wide projection on one side. Although hand mirror cells are often lymphoid in origin, immunophenotyping studies have revealed myeloid

lineage in some. It is likely that this morphologic form represents pseudopodia formation rather than a specific cell type.

Natural killer (NK) cell and NK-like lymphoproliferative disorders are rare. Large granular lymphocytes (LGLs) are a distinct subset of peripheral blood lymphocytes, normally comprising fewer than 15 percent. Morphologically, these cells are usually large, with variable amounts of pale blue cytoplasm and few distinct azurophilic granules. The nuclei appear mature. Phenotyping reveals either T (CD3+) or NK (CD3–, CD56+) cells. Historically, the lymphoproliferative disease of large granular lymphocytes has been defined by the presence of > 2,000/μL LGLs in the peripheral blood, persisting for longer than 6 months. This definition has been challenged because of the demonstration of typical clinical features in individuals with large granular lymphocytosis of smaller degree and, conversely, the heterogeneity of clinical features in cohorts of individuals who otherwise fit the definition. Unfortunately, there are presently no methods in general clinical use for investigating clonality in NK cell populations. Moreover, some of the clinical features classically associated with LGL leukemia may not be restricted to individuals in which the NK or T-cell expansion is clonal.

IMMUNOPHENOTYPING STUDIES IN THE DIAGNOSIS OF LEUKEMIA

Morphologic studies have the advantage of wide availability and have historically been used as the basis of leukemia diagnosis and classification. However, even with modern staining methods, the lineage and maturational stage of leukemic cells are often unable to be determined. Yet, such information is invaluable for informing treatment decisions and estimating prognosis in all adult leukemias. As an example of this, it is interesting to note how the ability to manufacture monoclonal antibodies directed at specific cellular antigens has extended diagnostic capabilities (immunophenotyping) while also providing the opportunity to treat patients with drugs directed selectively to leukemic cells.

An increasing array of monoclonal antibodies is available for the immunophenotypic diagnosis of the leukemias. For a detailed review of this topic, see Chapter 5.

Immunophenotyping with antibodies to hematopoietic (eg, CD45, the leukocyte common antigen) and nonhematopoietic antigens (eg, cytokeratin) is useful for investigating leukemic involvement of tissues other than bone marrow, where the differential diagnosis includes epithelial or connective tissue tumors. Antibodies to lineage-specific or -associated antigens, such as CD3, CD20, or anti-MPO, will support a T-cell, B-cell, or myeloid origin, respectively. For samples that can be analyzed as cell suspensions, flow cytometry is extremely useful because of the large number of available monoclonal antibody reagents and the ability to analyze several cellular characteristics simultaneously. In addition to lineage assignment, flow cytometry permits determination of the maturational stage of leukemic cells based on the pattern of expression of maturation-specific antigens. Evidence of malignancy is provided by the demonstration of disproportionately large numbers of cells with arrested maturation, aberrant antigen expression, or, in the case of B cells, clonal light-chain restriction. Flow cytometry is also useful for the rapid enumeration of hematopoietic cells. Monoclonal antibodies are currently under development for the direct detection of abnormal proteins produced as a result of translocations and other genetic lesions, such as the increased amounts of bcl-2 protein associated with t(14;18). The use of such antibodies in flow cytometry is likely to extend these studies to the detection of specific genetic abnormalities not only in acute leukemia but also in MDS, MPS, and other diseases. An interesting adaptation of flow cytometry is the demonstration of drug efflux from leukemic cells. This functional assay, which correlates with expression of the drug efflux protein P-glycoprotein, provides useful prognostic information in acute leukemia and in the future may be the basis for selection of specific chemotherapeutic drugs for individuals with acute leukemia. Flow cytometry has also been used to investigate cell-cycle turnover, to detect intracellular cytokines and putative oncogenes, and to measure apoptotic activity in cells; some of these applications, such as nuclear staining for cyclin D1 overexpression in mantle cell lymphoma, have already found their way into the clinical laboratory.

Flow Cytometry in Acute Leukemia

The major role of flow cytometry in the diagnosis of acute leukemia is in the differentiation of AML from ALL (Figure 3–23). This distinction cannot be accurately made by Wright-Giemsa staining in many cases, except when the presence of Auer rods is diagnostic of AML. Although immunohistochemical stains are capable of resolving this difficulty in most cases, minimally differentiated AML M0 and M7 present special difficulties because of the failure of the blasts associated with these subtypes to stain with MPO or SBB. Through flow cytometry, myeloid antigens such as CD33, CD13, and intracellular MPO can be clearly demonstrated to be associated with the blasts of M0 leukemia. Acute megakaryoblastic leukemia blasts uniquely stain positively for CD41 or CD61 by flow cytometry and characteristically lack MPO. Care must be taken in interpreting positive CD41 staining because monocytic blasts can exhibit false-positive staining through their affinity for contaminating platelets. The unique immunophenotype of APL (see Chapter 5) is helpful particularly in microgranular cases and in cases that lack the classic (15;17) translocation (see Chapter 6). Antibodies to CD11b, CD14, and CD64 are used to identify monocytic leukemia. The discrimination between monoblasts, promonocytes, and their more mature derivatives by flow cytometry may be difficult since the side scatter characteristics of these cells (proportional to cell granularity and complexity) merge smoothly across the entire spectrum.

There is currently no consensus on the terminology for leukemias that express both myeloid and lymphoid markers. It would seem reasonable to reserve the term "biphenotypic" for those extremely rare cases in which myeloid-restricted antigens (such as MPO, but not CD33 or CD13) are co-expressed with lymphoid restricted antigens (such as cytoplasmic CD22 or cytoplasmic CD3 but not CD19 or surface CD3). Bilineage leukemias might be described as those cases in which distinct myeloid and lymphoid blast cell subpopulations can be detected within one leukemic cell population. True acute undifferentiated leukemias lack lineage-specific antigen expression (MPO, intracytoplasmic CD22 or CD3). The majority

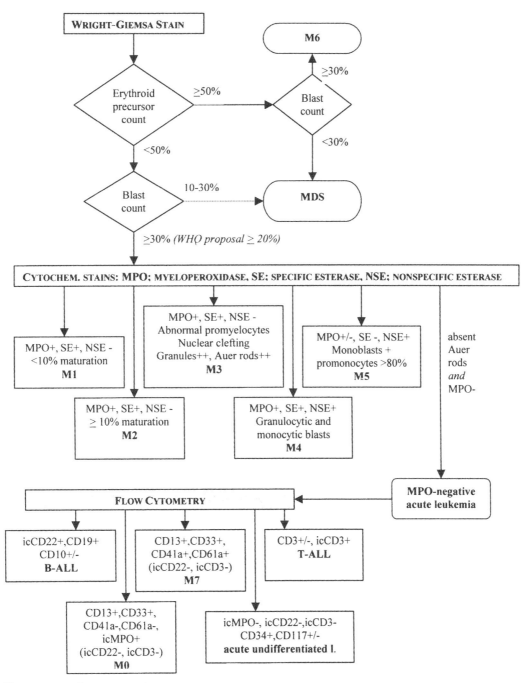

Figure 3–23. Combination of cytochemical stains and flow cytometry for acute leukemia diagnosis.

of these cases are positive for CD34 and human leukocyte antigen (HLA)-DR.

The acute lymphoid leukemias (ALLs) were the first to benefit from the introduction of monoclonal antibodies. Today, B- and T-lineage ALLs are categorized into immunophenotypic subsets according to their maturation stage-specific antigen expression patterns (see Chapter 5).

Aside from guiding modern treatment decisions at the time of diagnosis, flow cytometry is invaluable in evaluation of small blast populations found after treatment (minimal residual disease).[28] The antigen profile of the leukemic cells in the initial, diagnostic specimen provides the guidelines for the choice of antibodies when testing for residual blasts.

Flow Cytometry in Chronic Lymphoproliferative Disorders

Although the major role of flow cytometry in the evaluation of the chronic lymphoproliferative disorders is in the investigation of lineage and proof of clonality, disease-specific immunophenotypes have been delineated that allow the distinction between chronic lymphoid leukemia (CLL), prolymphocytic leukemia, leukemic phase of mantle cell lymphoma, and HCL (see Chapter 5). The diagnosis of B-cell CLL is based on the finding of more than 5,000/μL circulating lymphocytes that co-express CD5 with typical B-cell antigens such as CD19 or CD20. Patients with lymph node-based disease of the same phenotype as CLL, but who have lower degrees of lymphocytosis, are more properly classified as having small lymphocytic lymphoma; the distinction is important because different staging and treatment response criteria have historically been applied to the two diseases.[29] Flow cytometry is also often used to investigate the presence of antigens that are potential targets for monoclonal antibody-based therapy, such as CD20.

CYTOGENETIC STUDIES IN THE DIAGNOSIS OF LEUKEMIA

It is four decades since Nowell and Hungerford described the Philadelphia chromosome associated

with CML. Chromosomal banding techniques revealed later that the apparently truncated chromosome (22) is actually the result of a balanced translocation between chromosomes 9 and 22. Since then, numerous other chromosomal aberrations have been discovered in specific forms of leukemia, mainly translocations, deletions, and numeric abnormalities.[30] In addition, more cryptic abnormalities can now be demonstrated using the more sensitive methods of fluorescent in situ hybridization (FISH), Southern blotting, and PCR. The genes that are disrupted as a result of these lesions are being continuously probed using very sensitive molecular methods, including DNA sequencing. As a result, the mechanisms by which genetic aberrations cause leukemia are being elucidated, serving as targets of potential preventive and therapeutic strategies.

Because of their prognostic implication and because the information is essential in the assessment of treatment response and minimal residual disease after therapy, cytogenetic studies must be obtained routinely at the time of diagnosis. The results of cytogenetic studies may also influence the choice of postremission therapy. In the future, rationally designed drugs may be used to target the molecular lesions known to underlie the cytogenetic aberrations in leukemia. This approach has already proven successful with the use of ATRA and arsenic trioxide for patients with APL. See Chapter 6 for a detailed description of cytogenetic aberrations and their molecular consequences in leukemia.

MOLECULAR STUDIES IN THE DIAGNOSIS OF LEUKEMIA

Conventional cytogenetic studies, supplemented by FISH, are able to detect the majority of genetic lesions known to be important for the diagnosis of specific leukemic syndromes in adults. These studies, however, are limited in sensitivity and in the time needed to return test results. More sensitive and rapidly performed tests have therefore been applied to the diagnosis of specific molecular lesions in patients with leukemia, Southern blot analysis or PCR. In the future, as more rationally designed therapies targeted to specific genetic lesions become available, these tests will likely assume a greater role in the routine diagnostic evaluation of most leukemias.

Southern blot analysis is a hybridization technique used to identify DNA segments of varying length that have been separated by means of electrophoresis on a gel. The DNA fragments are produced by digestion with restriction endonucleases. After transfer of the DNA fragments to a membrane (usually nitrocellulose or nylon), labeled probes are used to detect the presence of specific DNA sequences in the various bands. Because restriction endonucleases cleave DNA at specific sites, clonally expanded DNA rearrangements form discrete bands that are distinct from the germline configuration. These bands must also be distinguished from normal genetic polymorphisms, which are also represented by discrete bands on Southern blot analysis. Southern blotting is reliable for the detection of clonal populations consisting of > 5 percent. Southern blotting has the advantage of being able to screen more effectively for chromosomal abnormalities where the translocation breakpoint has the possibility of lying anywhere within a wide span of DNA since, unlike PCR, the DNA sequence of regions flanking the breakpoints does not need to be known. Thus, for example, Southern blot analysis detects cases of 11q23 abnormalities that are difficult to detect using PCR because the breakpoints vary in location, necessitating the use of patient-specific rather than translocation-specific primers. The test is fairly tedious; most laboratories therefore batch samples, with a turnaround time of 2 to 3 weeks.

In contrast, PCR techniques have been successfully automated, and many laboratories are able to provide results in a few days. For an overview of the use of PCR in the diagnosis and monitoring of leukemias, see Chapter 6.

New Approaches to the Classification of Adult Leukemias

With recognition of the limited role of morphologic analysis in predicting clinical outcomes, newer classification systems are beginning to incorporate data from cytogenetic, molecular, and immunophenotyping studies in the initial evaluation of adult leukemias. The newer approaches also attempt to interpret pathologic data in the context of clinical information, yielding a composite diagnosis based

Table 3–7. WHO PROPOSALS FOR RECLASSIFIATION OF ACUTE LEUKEMIAS

Disease Group	Recommendation
AML and MDS	Define AML by blast count ≥ 20%; eliminate RAEB-t Recognize specific categories: AML with t(8;21) APL t(15;17) and variants AML with inv/t(16)(p13) AML with 11q23 breaks Consider multilineage dysplasia, history of MDS, or history of prior alkylating agent/topoisomerase II inhibitor therapy in classification Include cytogenetic information for prognostication within groups Retain MDS with multilineage dysplasia as distinct group
Lymphoid neoplasms	Eliminate FAB terms L1, L2, L3 Merge ALL and acute lymphoblastic lymphomas, retain "leukemia" Include cytogenetic information for prognostication within groups t(9:22), t(1;19), t(12;21), 11q23 abnormalities

on all that is known about specific disease entities. For example, by combining clinical, morphologic, and cytogenetic data for patients with MDS, a prognostic index, the International Prognostic Scoring System, has been devised that is more predictive of leukemic progression and overall survival than is provided by morphologic classification.[31,32] In a similar approach, authors of the Revised European and American Lymphoma System have proposed a classification for lymphoid neoplasms based on the integration of all known clinical, morphologic, phenotypic, and genetic features of disease entities.[33] The recent WHO proposals (Table 3–7) represent an attempt to extend this to nonlymphoid hematopoietic malignancies.[34] It is likely that such classification systems, based more fully on biologic correlates of disease rather than morphologic studies alone, will find increasing use among scientists and physicians seeking more innovative preventive and curative options for these challenging diseases.

REFERENCES

1. Greenlee RT, Hill-Harmon MB, Murray T, Thun M. Cancer statistics, 2001. CA Cancer J Clin 2001; 51:15–36.
2. Novik Y, Marino P, Makower DF, Wiernik PH. Familial erythroleukemia: a distinct clinical and genetic type

of familial leukemias. Leuk Lymphoma 1998; 30:395–401.

3. Lee EJ, Schiffer CA, Misawa S, Testa JR. Clinical and cytogenetic features of familial erythroleukaemia. Br J Haematol 1987;65:313–20.

4. Yuille MR, Houlston RS, Catovsky D. Anticipation in familial chronic lymphocytic leukaemia. Leukemia 1998;12:1696–8.

5. Perez-Encinas M, Bello JL, Perez-Crespo S, et al. Familial myeloproliferative syndrome. Am J Hematol 1994;46:225–9.

6. Lichtman MA. The relationship of excessive white cell accumulation to vascular insufficiency in patients with leukemia. Kroc Found Ser 1984;16:295–306.

7. Bennett JM, Catovsky D, Daniel MT, et al. Proposals for the classification of the acute leukaemias. French-American-British (FAB) Co-operative Group. Br J Haematol 1976;33:451–8.

8. Bennett JM, Catovsky D, Daniel MT, et al. Proposed revised criteria for the classification of acute myeloid leukemia. A report of the French-American-British Cooperative Group. Ann Intern Med 1985;103:620–5.

9. Byrd JC, Dodge RK, Carroll A, et al. Patients with t(8;21)(q22;q22) and acute myeloid leukemia have superior failure-free and overall survival when repetitive cycles of high-dose cytarabine are administered. J Clin Oncol 1999;17:3767–75.

10. Tallman MS. Therapy of acute promyelocytic leukemia: all-trans retinoic acid and beyond. Leukemia 1998; 12(Suppl 1):S37–40.

11. Dalton WT Jr, Ahearn MJ, Cork A, et al. Acute myelomonocytic leukemia associated with abnormalities of chromosome 16: a light and electron microscopic study. Hematol Pathol 1987;1:105–12.

12. Larson RA, Williams SF, Le Beau MM, Bitter MA, et al. Acute myelomonocytic leukemia with abnormal eosinophils and inv(16) or t(16;16) has a favorable prognosis. Blood 1986;68:1242–9.

13. Davey FR, Abraham N Jr, Brunetto VL, et al. Morphologic characteristics of erythroleukemia (acute myeloid leukemia; FAB-M6): a CALGB study. Am J Hematol 1995;49:29–38.

14. Mazzella FM, Kowal-Vern A, Shrit MA, et al. Acute erythroleukemia: evaluation of 48 cases with reference to classification, cell proliferation, cytogenetics, and prognosis. Am J Clin Pathol 1998;110:590–8.

15. Mertelsmann R, Tzvi Thaler H, To L, et al. Morphological classification, response to therapy, and survival in 263 adult patients with acute nonlymphoblastic leukemia. Blood 1980;56:773–81.

16. Sultan C, Deregnaucourt J, Ko YW, et al. Distribution of 250 cases of acute myeloid leukaemia (AML) according to the FAB classification and response to therapy. Br J Haematol 1981;47:545–51.

17. van't Veer MB. The diagnosis of acute leukemia with undifferentiated or minimally differentiated blasts. Ann Hematol 1992;64:161–5.

18. Nagai K, Kohno T, Chen YX, et al. Diagnostic criteria for hypocellular acute leukemia: a clinical entity distinct from overt acute leukemia and myelodysplastic syndrome. Leuk Res 1996;20:563–74.

19. Tuzuner N, Cox C, Rowe JM, et al. Hypocellular myelodysplastic syndromes (MDS): new proposals. Br J Haematol 1995;91:612–7.

20. Bennett JM, Catovsky D, Daniel MT, et al. Proposals for the classification of the myelodysplastic syndromes. Br J Haematol 1982;51:189–99.

21. Vallespi T, Imbert M, Mecucci C, et al. Diagnosis, classification, and cytogenetics of myelodysplastic syndromes. Haematologica 1998;83:258–75.

22. Stass SA, Pui CH, Melvin S, et al. Sudan black B positive acute lymphoblastic leukaemia. Br J Haematol 1984;57:413–21.

23. Bennett JM, Catovsky D, Daniel MT, et al. The morphological classification of acute lymphoblastic leukaemia: concordance among observers and clinical correlations. Br J Haematol 1981;47:553–61.

24. Michiels JJ. Diagnostic criteria of the myeloproliferative disorders (MPD): essential thrombocythaemia, polycythaemia vera and chronic megakaryocytic granulocytic metaplasia. Neth J Med 1997;51:57–64.

25. You W, Weisbrot IM. Chronic neutrophilic leukemia. Report of two cases and review of the literature. Am J Clin Pathol 1979;72:233–42.

26. Mauro FR, De Rossi G, Burgio VL, et al. Prognostic value of bone marrow histology in chronic lymphocytic leukemia. A study of 335 untreated cases from a single institution. Haematologica 1994;79:334–41.

27. Montserrat E, Villamor N, Reverter JC, et al. Bone marrow assessment in B-cell chronic lymphocytic leukaemia: aspirate or biopsy? A comparative study in 258 patients. Br J Haematol 1996;93:111–6.

28. Drexler HG. Classification of acute myeloid leukemias —a comparison of FAB and immunophenotyping. Leukemia 1987;1:697–705.

29. Cheson BD, Bennett JM, Rai KR, et al. Guidelines for clinical protocols for chronic lymphocytic leukemia: recommendations of the National Cancer Institute-sponsored working group. Am J Hematol 1988;29: 152–63.

30. Rowley JD. The critical role of chromosome transloca-

tions in human leukemias. Annu Rev Genet 1998; 32:495–519.

31. Maes B, Meeus P, Michaux L, et al. Application of the International Prognostic Scoring System for myelodysplastic syndromes. Ann Oncol 1999;10: 825–9.

32. Greenberg PL. Risk factors and their relationship to prognosis in myelodysplastic syndromes. Leuk Res 1998;22(Suppl 1):S3–6.

33. Jaffe ES, Krenacs L, Raffeld M. Classification of T-cell and NK-cell neoplasms based on the REAL classification. Ann Oncol 1997;8:17–24.

34. Harris NL, Jaffe ES, Diebold J, et al. The World Health Organization classification of hematological malignancies report of the Clinical Advisory Committee Meeting, Airlie House, Virginia, November 1997. Mod Pathol 2000;13:193–207.

4

Morphology of Adult Acute and Chronic Leukemias

M. KATHRYN FOUCAR, MD

The morphologic assessment of blood and bone marrow is a critical step in the diagnosis of adult acute and chronic leukemias. However, morphology alone is seldom the diagnostic "endpoint." Rather, the final diagnosis of an adult leukemia represents the synthesis of clinical, morphologic, immunophenotypic, and often genetic information that conveys not only diagnostic but prognostic information to guide clinical decision making. This chapter will review acute and chronic leukemias that affect adult patients with an emphasis on morphology, including both cytologic features of individual cells, morphologic features on bone marrow sections, and abnormalities, if any, in overall bone marrow architecture. General strategies will be presented to identify distinct clinicopathologic entities within the broad group of myeloid and lymphoid neoplasms.

For blood and bone marrow, morphologic review is an essential component in such basic diagnostic decisions as benign versus malignant. If malignant, morphology guides subsequent decisions such as acute versus chronic and myeloid versus lymphoid. This sequential systematic process should ultimately result in the delineation of distinct clinical pathologic entities that are segregated into standard classification systems. The two most commonly used classifications systems for adult acute leukemias are the French-American-British (FAB) and the newly proposed World Health Organization (WHO) classifications of B, T, and myeloid disorders (Tables 4–1 to 4–5).[1,2] The FAB classification system of acute leukemias as acute myelogenous leukemia (AML) M0 through AML M7 is based primarily on morphol-

ogy and cytochemistry with minimal immunophenotyping.[1,3,4] The FAB classification of acute lymphoblastic leukemias (ALLs) is also morphology based, delineating cases as ALL L1, ALL L2, and ALL L3. The FAB classification of chronic B and T leukemias focuses primarily on those disorders that involve peripheral blood and bone marrow (ie, predominantly leukemic process).[5] Similar to other FAB

Table 4–1. FRENCH-AMERICAN-BRITISH (FAB) CLASSIFICATION OF ACUTE AND CHRONIC LEUKEMIAS	
Acute myelogenous leukemia	**Acute lymphoblastic leukemia**
M0	L1
M1	L2
M2	L3
M3	
M3m	**B-Chronic Leukemias**
M4	CLL—common
M4eos	CLL—mixed
M5a, b	Prolymphocytic leukemia
M6a, b (proposed)	Hairy cell leukemia
M7	Hairy cell leukemia, variant
Other subtypes proposed	SLVL
	Leukemic phase of NHL
Chronic myelogenous leukemia	Lymphoplasmacytic lymphoma
Chronic, accelerated, and	Plasma cell leukemia
blast crisis phases	
Myelodysplastic syndromes	
Refracting anemia	**T-Chronic Leukemias**
Refractory anemia with ring	T-cell lymphocytosis
sideroblasts	T-prolymphocytic leukemia
RAEB	Adult T-cell leukemia/
Chronic myelomonocytic	lymphoma
leukemia	Sézary syndrome
RAEB in transformation	

CLL = chronic lymphocytic leukemia; SLVL = splenic lymphoma with villous lymphocytes; NHL = non-Hodgkin's lymphoma; RAEB = refractory anemia with excess blasts.
From Bennett et al.[1,3,5]

classification systems, the classification of chronic lymphoid leukemias uses limited immunophenotypic data, whereas morphologic features are emphasized.

The newly proposed WHO classification of lymphoid, natural killer (NK), and myeloid disorders is based on the systematic delineation of distinct clinical pathologic entities following a sequential process of first determining lineage and then stage of maturation of lymphoid and myeloid disorders.[2] Both leukemias and lymphomas are integrated into a single classification system reflecting the interrelationship between these processes (see Table 4–2). By convention, the distinction between a disorder designated as a leukemia and one designated as a lymphoma is often based on an arbitrary percentage of neoplastic cells within either bone marrow or peripheral blood, whereas other parameters, such as morphology, immunophenotype, and genotype, are identical. For example, chronic lymphocytic leukemia (CLL) and small lymphocytic lymphoma of B-cell type are derived from the same normal counterpart cell and differ only in disease distribution.[2] In the WHO classification system, the ALLs are designated as either precursor B-cell or precursor T-cell neoplasms, whereas the chronic B- and T-cell leukemias are admixed with numerous subtypes of peripheral B, T, and NK neoplasms (see Table 4–2). Those peripheral (mature) B- and T-cell neoplasms within the WHO classification system that are predominantly disseminated (ie, leukemic disorders) are listed in Table 4–3. Discussion in this chapter will focus on this more restricted compilation of chronic leukemic disorders. Finally, the acute and chronic myeloid disorders are segregated by WHO criteria into acute myeloid leukemias, myeloproliferative disorders, myelodysplastic/myeloproliferative diseases, and myelodysplastic syndromes (see Tables 4–4 and 4–5).[2] This chapter will emphasize those myeloid disorders that exhibit a leukemic blood picture (ie, leukocytosis with variable abnormalities of other lineages).

TABLE 4–2. PROPOSED WHO CLASSIFICATION OF LYMPHOID NEOPLASMS

B-cell neoplasms
 Precursor B-cell neoplasm
  Precursor B-lymphoblastic leukemia/lymphoma (precursor B-cell acute lymphoblastic leukemia)
 Mature (peripheral) B-cell neoplasms
  B-cell chronic lymphocytic leukemia/small lymphocytic lymphoma
  B-cell prolymphocytic leukemia
  Lymphoplasmacytic lymphoma
  Splenic marginal zone B-cell lymphoma (± villous lymphocytes)
  Hairy cell leukemia
  Plasma cell myeloma/plasmacytoma
  Extranodal marginal zone B-cell lymphoma of MALT type
  Nodal marginal zone B-cell lymphoma
  Follicular lymphoma
  Mantle-cell lymphoma
  Diffuse large B-cell lymphoma (two subtypes)
  Burkitt's lymphoma/Burkitt's cell leukemia

T-cell and NK cell neoplasms
 Precursor T-cell neoplasm
  Precursor T-lymphoblastic lymphoma/leukemia (precursor T-cell acute lymphoblastic leukemia)
 Mature (peripheral) T-cell neoplasms
  T-cell prolymphocytic leukemia
  T-cell granular lymphocytic leukemia
  Aggressive NK cell leukemia
  Adult T-cell lymphoma/leukemia (HTLV-1+)
  Extranodal NK/T-cell lymphoma, nasal type
  Enteropathy-type T-cell lymphoma
  Hepatosplenic gamma-delta T-cell lymphoma
  Subcutaneous panniculitis-like T-cell lymphoma
  Mycosis fungoides/Sézary syndrome
  Anaplastic large-cell lymphoma, T/null cell, primary cutaneous type
  Peripheral T-cell lymphoma, not otherwise characterized
  Angioimmunoblastic T-cell lymphoma
  Anaplastic large-cell lymphoma, T/null cell, primary systemic type

From Harris et al.[2]

APPROACH TO ACUTE AND CHRONIC LEUKEMIAS

There is a fundamental difference in the approach to disorders in which blasts predominate versus chronic leukemias in which either mature lymphoid or myeloid cells are abundant in blood and bone marrow. In acute leukemia, major diagnostic challenges include the determination of blast lineage and the exclusion of blastic look-alike disorders such as blastic mantle cell lymphoma. Morphology alone is not sufficient to distinguish all cases of ALL from AML. For lymphoid blasts, immunophenotype is essential in defining B-, T-, or NK cell lineage and stage of maturation. For AML, all types of immature myeloid elements must be successfully delineated to determine the number of lineages involved and to assess for evidence of maturation. Cytochemical stains are generally required to confirm lineage, whereas immunophenotyping and especially genetic assessment are needed to confirm many distinct

Table 4–3. DISSEMINATED/LEUKEMIC MATURE B- AND T-CELL DISORDERS (WHO)
B-cell neoplasms
B-cell CLL/SLL
Variant: with monoclonal gammopathy/plasmacytoid
differentiation
B-prolymphocytic leukemia
Hairy cell leukemia
Variant: hairy cell leukemia variant
Splenic lymphoma with villous lymphocytes
T-cell neoplasms
T-cell prolymphocytic leukemia, morphologic variants
Small cell
Cerebriform cell
Adult T-cell leukemia/lymphoma
T-cell granular lymphocytic leukemia
Sézary syndrome (mycosis fungoides)

From Harris et al.[2]

AML clinical subtypes. Indeed, current standard of practice includes the performance of cytogenetic/ molecular evaluation on all acute leukemias, whereas flow cytometric immunophenotyping is essential for diagnosis of all cases of ALL and many, but not all, cases of AML.

Table 4–4. PROPOSED WHO CLASSIFICATION OF ACUTE MYELOID LEUKEMIAS*
I. **Acute myeloid leukemias (AML) with recurrent cytogenetic translocations**
AML with t(8;21)(q22;q22), *AML1(CBFα)/ETO*
APL with t(15;17)(q22;q11-12) and variants, *PML/RARα*
AML with abnormal bone marrow eosinophils with
inv(16)(p13q22) or t(16;16)(p13;q11), *CBFβ/MYH11*
AML with 11q23 (*MLL*) abnormalities
II. **Acute myeloid leukemia with multilineage dysplasia**
With prior myelodysplastic syndrome
Without prior myelodysplastic syndrome
III. **Acute myeloid leukemia and myelodysplastic syndrome, therapy related**
Alkylating agent related
Epipodophyllotoxin related (some may be lymphoid)
Other types
IV. **Acute myeloid leukemia not otherwise specified**
AML minimally differentiated
AML without maturation
AML with maturation
AML with monocytic differentiation
Acute monocytic leukemia
Acute erythroid leukemia
Acute megakaryocytic leukemia
Acute basophilic leukemia
Acute panmyelosis with myelofibrosis

*Diagnosis of acute leukemia based on 20 percent blasts in blood or bone marrow; classification in progress.
APL = acute promyelocytic leukemia.
Data from Harris et al.[2]

In chronic leukemias, the morphologic distinction between a chronic myeloid versus a chronic lymphoid leukemia is virtually never a challenge. The various mature lymphoid and myeloid cells can be readily identified by review of the cytologic features on peripheral blood or bone marrow aspirate smears. Instead, the distinction between an atypical yet non-neoplastic process and a true clonal mature lymphoid or myeloid neoplasm is often the differential diagnostic challenge. For lymphocytic proliferations, flow cytometric immunophenotyping with selected molecular analyses for B- or T-cell clonality generally resolves problematic cases, whereas cytogenetic/molecular techniques are typically the preferred modality to distinguish atypical non-neoplastic myeloid disorders from the various clonal myeloproliferative and myelodysplastic processes. However, these specialized modalities do not resolve all cases.

IDENTIFICATION OF BLASTS AND OTHER IMMATURE ELEMENTS

The successful identification of various types of lymphoblasts, myeloid blasts, and other immature myeloid cells is essential in the diagnosis of acute leukemias (Table 4–6). Lymphoblasts must be distin-

Table 4–5. PROPOSED WHO CLASSIFICATION OF CHRONIC MYELOID NEOPLASMS*
Myeloproliferative diseases
Chronic myelogenous leukemia, Philadelphia chromosome
positive [(t(9;22)(q34;q11), *BCR/ABL*)]
Chronic neutrophilic leukemia
Chronic eosinophilic leukemia/hypereosinophilic syndrome
Chronic idiopathic myelofibrosis
Polycythemia vera
Essential thrombocythemia
Myeloproliferative disease, unclassifiable
Myelodysplastic/myeloproliferative diseases
Chronic myelomonocytic leukemia
Atypical chronic myelogenous leukemia
Juvenile myelomonocytic leukemia
Myelodysplastic syndromes
Refractory anemia
With ringed sideroblasts
Without ringed sideroblasts
Refractory cytopenia (myelodysplastic syndrome) with
multilineage dysplasia
Refractory anemia (myelodysplastic syndrome) with excess blasts
5q– syndrome
Myelodysplastic syndrome, unclassifiable

From Harris et al.[2]
*Classification in progress.

guished from the "family" of immature myeloid elements that includes myeloblasts, promyelocytes, monoblasts, promonocytes, erythroblasts, and megakaryoblasts.[6] For all cells categorized as "blasts," the key nuclear feature is dispersed, fine (ie, blastic) nuclear chromatin, whereas other nuclear features such as size, nuclear contours, and presence or absence of nucleoli vary by cell type (Figure 4–1). However, the diagnostician must be aware that some degree of chromatin condensation is still compatible with the designation "blast." In the author's experience, nuclear chromatin condensation is sometimes more prevalent in circulating blasts compared with those within the bone marrow in the same patient.

Several morphologic subtypes of lymphoblasts have been delineated; the FAB classification describes the types (L1, L2, L3), whereas the WHO recognizes two types (common and Burkitt's leukemia/lymphoma, a mature B-cell neoplasm that has by FAB convention been included within ALL).[1,2] Common-type (FAB L1, L2) lymphoblasts are characterized by a variably high nuclear to cytoplasmic ratio, finely dispersed nuclear chromatin, subtle convoluted nuclear contours, and variably prominent nucleoli. The FAB criteria distinguish L1 and L2 lymphoblasts by the greater amount of cytoplasm and more prominent nucleoli of L2 lymphoblasts, whereas the WHO lumps together these two types of

Table 4–6. MORPHOLOGIC FEATURES OF BLASTS AND OTHER IMMATURE CELLS

Type of Cell	Key Morphologic Features	Cytochemistry	Immunophenotypic Features
Lymphoblast (common type)	Moderately sized cells with generally finely dispersed chromatin and subtle nuclear convolutions Variable amounts of cytoplasm Variable prominence of nucleoli	PAS+	Precursor B and T subtypes
Burkitt's leukemia/ lymphoma	Moderate- to large-sized cells with round nuclear contours, moderately dispersed chromatin and generally inconspicuous nucleoli Moderate deeply basophilic and highly vacuolated cytoplasm	ORO+	Mature B cell
Myeloblast	Large nucleus with finely dispersed chromatin and variably prominent nucleoli Relatively high nuclear:cytoplasmic ratio with variable number of granules	SBB+, MPO+	HLA-DR, CD33, CD13, anti-MPO, CD34
Promyelocyte	Nuclear chromatin slightly condensed; nucleoli variably prominent; nucleus often eccentric and Golgi zone may be apparent Numerous cytoplasmic granules are more dispersed throughout cytoplasm; intense granularity in APL, common type	SBB+, MPO+	CD33, CD13, anti-MPO
Monoblast	Moderate to low nuclear:cytoplasmic ratio, nuclear chromatin finely dispersed with variably prominent nucleoli; nuclei round to folded Abundant, slightly basophilic cytoplasm containing fine granulation and occasional vacuoles	NSE+	HLA-DR, CD33, CD13, vCD14, CD4
Promonocyte	Slightly condensed nuclear chromatin; variably prominent nucleoli Abundant, finely granular blue/gray cytoplasm that may be vacuolated Very monocytic appearance with nuclear immaturity	NSE+	HLA-DR, CD33, CD13, CD14, CD4
Erythroblast	Relatively high nuclear:cytoplasmic ratio Nucleus round with slightly condensed chromatin; nucleoli variably prominent Moderate amounts of deeply basophilic cytoplasm that may be vacuolated	PAS+	Glycophorin A, hemoglobin A
Megakaryoblast	Highly variable morphologic features Often not recognizable without special studies May be lymphoid-appearing with high nuclear:cytoplasmic ratio Nuclear chromatin fine to variably condensed Cytoplasm may be scant to moderate, usually agranular or contain a few granules; blebbing or budding of cytoplasm may be evident Blasts may form cohesive clumps	PAS+	CD41, CD61, HLA-DR, v Factor VIII

PAS = Periodic acid–Schiff; ORO = Oil red O; SBB = Sudan black B; MPO = myeloperoxidase; APL = acute promyelocytic leukemia; NSE = nonspecific esterase; v = variable expression.
From Bennett et al.,[1,3,4] Foucar,[6] and Brunning and McKenna.[8]

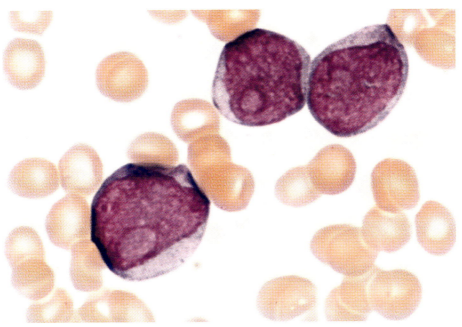

Figure 4–1. Several circulating blasts are evident in this peripheral blood smear from a patient with acute leukemia. Note finely dispersed nuclear chromatin and variably prominent nucleoli. Wright's stain (original magnification ×1,200).

lymphoblasts (Figures 4–2 and 4–3). These common-type lymphoblasts often have distinct cytoplasmic globules of periodic acid–Schiff (PAS)-positive material (Figure 4–4). Immunophenotyping studies, usually multicolor flow cytometric analyses, are required to determine B-, T-, or NK cell lineage and stage of maturation in ALL; leukemias generally parallel normal B- and T-cell stage of maturation, but aberrations and dysynchronous patterns of antigen expression are common (Table 4–7) (see Chapter 5).

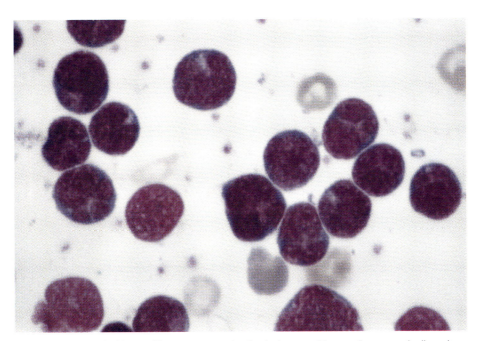

Figure 4–2. Lymphoblasts with scanty amounts of cytoplasm and inconspicuous nucleoli predominate in this bone marrow aspirate smear from a patient with acute lymphoblastic leukemia of FAB L1 type. Wright's stain (original magnification ×1,000).

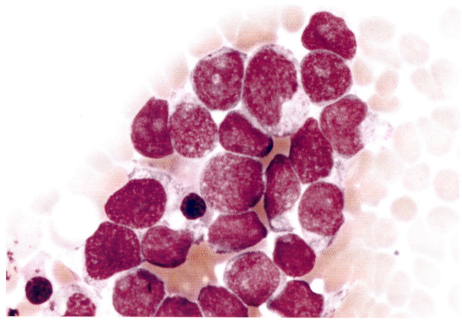

Figure 4–3. Lymphoblasts are more heterogeneous in this bone marrow aspirate smear from a patient with acute lymphoblastic leukemia FAB L2 type. Note more abundant amounts of cytoplasm and more conspicuous nucleoli. Wright's stain (original magnification ×1,000).

Although included by FAB convention within ALL, the Burkitt's leukemia/lymphoma cell or FAB ALL L3 lymphoblast is both morphologically distinctive and immunophenotypically mature.[7] These cells have round nuclear contours, variably dispersed nuclear chromatin with one to three incon-spicuous nucleoli, and moderate amounts of deeply basophilic and highly vacuolated cytoplasm (Figure 4–5). A starry sky pattern is often noted on bone marrow biopsy sections in these cases (see Figure 4–5). By cytochemical staining, the cytoplasmic vacuoles are lipid rich. Immunophenotyping reveals

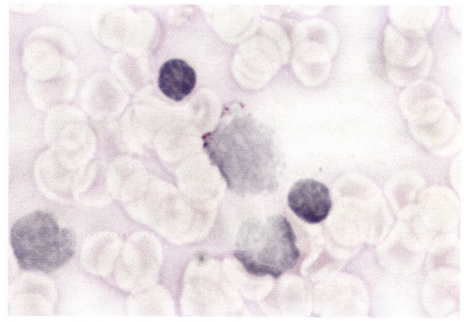

Figure 4–4. Globules of periodic acid–Schiff-positive material are present within the scanty cytoplasm in this case of acute lymphoblastic leukemia. Periodic acid–Schiff stain (original magnification ×1,000).

Table 4–7. NORMAL B AND T CELL MATURATION						
B-Cell Precursor Stages				**Pre-B Cell**	**Mature B Cell**	**Plasma Cell**
TdT	TdT	TdT	vTdT	vTdT	HLA-DR	CIg
HLA-DR	HLA-DR	HLA-DR	HLA-DR	HLA-DR	CD19	CD38
CD34	CD34	vCD34	CD19	CD19	CD20	vCD79a
CD79a	CD19	CD19	CD10	CD10	SIg	vCD20
vCD45	vCD10	CD10	CD20	CD20	CD22	vCD45
	cCD22	CD22	CD22	Cmu	CD79a	
	CD79a	CD79a	CD79a	CD22	CD79b	
	wCD45	wCD45	wCD45	CD79a	CD45	
				CD45		

T-Cell Precursors in Bone Marrow*		**Thymic Maturation Stages**				**Mature T Cell**
CD34	CD34	CD34	CD2	CD2		CD2
CD2	CD2	CD2	CD5	CD5		CD5
CD5	CD5	CD5	CD7	CD7		CD7
CD7	CD7	CD7	cCD3	CD3		CD3
CD38	CD38	CD38	CD1	CD1		CD4 or CD8
TdT	cCD3	cCD3	CD4,8	CD4,8		CD45
vCD3	TdT	CD1	CD45	CD45		
vcCD1	vCD1	CD4,8				
wCD45	wCD45	vTdT				
		CD4				
		wCD45				

*Represent 1 percent of CD34+ cells in pediatric bone marrow specimens.
From Dayton,[7] Brunning and McKenna,[8] and Foucar.[74]
TdT = terminal deoxynucleotidyl transferase; v = variable expression; CIg = cytoplasmic immunoglobulin; SIg= surface immunoglobulin; c = cytoplasmic expression; w = weak expression.

monoclonal surface light-chain expression, whereas markers of immaturity such as CD34 and terminal deoxynucleotidyl transferase (TdT) are generally absent (see Tables 4–6 and 4–7).

The morphologic classification of AML is more complex and problematic than ALL classification. A greater number of immature myeloid elements must be successfully identified in AML cases, paralleling normal multilineage myeloid hematopoiesis (see Table 4–6). In AML, either a single immature population may predominate or multilineage maturation may be appreciated, likely reflecting the stem cell versus committed progenitor cell of origin of the leukemic clone. The prototypic myeloblast has dispersed nuclear chromatin, variably prominent nucleoli, a variable nuclear configuration, and generally

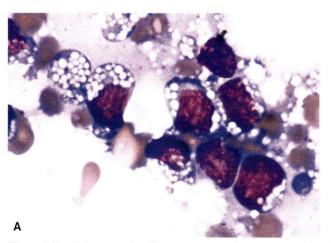
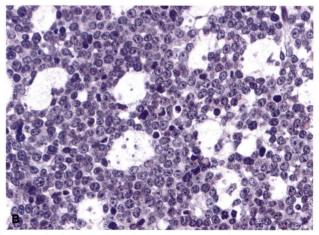

Figure 4–5. This composite of bone marrow aspirate smear and core biopsy section from a patient with Burkitt's leukemia (ALL L3) shows the typical cytologic features and starry sky pattern that is characteristic of this malignancy. Wright's (original magnification ×1,000) and hematoxylin and eosin stains (original magnification ×400). (Reproduced with permission from Foucar[75].)

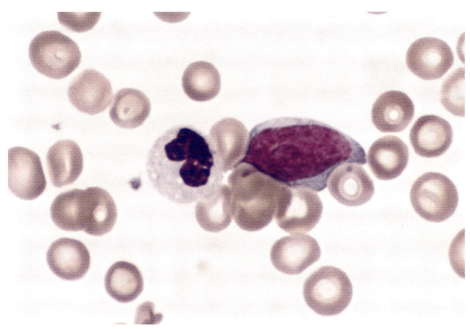

Figure 4–6. This peripheral blood smear from a patient with AML shows a circulating blast with dispersed chromatin, inconspicuous nucleoli, and moderate amounts of agranular cytoplasm. Wright's stain (original magnification ×1,200).

moderate amounts of agranular to minimally granular cytoplasm (Figure 4–6).[6,8,9] Myeloid maturation is obvious if Auer rods are appreciated, although either cytochemical stains or immunophenotype is generally required to confirm lineage (Figure 4–7). Immunophenotypic evidence of myeloid lineage includes pan myeloid antigen expression (CD13, CD33, cytoplasmic myeloperoxidase), whereas CD34 expression indicating immaturity is present on some but not all myeloblasts.

Maturation to the promyelocyte state is characterized by greater nuclear condensation, a paranuclear "hof" or Golgi zone, and greater numbers of more widely distributed cytoplasmic granules (Figure 4–8). Leukemic promyelocytes, especially those in acute promyelocytic leukemia, are often intensely granulated (Figure 4–9). These leukemic promyelocytes are characteristically intensely Sudan black B or myeloperoxidase positive and lack both human leukocyte antigen (HLA)-DR

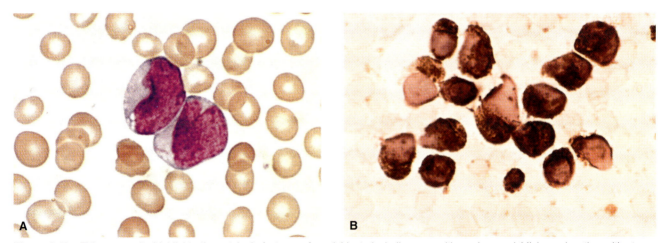

Figure 4–7. This composite highlights the cytologic features of myeloblasts including one with an Auer rod (*A*) in conjunction with strong cytoplasmic Sudan black B positivity (*B*) in this case of AML. Wright's (original magnification ×1,000) and Sudan black B stains (original magnification ×800).

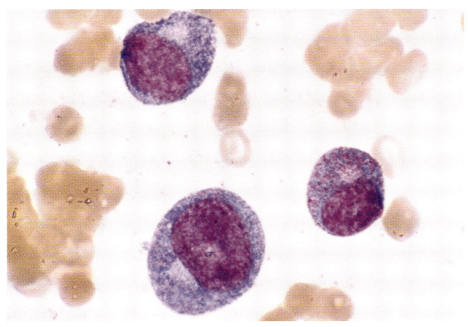

Figure 4–8. Benign promyelocytes are illustrated in this bone marrow aspirate smear. Note eccentric nucleus, prominent hof, and dispersed cytoplasmic granules. Wright's stain (original magnification ×1,200).

and CD34 expression reflecting maturation (see Figure 4–9)[6,9,10]

The hallmark of a monoblast is abundant, finely granulated cytoplasm that is diffusely nonspecific esterase positive by cytochemical stains (Figures 4–10 and 4–11).[6,8,9] The nucleus of monoblasts is characteristically round, whereas greater nuclear folding typifies maturation to a promonocyte. Monoblasts/promonocytes characteristically express HLA-DR and pan myeloid antigens, whereas CD34 is usually absent.

Like Burkitt's leukemia/lymphoma cells, erythroblasts are also characterized by round nuclear contours and moderate amounts of deeply basophilic, vacuolated cytoplasm (Figure 4–12) (see Table 4–6). However, these cells exhibit beaded or globular PAS positivity and can be delineated by either morphologically obvious maturation to more mature erythroid elements or hemoglobin A/glycophorin positivity by immunologic studies (Figure 4–13).[6]

Megakaryoblasts are often difficult to identify morphologically, especially if little maturation to

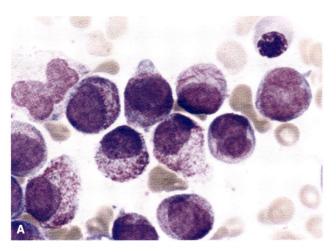
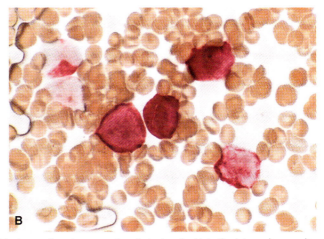

Figure 4–9. This composite illustrates the cytologic and cytochemical features of acute promyelocytic leukemia. Note the intensely granular cytoplasm (*A*), which is strongly positive by specific esterase positivity (*B*). Wright's and specific esterase stains (original magnification ×800).

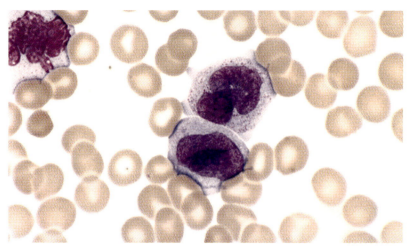

Figure 4–10. This peripheral blood smear from a patient with acute monocytic leukemia illustrates both a monoblast (lower cell) and a promonocyte (upper cell). Note dispersed chromatin and abundant amounts of cytoplasm. Wright's stain (original magnification ×800).

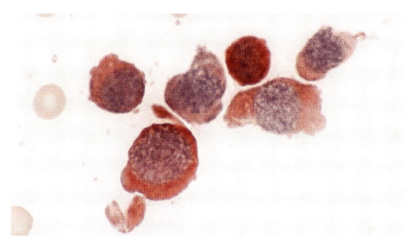

Figure 4–11. The majority of leukemic cells in this bone marrow aspirate smear are strongly nonspecific esterase positive in this case of acute monocytic leukemia. Nonspecific esterase stain (original magnification ×100).

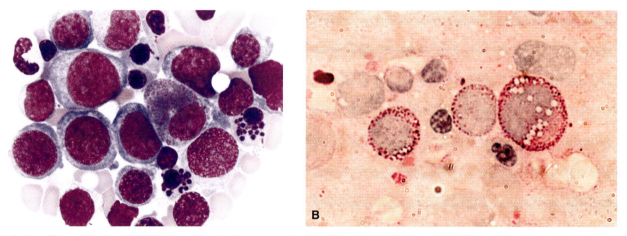

Figure 4–12. This composite highlights the cytologic (*A*) and cytochemical (*B*) features of acute erythroid leukemia. Note striking karyorrhexis of developing erythroid elements (*A*). Globules and diffuse periodic acid–Schiff (PAS) positivity is noted in these neoplastic erythroid elements (*B*). Wright's and PAS stains (original magnification ×800).

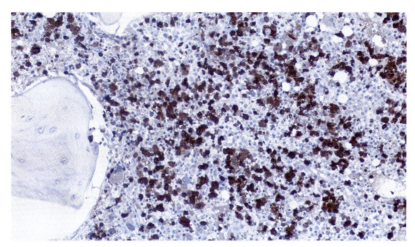

Figure 4–13. This hemoglobin A immunoperoxidase stain shows loss of normal colony formation in this bone marrow biopsy section from a patient with high-grade myelodysplasia/acute erythroid leukemia. Note predominance of individual large hemoglobin A-positive cells. Immunoperoxidase for hemoglobin A stain (original magnification ×400).

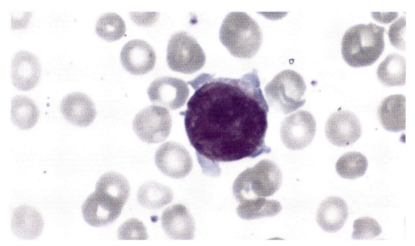

Figure 4–14. A circulating megakaryoblast is evident in this peripheral blood smear. Note cytoplasmic blebbing. Wright's stain (original magnification ×1,200).

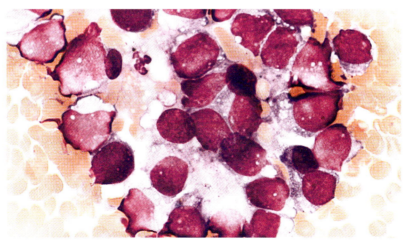

Figure 4–15. Clumped megakaryoblasts mimicking metastatic tumor are evident on this bone marrow aspirate smear from a patient with acute megakaryoblastic leukemia. Wright's stain (original magnification ×800). (Reproduced with permission from Foucar[6].)

more mature forms is evident. Megakaryoblasts range in appearance from lymphoblast-like cells with scant cytoplasm to clumped cells that resemble metastatic processes (Figures 4–14 and 4–15) (see Table 4–6).[6,11] Although cytoplasmic blebbing is a morphologic clue for megakaryoblasts, in the author's experience, blebbing is common in many other types of blasts and is therefore nonspecific. Immunophenotyping for expression of CD41 or CD61 is generally required to confirm the maturation of megakaryoblasts in a leukemic process (Figure 4–16)[4,12]

APPROACH TO ACUTE AND CHRONIC MYELOID DISORDERS

Microscopic Anatomy of Bone Marrow

To recognize and classify myeloid neoplasms, an understanding of the basic architecture and localization patterns in normal bone marrow is essential. Analogous to the immunoarchitecture of lymph node, the bone marrow is also organized into microenvironmental niches that support the various hematopoietic lineages.[13] Even though hematopoiesis may appear completely haphazard on aspirate smears and biopsy sections, microenvironmental niches of granulocytic, erythroid, and megakaryocyte precursors have been well defined. Alteration in this normal architecture is a feature of many myeloid neoplasms, especially more high-grade disorders.

The most immature granulocytic elements normally reside adjacent to bony trabeculae or around small-caliber blood vessels.[13,14] This localization pattern can be highlighted by immunoperoxidase staining for myeloperoxidase (Figure 4–17). Even though this microniche localization typifies normal granulopoiesis, CD34 staining for blasts on normal bone marrow sections tends to reveal very low numbers of apparently randomly distributed, individually dispersed, positive cells that do not segregate to paratrabecular or perivascular areas. Depending on patient age, fewer than one CD34-positive cell per high-power field is physiologic (personal observation).

Erythropoiesis is characterized by well-delineated colony formation; these colonies are apparently randomly distributed and do not localize to paratrabecular regions.[15] Erythropoiesis can be highlighted by immunoperoxidase staining for hemoglobin A (Figure 4–18). Colonies become confluent in both non-neoplastic and neoplastic disorders associated with marked erythroid hyperplasia. However, in the author's experience, the identification of a prominent pattern of poor colony formation with individually dispersed hemoglobin A-positive cells is more commonly encountered in neoplastic processes, especially myelodysplasia.[16]

Megakaryocyte maturation occurs by a process of endomitosis characterized by successive deoxyribonucleic acid (DNA) synthesis with nuclear lobulation without actual mitoses.[17] Consequently, these multilobulated megakaryocytes have an increased DNA content. Although the distribution of megakaryocytes appears random on bone marrow biopsy

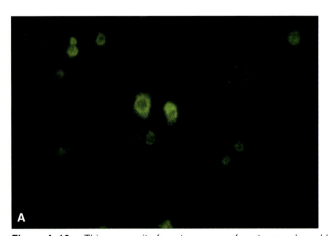
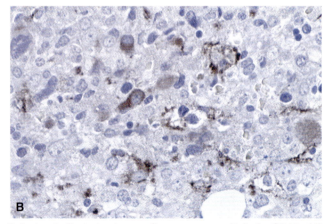

Figure 4–16. This composite from two cases of acute megakaryoblastic leukemia illustrates immunofluorescence positivity for CD41a (*A*) and immunoperoxidase positivity for factor VIII (*B*). Immunofluorescence for CD41a and immunoperoxidase for factor VIII stains (original magnification ×900).

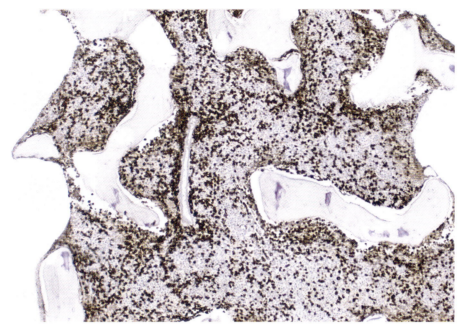

Figure 4–17. Immunoperoxidase staining for myeloperoxidase shows strong positivity adjacent to bony trabeculae and surrounding blood vessels in this normal bone marrow core biopsy section. Immunoperoxidase for myeloperoxidase stain (original magnification ×300).

sections, these cells are perisinusoidal, and platelets are released directly into these sinuses from megakaryocyte cytoplasm that protrudes through the sinus wall.[18] Although mature megakaryocytes are readily identifiable by hematoxylin and eosin stain, the delineation of more immature megakaryocytic elements is enhanced by immunoperoxidase staining for CD31, CD41, CD61, and, less consistently, Factor VIII (Figure 4–19).[12]

Overview of Clonal Myeloid Disorders

Myeloid disorders are clonal hematopoietic neoplasms that manifest a broad range of clinical,

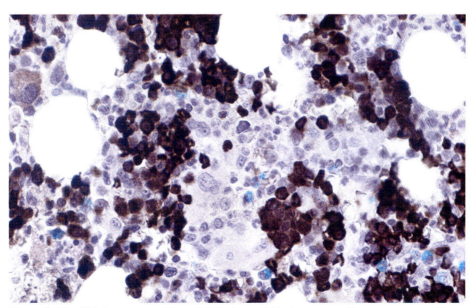

Figure 4–18. This immunoperoxidase stain for hemoglobin A on a normal bone marrow core biopsy section shows prominent colony formation. Immunoperoxidase for hemoglobin A stain (original magnification ×800). (Reproduced with permission from Foucar[21].)

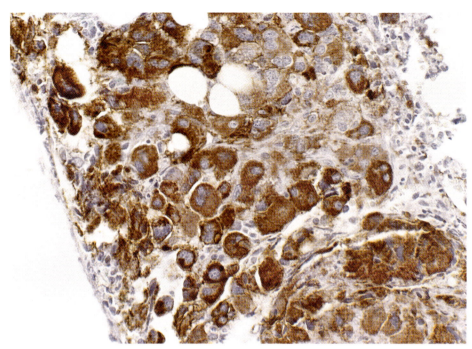

Figure 4–19.   Immunoperoxidase for CD31 shows a striking predominance of megakaryoblasts and more mature megakaryocytic elements in this case of acute megakaryoblastic leukemia. Immunoperoxidase for CD31 stain (original magnification ×600).

hematologic, and biologic features. These disorders can be classified using traditional classification schemes, especially the FAB proposals, or the newly developed WHO system that emphasizes lineage and stage of maturation first, followed by the delineation of unique clinicopathologic entities within this framework (see Tables 4–4 and 4–5).[2] At this time, the WHO proposal includes four general categories of myeloid disorders:

1. Myeloproliferative disorders
2. Myelodysplastic/myeloproliferative disorders
3. Myelodysplastic syndromes (MDSs)
4. Acute myeloid leukemias

All of these diverse acute and chronic myeloid neoplasms can be broadly categorized as either acute or chronic leukemic processes, and these disorders predominate in adults.

Chronic Myeloproliferative Disorders

Chronic myeloproliferative disorders (CMPDs) are characterized by an unregulated, sustained, excess production of one or more mature peripheral blood elements with a typical bone marrow picture of hypercellularity, intact maturation, and minimal dyspoiesis.[19–21] These disorders have an incidence rate of approximately 1 per 100,000 population. Patients with CMPD characteristically present with unexplained splenomegaly, variable hepatomegaly, and a variety of other symptoms such as malaise, fatigue, and weight loss. The typical hematologic findings that should prompt consideration of a CMPD are listed in Table 4–8. Unexplained single or multilineage cytosis seen in conjunction with a hypercellular bone marrow within intact maturation, atypical megakaryocytic hyperplasia, and dilated sinuses typifies a CMPD.[19–21]

These CMPD are generally segregated by the predominant cell type that is excessively produced, such as polycythemia vera (erythrocytosis) or essential thrombocythemia (thrombocytosis).[22] The CMPD with a prototypic chronic leukemic blood and bone marrow picture (ie, leukocytosis) is chronic myelogenous leukemia (CML). Chronic myelogenous leukemia is distinct from all other CMPD in that a specific reciprocal translocation, t(9;22) (q34;q11), producing a *BCR/ABL* fusion gene, is the defining hallmark of this disease and is present in virtually all cases.[20,23] Chronic myeloge-

Table 4–8. HEMATOLOGIC FEATURES USUALLY INDICATIVE OF A CHRONIC MYELOPROLIFERATIVE DISORDER

Blood	Bone Marrow
Unexplained increase in mature blood element(s) (erythrocytes, leukocytes, or platelets)	Hypercellular
Lack of toxic changes in neutrophils	Multilineage hyperplasia with predominance of mature forms
Multilineage abnormalities	Increased megakaryocytes, usually clustered and dyspoietic/pleomorphic
Basophilia	Dilated sinuses with intravascular hematopoiesis
Left shift, including occasional blasts	Unexplained fibrosis
Nucleated erythroid elements	Unexplained osteosclerosis
No significant dyspoiesis of neutrophils, monocytes	No increase in blasts
Teardrop erythrocytes (some cases)	No significant dyspoiesis except for megakaryocytes
Dyspoietic eosinophils (occasional cases)	
Enlarged, atypical platelets	

From Dickstein and Vardiman,[19] Anastasi and Vardiman,[20] and Foucar.[21]

nous leukemia is also distinct from all other CMPD in terms of clinical course. Clonal evolution of CML into blast crisis is a consistent feature of this disease, whereas blast crisis is an infrequent, likely therapy-related, phenomenon in other CMPD.[24,25]

Chronic myelogenous leukemia accounts for about 20 percent of all leukemias in adults; middle-aged patients are most commonly affected, and there is a slight male predominance.[23] The peripheral blood and bone marrow features of CML are highlighted on Table 4–9 (Figures 4–20, 4–21, and 4–22).

Although most patients with CML experience an initial indolent disease course, the vast majority of these patients develop a more aggressive disease characterized by a progressive increase in blasts. The proposed stages of evolution of CML are listed in Table 4–9 and include the chronic phase, the accelerated phase, and blast crisis. Although most cases of blast crisis consist of AMLs or ALLs, virtually any hematopoietic element may be involved in a blast crisis, and multilineage features may be appreciated (Figures 4–23 and 4–24).[20,24]

Hybrid Myelodysplastic/ Myeloproliferative Disorders

The WHO system proposes that hybrid myelodysplastic/myeloproliferative disorders such as chronic myelomonocytic leukemia (CMML) be distinguished from both CMPD and myelodysplastic syndromes.[2] Chronic myelomonocytic leukemia in adults is characterized by leukocytosis with typically both monocytosis and neutrophilia. Left shift may be present, and dyspoiesis, especially of neutrophils and mono-

Table 4–9. HEMATOLOGIC AND MORPHOLOGIC FEATURES OF CHRONIC MYELOGENOUS LEUKEMIA

Chronic phase
Blood
 Markedly elevated white blood cell count; pronounced nondysplastic neutrophilia with left shift (blasts < 5%)
 Absolute basophilia
 Normal mature erythrocytes; occasional normoblasts
 Thrombocytosis with enlarged platelets
 Circulating megakaryocytes and fragments may be evident
Bone marrow
 Marked hypercellularity
 Pronounced granulocytic hyperplasia with normal localization of immature forms
 Although variable, many cases exhibit pronounced increase and clustering of megakaryocytes
 Megakaryocytes often small and mononuclear
 Dyspoiesis, except for megakaryocytes, minimal or absent
 Variable reticulin fibrosis, if present, is usually mild

Accelerated phase*
Inconsistently defined; characterized by rising blast counts, progressive dyspoiesis and leukocytosis, progressive cytopenias, increasing basophilia, progressive bone marrow fibrosis, progressive splenomegaly, and refractoriness to therapy
Blasts 10–20%
Increased layers of immature myeloid cells adjacent to bony trabeculae and around blood vessels
Clonal evolution common by cytogenetic studies
May progress to blast crisis

Blast crisis*
Blasts exceed 20% in blood or bone marrow, or intra-extramedullary focus of blasts
Cytologic dysplasia in blood and bone marrow, progressive cytopenias, variable increasing splenomegaly, and increasing basophilia
Acquired pseudo Pelger-Huët anomaly of neutrophils found in 15% of cases at onset of blast crisis
Clonal evolution frequently documented by cytogenetic studies
Develops approximately 3–7 years after disease onset

*Suggested blast percentage for acute leukemia reduced from 30 to 20% in WHO proposal.
From Anastasi and Vardiman,[20] Foucar,[21] Thijsen et al.,[23] and Kantarjian et al.[24]

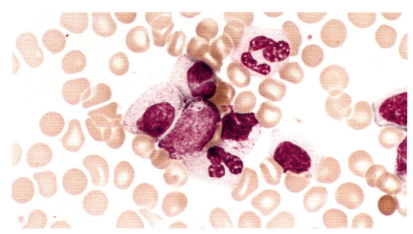

Figure 4–20. This peripheral blood smear from a patient with marked leukocytosis shows a left shift including circulating myeloblasts, although mature neutrophils predominate in this case of chronic myelogenous leukemia. Note basophil. Wright's stain (original magnification ×800).

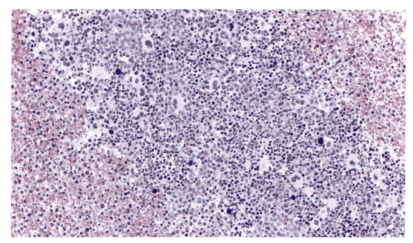

Figure 4–21. This bone marrow clot section shows 100 percent cellularity in this case of chronic myelogenous leukemia. Note increased numbers of megakaryocytes, which are generally small in size. Hematoxylin and eosin stain (original magnification ×200).

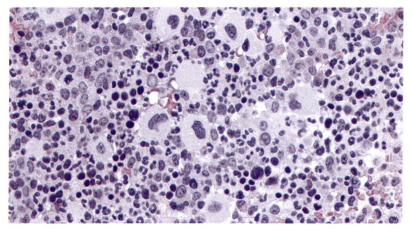

Figure 4–22. This high-power magnification of a bone marrow clot section from a patient with chronic myelogenous leukemia illustrates markedly increased megakaryocytes, many of which have a mononuclear nucleus. Hematoxylin and eosin stain (original magnification ×400).

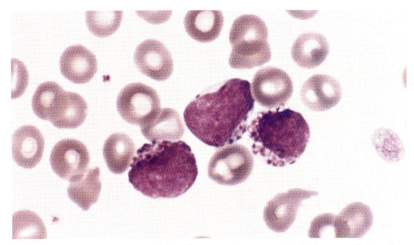

Figure 4–23. This peripheral blood smear shows markedly increased immature basophils in this case of basophilic blast crisis of chronic myelogenous leukemia. Wright's stain (original magnification ×1,000).

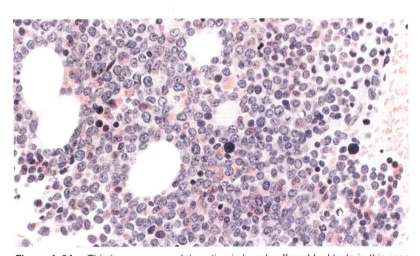

Figure 4–24. This bone marrow clot section is largely effaced by blasts in this case of myeloid blast crisis of chronic myelogenous leukemia. Note residual small mononuclear megakaryocytes. Hematoxylin and eosin stain (original magnification ×300).

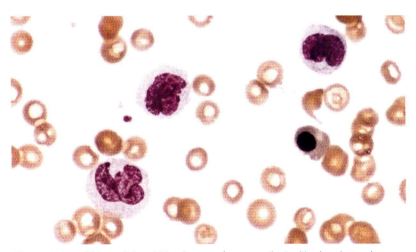

Figure 4–25. This peripheral blood smear from a patient with chronic myelomonocytic leukemia reveals increased numbers of circulating monocytes, marked anemia, and circulating erythroblasts. Wright's stain (original magnification ×800).

cytes, may be evident (Figure 4–25).[26,27] The bone marrow is characteristically hypercellular; megakaryocyte abnormalities may be present, and greater cytologic immaturity may be evident compared to blood. The disease course of CMML is variable, and no currently recognized genetic features typify this disorder.

Myelodysplastic Syndromes

Myelodysplastic syndromes are clonal stem cell disorders that are characterized by single or multilineage dysplasia, cytopenias, ineffective hematopoiesis, and intact maturation with a variable increase in blasts. High-grade myelodysplastic disorders and AML may represent a biologic continuum that likely results from a stepwise accumulation of genetic lesions following the initial development of clonal hematopoiesis.[28] A hallmark of MDS is ineffective hematopoiesis characterized by sustained cytopenias with paradoxical hypercellularity in the bone marrow.[29,30]

Myelodysplastic syndromes can occur in patients of all ages, but these disorders clearly predominate in adults, especially elderly patients.[30,31] The incidence of MDS increases remarkably with age, and among elderly patients, MDS is more common than AML.[32] Myelodysplasia can occur de novo or secondary to occupational, environmental, and iatrogenic exposures.[33,34]

The prototypic features of MDS in blood and bone marrow are listed on Table 4–10. Patients characteristically present with cytopenias, often pancytopenia. Multilineage dysplasia is common, especially in high-grade processes (Figure 4–26). The bone marrow is characteristically hypercellular with single/multilineage dysplasia (Figure 4–27). The blast count ranges

from normal to moderately increased, and both erythroid and granulocytic architectural aberrations may be apparent, especially by immunohistochemical staining (Figures 4–28 and 4–29). Although highly variable, the bone marrow is characteristically hypercellular. Megakaryocytes may be increased, clustered, and atypical. The disease course in MDS is highly variable; patients with low-grade processes may experience prolonged survival, whereas death from either bone marrow failure or evolution to AML is characteristic in patients with high-grade MDS.[35]

Acute Myelogenous Leukemia

Acute myelogenous leukemia is a clonal hematopoietic disorder characterized by the predominance of immature cells capable of minimal, if any, maturation. An acute myeloid leukemia can be derived from progenitors of any hematopoietic cell, and multilineage differentiation may be noted. Acute myelogenous leukemia can occur in patients of all ages, but it is clearly more prevalent in adults.[36] Although rare, most congenital leukemias are myeloid in origin.[37] The incidence of AML is low throughout childhood and early adulthood, although the proportion of cases of acute leukemia that are myeloid steadily increases during these years. Approximately 70 to 80 percent of cases of acute leukemia in adults are myeloid, and the incidence of AML increases substantially with advanced patient age.[38]

Factors linked to an increased incidence of AML include constitutional genetic disorders, acquired bone marrow diseases, smoking, occupational and environmental exposures, and therapeutic agents.[39,40] Numerous studies have documented the increased incidence

Table 4–10. BLOOD AND BONE MARROW FINDINGS SUGGESTIVE OF MYELODYSPLASIA	
Blood	**Bone Marrow**
Single or multilineage cytopenias*	Hypercellularity (ineffective hematopoiesis)
Left shift with myeloblasts (< 20%)	Increased blasts (< 20%)
Single or multilineage dysplasia	Single or multilineage dysplasia
Neutrophils with hypogranular cytoplasm and/or nuclear segmentation abnormalities	Loss of normal localization of immature granulocytic elements (some cases)
Erythrocyte dyspoiesis with nucleated forms	Loss of normal erythroid colony formation (some cases)
Enlarged, hypogranular platelets; other platelet abnormalities	Increased, dysplastic, clustered megakaryocytes
	Ring sideroblasts, coarse iron granules in erythroid cells (some cases)

*Cytopenias unexplained by clinical findings or laboratory evaluation.
From Foucar.[29]

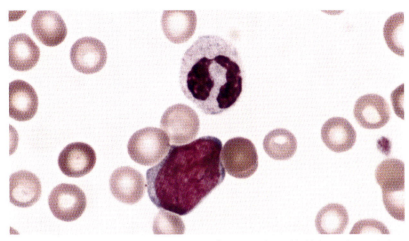

Figure 4–26.   This peripheral blood smear from a patient with high-grade myelodysplasia evolving into acute myelogenous leukemia shows marked anemia, occasional hypogranular platelets, dyspoietic neutrophils, and circulating myeloblasts. Wright's stain (original magnification ×1,000).

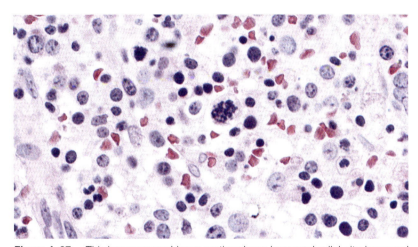

Figure 4–27.   This bone marrow biopsy section shows increased cellularity, increased immature elements, and dysplastic megakaryocytes in this patient with high-grade myelodysplasia. Hematoxylin and eosin stain (original magnification ×400).

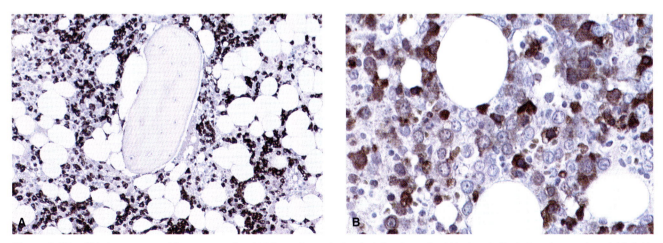

Figure 4–28.   This immunoperoxidase composite of high-grade myelodysplasia/acute erythroid leukemia illustrates abnormal myeloid distribution (*A*) and abnormal erythroid distribution with poor colony formation (*B*) by immunoperoxidase staining for myeloperoxidase and hemoglobin A (original magnification ×200 and ×400).

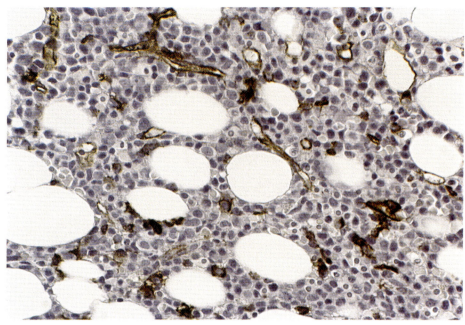

Figure 4–29.   Both increased CD34-positive blasts and a marked increase in vascularity are apparent on this bone marrow biopsy section from a patient with high-grade myelodysplasia. Immunoperoxidase for CD34 stain (original magnification ×300).

of AML in patients receiving chemotherapy, especially alkylating agents or topoisomerase II inactivators.[40–42]

By combining morphology with cytochemical assessment, the lineage and stage of maturation of most AML cases can be determined (Figures 4–30 and 4–31). Immunophenotyping is a useful ancillary study that can also be helpful in defining lineage and stage of maturation (Figure 4–32). In addition, immunophenotyping is essential in identifying minimally differentiated myeloid leukemias in which neither morphology nor cytochemical stains are definitive, so-called AML M0 by FAB criteria.[43] Immature megakaryoblastic elements are also best documented by immunologic techniques (see Figure 4–16).

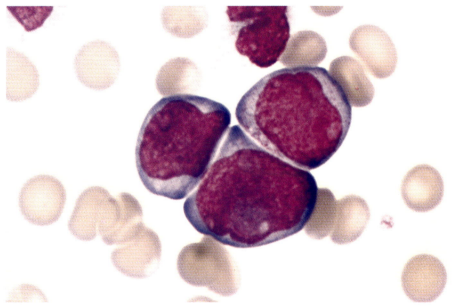

Figure 4–30.   Circulating myeloblasts are abundant in this peripheral blood smear from a patient with acute myelogenous leukemia. Wright's stain (original magnification ×1,200).

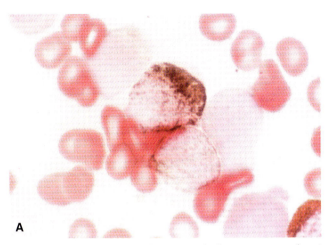
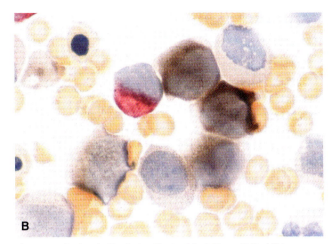

Figure 4–31. This cytochemical composite from two cases of acute myelogenous leukemia illustrates Sudan black B positivity (*A*) in a case of acute myelogenous leukemia, whereas both specific and nonspecific esterase positivity are illustrated in a case of acute myelomonocytic leukemia (*B*). Sudan black B and combined esterase stains (original magnification ×1,000).

As described earlier, AMLs can be classified by using either FAB or WHO criteria.[1,2] Although some overlap exists between these two proposals, there are several significant differences. The FAB classification system for AML is based almost exclusively on morphology and cytochemistry and is purely a lineage-based system. A requirement of 30 percent blasts or 30 percent nonerythroid blasts is used to define the separation between AML and high-grade MDS (Table 4–11).[1,3] In contrast, the WHO proposal attempts to define biologic subtypes of AML based on genetics or "surrogates" for genotype such as background dysplasia of mature cells and antecedent chemotherapy (see Table 4–4).[2] When there are insufficient data to categorize an AML into the three biologic groups of AML with recurrent cytogenetic translocations, AML with multilineage dysplasia, and therapy-related AML, then the WHO defaults to a traditional lineage-based classification system that largely parallels the FAB system.[2]

Morphologic Features of Acute Myelogenous Leukemia Subtypes

Minimally Differentiated Acute Myelogenous Leukemia (FAB AML M0)

Morphologic features of this AML subtype are nondescript, and immunophenotyping is required to confirm that the leukemia is derived from the myeloid lineage(s).[43] The bone marrow core biopsy typically shows hypercellularity; blasts predominate, and there is characteristically no evidence of maturation.

Acute Myelogenous Leukemia without Maturation (FAB AML M1)

The presence of usually sparse cytoplasmic granules, occasional Auer rods, and Sudan black B/myeloperoxidase positivity allows recognition of this AML subtype by standard morphologic/cytochemical assessment (see Figure 4–7).

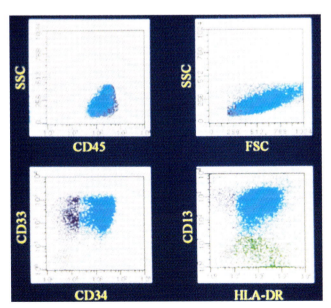

Figure 4–32. This flow cytometric composite histogram illustrates the immunophenotypic profile of a case of acute myelogenous leukemia characterized by weak CD45 expression in conjunction with expression of CD13, CD33, HLA-DR, and CD34 in this prototypic case of acute myelogenous leukemia.

Acute Myelogenous Leukemia with Maturation (FAB AML M2)

Myeloid lineage derivation is obvious by standard morphologic assessment, and Sudan black B/myeloperoxidase positivity is often moderately intense in many of the blasts (Figure 4–33).

Some cases that fulfill criteria for this AML subtype exhibit a distinct genotype, t(8;21)(q22;q22), which is linked to a variety of unique morphologic and immunophenotypic features (Table 4–12). The distinctive morphologic features include long-tapered Auer rods and a homogeneous salmon pink cytoplasm with a basophilic margin (Figure 4–34).[44] Aberrant CD56 and/or CD19 expression is commonly detected on these immature myeloid cells in this genotypic subset of AML with maturation.[45]

Acute Promyelocytic Leukemia (FAB AML M3 and M3m)

Intense cytoplasmic granulation obscuring the nucleus is typical in the promyelocytes that predominate in the common type of acute promyelocytic leukemia (Figure 4–9). The microgranular variant of acute promyelocytic leukemia is also distinct, exhibiting marked nuclear folding/lobulation and subtle, if any, perceptible cytoplasmic granulation (Figure 4–35).[46,47] By cytochemical staining, both subtypes exhibit intense uniform Sudan black B/myeloperoxidase positivity. Acute promyelocytic leukemia demonstrates the strongest association between lineage-based classification and genotype in that t(15;17)(q22;q11-12) is present in virtually all cases of common type and microgranular acute promyelocytic leukemia (see Table 4–12).[48]

Table 4–11. FAB CLASSIFICATION OF ACUTE MYELOGENOUS LEUKEMIA*	
Subtype	**Definition***
AML M0	≥ 30% blasts < 3% Sudan black B/myeloperoxidase positivity Myeloid antigen expression by immunophenotyping or myeloperoxidase expression by electron microscopy
AML M1	≥30% blasts ≥3% Sudan black B/myeloperoxidase positivity in blasts < 10% cells exhibiting maturation beyond blast stage
AML M2	≥ 30% blasts ≥ 3% Sudan black B/myeloperoxidase positivity in blasts > 10% granulocytic cells exhibiting maturation beyond blast stage < 20% monocytic cells
AML M3	≥ 30% blasts + hypergranular promyelocytes[†] Intense myeloperoxidase/Sudan black B reaction in virtually all cells
AML M3m	Same criteria, except that granules within most promyelocytes very inconspicuous and nuclei highly grooved and reniform
AML M4	Monocytosis (≥ 5 × 10⁹/L); increased lysozyme ≥ 30% myeloblasts + monoblasts + promonocytes > 20% Sudan black B/myeloperoxidase positive cells > 20% nonspecific esterase positive cells
AML M4 eos	Same criteria as AML M4 plus abnormal eosinophils in bone marrow
AML M5 a, b	≥ 30% myeloblasts + monoblasts + promonocytes < 20% Sudan black B/myeloperoxidase positive cells > 80% nonspecific esterase positive cells Monoblasts predominate in M5a Promonocytes predominate in M5b
AML M6 a, b	≥ 30% of nonerythroid cells are myeloblasts > 50% erythroid elements Erythroblasts predominate (suggested AML M6b category)
AML M7	≥ 30% blasts (myeloblasts + megakaryoblasts) > 30% megakaryocytic elements defined by immunophenotyping or ultrastructural electron microscopy

FAB = French-American-British.
*FAB requires 30% blasts (nonerythroid) in bone marrow for diagnosis of acute leukemia.
[†]Promyelocytes usually predominate in AML M3.
From Bennett et al.,[1,3,4,43] Foucar,[6] and Brunning and McKenna.[8]

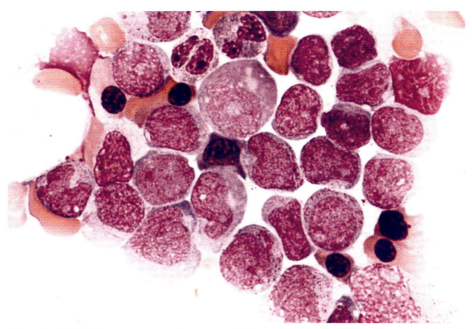

Figure 4–33. This bone marrow aspirate smear is from a patient with acute myelogenous leukemia with maturation. Note occasional neutrophils. Wright's stain (original magnification ×1,000).

Table 4–12. MORPHOLOGIC CYTOCHEMICAL AND IMMUNOPHENOTYPIC FEATURES OF BIOLOGIC SUBTYPES OF AML

Cytogenetics	Morphology	Morphology Caveats	Cytochemistry	Immunophenotype	Molecular
t(15;17) (q22;q11-12)	Classic APL: hypergranular blasts and numerous promyelocytes, many with Auer rod bundles Microgranular variant: folded nucleus and moderately abundant cytoplasm resembling immature monocytes	Only rare circulating blasts may be present in classic form	Intense SBB positivity	Myeloid ag+, CD34-, HLA-DR-, M3v: CD2+	*PML/RAR* fusion gene
t(8;21) (q22;q22)	Significant myeloid maturation. Prominent tapered Auer rods. Salmon pink granules surrounded by basophilic rim in more mature myeloid elements.	Blast percentage may be < 30% leading to mistaken diagnosis of MDS	Many SBB/MPO positive cells; less uniform intensity than APL	Myeloid ag+, CD34+, usually CD19+, CD56+	*AML/ETO* fusion gene
Inv(16) (p13q22)	Myelomonocytic blasts; dysplastic eosinophils with characteristic mixed eosinophil/basophil granules in cytoplasm	Very low percentage of abnormal eosinophil may be seen in AML with deletions of chromosome 16, other abnormalities	Eosinophils: PAS+, chloroacetate esterase +	Myeloid ag+, variable expression of CD34, CD2	*CBFβ/MYH11* fusion gene
t(11q23)	Acute monoblastic leukemias predominate including congenital AML and topoisomerase II inhibitor therapy-related AMLs	Other morphologic subtypes occasionally noted	NSE positivity	Myeloid ag+, may be CD4+, CD14+ but not specific	*MLL* fusion with multiple partner genes
Structural abnormalities including −5/del(5q) −7/del(7q)	Multilineage dysplasia and multilineage involvement in leukemia; some cases alkylating agent therapy related	Blast percentage highly variable, bone marrow fibrosis may interfere with aspiration	Variable depending on lineages involved	Myeloid ag+, variable CD34 expression	Loss of genetic material

AML = acute myelogenous leukemia; APL = acute promyelocytic leukemia; SBB = Sudan black B; ag = antigen; MDS = myelodysplasia; MPO = myeloperoxidase; PAS = periodic acid–Schiff; NSE = nonspecific esterase.
From Foucar[6] and Foucar and Leith.[58]

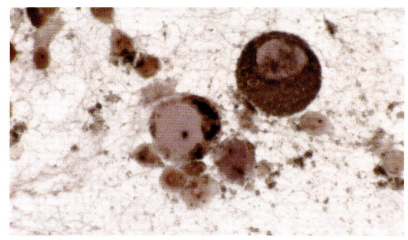

Figure 4–34.   Blasts with variable sudanophilia are evident in this bone marrow aspirate smear from a patient with acute myelogenous leukemia with maturation and t(8;21). Sudan black B stain (original magnification ×1,000).

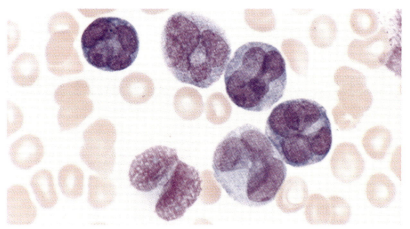

Figure 4–35.   This peripheral blood smear from a patient with microgranular acute promyelocytic leukemia shows leukocytosis in conjunction with leukemic cells that exhibit marked nuclear folding and minimal, if any, apparent granulation. Wright's stain (original magnification ×1,000).

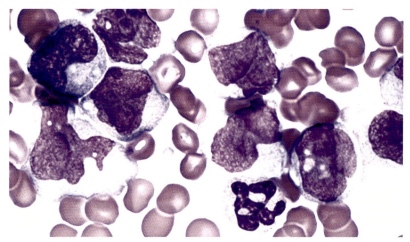

Figure 4–36.   This bone marrow aspirate smear is from a patient with acute myelomonocytic leukemia. Note immature monocytes and dysplastic neutrophils. Wright's stain (original magnification ×1,000).

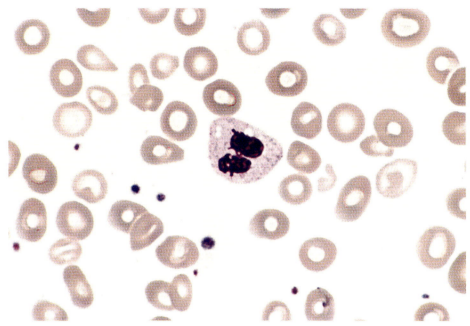

Figure 4–37. A hypogranular neutrophil with a pseudo Pelger-Huët nucleus is evident in this peripheral blood smear. Note abnormal erythrocytes. Wright's stain (original magnification ×1,000).

Acute Myelogenous Leukemia with Monocytic Differentiation (FAB AML M4)

Both immature myeloid and monocytic elements comprise this AML subtype (Figure 4–36). This "dual-lineage" maturation is generally confirmed by morphologic and cytochemical assessment. The more mature elements of both the myeloid and monocytic lineages often exhibit dysplastic features such as hypogranular cytoplasm and nuclear hyposegmentation of neutrophils (Figure 4–37).

One subset of AML with monocytic differentiation is defined by inv(16) (p13q22) or related translocations; this acute myelomonocytic leukemia

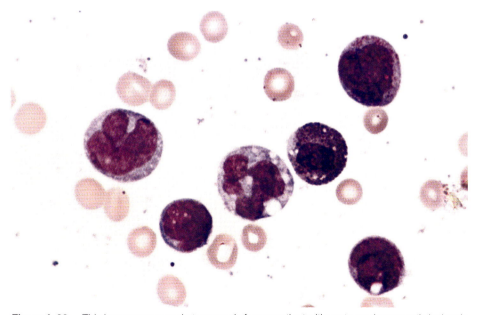

Figure 4–38. This bone marrow aspirate smear is from a patient with acute myelomonocytic leukemia and inv(16) and illustrates dysplastic eosinophils. Wright's stain (original magnification ×1,000).

also exhibits bone marrow eosinophilia (see Table 4–12)[10,49] These eosinophils contain mixed eosinophil-basophil granules (Figure 4–38).

Acute Monocytic Leukemia (FAB AML M5a, b)

Immature monocytes predominate in this leukemia subtype (see Figure 4–10). The most immature monocytic elements have round nuclear contours, whereas early maturation is associated with nuclear lobulation. Diffuse cytoplasmic nonspecific esterase positivity is typical in these monocytic leukemias (see Figure 4–11). Bone marrow core biopsy sections are characteristically packed with leukemic cells that exhibit round to folded nuclei and abundant cytoplasm.

Some cases of acute monocytic leukemia have a unique cytogenetic aberration, 11q23 gene rearrangement with multiple partner genes (see Table 4-12).[50] These 11q23-associated monocytic leukemias have several clinicopathologic associations. For example, congenital monocytic leukemias often have t(11q23). Likewise, therapy-related monocytic leukemias following topoisomerase II inhibitor therapy are typically t(11q23) associated.[51]

Acute Erythroid Leukemia (FAB AML M6)

Cases of acute erythroid leukemia demonstrate a variable morphologic appearance. Although most cases are characterized by increased myeloblasts and dysplastic erythroid elements, occasional cases demonstrate a marked predominance of immature erythroid elements (Figures 4–12, 4–39).[52] Multilineage maturation is generally readily apparent on core biopsy sections.

Acute Megakaryocytic Leukemia (FAB AML M7)

The morphologic appearance of acute megakaryocytic leukemia is highly variable, and immunophenotyping is generally required to identify the most immature forms (see Figures 4–14, 4–15, and 4–16). Clumping, multinucleation, and cytoplasmic membrane blebbing are all morphologic features of megakaryoblasts.[6] In some cases, myeloblasts are also increased, whereas a more homogeneous population of megakaryoblasts is evident in other cases. Fibrosis may be evident on bone marrow core biopsy sections (Figure 4–40).

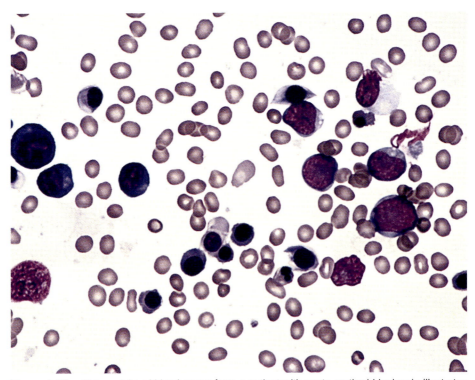

Figure 4–39.   This peripheral blood smear from a patient with acute erythroid leukemia illustrates abundant circulating myeloblasts and erythroblasts. Wright's stain (original magnification ×800).

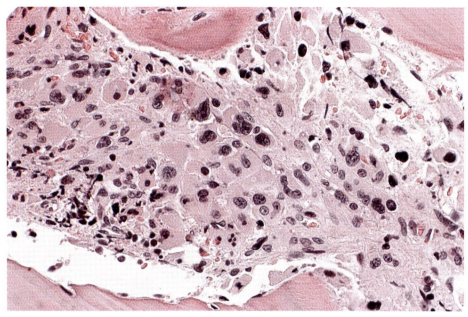

Figure 4–40. This bone marrow biopsy section from a patient with acute megakaryoblastic leukemia shows a predominance of immature megakaryocytic elements in association with fibrosis. Hematoxylin and eosin stain (original magnification ×400).

Acute Myeloid Leukemia with Multilineage Dysplasia

Dyspoiesis of mature granulocytic, erythroid, and megakaryocytic elements is seen in conjunction with increased myeloblasts in these cases. Trilineage aberrations are also apparent on bone marrow aspirate and core biopsy sections. Patients with AML with multilineage dysplasia may have antecedent myelodysplasia. Cytogenetic studies often reveal numeric abnormalities, and the cases are typically resistant to therapy (see Table 4–12).[53,54]

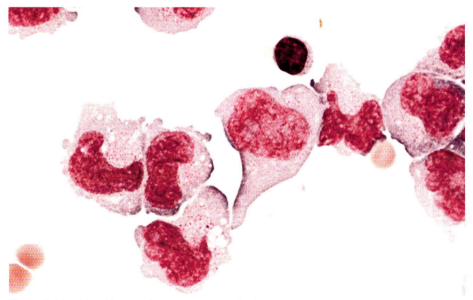

Figure 4–41. Monoblasts and promonocytes predominate in this bone marrow aspirate smear from a patient with acute monoblastic leukemia associated with an 11q23 translocation. Wright's stain (original magnification ×1,000).

Therapy-Related
Acute Myelogenous Leukemia

Both alkylating agent and topoisomerase II inhibitor therapies are linked to the development of secondary leukemia and myelodysplasia. The prototypic alkylating agent therapy-related AML is preceded by a brief myelodysplastic phase, characterized by multilineage dysplasia in blood and bone marrow, and associated with numeric cytogenetic abnormalities (see Table 4–12).[40,55] In contrast, acute leukemias that follow topoisomerase II inhibitor therapy are classically abrupt in onset and monoblastic/monocytic (Figure 4–41).[51] However, some topoisomerase II inhibitor-related cases demonstrate other morphologic and genotypic aberrations.[56–58]

APPROACH TO ACUTE
AND CHRONIC LYMPHOID LEUKEMIAS

Chronic lymphoproliferative disorders (CLPDs) are a diverse group of B- and T-cell neoplasms that are characterized by intact maturation, whereas maturation failure typifies ALL. Although this chapter will emphasize the morphologic features of acute and chronic lymphoid leukemias, immunophenotypic studies to define lineage and stage of maturation are essential in the diagnosis and classification of these neoplasms. The stages of B- and T-cell maturation are listed in Table 4–7, and an immunophenotypic profile can be used to delineate many different subtypes of chronic B- and T-cell disorders. For both acute and chronic lymphoid neoplasms, the final diagnosis represents an integration of clinical, morphologic, and immunophenotypic features.

Chronic Lymphoproliferative Disorders

Those mature B-, T-, and NK cell neoplasms that manifest with a leukemic blood and bone marrow picture are listed in Table 4–3. Although discussion will be restricted to these leukemic disorders, the diagnostician must be aware that many other mature B-cell lymphomas can occasionally manifest with predominant blood and bone marrow disease.

Chronic Lymphocytic Leukemia

Chronic lymphocytic leukemia (CLL) is by far the most common CLPD encountered in clinical practice. Patients are usually middle aged to elderly, and many cases are incidentally detected by complete blood count. The circulating lymphocytes tend to be small and monotonous and exhibit round nuclear contours with highly condensed nuclear chromatin (Figure 4–42) (Table 4–13).[59–61]

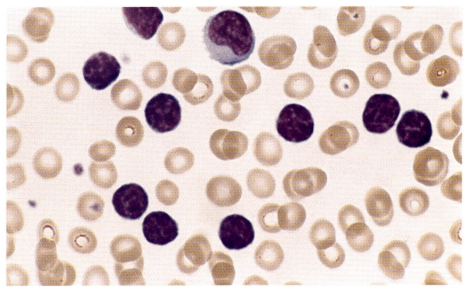

Figure 4–42.   A marked leukocytosis with a predominance of monotonous, small, mature lymphocytes with highly condensed nuclear chromatin is evident in this peripheral blood smear from a patient with chronic lymphocytic leukemia. Wright's stain (original magnification ×1,000).

Table 4–13. MORPHOLOGIC FEATURES OF CHRONIC LYMPHOPROLIFERATIVE DISORDERS IN BLOOD AND BONE MARROW

Disorders	White Blood Cell Count	Morphologic Features	Histologic Features in Bone Marrow
B-Cell Disorders			
Chronic lymphocytic leukemia	Usually elevated (modest)	Small lymphocyte with condensed nuclear chromatin and inconspicuous nucleoli, cytoplasm usually scant	Focal, nonparatrabecular infiltrates Occasionally diffuse
B-prolymphocytic leukemia	Markedly elevated	Usually homogeneous cells with huge central nucleoli, round nuclear contours, and variable amounts of cytoplasm	Diffuse, occasionally nodular
Hairy cell leukemia	Usually decreased	Moderately sized cells with "spongy" chromatin, oval to folded nuclei, and moderate to abundant cytoplasm with shaggy contours	Diffuse or subtle interstitial pattern Bone marrow may be hypocellular
Splenic lymphoma with villous lymphocytes	Mildly to moderately elevated	Maybe plasmacytoid, variable cytologic features; may exhibit bipolar cytoplasmic projections	Nodular, intrasinusoidal
T-cell disorders			
T-prolymphocytic leukemia	Markedly elevated	Variable; some cases have prominent central nucleoli, others "knobby"-appearing nuclei	Usually diffuse
Adult T-cell leukemia/ lymphoma	Usually markedly elevated	Marked, coarse nuclear lobulations apparent at low-power magnification; nuclear chromatin condensed	Usually diffuse
T-cell granular lymphocytic leukemia	Variable, modest lymphocytosis	Cytologically bland cells with round nuclear contours and moderate amounts of cytoplasm containing a few coarse granules	Patchy, usually subtle infiltrates
Sézary syndrome (mycosis fungoides)	Variable	Condensed chromatin with subtle cerebriform nuclear contours	Patchy, variably subtle infiltrates

From Kroft et al.,[59] Foucar,[60,61] Jennings and Foon,[62] and Moreau et al.[63]

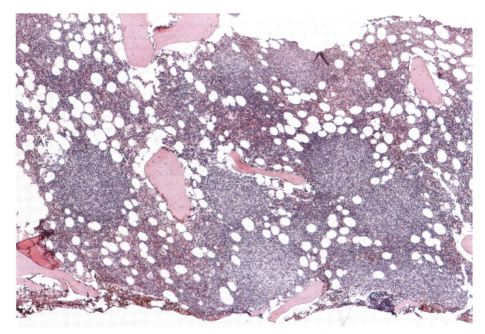

Figure 4–43. This low-power photograph of a bone marrow core biopsy from a patient with chronic lymphocytic leukemia illustrates numerous nonparatrabecular nodular leukemic infiltrates. Hematoxylin and eosin stain (original magnification ×200). (Reproduced with permission from Foucar[61].)

Table 4–14. CLASSIC IMMUNOPHENOTYPIC PROFILE OF LEUKEMIC B- AND T-CELL CHRONIC LYMPHOPROLIFERATIVE DISORDERS*

B-Cell Disorders	SIg	CD19	CD20	CD22	CD79b	CD23	CD25	CD5	FMC7	CD11c	CD10
Chronic lymphocytic leukemia	W	+	W	W	−	+	±	+	±	W	−
Prolymphocytic leukemia	+	+	+	+	+	−	−	±	+	−	−
Hairy cell leukemia[†]	+	+	+	+	−	±	+	−	+	+	±
Splenic lymphoma with villous lymphocytes[†]	+	+	+	+	+	−	−	±	+	±	−
Mantle cell lymphoma	+	+	+	+	+	−	−	+	+	−	−
Follicular lymphoma	+	+	+	+	+	±	−	−	+	−	+

T-Cell Disorders	CD3	CD2	CD4	CD5	CD7	CD8	CD16	CD25	CD56	CD57
Large granular lymphocytosis—T	+	+	−	+	±	+	+	NA	±	+
Large granular lymphocytosis—NK	−	+	−	+	−	−	+	NA	+	−
T-prolymphocytic leukemia	+	+	+	+	+	−	−	±	−	−
Adult T-cell leukemia	+	+	+	+	−	−	−	+	−	−
Sézary syndrome/mycosis fungoides	+	+	+	+	−	−	−	−	−	−

W = weak expression; NK = natural killer cell; NA = not available.
*Variations in classic profile described.
[†]Expression of DBA-44 by immunoperoxidase techniques also a feature of immunophenotypic profile of hairy cell leukemia and a fair number of cases of splenic marginal zone lymphoma with villous lymphocytes.
From Kroft et al.[59] and Morea et al.[63]

Bone marrow aspirate smears typically reveal a mature lymphocytosis; these cells generally are morphologically similar to the circulating lymphocytes. On bone marrow biopsy sections, several patterns of infiltration by CLL have been described, the most common of which are focal, nonparatrabecular infiltrates that are readily identifiable at low-power examination (Figure 4–43).[59–61] These nodular lesions consist of discrete, densely packed collections of leukemia cells that characteristically demonstrate round nuclear contours and scant cytoplasm. Mitotic activity is minimal. Rarely, proliferation foci are evident on bone marrow biopsy sections. A diagnosis of CLL is generally confirmed by flow cytometric immunophenotyping, and the characteristic surface antigen profile of this mature leukemia subtype is listed on Table 4–14.[59–63]

Over time, well-recognized types of transformation of CLL have been delineated. The most common of these include prolymphocytoid transforma-

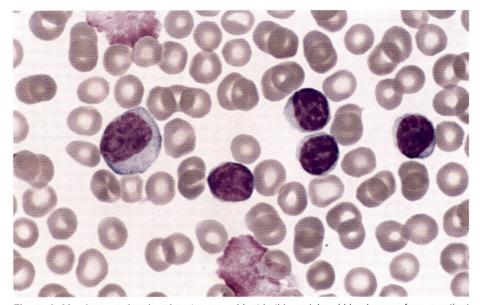

Figure 4–44. Increased prolymphocytes are evident in this peripheral blood smear from a patient with long-standing chronic lymphocytic leukemia. Wright's stain (original magnification ×1,000).

tion and the development of large cell lymphoma, so-called Richter's transformation.[61,64,65] Prolymphocytoid transformation is characterized by the progressive increase in circulating prolymphocytes and is generally associated with a more adverse outcome (Figure 4–44). The development of large cell lymphoma in patients with established CLL (Richter's syndrome) is generally characterized by the abrupt onset of symptomatology, progressive adenopathy, and progressive organomegaly. The bone marrow is an infrequent site of involvement by Richter's transformation, but these large B lymphoma cells can occasionally be identified in bone marrow specimens. The clinical course of Richter's transformation of CLL is generally aggressive.

B-Prolymphocytic Leukemia

B-prolymphocytic leukemia (B-PLL) generally affects elderly men who present with a marked lymphocytosis and splenomegaly. The absolute lymphocyte count often exceeds 100,000/mm³ and consists of a relatively homogeneous population of intermediate to large cells with moderate amounts of cytoplasm and round nuclei containing central prominent nucleoli (Figure 4–45).[60,61,64] Bone marrow examination generally reveals extensive effacement by the leukemic infiltrate, which exhibits either a

diffuse or mixed nodular and diffuse pattern of infiltration. The central prominent nucleoli of these prolymphocytes can be appreciated on bone marrow sections. The immunophenotypic profile of this distinctive chronic B lymphoproliferative disorder is listed in Table 4–14. Mantle cell lymphoma must be excluded from consideration by genetic or immunologic studies.

Hairy Cell Leukemia

Hairy cell leukemia (HCL) characteristically affects middle-aged to elderly patients who present with splenomegaly and pancytopenia. The leukopenia that characterizes HCL is unique among the B- and T-cell CLPDs, which are generally characterized by an absolute lymphocytosis.[59-61] Either single or multilineage cytopenias dominate blood findings in patients with HCL. Both neutropenia and especially monocytopenia are characteristic in HCL.

Careful review of the peripheral blood smear is essential in identifying the low numbers of circulating hairy cells (Figure 4–46). Both nuclear and cytoplasmic features contribute to the prototypic HCL morphology. The nuclei of hairy cells tend to be round or slightly folded and exhibit a dispersed "spongy" chromatin configuration, whereas cytoplasm is moderate to abundant and demonstrates cir-

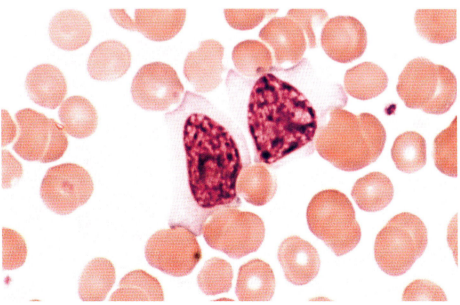

Figure 4–45.   This peripheral blood smear is from a patient with de novo prolymphocytic leukemia associated with a markedly increased leukocyte count. Wright's stain (original magnification ×1,200).

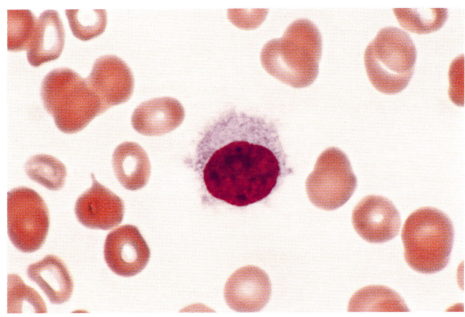

Figure 4–46.   A rare circulating hairy cell is evident in this peripheral blood smear from a patient who presented with pancytopenia. Wright's stain (original magnification ×1,200).

cumferential hairy projections. The identification of strong tartrate-resistant acid phosphatase cytoplasmic positivity in at least a portion of the hairy cells is a hallmark of HCL.[61]

Although the bone marrow is frequently inaspirable due to reticulin fibrosis, the bone marrow biopsy is invaluable in establishing a diagnosis of HCL. Unlike virtually all other CLPDs, discrete nodular infiltrates of leukemia are extremely unusual in HCL. Instead, bone marrow biopsy sections reveal either subtle patchy infiltrates of hairy cells or a diffuse interstitial pattern of infiltration. The fact that up to one-third of cases of HCL are associated with marked overall hypocellularity makes the recognition of these subtle infiltrates even more problematic (Figure 4–47).[61] Staining of the bone marrow biopsy sections with a pan B-cell antigen such as CD20 or CD79a greatly enhances the

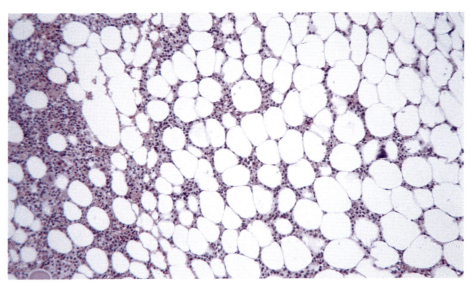

Figure 4–47.   This bone marrow core biopsy section is taken from an elderly patient who presented with hypocellular hairy cell leukemia. The leukemic infiltrates are particularly subtle. Hematoxylin and eosin stain (original magnification ×300).

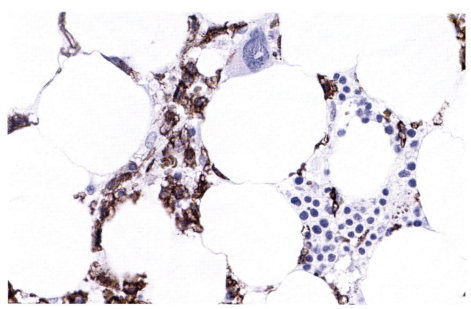

Figure 4–48. Immunoperoxidase staining for CD20 highlights the subtle hairy cell infiltrates in this case of hypocellular hairy cell leukemia. Immunoperoxidase for CD20 stain (original magnification ×400).

identification of these subtle infiltrates (Figure 4–48). Because of abundant cytoplasm, HCL infiltrates in bone marrow biopsy sections are characterized by widely spaced nuclei that are round to oval and exhibit little, if any, mitotic activity. Occasionally, hairy cells can demonstrate a distinctly spindled appearance on bone marrow biopsy sections.

Although multiple morphologic subtypes of HCL have been described, the HCL variant designation generally refers to a disorder characterized by features overlapping between B-PLL and HCL.

These patients present with a leukocytosis, and the circulating leukemia cells exhibit prominent central nucleoli and hairy cytoplasmic projections.

The classic immunophenotypic profile of HCL is listed in Table 4–14.[61–63]

Splenic Lymphoma with Villous Lymphocytes

Even though primary splenic marginal zone lymphoma with villous lymphocytes (SLVL) is a recognized subtype of non-Hodgkin's lymphoma, this disorder is

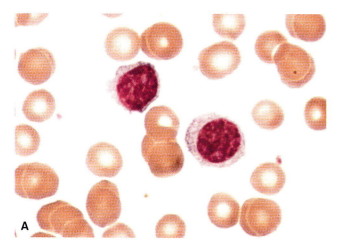
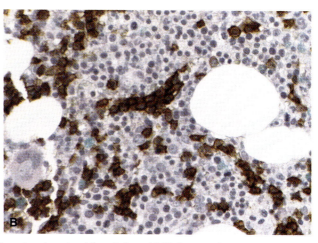

Figure 4–49. This composite photomicrograph illustrates circulating villous lymphocytes (*A*) and sinusoidal infiltrates of villous lymphocytes highlighted by CD20 staining in a core biopsy section (*B*) in a case of splenic lymphoma with villous lymphocytes involving peripheral blood and bone marrow. Wright's (original magnification ×1,000) and immunoperoxidase for CD20 stains (original magnification ×200).

included within the discussion of chronic leukemias because of the frequent leukemic manifestations at presentation.[66] Splenic lymphoma with villous lymphocytes typically affects elderly men who present with splenomegaly. The peripheral blood exhibits a moderate absolute lymphocytosis; mild anemia and thrombocytopenia may also be appreciated. The circulating neoplastic lymphocytes in SLVL demonstrate morphologic heterogeneity and include plasmacytoid forms and lymphoid cells with distinct bipolar villous projections of the cytoplasm (Figure 4–49).[66]

Bone marrow examination can be useful in distinguishing SLVL from other B-CLPD cells, especially HCL. The bone marrow infiltrates in SLVL are generally focal and discrete; recently, intrasinusoidal infiltrates have also been identified within the bone marrow (see Figure 4–49). The characteristic immunophenotypic profile of this B-CLPD is listed in Table 4–14.[67]

T-Cell Prolymphocytic Leukemia

Analogous to B-CLPDs, there are several types of leukemic T-CLPDs. In contrast to B-CLPDs, all of these T-cell disorders are encountered infrequently in clinical practice, with the exception of T-large granular lymphocytosis (T-LGL).

The current WHO recommendation is that disorders formerly termed T-CLL and T-PLL be merged into a single entity, T-PLL.[2,68] Patients with T-PLL present with clinical manifestations that are generally similar to the B-cell counterpart in that most patients are elderly men who present with splenomegaly and leukocytosis, although clinical heterogeneity has been noted. Cases of T-PLL exhibit a spectrum of morphologic subtypes; some cases are morphologically identical to B-PLL and demonstrate huge central nucleoli.[61,68,69] More commonly, the morphologic features are more heterogeneous and nucleoli are inconspicuous (Figure 4–50). In these cases of T-PLL, the nuclei may exhibit more nuclear irregularity, condensed nuclear chromatin, and inconspicuous nucleoli. Some cases are indistinguishable morphologically from T-CLL. The immunophenotypic profile of this mature T-cell neoplasm that is characteristically of helper subtype is listed in Table 4–14.

T-Large Granular Lymphocytosis

Normally, only a small proportion of peripheral blood lymphocytes contain coarse cytoplasmic azurophilic granules, so-called LGLs. Cells exhibiting this distinct morphologic appearance consist

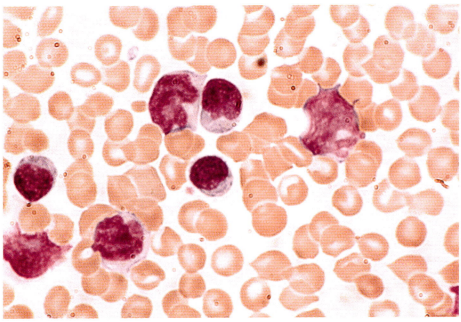

Figure 4–50.   A marked leukocytosis is evident in this peripheral blood smear from a patient with T-prolymphocytic leukemia. Note nuclear irregularity. Wright's stain (original magnification ×1,000).

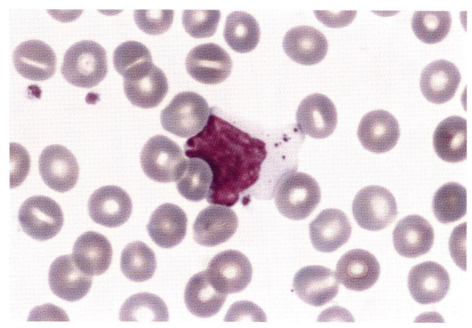

Figure 4–51. A prototypic large granular lymphocyte is evident in this peripheral blood smear. Wright's stain (original magnification ×1,600).

largely of either T cytotoxic/suppressor or true NK cells. Large granular lymphocytes are transiently increased in a wide variety of disorders, especially in patients with viral infections or immune aberrations.[61,70] Rare patients develop sustained increases in LGLs, so-called large granular lymphocytosis. In these patients, increased numbers of LGLs can be appreciated within peripheral blood, bone marrow aspirate smears, and on bone marrow biopsy sections (Figure 4–51). Circulating LGLs are generally morphologically unremarkable, resembling their normal counterparts. Bone marrow infiltrates in T-LGL are often very subtle and best highlighted by immunoperoxidase staining for pan T-cell antigens.

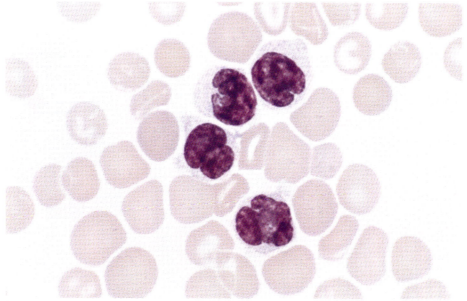

Figure 4–52. This peripheral blood smear from a case of nonendemic adult T-cell leukemia/lymphoma shows a striking leukocytosis with marked nuclear irregularities. Wright's stain (original magnification ×1,000).

Rare cases of LGL are derived from true NK cells and exhibit more variable morphologic features and a generally more aggressive disease course.[61] The immunophenotypic profile of T-LGL derived from cytotoxic/suppressor cells is listed in Table 4–14.

Adult T-Cell Leukemia Lymphoma

Adult T-cell leukemia lymphoma (ATLL) is a distinctive mature T-cell neoplasm originally described in Japanese patients about 20 years ago.[71] Subsequent studies have documented the unique worldwide geographic distribution of this rare leukemic disorder that is caused by human T-cell leukemia virus type 1 (HTLV-1). Although leukemias were initially recognized, the spectrum of HTLV-1–related disease is quite broad. This discussion will focus only on patients who present with a leukemic blood picture.

A striking leukocytosis with a predominance of morphologically abnormal circulating lymphoid cells characterizes the leukemic subtype of ATLL.[61,72] These lymphoid cells show pronounced nuclear irregularity with coarse lobulations and cloverleaf forms that can be appreciated on low- to medium-power microscopic review (Figure 4–52). Heterogeneity of both overall cell size and nuclear configurations is common. The chromatin of these cells tends to be coarsely clumped, and nucleoli are either absent or inconspicuous. The amount of cytoplasm is variable. The bone marrow generally exhibits a diffuse pattern of infiltration, and the immunophenotypic profile of this mature T-cell neoplasm generally derived from helper lymphocytes is listed in Table 4–14.

Sézary Syndrome/Mycosis Fungoides

Sézary syndrome (SS) and mycosis fungoides (MF) are closely related disorders that comprise the bulk of cutaneous T-cell lymphomas. Only a subset of patients with cutaneous T-cell lymphoma exhibit a leukemic blood picture; this phenomenon occurs more frequently in patients with SS.[61,73]

The peripheral blood picture is quite variable in SS/MF patients who develop peripheral blood involvement. In some patients, the circulating neoplastic lymphocytes are quite inconspicuous and the overall hemogram is essentially normal, whereas other patients develop a striking leukocytosis with a predominance of circulating abnormal forms. The cytologic features of the circulating cells are similar in both of these circumstances. The nuclear:cyto-

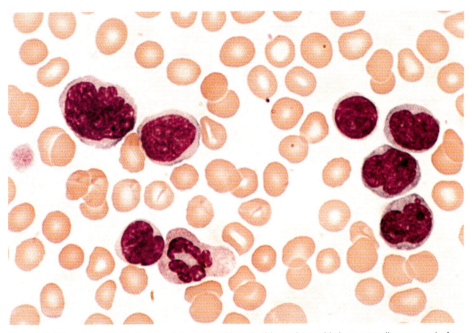

Figure 4–53. A frankly leukemic picture is evident in this patient with long-standing mycosis fungoides/Sézary syndrome. Note variability in overall nuclear size and subtle cerebriform nuclear configurations. Wright's stain (original magnification ×1,000). (Courtesy of Dr. C. Sever.)

Table 4–15. ACUTE LYMPHOID LEUKEMIAS

French-American-British
ALL L1
  High nuclear:cytoplasmic ratio; subtle nuclear
    irregularities; fine to slightly condensed chromatin
ALL L2
  Variable nuclear size, nucleoli generally conspicuous,
    moderate amounts of cytoplasm
ALL L3
  Homogeneous population of cells with round nuclear
    contours, inconspicuous nucleoli, and moderate amounts
    of deeply basophilic, vacuolated cytoplasm

World Health Organization
  Precursor B-cell acute lymphoblastic leukemia
    (cytogenetic subgroups)
    t(9;22)(q34;q11); *BCR/ABL*
    t(v;11q23); *MLL* rearranged
    t(1;19)(q23;p13) *E2A/PBX1*
    t(12;21)(p12;q22) *ETV/CBF-α*
  Precursor T-cell acute lymphoblastic leukemia
  Burkitt's cell leukemia

From Bennett et al.,[1] Harris et al.,[2] Brunning and Mckenna,[8] and Foucar.[74]

plasmic ratio is generally high, and the cytoplasm is typically basophilic and agranular. The nuclei are dark staining and exhibit a subtle cerebriform configuration best appreciated under high-power microscopic examination (Figure 4–53). Circulating SS/MF cells range in size from slightly larger than normal lymphocytes to markedly enlarged.

As predicted from this marked range in peripheral blood involvement, the bone marrow features in patients with SS/MF are highly variable.[61] In some patients, only subtle, inconspicuous infiltrates of SS/MF cells are present; these can be best appreciated by immunoperoxidase staining for pan T-cell antigens. In contrast, other patients may exhibit more overt and extensive bone marrow replacement. The immunophenotypic features of this mature T-cell neoplasm that is generally comprised of helper lymphocytes are listed in Table 4–14.

Acute Lymphoblastic Leukemias

Acute lymphoblastic leukemia is a clonal B- or T-cell neoplasm derived from immature lymphoid cells that correspond approximately to normal B or T precursor cells (see Table 4–7).[74] Acute lymphoblastic leukemia can occur at any age but predominates in children; approximately 20 percent of adult acute leukemias are lymphoid. The foundation for establishing a diagnosis of ALL is the successful determination of lineage and stage of maturation of the abnormal infiltrate, usually within blood or bone marrow.[75–78] In addition to flow cytometric immunophenotyping, it is essential to perform cytogenetic analyses on cases of ALL; the recent

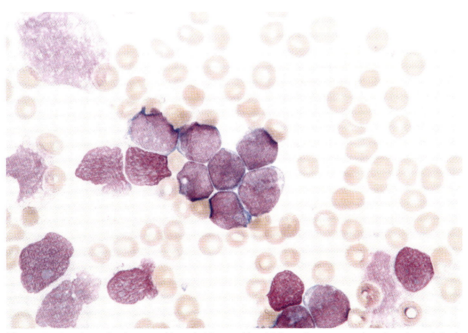

Figure 4–54. A predominance of lymphoblasts with a high nuclear to cytoplasmic ratio and finely dispersed nuclear chromatin is evident on this bone marrow aspirate smear. Wright's stain (original magnification ×1,000).

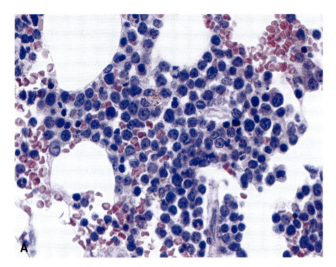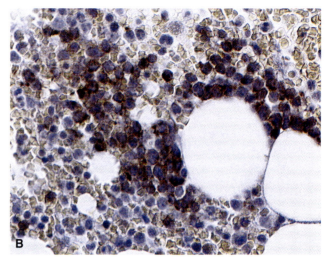

Figure 4–55.   This composite illustrates bone marrow infiltration by acute lymphoblastic leukemia in hematoxylin and eosin stain sections (*A*) and by immunoperoxidase for CD34 staining highlighting a focus of blasts (*B*) (original magnification ×300).

WHO classification of ALL incorporates genotype into the classification system (Table 4–15)[2,74]

Although the blood findings are variable, most patients with ALL present with evidence of bone marrow failure, resulting in severe hematopoietic cytopenias. In conjunction with these cytopenias, circulating leukemic cells are generally evident; some patients present with a striking lymphocytosis.

Cases of ALL can be classified according to the traditional FAB classification system or the recently proposed WHO classification system that attempts to identify specific clinical pathologic entities within the broad group of ALL (see Tables 4–1, 4–2, and 4–15).

The morphologic features of lymphoblasts are highlighted on Tables 4–6 and 4–15. Both within the peripheral blood and bone marrow aspirate smears, lymphoblasts in adult patients with ALL generally exhibit finely dispersed nuclear chromatin, convoluted nuclear contours, variably conspicuous nucleoli, and variable amounts of cytoplasm (Figure 4–54). Burkitt's leukemia/lymphoma or ALL L3 by FAB criteria is only rarely encountered in adults and is most frequently associated with underlying acquired immunodeficiency syndrome (AIDS).[74] These Burkitt's leukemia/lymphoma cells are morphologically distinctive with round nuclear contours, inconspicuous nucleoli, and moderate amounts of distinctly basophilic cytoplasm containing numerous prominent cytoplasmic vacuoles (see Figure 4–5).

On bone marrow biopsy sections, virtually the entire hematopoietic cavity is typically infiltrated by lymphoblasts.[74] The nuclei of these blasts on tissue sections are often closely juxtaposed secondary to the scant amounts of cytoplasm in these cells. The nuclei are round to convoluted and exhibit finely dispersed, stippled chromatin. Nucleoli are variable but generally inconspicuous. Mitotic activity may be brisk, and tingible body macrophages are occasionally noted (Figure 4–55). In contrast, the appearance of Burkitt's leukemia/lymphoma on bone marrow biopsy sections is quite distinctive. These leukemic cells on sections are generally homogeneous and have round nuclear contours with one to three small basophilic nucleoli. Mitotic activity is generally abundant, and a starry sky pattern may be identified, similar to that seen in other tissues involved by Burkitt's lymphoma.

Other less common findings on bone marrow sections of ALL include reticulin fibrosis, necrosis, and bony abnormalities such as osteopenia.[74] All of these features are encountered in only a minority of bone marrow specimens obtained in patients. Resolution of fibrosis and bony changes generally occurs after successful induction chemotherapy.

CONCLUSION

Although morphology forms the foundation for the approach to both the acute and chronic leukemias in adult patients, the final diagnosis in these diverse types of leukemia is generally dependent on the integration of morphology, clinical findings, immunophenotype, and genotype. Recently proposed classification systems for both acute and chronic leukemias emphasize the systematic approach to these disorders that focuses on lineage and stage of maturation followed by the delineation of distinct clinical pathologic entities whenever feasible. In addition to cytologic features, evaluation of overall bone marrow architecture has utility in patients with acute and chronic leukemias, especially those with chronic myeloid disorders such as myelodysplasia and chronic myeloproliferative processes.

REFERENCES

1. Bennett JM, Catovsky D, Daniel MT, et al. Proposals for the classification of the acute leukaemias. French-American-British (FAB) Co-operative Group. Br J Haematol 1976;33:451–8.

2. Harris NL, Jaffe ES, Diebold J, et al. World Health Organization classification of neoplastic diseases of the hematopoietic and lymphoid tissues. Report of the Clinical Advisory Committee Meeting-Airlie House, Virginia, November 1997. J Clin Oncol 1999;17:3835–49.

3. Bennett JM, Catovsky D, Daniel MT, et al. Proposed revised criteria for the classification of acute myeloid leukemia. A report of the French-American-British Cooperative Group. Ann Intern Med 1985;103:620–5.

4. Bennett JM, Catovsky D, Daniel MT, et al. Criteria for the diagnosis of acute leukemia of megakaryocyte lineage (M7). A report of the French-American-British Cooperative Group. Ann Intern Med 1985;103:460–2.

5. Bennett JM, Catovsky D, Daniel MT, et al. Proposals for the classification of chronic (mature) B and T lymphoid leukaemias. French-American-British (FAB) Cooperative Group. J Clin Pathol 1989;42:567–84.

6. Foucar K. Acute myelogenous leukemia. In: Bone marrow pathology. 2nd ed. Chicago: ASCP Press; 2001. p. 263–312.

7. Dayton VD, Arthur DC, Gajl-Peczalska KJ, Brunning R. L3 acute lymphoblastic leukemia. Comparison with small noncleaved cell lymphoma involving the bone marrow. Am J Clin Pathol 1994;101:130–9.

8. Brunning RD, McKenna RW. Acute leukemias. In: Brunning RD, McKenna RW, editors. Tumors of the bone marrow. Vol. 9. Third Series, Fascicle 9. Washington, DC: Armed Forces Institute of Pathology; 1994. p. 19–142.

9. Taylor CG, Stasi R, Bastianelli C, et al. Diagnosis and classification of the acute leukemias: recent advances and controversial issues. Hematopathol Mol Hematol 1996;10:1–38.

10. Casasnovas RO, Campos L, Mugneret F, et al. Immunophenotypic patterns and cytogenetic anomalies in acute non-lymphoblastic leukemia subtypes: a prospective study of 432 patients. Leukemia 1998;12:34–43.

11. Pui CH, Rivera G, Mirro J, et al. Acute megakaryoblastic leukemia. Blast cell aggregates simulating metastatic tumor. Arch Pathol Lab Med 1985;109:1033–5.

12. Brown DC, Gatter KC. The bone marrow trephine biopsy: a review of normal histology. Histopathology 1993;22:411–22.

13. Naeim F. Topobiology in hematopoiesis. Hematol Pathol 1995;9:107–19.

14. Foucar K. Hematopoiesis and morphologic review of bone marrow. In: Bone marrow pathology. 2nd ed. Chicago: ASCP Press; 2001. p. 1–29.

15. Wickramasinghe SN. Bone marrow. In: Sternberg SS, editor. Histology for pathologists. New York: Raven Press; 1992. p. 1–31.

16. Scott J, Moore J, Dean T, et al. Utility of bone marrow architecture in the diagnosis of myelodysplasia (MDS) [abstract]. Mod Pathol 2000;13:163.

17. Vitrat N, Cohen-Solal K, Pique C, et al. Endomitosis of human megakaryocytes are due to abortive mitosis. Blood 1998;91:3711–23.

18. Sieff CA, Nathan DG, Clark SC. The anatomy and physiology of hematopoiesis. In: Nathan DG, Orkin SH, editors. Hematology of infancy and childhood. Vol. 1. Philadelphia: WB Saunders; 1998. p. 161–236.

19. Dickstein JI, Vardiman JW. Hematopathologic findings in the myeloproliferative disorders. Semin Oncol 1995;22:355–73.

20. Anastasi J, Vardiman JW. Chronic myelogenous leukemia and the myeloproliferative disorders. In: Knowles DM, editor. Neoplastic hematopathology. Baltimore: Williams & Wilkins; 2000. p. 1745–90.

21. Foucar K. Chronic myeloproliferative disorders. Bone marrow pathology. 2nd ed. Chicago: ASCP Press; 2001. p. 175–223.

22. Murphy S. Diagnostic criteria and prognosis in polycythemia vera and essential thrombocythemia. Semin Hematol 1999;36:9–13.

23. Thijsen S, Schuurhuis G, van Oostveen J, Ossenkoppele G. Chronic myeloid leukemia from basics to bedside. Leukemia 1999;13:1646–74.

24. Kantarjian HM, Giles FJ, O'Brien SM, Talpaz M. Clinical course and therapy of chronic myelogenous leukemia with interferon-alpha and chemotherapy. Hematol Oncol Clin North Am 1998;12:31–80.

25. Griesshammer M, Heinze B, Hellmann A, et al. Chronic myelogenous leukemia in blast crisis: retrospective analysis of prognostic factors in 90 patients. Ann Hematol 1996;73:225–30.

26. Bennett JM, Catovsky D, Daniel MT, et al. The chronic myeloid leukaemias: guidelines for distinguishing chronic granulocytic, atypical chronic myeloid, and chronic myelomonocytic leukaemia. Proposals by the French-American-British Cooperative Leukaemia Group. Br J Haematol 1994;87: 746–54.

27. Michaux JL, Martiat P. Chronic myelomonocytic leukaemia (CMML)—a myelodysplastic or myeloproliferative syndrome? Leuk Lymphoma 1993;9:35–41.

28. Willman CL. Molecular genetic features of myelodysplastic syndromes (MDS). Leukemia 1998;12 (Suppl 1):S2–6.

29. Foucar K. Myelodysplastic syndrome. In: Bone marrow pathology. 2nd ed. Chicago: ASCP Press; 2001. p. 225–61.

30. Parker JE, Mufti GJ. Ineffective haemopoiesis and apoptosis in myelodysplastic syndromes. Br J Haematol 1998;101:220–30.

31. Head DR. Revised classification of acute myeloid leukemia. Leukemia 1996;10:1826–31.

32. Radlund A, Thiede T, Hansen S, et al. Incidence of myelodysplastic syndromes in a Swedish population. Eur J Haematol 1995;54:153–6.

33. West RR, Stafford DA, Farrow A, Jacobs A. Occupational and environmental exposures and myelodysplasia: a case-control study. Leuk Res 1995;19:127–39.

34. Rigolin GM, Cuneo A, Roberti MG, et al. Exposure to myelotoxic agents and myelodysplasia: case-control study and correlation with clinicobiological findings. Br J Haematol 1998;103:189–97.

35. Greenberg P, Cox C, LeBeau MM, et al. International scoring system for evaluating prognosis in myelodysplastic syndromes. Blood 1997;89:2079–88.

36. Willman CL. Molecular evaluation of acute myeloid leukemias. Semin Hematol 1999;36:390–400.

37. Weinstein HJ. Acute myelogenous leukemia in infants and children. In: Henderson ES, Lister TA, Greaves MF, editors. Leukemia. Philadelphia: WB Saunders; 1996. p. 509–12.

38. Hoff PM, Pierce S, Estey E. Comparison of acute myeloid leukemia patients at MD Anderson: 1982–1986 vs 1992–1996. Leukemia 1997;11:1997–8.

39. Bhatia S, Neglia JP. Epidemiology of childhood acute myelogenous leukemia. J Pediatr Hematol Oncol 1995;17:94–100.

40. Thirman MJ, Larson RA. Therapy-related myeloid leukemia. Hematol Oncol Clin North Am 1996; 10:293–320.

41. Tallman MS, Gray R, Bennett JM, et al. Leukemogenic potential of adjuvant chemotherapy for early-stage breast cancer: the Eastern Cooperative Oncology Group experience. J Clin Oncol 1995;13:1557–63.

42. Greaves MF. Aetiology of acute leukaemia. Lancet 1997;349:344–9.

43. Bennett JM, Catovsky D, Daniel MT, et al. Proposal for the recognition of minimally differentiated acute myeloid leukaemia (AML-MO). Br J Haematol 1991;78:325–9.

44. Nakamura H, Kuriyama K, Sadamori N, et al. Morphological subtyping of acute myeloid leukemia with maturation (AML-M2): homogeneous pink-colored cytoplasm of mature neutrophils is most characteristic of AML-M2 with t(8;21). Leukemia 1997;11:651–5.

45. Khalidi HS, Medeiros LJ, Chang KL, et al. The immunophenotype of adult acute myeloid leukemia: high frequency of lymphoid antigen expression and comparison of immunophenotype, French-American-British classification, and karyotypic abnormalities. Am J Clin Pathol 1998;109:211–20.

46. Neame PB, Soamboonsrup P, Leber B, et al. Morphology of acute promyelocytic leukemia with cytogenetic or molecular evidence for the diagnosis: characterization of additional microgranular variants. Am J Hematol 1997;56:131–42.

47. Bennett JM, Catovsky D, Daniel MT, et al. A variant form of hypergranular promyelocytic leukaemia (M3). Br J Haematol 1980;44:169–70.

48. Melnick A, Licht JD. Deconstructing a disease: RAR-alpha, its fusion partners, and their roles in the pathogenesis of acute promyelocytic leukemia. Blood 1999;93:3167–215.

49. Le Beau MM, Larson RA, Bitter MA, et al. Association of an inversion of chromosome 16 with abnormal marrow eosinophils in acute myelomonocytic leukemia. A unique cytogenetic-clinicopathological association. N Engl J Med 1983;309:630–6.

50. DiMartino JF, Cleary ML. MLL rearrangements in haematological malignancies: lessons from clinical and biological studies. Br J Haematol 1999; 106:614–26.

51. Pui CH, Behm FG, Raimondi SC, et al. Secondary acute myeloid leukemia in children treated for acute lymphoid leukemia. N Engl J Med 1989;321: 136–42.

52. Mazzella FM, Kowal-Vern A, Shrit MA, et al. Acute erythroleukemia: evaluation of 48 cases with reference to classification, cell proliferation, cytogenetics, and prognosis. Am J Clin Pathol 1998;110: 590–8.

53. Gahn B, Haase D, Unterhalt M, et al. De novo AML with dysplastic hematopoiesis: cytogenetic and prognostic significance. Leukemia 1996;10:946–51.

54. Kuriyama K, Tomonaga M, Matsuo T, et al. Poor response to intensive chemotherapy in de novo

acute myeloid leukaemia with trilineage myelodysplasia. Br J Haematol 1994;86:767–73.

55. Pedersen-Bjergaard J, Pedersen M, Roulston D, Philip P. Different genetic pathways in leukemogenesis for patients presenting with therapy-related myelodysplasia and therapy-related acute myeloid leukemia. Blood 1995;86:3542–52.

56. De Renzo A, Santoro LF, Notaro R, et al. Acute promyelocytic leukemia after treatment for non-Hodgkin's lymphoma with drugs targeting topoisomerase II. Am J Hematol 1999;60:300–4.

57. Bigoni R, Cuneo A, Roberti MG, et al. Therapy-related adult acute lymphoblastic leukemia with t(4;11)(q21;q23): MLL rearrangement, p53 mutation and multilineage involvement. Leukemia 1999;13:704–7.

58. Foucar K, Leith C. Acute leukemias. In: Collins R, Swerdlow WS, editors. Pediatric hematopathology. Churchill Livingston; 2001.

59. Kroft SH, Finn WG, Peterson LC. The pathology of the chronic lymphoid leukaemias. Blood Rev 1995;9:234–50.

60. Foucar K. Chronic lymphoid leukemias and lymphoproliferative disorders. Mod Pathol 1999;12:141–50.

61. Foucar K. Chronic lymphoproliferative disorders. In: Bone marrow pathology. 2nd ed. Chicago: ASCP Press; 2001. p. 367–405.

62. Jennings CD, Foon KA. Recent advances in flow cytometry: application to the diagnosis of hematologic malignancy. Blood 1997;90:2863–92.

63. Moreau EJ, Matutes E, A'Hern RP, et al. Improvement of the chronic lymphocytic leukemia scoring system with the monoclonal antibody SN8 (CD79b). Am J Clin Pathol 1997;108:378–82.

64. Foucar K. B-chronic lymphocytic leukemia and prolymphocytic leukemia. In: Knowles DK, editor. Neoplastic hematopathology. Baltimore: Williams and Wilkins; 2000. p. 1505–30.

65. Oscier D. Chronic lymphocytic leukaemia. Br J Haematol 1999;105(Suppl 1):1–3.

66. Troussard X, Valensi F, Duchayne E, et al. Splenic lymphoma with villous lymphocytes: clinical presentation, biology and prognostic factors in a series of 100 patients. Br J Haematol 1996;93:731–6.

67. Matutes E, Morilla R, Owusu-Ankomah K, et al. The immunophenotype of splenic lymphoma with villous lymphocytes and its relevance to the differential diagnosis with other B-cell disorders. Blood 1994;83:1558–62.

68. Bartlett NL, Longo DL. T-small lymphocyte disorders. Semin Hematol 1999;36:164–70.

69. Garand R, Goasguen J, Brizard A, et al. Indolent course as a relatively frequent presentation in T-prolymphocytic leukaemia. Br J Haematol 1998;103:488–94.

70. Sood R, Stewart CC, Aplan PD, et al. Neutropenia associated with T-cell large granular lymphocyte leukemia: long-term response to cyclosporine therapy despite persistence of abnormal cells. Blood 1998;91:3372–8.

71. Uchiyama T. Adult T-cell leukemia. Blood Rev 1988;2:232–8.

72. Tsukasaki K, Imaizumi Y, Tawara M, et al. Diversity of leukaemic cell morphology in ATL correlates with prognostic factors, aberrant immunophenotype and defective HTLV-1 genotype. Br J Haematol 1999;105:369–75.

73. Diamandidou E, Cohen PR, Kurzrock R. Mycosis fungoides and Sézary syndrome. Blood 1996;88:2385–409.

74. Foucar K. Acute lymphoblastic leukemia. In: Bone marrow pathology. 2nd ed. Chicago: ASCP Press; 2001. p. 485–514.

75. Moore TA, Zlotnik A. T-cell lineage commitment and cytokine responses of thymic progenitors. Blood 1995;86:1850–60.

76. Lucio P, Parreira A, van den Beemd MW, et al. Flow cytometric analysis of normal B cell differentiation: a frame of reference for the detection of minimal residual disease in precursor-B-ALL. Leukemia 1999;13:419–27.

77. Spits H, Lanier LL, Phillips JH. Development of human T and natural killer cells. Blood 1995;85:2654–70.

78. Dworzak MN, Fritsch G, Froschl G, et al. Four-color flow cytometric investigation of terminal deoxynucleotidyl transferase-positive lymphoid precursors in pediatric bone marrow: CD79a expression precedes CD19 in early B-cell ontogeny. Blood 1998;92:3203–9.

5

Immunophenotyping of Adult Leukemia

ELISABETH PAIETTA, PhD

Modern laboratory techniques represent an integral part of today's work-up and management for any patient presenting with leukemia. The hematopoietic malignancies offer an excellent example of how the application of special laboratory techniques has advanced the role of cytobiology to a highly practical level in terms of patient diagnosis, management, and, ultimately, prognosis.

VALUE OF IMMUNOPHENOTYPING IN THE CLASSIFICATION OF LEUKEMIAS

There are several major reasons why immunophenotyping is essential in the laboratory assessment of every leukemia patient, starting at the time of diagnosis and continuing through remission and, if applicable, relapse. By no means, however, should immunophenotyping be the only diagnostic tool employed. It must be emphasized that only a multifaceted laboratory approach that combines morphology, immunophenotyping, and cytogenetic and selected molecular analyses provides the scientific information essential for optimal care of patients.

DIAGNOSIS

Immunophenotypic evidence of differentiation defects or maturation arrest provides first clues to the lineage affiliation of a leukemia population. Lineage affiliation, in turn, will determine treatment options, as will certain immunophenotypic findings that have proven prognostic implications. Although phenotyping is feasible on frozen sections from bone marrow biopsies and even on paraffin sections, flow cytometric testing of bone marrow aspirates or heparinized peripheral blood is the preferred method. Flow cytometry allows the accurate delineation of antigen profiles that constitute the aberrant leukemic phenotype. Since normal and leukemic cells share the same hematopoietic antigens, demonstrating antigen combinations or disease subtype-specific antigen expression patterns, rather than single antigens, is the major focus of immunophenotyping.

Exceptions to the statement that leukemia-specific antigens do not exist are pathognomonic novel proteins that are generated as the result of disease subtype-specific chromosomal translocations. Antibodies to a few of these unique proteins have been produced but have been studied as therapeutic rather than diagnostic reagents.

Immunophenotyping goes beyond the classic morphologic classification of the leukemias as it eliminates subjective judgment and relies on reproducible biologic measurements and interpretations. Given that the morphology-based French-American-British (FAB) system was the first leukemia classification system, several current clinical trials still require a diagnosis based on morphology and cytochemistry and use immunologic markers to supplement rather than determine diagnosis. This has led to numerous publications on aberrant phenotypes when myeloid antigens were detected on blasts with lymphoid morphology and vice versa and their clinical responsiveness. Although we now know that lineage overlap does exist in leukemia, many of these reports were based on false assumptions. The fact is that leukemia immunophenotypes show no or little (the exception being M3 acute promyelocytic leukemia [APL]) correlation with the morphology- and cytochemistry-based subclasses in the FAB system. Antigen expression patterns cross the borders between FAB subclasses. Morphology and immunophenotyping constitute two distinct means of leukemia cell characterization providing diverse information. For instance, in a patient with differentiated acute myeloid leukemia (AML), morphologic examination may report the presence of Auer rods, a cellular feature not seen by immunophenotyping. In that patient, immunologic analysis may demonstrate combined expression of CD19 (a B-cell–associated antigen) and CD56 (a natural killer [NK] cell marker) on otherwise typical myeloblasts, a pattern associated with the chromosomal (8;21) translocation. This patient will be diagnosed as AML with t(8;21), which will predict this patient's prognosis.

The ultimate goal of an immunophenotypic classification system is classification based on prognosis. Whether immunophenotyping alone contributes to clinical prognosis (eg, in the case of CD11b+ AML or NK cell AML) or whether it is used for pre-screening, which may curtail cytogenetic or molecular testing (eg, with CD19/CD56 in AML with t[8;21] or CD25 in Philadelphia [Ph] chromosome-positive acute lymphocytic leukemia [ALL]), immunophenotyping focuses on the diagnosis of leukemia phenotypes with prognostic implications or specific treatment requirements.

PROGNOSIS

Proposals for the prognostic implications of leukemia immunophenotyping are varied. Unfortunately, their reproducibility has been limited when single antigens are concerned. For instance, expression of CD7 by leukemic myeloblasts has been repeatedly associated with poor prognosis in some studies but not in others. Reasons for such discrepancies lie in the premature publication of data, based on small cohorts of patients, in the analysis of heterogeneous groups of patients (ie, not stratified by cytogenetic findings or age) and in the use of arbitrary rather than biologically determined cutoff points for defining antigen positivity. Various com-

puter-aided models have recently been developed that address these pitfalls and promise to enhance the prognostic significance of immunophenotyping.[1,2]

PHENOTYPE-SPECIFIC THERAPY

That phenotype-specific therapy should be the ultimate goal in leukemia management is demonstrated by the success of retinoic acid treatment in APL.[3] This disease exemplifies the importance of detailed immunophenotyping in recognizing subtle differences in antigen expression that may translate into major differences in therapeutic responsiveness of patients. The association of certain antigens with cytogenetic abnormalities of proven prognostic implication provides another step toward achieving that goal (eg, CD19/CD56 expression in AML with t[8;21], an AML subtype with particular sensitivity to high-dose cytosine arabinoside). Although the goal is to develop new or better therapeutic agents on a more mechanistic basis, as was the case in APL, it is important to continue to identify leukemia subtypes with established clinical relevance, even though the therapeutic consequences may currently be unknown (eg, CD11b-positive AML or undifferentiated AML).

MINIMAL RESIDUAL DISEASE

Establishing the specific antigen profile or immunologic fingerprint of a leukemic cell population in individual patients at the time of presentation will allow monitoring of disease activity by serial immunophenotyping.[4] During clinical and hematologic complete remission, the detection of minimal residual disease (MRD) may prompt the clinician to initiate reinduction therapy or undertake other therapeutic measures such as immunomodulatory interventions. Conversely, occult leukemia can be discovered in stem cell harvests, which may encourage purging or be correlated with the patient's clinical course after transplant. The complexity of most leukemic antigen profiles facilitates the recognition of low-level disease among predominantly normal hematopoiesis.[5] One caveat to keep in mind when acute leukemias are monitored is the appearance of increased normal precursor cells in recovering bone marrow after chemotherapy. These cells may be mistaken for persistent leukemia if the leukemic immunophenotype resembled that of normal precursor cells. For example, we and others have seen fluctuating numbers of terminal deoxynucleotidyl transferase (TdT)-positive lymphoblasts in marrows of patients with ALL in remission that did not correlate with disease activity or prognosis. In such cases, the detail and sophistication of immunophenotypic analysis executed at diagnosis will pay off and reveal crucial differences between rare leukemic cells and normal regeneration. Depending on diagnosis, limited antibody studies may occasionally suffice for the detection of MRD. Even with the most sophisticated flow cytometric analyses, however, we must admit to the limitations of immunologic MRD in terms of sensitivity, which is clearly inferior to the level achieved by molecular techniques. However, given that several studies have suggested significant correlations between immunologic MRD status and clinical outcome, this lesser sensitivity may not necessarily represent a negative aspect but rather an advantage. Whether molecular remission is the clinically significant goal that treatment must aim for or whether immunologic remission is sufficient for long-term disease-free survival or even cure is still a matter of controversy.

RELAPSE

Early prediction of relapse based on a patient's original immunophenotype may be complicated by changes in antigen expression patterns at the time of recurrence. The literature suggests that ALL phenotypes are quite sturdy, whereas relapsed AML phenotypes differ frequently from original diagnostic findings. In our experience, antigen profiles are surprisingly robust in the majority of leukemia patients who relapse. In ALL, the most common change was a loss or gain of CD10, suggesting a less or more differentiated immunophenotype, respectively. On the other hand, leukemia-specific expression of myeloid markers by the lymphoblasts was usually maintained. The same was true in AML, where relapse cells may present with a lesser or greater degree of myeloid or monocytic differentiation, whereas leukemia-specific features such as expres-

sion of lymphoid antigens by the myeloblasts were conserved. Whether relapse is suspected or already clinically confirmed, it is recommended to re-employ the same detailed antibody panels used at the time of presentation to account for possible deviations from the initial phenotype and to be prepared for unexpected immunophenotypic diagnoses, such as in the case of secondary myeloid leukemia after chemotherapy for a primary lymphoid malignancy.

FLOW CYTOMETRY

The principle behind multiparameter flow cytometry is the simultaneous measurement of physical (eg, estimated size and cytoplasmic granularity) and fluorescent parameters of single cells as they pass through the focused beam of a laser. Cells are stained with one or several antibodies that are conjugated to different fluorochromes (eg, fluorescein isothiocyanate [FITC], phycoerythrin [PE]). When an antibody (ie, fluorochrome) binds to a cell, the fluorescent dye is excited to a higher energy state as the cell passes through the laser beam, and the presence and intensity of the emitted fluorescence signal are detected and recorded. Since cells are simultaneously exposed to fluorochromes that emit light at distinct wavelengths, the different colors of these fluorochromes can be recorded separately. Per minute, 10,000 to 100,000 cells or events can be recorded, and their nonfluorescent light-scattering and fluorescent properties are subsequently selectively analyzed.

Gating on Leukemic Cells

It cannot be emphasized enough that immunophenotypic data must be derived from gated leukemic cells. As was discussed earlier, there are no leukemia-specific antigens, only leukemia-specific antigen expression patterns. When employing flow cytometric analysis of peripheral blood or bone marrow for leukemia immunophenotyping, it is therefore important to be able to separate the leukemic cells from normal hematopoiesis. This is particularly true when small numbers of blast cells are to be localized among a majority of normal hematopoietic cells, for instance, at the time of clinical remission when the detection of MRD or early relapse may alter the clinical management of a patient. Figure 5–1 illustrates how a small subpopulation of blasts can be selected from the heterogeneous mononuclear cell fraction of a bone marrow. In the example chosen, the dot plot (with each dot representing one cell) of the myeloid and lymphoid populations in this bone marrow demonstrates a normal distribution of cells with regard to size and granularity (A). Based on these physical characteristics, nonviable cells and debris can be gated from the population of interest (Gate R1). To reveal subpopulations, for instance, blast cells, which cannot be distinguished from the normal cells based on nonfluorescent, light-

scatter characteristics, the whole cell population is exposed to an antibody chosen to select the cell type of interest. For instance, in Figure 5–1, we chose CD34, an antibody that stains hematopoietic precursor cells and is expressed by a large percentage of acute leukemias. Flow analysis of CD34 fluorescence in a contour plot (B) reveals a small population of immature, CD34-expressing hematopoietic cells that can now be selected by a second gate (Gate R2) and analyzed separately from CD34-negative cells. Given that CD34 is shared by both normal and leukemic cells, the CD34-expressing cells must be characterized further for their antigen expression

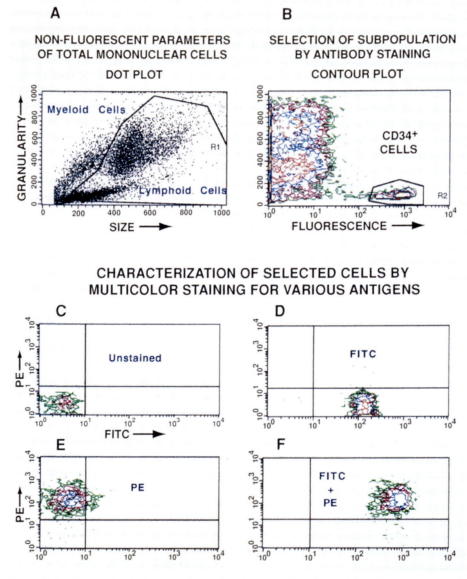

Figure 5–1. Concept of leukemia cell detection by flow cytometry and their immunophenotypic characterization.

pattern. Again, the entire cell population is exposed to additional antibodies, but analysis is restricted to cells of interest. Antibodies conjugated to fluorochromes different from those used for CD34 detection (eg, FITC and PE) are subsequently tested to reveal the immunophenotype of cells selected based on CD34 expression. Autofluorescence and fluorescence caused by nonspecific binding of control immunoglobulins (Igs) define the "negative" or "unstained" cell population (C). In the presence of one FITC-conjugated and one PE-conjugated specific antibody, cells may bind the FITC-conjugated antibody alone and appear only in the lower right quadrant, with increasing fluorescence along the X-axis (D), or cells may stain only with the PE-conjugated antibody and appear in the upper left quadrant with increasing fluorescence along the Y-axis (E), or cells may bind both antibodies and appear in the upper right quadrant (F).

Thus, flow cytometry is more efficient than conventional fluorescent microscopy in terms of cell numbers analyzed and the multiplicity of parameters recorded; it is more sensitive in detecting differences in fluorescence intensities among cell subpopulations that may be exploited diagnostically, and it is more sensitive in detecting small numbers of abnormal cells. Provided that the antibodies tested are chosen with knowledge of hematopoietic antigen expression patterns and that interpretations are left in the hands of experienced immunobiologists, this approach will yield a diagnostic or informative immunophenotype in nearly 100 percent of cases. Moreover, there are strong implications for using the flow cytometer for performing functional assays that reflect clinically relevant biologic cell properties, such as multidrug resistance or apoptosis.

CHOICE OF ANTIBODIES

Seven International Workshops on Human Leukocyte Differentiation Antigens, the last one held in 2000, have defined 247 clusters of differentiation (CDs). Proceedings of the 6th Workshop are the latest published to date.[6] Each cluster contains more than one antibody found to recognize the same antigen. The hierarchy of CDs follows the timeline of their designation. Since early antibodies were directed predominantly against lymphoid antigens, the first CDs cover mostly T- and B-lymphoid antigens. The choice of antibodies tested depends on the purpose of the analysis. Using smaller diagnostic antibody panels will limit costs more efficiently than the use of research panels that aim at defining new leukemia subsets or discerning novel prognostic markers. Table 5–1 summarizes the various classes of antibodies and antigens that may be useful in the characterization of leukemias. To keep matters simple, some antigens are represented by their functional designation only (eg, activation antigens); others are listed in the context of a certain hematopoietic cell lineage, indicating that they may be useful in defining lineage affiliation. There is substantial overlap in antigen expression between cell lineages so that the majority of antibody/antigens should be considered lineage associated rather than lineage specific.

For the clinical laboratory focusing predominantly on leukemia diagnosis, the overabundance of antibodies clustered, most of them commercially

Table 5–1. ANTIBODIES (CDs) AND ANTIGENS IN LEUKEMIA IMMUNOPHENOTYPING				
Lineage-Uncommitted	**Myeloid**	**Lymphoid**	**Erythroid/Megakaryocytic**	**Natural Killer Cells**
CD34	MPO	TdT	CD71	CD56
HLA-DR	CD117	CD1-10	CD36	CD57
CD38	CD33	CD19-24	H-ag	CD16
Activation antigens	CD13	CD40	Glycophorin	
Adhesion molecules	CD65s	CD74	CD31	
Drug resistance	CD15(s)	CD79a	CD41	
Leukocyte antigens (CD45,CD52)	CD11b	CD79b	CD42	
	CD14	CD103	CD61	
	CD64	CD138		
	CD68			
	Lactoferrin			

H-ag = bloodgroup-H antigen; MPO = myeloperoxidase.

available, may be tempting but financially oppressive. In the chronic leukemias, lineage overlap is less of a concern, and, despite some degree of variability, consensus exists regarding immunophenotypic features diagnostic of certain disease entities. In the acute leukemias, a minimal antibody panel, as illustrated in Figure 5–2, will reliably distinguish between myeloid and lymphoid leukemia. The overlapping circles reflect shared antigen expression between lineages, and only few markers appear to be lineage specific. Those are myeloperoxidase (MPO) for the myeloid series and intracytoplasmic CD3 for the T- and intracytoplasmic CD22 for the B-cell lineage. The reliability of these markers for their respective lineages has been established beyond question. Although such a skeleton panel will be helpful when limited material is available for testing or under extreme time or financial constraints, clinically essential subtype characterizations, such as the differentiation of APL from natural NK cell AML (NK-AML), will not be accomplished.

EXPRESSION OF PRESUMED LINEAGE FOREIGN ANTIGENS IN LEUKEMIA

As we discussed in the previous section, there are several lineage-affiliated but only few lineage-specific antigens. If a given leukemia population is assigned to a certain cell lineage based on the presence of a lineage-specific antigen (eg, cytoplasmic CD22 defining B-lineage ALL), how should one interpret the simultaneous presence of one or more antigens affiliated with another cell lineage (eg, CD33)? The nomenclature for leukemias expressing lineage-foreign antigens is highly variable. The European Group for the Immunological Characterization of Leukemias (EGIL) established a scoring system for the definition of biphenotypic leukemias that assigns a point value to every lineage-foreign antigen.[7] Although an interesting attempt to standardize the interpretation of flow cytometry results, this system, established several years ago, does not incorporate our current knowledge of antigenic diversity among the leukemias. For instance, expression of two myeloid antigens (eg, CD13 and CD33) by ALL blast cells is not at all uncommon and should never yield a diagnosis of biphenotypic leukemia. However, this is exactly what the EGIL system would imply.

Before any discussion of lineage-foreign antigen expression can be entertained, it is essential to demonstrate that a lineage-foreign antigen is actually expressed by the leukemic blast cells. Furthermore, the use of arbitrary cutoff points for the definition of biphenotypic leukemias is discouraged. If we limit our data collection to the leukemic cell population by identifying the blast cells based on anti-

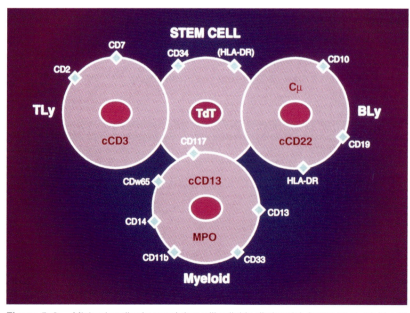

Figure 5–2. Minimal antibody panel that will reliably distinguish between myeloid and lymphoid leukemias.

gen expression, then the observation of any percentage of cells expressing a lineage-foreign antigen is noteworthy. Whether this observation is of clinical relevance and may eventually lead to the definition of a new leukemia subtype will depend on the result of retrospective analyses of large numbers of patients. Until the prognostic significance of certain lineage-foreign antigens is proven, we should record our immunophenotypic observations without altering the basic diagnosis. For example, a case of AML expressing CD7 and TdT should be described as such; we already have sufficient data to dismiss a prognostic significance of TdT expression in AML; that of CD7 is still under investigation.

ACUTE VERSUS CHRONIC LEUKEMIAS

The degree of cellular maturation constitutes the major biologic difference between the acute and chronic leukemias. Immaturity and aggressive clinical course are hallmarks of the acute leukemias, whereas the term *chronic* is synonymous with a more mature stage of lymphoid or myeloid differentiation. For some of the major established leukemia subtypes, normal counterparts have been tentatively postulated, although such grouping according to normal developmental stages remains debatable. Although understanding the relationship between leukemic and normal hematopoiesis may assist in the categorization of the leukemias, there is currently no evidence that it will advance treatment strategies.

ACUTE LEUKEMIAS

The categorization of the acute leukemias according to antigen expression patterns relies on the finding of lineage-associated antigens on the cell surface or in the cytoplasm. With the introduction of antibodies to the earliest lineage-committed antigens known to date, the number of leukemias that resist lineage assignment has decreased to less than 1 percent.

Lineage-Negative or Truly Undifferentiated Acute Leukemia

Truly undifferentiated, lineage-antigen negative stem cell leukemia, expressing only CD34, human leuko-

cyte antigen (HLA)-DR, and occasionally CD7 or TdT, is exceedingly rare (< 1% of acute leukemias) and bears no relationship to the morphologic diagnosis of undifferentiated AML (FAB M0). Most cases of presumed immunologically undifferentiated acute leukemia can be reclassified to a certain cell lineage by more precise testing, particularly for the intracytoplasmic antigens MPO, CD3, and CD22. Detection of one of these antigens in the undifferentiated blast cells is sufficient for diagnosis. Of additional help may be CD117, an antigen assigned to the myeloid lineage. However, we have seen CD117 expression in rare, very immature T-lymphoid leukemias recognized only by the presence of intracytoplasmic CD3. Clinical information is limited; however, this immunophenotype does not appear to confer an adverse prognosis.

Acute Lymphocytic Leukemia

The simple classification into early, more immature, and late ALL subtypes no longer bears strong prognostic significance. Despite many years of immunophenotyping adult ALL, several questions have remained unanswered—for instance, the question of whether myeloid antigen expression on the lymphoblasts may have any impact on disease outcome. Originally thought to be a rare occurrence, the more myeloid antigens are tested, the more they are detected on lymphoid leukemic cells. In a large intergroup trial of adult ALL, we found the expression of one or more myeloid antigens in the majority of patients. Any conclusions regarding the clinical significance of this observation have to await closure of the study. Based on the results of these statistical analyses, we will define new ALL subtypes characterized by specific antigen expression patterns with prognostic significance.

Cytogenetic (eg, Ph positivity, t[4;11]) and particularly molecular evidence (eg, *BCR/ABL, AF4/MLL* fusion genes) are increasingly used for predicting outcome in ALL. Certain antigens or patterns of antigen expression have been associated with some of these genetic aberrations (eg, CD25 expression with Ph-positive ALL).[8] As a result, immunophenotypic prescreening of ALL patients for favorable or unfavorable molecular genetic features may soon become routine. Table 5–2 summarizes cytogenetic abnormalities that are associated with specific immunophenotypic features in B-lineage ALL and that are discussed in more detail below. With this in mind, antibody panels in ALL typing should exceed those used for standard diagnosis to allow for retrospective analyses that might reveal hitherto undisclosed associations between immunophenotypic features and specific genetic defects.

Antigen-Specific Receptors in ALL

The multitude of specific antigen recognition by mature lymphocytes is mediated by surface-bound Igs on B cells and T-cell receptors (TCR) on T cells. Normal rearrangements occur between the variable (V), diverse (D), joining (J), and constant (C) segments of these genes. During recombination, nucleotides can be randomly deleted from the germline gene segments or inserted, probably through the activity of TdT polymerase. This creates a unique DNA sequence that is specific for each individual lymphocyte and its progeny and, therefore, provides a clone-specific genetic marker that assists in the detection of monoclonality and the monitoring of MRD in ALL.

The Igs consist of pairs of disulfide-linked heavy and light chains. Each lymphocyte will only express either kappa or lambda light chains. Monoclonality of a given B-cell population for Ig light-chain expression suggests a malignant process.

Mature T lymphocytes express either a TCR composed of alpha and beta subunits (majority of T cells) or of gamma and delta chains (< 1 to 20% of T cells), which can be detected with specific antibodies. Typically, CD3-positive gamma/delta T lymphocytes lack both CD4 and CD8 expression, whereas virtually all CD3-positive alpha/beta T cells express either CD4 or CD8.

Immunoglobulin heavy-chain or TCR gene rearrangements are not diagnostic of B- or T-lineage ALL as cross-lineage somatic gene rearrangements occur in 10 to 15 percent of cases. Chromosomal aberrations that involve Ig or TCR loci are predictive of the immunophenotype. The Ig heavy-chain locus is at 14q32, Ig kappa maps to 2p12, and Ig lambda to 22q11, and the TCR-alpha and delta genes are located on chromosome 14q11, the TCR-beta genes on chromosome 7q35, and the TCR-gamma genes on chromosome 7p14.

ALL Subtypes

The separation into B- and T-lineage ALL relies on the expression of respective lineage-associated antigens. Antigens shared by T- and B-ALL subtypes, such as TdT, CD45, CD34, and HLA-DR, are those expressed by the lymphoid stem cell.

Terminal Deoxynucleotidyl Transferase. Terminal deoxynucleotidyl transferase detection was one of the first diagnostic tools in ALL and was initially thought to be lymphoid specific. More recently, TdT has been described in a large proportion of patients with AML. Differences in the staining intensity for TdT, detectable only by flow cytometry, allow the distinction between TdT expression in ALL and AML.[9] Because of the weak staining pattern of TdT in AML, the choice of antibodies in flow cytometric TdT analysis is crucial. Only monoclonal, directly fluorochrome-conjugated anti-TdT antibody is recommended.

Figure 5–3 illustrates the distribution of TdT in the various cell lineages. Although restricted to

Table 5–2. CYTOGENETIC ABNORMALITIES WITH SPECIFIC IMMUNOPHENOTYPIC FEATURES IN B-LINEAGE ALL				
Parameter	t(4;11), (q21;q23)	t(9;22)(q34;q11)	t(1;19)(q23;p13)	t(8;14)(q24;q32), t(2;8)(p11;q24), t(8;22)(q24;q11)
Phenotype	Pre-pre-B (CD10⁻) CD15⁺	Early pre-B (CD10⁺) My Ag+,CD34+,CD25+	Pre-B CD34⁻,CD20±	Mature B CD34⁻,TdT⁻
Molecular consequence	*AF4/MLL* fusion gene	*BCR/ABL* fusion gene	*PBX/E2A* fusion gene	c-myc proto-oncogene under Ig gene control
Prognosis	Poor	Poor	Poor	Poor

My Ag = myeloid antigen.

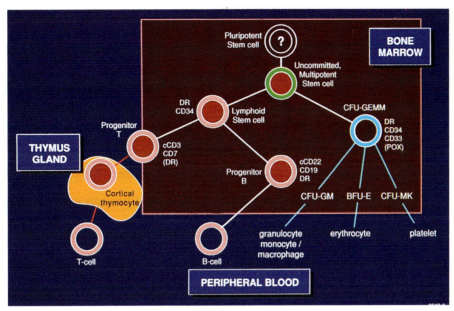

Figure 5–3. TdT distribution in normal hematopoietic cells. Red-colored schematic nuclei represent TdT positivity.

immature lymphoid committed cells and lost with lymphoid maturation, TdT-, CD34-, and HLA-DR-positive cells are part of the multipotent stem cell pool and may represent progenitors of TdT-positive myeloid leukemias.

CD45. The common leukocyte antigen CD45 is expressed by the majority of cases with B-lineage ALL, across all subtypes. However, a small percentage of patients at variable differentiation stages have low or absent CD45, which is a unique finding among the leukemias. Although most data on the prognostic significance of this finding are available from pediatric studies, it is noteworthy that lack of CD45 is associated with chromosomal hyperdiploidy, lower white blood cell counts, and favorable prognosis.

CD34. CD34 is variably expressed throughout B- and T-lineage ALL. As a general rule, the more mature subtypes demonstrate decreased or infrequent CD34 expression (eg, mature B-ALL). Whether CD34 truly represents an adverse prognostic factor in B-lineage ALL, as suggested by some small studies, awaits confirmation from large multivariate analyses.

HLA-DR. HLA-DR is expressed through all developmental stages of B lymphocytes until the most mature plasma cell stage, which is HLA-DR negative. The same is true for B-lineage ALL. HLA-DR is detected occasionally in T-lineage ALL,

mostly of the more immature type, consistent with the brief expression of this antigen by normal early T-cell progenitor cells; no impact on outcome is associated with this HLA-DR expression.

Myeloid Antigens in ALL. The incidence of myeloid antigen expression in ALL increases with the number of myeloid antigens tested. The two most frequently tested antigens, CD33 and CD13, are detected on approximately 10 percent of ALLs. As a rule, the occurrence of myeloid antigens decreases with increasing lymphoid maturation.

A comprehensive study of myeloid antigens in ALL should include CD65s in addition to CD33 and CD13 as the presence of all three antigens would question the diagnosis of a lymphoid leukemia. The possibility of AML must be considered, particularly in patients with presumed very immature T-ALL (or pro-T ALL) with expression of CD7 as the sole T antigen. The poor prognosis of these patients in pediatric trials may be the result of misdiagnosis.

The CD15 molecule was the first myelomonocytic antigen ever described on TdT-positive leukemic lymphoblasts (Figure 5–4). Prior to the routine use of flow cytometry, we demonstrated double-staining for nuclear TdT and surface staining with CD15 antibody VIM-D5, under the fluorescence microscope. Such expression of myeloid antigens on the surface of otherwise immunophenotypi-

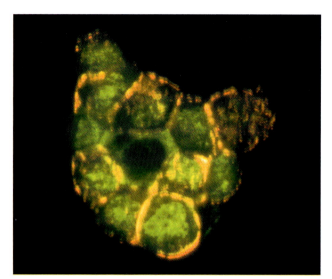

Figure 5–4. Double-staining of leukemic lymphoblasts for intranuclear TdT (green color) and surface CD15 molecule (red color) (original magnification ×400).

cally unquestionable ALL cells is seen much more often than true biclonality with a distinct myeloid leukemia component contributing to a predominantly lymphoid leukemia.

To date, myeloid antigen expression has not affected survival in any of the larger adult or pediatric studies. In the absence of convincing evidence to the contrary, we recommend refraining from confusing the classification of ALL by introducing the term *biphenotypic leukemia*, based on selected myeloid antigen expression. Practical guidelines for the interpretation of myeloid antigen expression in ALL may need to be modified in the future if one or more

myeloid antigens are found to be associated with outcome or with a particular ALL subtype (eg, as defined by a specific cytogenetic or molecular aberration).

The major B- and T-cell–related ALL immunophenotypes are depicted in Figures 5–5 and 5–6, respectively. Their designation as pro, pre, immature or mature, early or late refers to antigen expression patterns observed during early or later normal lymphopoiesis. Recommendations for leukemia subtype nomenclature may vary among treatment centers and have changed over the years; however, the major prognostic conclusions are identical.

B-Lineage ALL Subtypes

As shown in Figure 5–5, the most immature B-lineage ALL is often characterized by the sole expression of intracytoplasmic CD22 in the absence of B-surface markers. Another intracytoplasmic marker of early B-cell differentiation is CD79a, a polypeptide involved in the intracellular signaling that eventually leads to surface Ig expression. This stage is variably termed pro-B, pre–pre-B, null-cell, B1 stage, or CD10-negative early pre-B ALL. The cells contain nuclear TdT. Occasionally, surface CD19 and/or CD24 are detected in support of a B-lineage affiliation. The important feature is absence of CD10. Approximately 10 percent of adult ALLs present with this phenotype. Early trials suggested a poorer outcome with CD10-negative than CD10-positive early pre-B ALL. It appears from the more

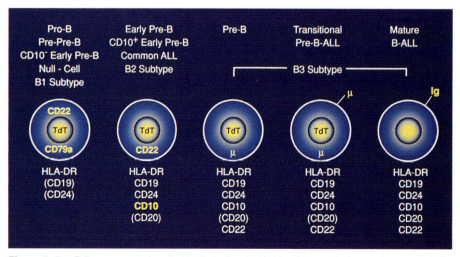

Figure 5–5. B-lineage acute lymphoblastic leukemia (ALL) subtypes. Antigens characteristic for each subtype are in yellow.

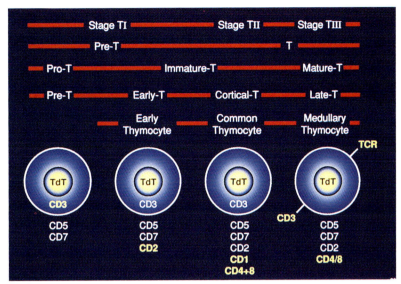

Figure 5–6. T-lineage acute lymphoblastic leukemia (ALL) subtypes. Antigens characteristic for each subtype are in yellow. In most mature T-ALL, TdT may be absent.

recent literature that this difference is diminishing with intensified postremission treatment, even in cases displaying unfavorable cytogenetic abnormalities such as t(4;11)(q21;q23) or its molecular equivalent (*AF4/MLL* fusion transcripts). The t(4;11) is included in Table 5–2, which describes the most prominent features of the major cytogenetic groups in B-lineage ALL.

Expression of CD10 is the cardinal diagnostic finding in early pre-B ALL or B2-stage ALL, previously called common ALL. This is the most common ALL subtype in adults. A substantial fraction of these patients, most of them older in age, will present with the (9;22)(q34;q11) translocation (Ph-positive ALL), which, in all clinical trials reported to date, predicts for poor disease-free survival. Frequently, Ph-positive lymphoblasts express myeloid antigens and are invariably positive for CD34. We have demonstrated that lymphoblasts expressing CD25, the alpha chain of the interleukin-2 receptor, have a high probability of having the Ph chromosome or its molecular equivalent (*BCR/ABL* transcripts).[8] This predictive value of CD25 for the most important negative prognostic indicator in ALL translates into a clinically useful prescreening tool that is quick and inexpensive. A very small percentage of patients with early pre-B ALL contain *TEL/AML1* transcripts that result from cryptic (12;21)(p12;q22) translocation. Despite its low

incidence, this finding is noteworthy since the *TEL/AML1* fusion is the most common genetic abnormality in pediatric ALL and is associated with a good prognosis.

Pre-B ALL is defined by the presence of cytoplasmic IgH (cμ). Its reputation as a poor prognostic indicator appears to result from its frequent (approximately 25% of all pre-B cases) association with t(1;19)(q23;p13), a translocation that at the molecular level results in the creation of the *PBX/E2A* fusion gene. Blast cells with this translocation commonly lack CD34 and often lack CD20. Again, modern treatment strategies have improved the outcome in this disease subtype. More African Americans have been reported to present with this subtype than with early pre-B ALL.

An intermediate stage between pre-B and mature B-ALL is the most recently characterized subtype of transitional pre-B ALL. Lymphoblasts express both intracytoplasmic and surface μ Ig heavy chains without associated Ig light chains. This subtype confers a good prognosis.

Mature B-cell ALL is uncommon in adult ALL (< 10%). As a sign of maturity, cells are negative for TdT but express surface Ig. Because of shared morphologic, immunologic, cytogenetic, and clinical features, mature B-ALL is often considered a leukemic phase of Burkitt's lymphoma. Frequent cytogenetic abnormalities involve translocations with breakpoints near Ig heavy- or light-chain gene loci, such as t(8;14)(q24;q32). In all of these translocations, the c-myc proto-oncogene on chromosome 8 is brought under the control of the involved Ig gene locus (eg, in the case of the t[8;14], under the control of the Ig heavy-chain locus [14q32]). As a result of these gene rearrangements, c-myc expression is deregulated. Improvement in therapy has alleviated the poor prognosis of patients with mature B-ALL, but remission rate and remission duration are still inferior to other ALL subtypes in most clinical trials.

T-Lineage ALL Subtypes

Approximately 20 percent of adult ALL patients present with T-cell immunophenotype. Although T-lineage ALLs appear to do better clinically than B-lineage ALLs overall in some studies, differences have become smaller with the intensification of postremission therapy. As illustrated in Figure 5–6, multiple schemes exist for the categorization of T-lineage ALL. The earliest stage is recognized by the presence of intracytoplasmic CD3, which, in the absence of additional T markers, is diagnostic of T-ALL. The T-cell–associated CD7 antigen alone is not sufficient to make this diagnosis since CD7 is an antigen of early uncommitted hematopoietic precursor cells and is frequently expressed by immature myeloid leukemias. The First Morphologic, Immunologic and Cytogenetic (MIC) Working Classification of ALL suggested dividing T-lineage ALL into T-precursor and T-mature ALL, based only on CD2 expression. More commonly, further subdivisions are made to account for the expression of CD1 and, eventually, the expression of membrane CD3 in the most mature subtype. None of these subgroups, however, differ in outcome. The same is true for the rare subtype of TCR-gamma/delta T-ALL, which is usually positive for surface CD3, CD1, and TdT. It is of interest that TCR-gamma/delta is more often used in T-ALL than TCR-alpha/beta, whereas the opposite is the case with normal T lymphocytes or T-cell lymphoblastic lymphoma.

The one immunophenotypic marker that continues to have prognostic implications in T-ALL in terms of disease-free survival is CD10. During normal T lymphopoiesis, CD10 is transiently expressed at an early stage. CD10-positive T-ALL is often positive for CD1 and rarely for membrane CD3. It is of interest in this context that in normal T lymphocytes, CD10 is a marker for T cells undergoing apoptosis.

CD56-Positive ALL (NK-ALL)

The incidence of CD56-positive ALL is very low.[10] The majority of cases reported to date demonstrate antigenic characteristics typical of early T lymphocytes, such as cytoplasmic CD3, concomitantly with the NK cell marker CD56 but not CD16 or CD57. This is not surprising, given the common developmental pathway of NK cells and T lymphocytes. However, there are occasional cases of CD56-positive non–T-ALL. Outcome information is variable so that the definition of CD56-positive ALL as a distinct entity remains provisional.

Immunologic Minimal Residual Disease in ALL

In a high percentage of patients with ALL, antigenic aberrations of the blast cells constitute an immunophenotypic fingerprint or signature that allows monitoring of the disease at a subclinical level. Figure 5–7 exemplifies detection of MRD in the remission bone marrow of a patient whose immunophenotype fluctuated between Ph-, CD34-, and CD10-positive and CD34-positive, CD10-negative early pre-B and pre–pre-B ALL, respectively, throughout the course of disease. In this case, the immunophenotypic fingerprint relied on co-expression of the myeloid antigen CD13 with B-cell antigens and on the expression of CD25, a surrogate marker for the Ph chromosome.

In CD34-positive leukemias, the primary antibody of choice for detecting low-level blast cells is CD34. Subsequently, however, cells caught in the CD34 gate must be carefully examined to ensure their leukemic nature. Table 5–3 illustrates this in a patient with CD34-, TdT-, CD7-, and CD8-positive T-ALL in hematologic remission. Following therapy, 2 percent of mononuclear cells expressed CD34 and CD7, suspicious of residual leukemia. Flow cytometric analysis of these CD34-positive cells, however, identified them as normal myeloid precursor cells, positive for CD117 and CD33 and negative for TdT.

As discussed earlier, potential pitfalls of immunologic MRD result from insufficient sensitivity levels or therapy-induced changes in the immunophenotypic fingerprint of a given ALL. Still, considering the likely clinical implications of a positive finding, serial flow cytometric testing should be routine in patients with ALL.

Acute Myeloid Leukemia

There is still reluctance among clinical investigators to accept that immunophenotypic patterns, which can often be supplemented with cytogenetic or molecular information, provide a more informative and above all prognostically more relevant classification of AML than does the morphology-based FAB system. Table 5–4 summarizes characteristic antigenic features associated with certain cytogenetic abnormalities. Only by basing subgrouping on reliable and reproducible laboratory parameters will we achieve the ultimate goal of diagnostic consensus and confidence in the majority of cases. Figure 5–8 portrays the major subtypes of AML, undifferentiated AML, differentiated AML, APL, acute myelomonocytic leukemia (AMML), and

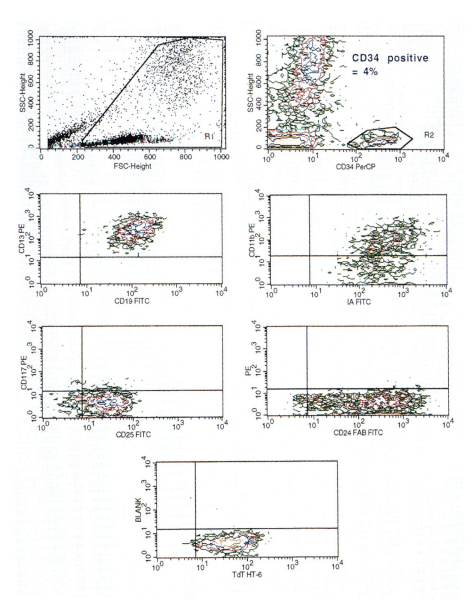

Figure 5–7. Flow cytometric detection of minimal residual disease in a patient with acute lymphoblastic leukemia. Immature cells were selected based on their expression of CD34. Their antigen profile confirms that they are indeed residual lymphoblasts.

Table 5–3. FLOW CYTOMETRIC EVALUATION OF A BONE MARROW FOR MINIMAL RESIDUAL DISEASE IN A PATIENT WITH T-LINEAGE ALL

Disease Status	% CD34	% Antigen Expression in CD34 Gate						
		TdT	CD117	CD7	CD5	CD8	CD33	HLA-DR
Presentation	85	99	0	99	99	90	0	8
Remission	2	0	95	85	0	0	99	99

acute monocytic leukemia (AMOL). Although this nomenclature appears to parallel that of the FAB system, there is very limited concordance between the morphologic and the immunophenotypic features in these subgroups. Incorporated in this figure are novel AML diagnoses that rely exclusively on antigen expression patterns, are sometimes associated with specific cytogenetic abnormalities, and are of clinical relevance, such as NK-AML or CD19- and CD56-positive AML with t(8;21).

Undifferentiated AML

This form of AML is poorly defined. This is explained by the unfortunate fact that minimally differentiated morphology, designated FAB AML M0 in 1991, is used as the primary feature to recognize this subtype. Subsequently, antigenic characteristics were established. The diagnosis of AML M0 demands expression of CD13 and/or CD33, as myeloid markers, and negativity for histochemical MPO activity, as a sign of myeloid immaturity. However, it does not require MPO positivity by antibody staining or negativity for intracytoplasmic CD3 and CD22, the only reliable indicators of an affiliation with the lymphoid lineage. Under these original guidelines, lymphoid leukemias may be included into this subtype.

The proportion of M0 in AML ranges from 2 to 5 percent. Although immunophenotypically hetero-

geneous, certain antigens are observed more frequently in AML M0 than in other FAB types. These are CD34, TdT, and, in some studies, CD7 and the multidrug resistance molecule P-glycoprotein, all antigens associated with a stem cell phenotype. Recurrent cytogenetic abnormalities are trisomy 13, partial or complete loss of chromosomes 5 and 7, and/or a high level of complexity. The likelihood of failing to respond to induction chemotherapy is known to increase significantly with the degree of combined P-glycoprotein/CD34 expression, and this antigen pattern is significantly more likely to occur in patients with monosomy 5 or 7 and/or deletion of the long arm of chromosome 5 or 7. In summary, the poor outcome in AML M0 may be linked to an immature phenotype, positive multidrug resistance status, unfavorable cytogenetics, and older age.

To establish an immunophenotypic subtype, criteria must be based on antigen expression, not on morphologic appearance. We therefore suggest basing the definition of undifferentiated AML on low expression of the myeloid antigen CD65s, which, in normal myelopoiesis, appears at a later stage than CD33 or CD13. Patients with low CD65s AML are older, present with immature morphology (high incidence of M0/M1), and show increased expression of CD34, CD117, and TdT and low expression of MPO and CD15, signs of decreased myeloid maturation compared with differentiated AML.

Table 5–4. ASSOCIATIONS BETWEEN CYTOGENETICS AND ANTIGENS IN AML

Cytogenetics	Antigens										
	Pgp	CD34	CD117	HLA-DR	CD11a	CD7	CD2	CD19	CD56	CD4	TdT
-5/5q-;-7/7q-	+	+	+	+	+	+	–	–	–	+	+
t(8;21)(q22;q22)	–	+	+	+	–	–	–	+	+	+	+
t(15;17)(q22;q11.2)	–	–	+	–	–	–	(+)	–	–	–	–
inv(16)(p13q22)	–	(+)	(+)	+	+	–	+	–	–	+	+
t(9;22)(q34;q11)	(+)	+	+	+	+	–	–	(+)	–	–	+

Positivity and negativity in this table refer to characteristic findings only. See text for more detailed descriptions.
Pgp = P-glycoprotein as established by antibodies to surface epitopes.

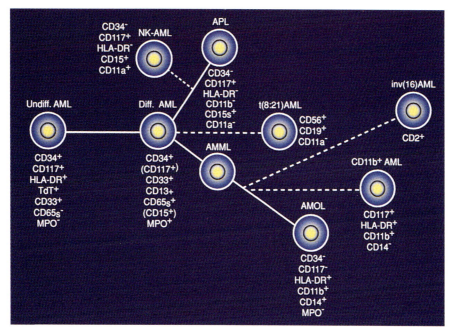

Figure 5–8. Immunophenotypic subtypes in acute myeloid leukemia (AML). Undiff. AML = undifferentiated AML; Diff. AML = differentiated AML; APL = acute promyelocytic leukemia; NK-AML = natural killer cell AML; AMML = acute myelomonocytic leukemia; AMOL = acute monocytic leukemia; MPO = myeloperoxidase; TdT = terminal transferase. Dotted lines connect novel AML subtypes, which are characterized only by immunophenotype and/or cytogenetic abnormality with the major established AML subtypes. MPO in undifferentiated AML may be positive or negative by antibody staining.

Differentiated AML

Four myeloid antigens determine the diagnosis of differentiated AML: MPO, CD33, CD13, and the key antigen, CD65s. Of the more mature myeloid antigens, CD15 may be present, but CD11b is typically absent, as is the monocytic CD14 antigen. Positivity for CD34, CD117, and HLA-DR is common.

CD56- and CD19-Positive AML with t(8;21)

The simultaneous expression of the NK marker CD56 and the B-lymphoid–associated CD19 antigen is a pattern characteristic of AML cells containing the (8;21)(q22;q22) translocation and found in > 50 percent of cases with this cytogenetic aberration.[11] This subtype is not to be confused with CD56-positive NK-AML. Figure 5–9 illustrates an example of a typical flow cytometry picture obtained in the case of CD56- and CD19-positive AML. Although most common in differentiated AML, this phenotype has also been described in immunophenotypically more immature AML (ie, with low MPO and/or CD65s reactivity).

The adhesive properties of CD56, the neural cell adhesion molecule, may contribute to the increased likelihood of extramedullary disease (granulocytic sarcomas) in t(8;21) AML.[12] Baer and colleagues[13] reported shorter remission duration and survival in t(8;21) patients with CD56 expression when compared with those who were CD56 negative. When treatment included high-dose cytosine arabinoside, the prognostic implication of CD56 expression was no longer observed.[14] Additional immunophenotypic characteristics include the absence of another NK marker, CD16, high expression of CD34, frequent finding of TdT- and CD4-positive blasts, and low or absent staining for CD11a. CD11a, a leukocyte adhesion molecule, is expressed by all other AML subtypes, with the exception of APL.

The uniqueness of the CD56- and CD19-positive immunophenotype makes it possible to predict the cytogenetic abnormality with great certainty. It also makes this AML subtype a model for monitoring immunologic MRD and a valuable asset to the molecular detection of minimal disease (*AML1/ETO* fusion gene).

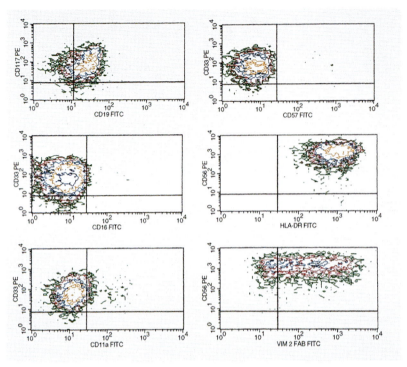

Figure 5–9.   Characteristic antigen profile in a patient with t(8;21) AML. The antigen expression pattern of gated CD34-positive blast cells is shown.

CD11b-Positive AML

CD11b-positive AML is defined by expression of CD11b, an immature monocytic antigen, in the absence of the mature monocytic antigen CD14, on myeloid blast cells.[15] Co-expression of CD11b and HLA-DR is essential to separate CD11b-positive blast cells from mature myeloid cells at and beyond the myelocyte/metamyelocyte stage. This subtype is derived from a response-driven analysis of patients with AML. When compared to AMOL or AML overall, CD11b-positive AML has an impaired prognosis with respect to achievement of complete remission and survival that cannot be explained by age, multidrug resistance status, or cytogenetic abnormalities (Table 5–5). Compared with CD14-positive monocytic leukemia, CD11b-positive leukemia cells show higher expression of CD117

and decreased CD15, both indicators of a more immature stage of differentiation. Although CD117 alone no longer qualifies as a prognostic marker in AML, overall myeloid maturation remains a most significant predictor for outcome.

Acute Promyelocytic Leukemia

Acute promyelocytic leukemia is the paradigm for a disease in which accurate diagnosis is of crucial clinical significance because of its sensitivity to all-*trans* retinoic acid. The diagnostic laboratory finding in APL is the chromosomal (15;17)(q22;q11.2) translocation or the detection of its molecular equivalent, the *PML/RARα* fusion gene.[16] A unique immunophenotype is associated with both the hypergranular and the microgranular variants of this genotype. Its basic characteristics comprise negativity for CD34 and HLA-DR. More recently, non-APL phenotypes have been identified that show these very same antigenic features (eg, NK-AML). This has made it necessary to expand the immunophenotypic definition of APL (Figure 5–10). Added distinctive features of this myeloid phenotype are low or absent P-glycoprotein, low or absent CD11a,

Table 5–5. CD56 EXPRESSION IN APL WITH t(15;17)	
Range	0–99% of leukemic promyelocytes
Median	12% of leukemic promyelocytes
> 20% CD56⁺ leukemic promyelocytes	40% of patients
Prognosis	Poor?

From Murray et al,[18] and the unpublished experience of the author.

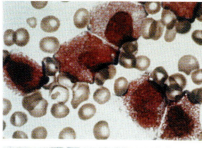
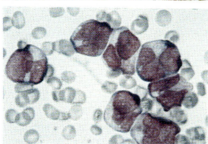

REFINED APL IMMUNOPHENOTYPE

Myeloid	
CD34	Low
HLA-DR	Low
P-Glycoprotein	Low
CD11a	Low
CD15	Low
CD15s	High
CD117	High

Figure 5–10. Refined immunophenotype of acute promyelocytic leukemia (APL), which corresponds to both FAB M3 (top morphology) and FAB M3v (bottom morphology) disease (original magnification ×1,200, Wright-Giemsa stain). (The morphology image is courtesy of Dr. John Bennett, University of Rochester, Rochester, NY.)

expression of a sialylated form of the CD15 molecule, and positivity for CD117.

Appearance of CD15, the Le^x-carbohydrate epitope, characterizes the promyelocytic stage during normal hematopoiesis. In contrast to APL cells, normal promyelocytes express asialo-CD15, which can be revealed by differential reactivity with CD15 and CD15s antibodies (Figure 5–11).[17] This distinctive staining pattern of CD15 antibodies with normal and leukemic promyelocytes can be exploited for the evaluation of remission bone marrows in patients with APL.

Although CD56 expression in a suspected case of APL must raise the question of NK-AML (see below), leukemic promyelocytes can express this antigen (Table 5–6). The limited data available suggest that CD56 may be an indicator of poor treatment outcome in APL.[18] An increased incidence of the short over the long isoform of *PML/RARα* has been implied but awaits confirmation from larger studies. The same applies to the proposed association between the short form and expression of the T-lymphocyte antigen CD2.

Natural Killer Cell or CD56-Positive AML

CD56 and lack of sensitivity to all-*trans* retinoic acid were the first indications for a non-APL diagnosis in

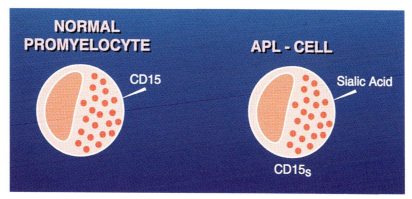

Figure 5–11. Differential expression of the CD15 molecule in normal and leukemic promyelocytes.

Table 5–6. IMMUNOPHENOTYPE OF NORMAL MAST CELLS AND BASOPHILS

Antigen	Mast Cell	Basophil
CD117 (c-kit)	+	–
cCD68 (lysosomal protein)	+	–
CD11b (CR3, integrin)	–	+
CDw17 (lactoceramide)	–	+
CD25 (IL-2Rα)	–	+
CD35 (CR1)	–	+
CD121b (IL-1Rα)	–	+
CD123 (IL-3Rα)	–	+

All antigens but CD68 are surface associated.
IL-2Rα = α-chain of the interleukin-2 receptor; IL-1Rα = α-chain of the interleukin-1 receptor; IL-3Rα = α-chain of the interleukin-3 receptor; CR3 = C3bi receptor; CR1 = C3b/4b receptor.

some patients with microgranular morphology and APL-like immunophenotype.[19] Subsequently, absence of t(15;17) confirmed this suspicion. Figure 5–12 summarizes the immunophenotypic characteristics of NK-AML, wherein those features distinct from APL are highlighted. Expression of CD11a may be the most reliable marker for this disease subtype.

Acute Myelomonocytic and Monocytic Leukemia

When a fraction of the myeloid leukemia population expresses CD14, the prototype monocytic antigen, it will be reflected in the diagnosis of AMML or AMOL. Typically, cells are doubly positive for HLA-DR and CD11b, an antigen expressed earlier than CD14 during monocytic differentiation. CD34 and CD117 reactivity are usually absent. Among lymphoid antigens, CD7 is frequently detected and may be associated with a worse prognosis. CD4, a differ-

entiation antigen of T-helper lymphocytes, shows a higher incidence of expression in monocytic than other nonlymphoid leukemias, representing mature monocytic differentiation. The presence of this antigen, however, has also been reported in immature hematopoietic progenitors; these may be the normal counterpart of CD4-positive AML with high CD34-positive expression, such as t(8;21) AML. In contrast to CD4 in lymphocytes, CD4 in nonlymphocytic cells is not associated with tyrosine kinase activity, and its biologic relevance remains speculative.

Surface expression of CD64 and intracytoplasmic CD68 can be helpful in the recognition of monocytic leukemias. Differential expression of the B-lymphoid–associated CD24 antigen can also be useful as follows: normal mature monocytes lack CD24, whereas leukemic monocytes are frequently CD24 positive; however, normal myeloid cells are CD24 positive, whereas leukemic myeloid cells are CD24 negative.[20]

CD2-Positive AML with inv(16)

The T-cell–associated CD2 antigen is found on significantly more blast cells in patients with the inv(16)(p13q22) cytogenetic abnormality than in myelomonocytic leukemias without the inversion.[21] CD2 expression is correlated with both monocytic markers, CD11b and CD14. In patients with missing or equivocal chromosomal and molecular analysis, this immunophenotypic peculiarity can be a helpful diagnostic indicator for this AML subtype with excellent prognosis.

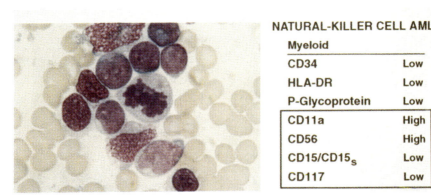

NATURAL-KILLER CELL AML

Myeloid	
CD34	Low
HLA-DR	Low
P-Glycoprotein	Low
CD11a	High
CD56	High
CD15/CD15s	Low
CD117	Low

Figure 5–12. Immunophenotypic characteristics of natural killer cell AML. Features useful in distinguishing NK-AML from APL are emphasized (original magnification × 1,200, Wright-Giemsa stain). (The morphology image is courtesy of Dr. John Bennett, University of Rochester, Rochester, NY.)

Ph-Positive AML

The incidence of the (9;22) translocation in immunophenotypically characterized AML is exceedingly low (< 1 %).[22] An immature myeloid phenotype and expression of variable lymphoid-associated antigens are common. Response to conventional chemotherapy is poor.

Leukemias Involving the Basophil or Mast Cell Lineage

Dysregulation of the basophil or mast cell lineage is frequently found in combination with pluripotent stem cell disorders, such as chronic myeloid leukemia and myeloproliferative disease.[23] Certain forms of AML are associated with prominent basophilia or eosinophilia: inv(16) is marked by atypical eosinophils with basophilic granulation; the (6;9)(p23;q14) translocation occurs with basophilia and so does trisomy 21, and a basophilic variant of APL with t(15;17) has been described.

Acute basophilic or mast cell leukemia is very rare. The two cell types share metachromatic staining properties. According to their cell of origin and immunophenotype, however, mast cells are related more closely to the monocytic lineage, whereas basophils are circulating granulocytes. Table 5–6 compares the most characteristic antigenic features of normal mast cells and basophils. They may serve as guidelines for their discrimination when they present as leukemia. Care has to be taken, however, as crossover of presumably specific antigens for one or the other cell type in leukemic cell lines has been reported. Major discrepancies in cytokine receptor expression reflect differential growth factor requirements of these cells.

Acute Erythroid and Megakaryocytic Leukemia

Because some overlap exists in antigen expression patterns during normal erythro- and megakaryocytopoiesis,[20] these two developmental pathways are presented together in Figure 5–13. Most acute erythroid leukemias (AELs) lack the early progenitor cell antigens CD34 and HLA-DR and stain with CD36 antibody, but do not yet express glycophorin A. This suggests that these leukemias correspond to the proerythroblast stage. Although CD36, reactive with platelet glycoprotein IV (GP IV), is also expressed on normal megakaryoblasts, the demonstration of CD71 will confirm the erythroid nature of these blast cells. Antibody to the bloodgroup H antigen, the precursor structure of ABO bloodgroup substances, frequently identifies AEL cells that are

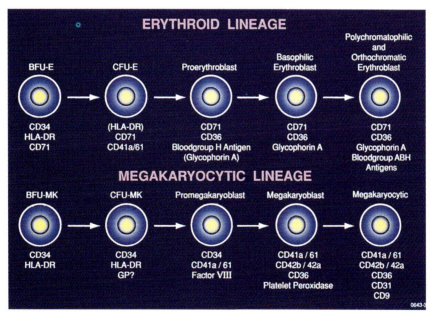

Figure 5–13. Antigen expression during normal erythro- and megakaryocytopoiesis. GP = platelet glycoproteins.

too immature to express glycophorin A. Bloodgroup H antigen has also been detected on myeloid cells from cases of AML and CML. Myeloblasts that may comprise a substantial component of AEL leukemia populations can be distinguished from the erythroid blasts based on their staining for MPO, CD33, CD13, and other myeloid antigens.

Negativity for MPO in the absence of lymphoid markers and without evidence for mature monocytic differentiation is the best indication for the diagnosis of acute megakaryocytic leukemia (AMegL). Antibodies to platelet-specific GPs permit the immunophenotypic characterization of AMegL. The most immature subtype corresponds to the level of megakaryocyte colony-forming units with expression of CD34 and CD41a/CD61 (GPIIb/IIIa) without demonstrable platelet peroxidase activity. With the acquisition of additional GPs (GPIb/IX or CD42b/CD42a and GPIV or CD36), CD34 is lost in the more mature forms of AMegL. Because mature platelets, expressing platelet GPs on their surface, can adhere to blast cells in AMOL, negativity for CD14 is an absolute requirement for the diagnosis of AMegL.

CHRONIC LYMPHOID LEUKEMIAS

Modern lymphoma classification invariably includes immunophenotypic criteria.[24–26] This section on chronic lymphoid neoplasms is divided into neoplasms of the B- and the T-cell lineage. Both phenotypes can be encountered in chronic lymphocytic (CLL) and prolymphocytic leukemia (PLL), although the B-cell phenotype is much more common in both. Hairy cell leukemia (HCL) and plasma cell leukemia are part of the B-cell neoplasms. The leukemic variant of Burkitt's lymphoma was discussed under mature B-cell ALL. According to the International Lymphoma Study Group and prompted by the common developmental pathway of NK cells and T lymphocytes, chronic lymphatic leukemias of NK cell type are discussed together with large granular lymphocyte leukemia of the T-cell type. Antigenic differences between chronic leukemias and non-Hodgkin's lymphomas in leukemic phase will be alluded to when they are essential for differential diagnosis.

These are all diseases of intermediately differentiated or mature lymphocytes.[27] In particular for chronic B-cell neoplasms, pronounced antigenic characteristics exist that allow clear distinctions between the subtypes. Common to the B-cell leukemias is monoclonal expression of surface Ig. In conjunction with distinct marker profiles, this monoclonality can be exploited for the detection of MRD. Flow cytometry is the ideal technology for the detection of B-cell clonality.

Chronic Leukemias of B-Cell Phenotype

B-Cell Chronic Lymphocytic Leukemia

Immunophenotyping is essential in discriminating CLL from reactive lymphocytosis or other non-Hodgkin's lymphomas in leukemic phase. Antigen profiles in B-CLL, B-PLL, classic HCL, and mantle cell lymphoma (MCL) are compared in Table 5–7.

The majority of cases of CLL are of B-cell phenotype and present with a typical antigen profile: the cells co-express the B-cell marker CD19 and the T-cell marker CD5. The only other B-cell leukemia or lymphoma that expresses CD5 is MCL (except for rare HCL variants). In contrast to B-CLL, MCL cells lack CD23. Furthermore, although positivity for CD25 and CD11c is common in B-CLL, these two markers are usually absent in MCL. Lack of CD11c expression may be seen in advanced-stage B-CLL and is often associated with strong CD44 expression. This observation suggests that these

Table 5–7. IMMUNOPHENOTYPIC DIFFERENCES BETWEEN CLASSIC B-CHRONIC LYMPHOCYTIC LEUKEMIA (B-CLL), B-PROLYMPHOCYTIC LEUKEMIA (B-PLL), HAIRY CELL LEUKEMIA (HCL), AND MANTLE CELL LYMPHOMA (MCL)

Antigen	B-CLL	B-PLL	HCL	MCL
B-antigens				
Immunoglobulins	±	+	++	+
CD20/CD22	±	+	+	+
CD23	+	+	−	−
CD24	+	+	±	+
T-antigens				
CD5	+	−	−	+
Activation and other antigens				
CD25	+	−	+	−
CD11c	+	±	+	−
CD38	−	±	+	±
CD103	−	−	+	−
FMC-7	−	+	+	+

adhesion molecules and their putative role in cell-cell or cell-stroma interactions may be of biologic significance in B-CLL.[28] Although some reports suggest that lack of CD43 expression in B-CLL may be another discriminatory parameter between B-CLL and MCL, we and others have not been able to confirm these data. The fluorescence intensity of staining for two other B-cell markers, CD20 and CD22, is much weaker in B-CLL than in normal B lymphocytes or lymphomas of other types, and CD22 may even be undetectable. Other B-lineage antigens, such as CD24 and CD40, are present, thus confirming the B-cell nature of these cells. CD10 is absent, which is useful for distinguishing B-CLL from follicular lymphoma in leukemic phase.

Data on the expression of CD79, another reliable B-cell marker, in B-CLL compared with other B-cell neoplasms is controversial. CD79 comprises two polypeptide chains, CD79a (mb-1) and CD79b (B29), which form a disulfide-linked complex with Ig in the B-cell membrane. Depending on the antibodies selected to react with the CD79 subunits, differential surface and cytoplasmic expression patterns of CD79a and CD79b in B-CLL versus MCL and HCL have been described. Because in paraffin sections, specimens from both B-CLL and MCL stain with anti-CD79a antibodies, CD79a has been suggested as a pan B-cell marker. However, when using an antibody to a surface epitope of CD79a (clone ZL7.4), B-CLL cells are reported negative for CD79a, whereas MCL cells remain positive.[29] As a word of caution, B-PLL cells may also express CD79a on the cell surface and may also carry the MCL-typical t(11;14) cytogenetic aberration so that other immunophenotypic findings, such as absence of CD23, must be present to confirm the diagnosis of MCL in CD79a surface-positive cases.

In many cases of B-CLL, only a small percentage of cells express CD38, an antigen expressed widely by lymphoid and myeloid precursor cells, activated lymphocytes, and plasma cells. Whereas most studies have shown that the prognostic significance of immunophenotyping in B-CLL is rather low, a recent study suggested that patients displaying high percentages of CD38-positive cells ($\geq 30\%$) responded more poorly to chemotherapy and had shorter survival than patients with lower CD38 expression.[30] Whether strong CD38 expression correlates with an unmutated Ig V_H gene status, another indicator of aggressive disease in B-CLL,[31] remains to be confirmed.[32]

Monoclonality for surface Ig light chain is the strongest indication for malignancy in B-cell lymphocytosis. This means that a population of lymphocytes in B-CLL will consist of cells that are restricted to either kappa or lambda Ig light-chain expression on their surface, whereas cells in a population of normal B lymphocytes demonstrate dominant kappa expression and 30 to 40 percent of cells with lambda chains. Absolutely essential for immunologic Ig light-chain determination is the removal of plasma proteins from the staining process. Figure 5–14 demonstrates the inhibitory effect of whole, unwashed blood on the flow cytometric detection of surface kappa light chains in a patient with B-CLL. Weak intensity of fluorescence staining for Igs is typical of B-CLL cells, and lack of detectable surface Ig light chain by flow cytometry is not uncommon in this disease. We have recently found that the choice of antibodies is critical in the detection of surface Ig light chain on B-CLL cells and that several cases initially thought to lack demonstrable Ig light-chain expression are found to have monoclonal kappa or lambda expression when polyclonal rather than monoclonal antibodies are used. In terms of surface Ig heavy chains, expression is faint, and cells are most commonly IgM positive and sometimes IgD positive. A composite of flow cytometric findings typical for B-CLL is shown in Figure 5–15. Note the weak staining for CD38 and CD22, lack of FMC-7 expression, and low-intensity, monoclonal surface lambda light-chain expression, immunophenotypic findings that differ strikingly from those in PLL (Figure 5–16).

Atypical, CD5-negative B-CLL may be a distinct entity. On the other hand, given that CD5-negative B-CLL often shares antigenic features with B-PLL, and the fact that CD5 negativity is more common in advanced-stage disease, CD5-negative B-CLL may represent an interim stage between B-CLL and B-PLL.

Prolymphocytic Leukemia of B-Cell Phenotype

B-PLL cells are typically CD5 negative, are more often positive for CD22 and CD38 than B-CLL,

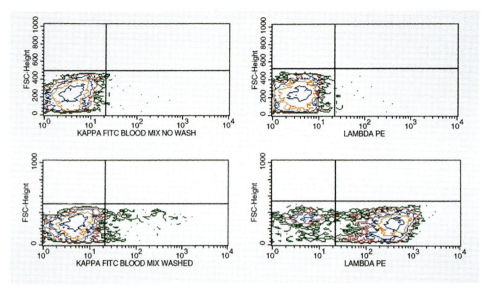

Figure 5–14. The presence of plasma proteins inhibits detection of surface immunoglobulin light chains on B-CLL cells. In the upper row of contour plots, whole, unwashed blood is used and neither kappa nor lambda light chains are detected on the cell surface. In the lower row of contour plots, the same blood is washed free of plasma proteins, which allows for the demonstration of monoclonal lambda light-chain expression.

demonstrate stronger surface Ig light-chain staining than B-CLL cells, lack CD25 and CD11c, and express FMC-7. Figure 5–16 demonstrates these characteristic immunophenotypic findings. FMC-7 was the first and, to date, last monoclonal antibody found to distinguish between B-CLL and B-PLL cells. It also reacts with HCL and MCL but not with cells derived from B-cell precursors. Expression of FMC-7 on cells from a patient with otherwise immunologically typical B-CLL, without clinical evidence of transformation toward B-PLL, is often accompanied by the appearance of larger, more

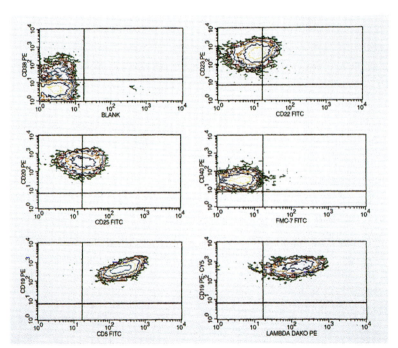

Figure 5–15. Antigen expression pattern typical of B-cell chronic lymphocytic leukemia.

immature-looking prolymphocytic cells and should be viewed as a potential early laboratory marker for disease progression.

Hairy Cell Leukemia

The cells in HCL have two rather unique features, morphology and expression of tartrate-resistant acid phosphatase (TRAP). As a result, the immunophenotype, although unique as well, usually falls only under confirmatory diagnostic criteria. However, immunophenotyping does distinguish HCL from other uncommon neoplasms, particularly monocytoid B-cell lymphoma, or lymphoproliferative disorders that may demonstrate weak TRAP staining, and it will detect small numbers of hairy cells in the peripheral blood or bone marrow after treatment. Hairy cell leukemia cells are rather mature B lymphocytes that have antigenic features of late-stage differentiation (absence of CD21) and B- but also T-cell activation.[33,34] In fact, TRAP expression may reflect stimulation as exposure of B-CLL cells with phorbol ester can induce this enzyme. Hairy cell leukemia cells express B-cell antigens such as CD19, CD22, and weakly CD20 but may lack CD24, which is normally lost with B-cell activation,

whereas they have gained CD72, another marker of B-cell activation. Fluorescence intensity of monoclonal surface Igs is characteristically strong, and IgG is found more often than IgM/IgD. In further contrast to B-CLL, HCL cells are negative for CD5 and CD23, whereas CD25 and CD11c, antigens also found in B-CLL, and FMC-7, the antigen characteristic of P-CLL, are typically present in HCL. Although HCL cells do not demonstrate features of plasmacytoid differentiation, they do express PCA-1, an antigen typical of plasma cells. The diagnostic marker of HCL is the integrin CD103. CD103 antibodies, such as the prototype antibody B-ly-7, do not react with other lymphoid malignancies, except for some rare, intestinal T-cell and splenic marginal zone B-cell lymphomas. CD103 is expressed on normal in vitro activated CD8-positive T cells, intraepithelial T cells of the gut, and a small subset of normal peripheral blood B lymphocytes. Due to its specificity, CD103 is a sensitive marker for detection of MRD in HCL.

Immunophenotypically variant forms of HCL (HCL-V) have been associated with resistance to interferon-α therapy. Hairy cell leukemia-V cells may be TRAP negative and negative for surface Igs and CD25, the alpha-chain of the interleukin-2

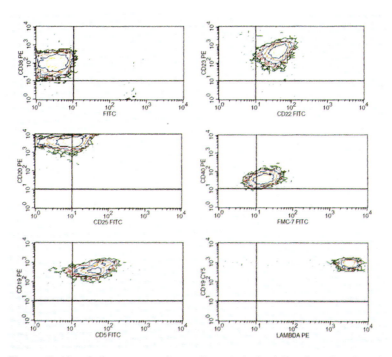

Figure 5–16. Antigen expression pattern typical of B-cell prolymphocytic leukemia.

receptor, or positive for CD5. It has been suggested that HCL-V may represent an intermediate between HCL and B-PLL. Interestingly, CD25-negative HCL-V cells still express CD122, the beta-chain of the interleukin-2 receptor, as do classic HCL cells.

Primary Plasma Cell Leukemia

Circulating monoclonal plasma cells are not uncommon in multiple myeloma (MM) and have been proposed as indicators of active disease and poor survival. The FAB group for the classification of chronic (mature) B and T lymphoid leukemias proposed that the term primary plasma cell leukemia (PCL) be restricted to a de novo presentation in leukemic phase. Others, however, have used PCL more loosely to define significantly elevated numbers of circulating plasma cells. Despite extensive overlap, some antigenic differences have been described to exist between the two disease entities. Malignant plasma cells from both conditions differ markedly in their immunophenotype from normal plasma cells or malignant B lymphocytes of intermediate-stage differentiation (eg, B-CLL) (Table 5–8).

Like normal plasma cells, plasma cells in MM and PCL have lost most surface B-lineage antigens, with the exception of CD138. Together with CD38 and intracytoplasmic Igs, CD138 identifies plasma cells and can be used to deplete malignant plasma cells from stem cell harvests prior to autografting. Immunoglobulins are monoclonal. Low proliferative activity, reflected in the Plasma Cell Labeling Index, may be associated with improved survival (Figure

5–17). In contrast to normal plasma cells, malignant plasma cells lack the leukocyte common antigen CD45, whereas CD38, which is down-regulated in lymphocytes of intermediate differentiation stage (eg, B-CLL), is expressed strongly on plasma cells from MM and PCL. CD10 is detected in a small percentage of patients with either diagnosis and may confer adverse prognosis. HLA-DR, although expressed throughout B-lymphocyte differentiation, is generally absent, especially in PCL. Particularly at their most mature stage, malignant plasma cells express unique adhesion molecules, such as CD56, CD44, CD49, and CD54, which may be linked to extramedullary homing properties of these cells. CD56 positivity is used to distinguish malignant plasma cells from monoclonal gammopathy of undetermined significance. Interestingly, CD117, the receptor for the stem cell factor c-kit, which is consistently found on the surface of plasma cells in MM, may be absent in PCL.[35]

Detection of Immunologic MRD in Chronic B-Cell Neoplasms

Because of the uniqueness and specificity of antigen profiles in chronic B-cell neoplasms, MRD can be detected by multicolor flow cytometry. This laboratory approach has increasing significance in the clinical management of these patients as more effective therapeutic agents and modalities are employed. For instance, monoclonal leukemia cells have been found to contaminate peripheral blood stem cell harvests, detectable only by sensitive flow cytometric technique. Sensitivity levels of 1 malignant cell in 10,000 can be achieved by increasing the number of antigens tested simultaneously and by including quantitative measurements of antigen expression into the analysis.

Chronic Leukemias of T-Cell Phenotype

As with the B-cell chronic leukemias, the advanced maturation stage of the malignant T cells distinguishes these neoplasms from T-cell precursor leukemias, such as pre-T ALL or lymphoblastic lymphoma in leukemic phase. Typically, chronic T-cell leukemias express CD3 on the cell surface, have either a CD4 or a CD8 phenotype, and lack CD1a as well as intranuclear TdT. With

			Table 5–8. DIAGNOSTICALLY MOST USEFUL IMMUNOPHENOTYPIC DIFFERENCES BETWEEN NORMAL AND MALIGNANT PLASMA CELLS AND MALIGNANT B LYMPHOCYTES OF INTERMEDIATE STAGE DIFFERENTIATION		
Antigen	Normal Plasma Cells	MM/PCL	Intermediate Stage
CD45	+	–	+
CD38	+	+	–
HLA-DR	–	–	+
CD19	–	–	+
Ig*	Intracytoplasmic	Intracytoplasmic	Surface
CD56	–	+	–
CD117	–	+	–

*Immunoglobulin heavy and light chains.

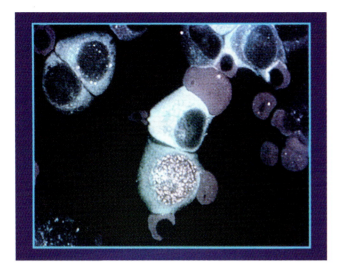

Figure 5–17. The image represents a labeled plasma cell with cytoplasmic Ig stained with fluorescein-conjugated anti-kappa and a bromodeoxyuridine-labeled nucleus, the strategy employed for measuring the proliferative activity or Plasma Cell Labeling Index (original magnification ×756). (Courtesy of Dr. Philip Greipp, Mayo Clinic, Rochester, MN.)

the exception of the NK cell neoplasms, which lack TCR expression, and the exceedingly rare hepatosplenic gamma/delta lymphoma in leukemic phase, chronic T-cell leukemias express alpha/beta TCR molecules. Even in the presence of a restricted CD4 or CD8-only phenotype, evidence for clonality of the malignant T-cell population depends on the demonstration of clonal TCR gene rearrangements by molecular techniques. Genetic clonality is the laboratory tool of choice for detecting MRD in these diseases. Differences in the expression pattern of lymphoid antigens are much more subtle in the chronic T-cell than the B-cell leukemias and are thus diagnostically of less importance. The diagnostically most helpful immunophenotypic differences between T-CLL/PLL, large granular lymphocyte leukemia of the T-cell (T-LGL) or the NK cell type (NK-LGL), and adult T-cell leukemia/lymphoma (ATLL) will be discussed.

Chronic Lymphocytic and Prolymphocytic Leukemia of T-Cell Phenotype

Whereas T-CLL is very rare,[36] T-PLL can amount to up to 20 percent of PLL cases.[24] The cells usually express all pan T antigens (CD3, CD5, CD2, CD7) and more often demonstrate a CD4 than a CD8 phenotype. Immunophenotypically, it will not be possi-

ble to distinguish T-CLL from the leukemic phase of peripheral T-cell lymphoma.

Large Granular Lymphocyte Leukemia of T- or NK Cell Phenotype

These two forms of LGL are biologically related.[37,38] Typical T-LGL is positive for CD3 and the NK cell-associated markers CD16 and CD57 but negative for the NK marker CD56. Natural killer LGL cells are characterized by CD56 expression and absence of CD57, CD3, and TCR proteins, so that clonality cannot be easily established. The extent to which other pan T markers are present varies in the literature. A variant form of T-LGL with a more aggressive course has been described expressing CD56 in addition to CD3. Given the proven common developmental pathway for T lymphocytes and NK cells, these overlapping immunophenotypic presentations are not surprising.

Adult T-Cell Leukemia/Lymphoma

Adult T-cell leukemia cells express T-cell–associated antigens CD5, CD2, and CD3 but typically lack CD7. Most cases are CD4 positive, and expression of CD25 distinguishes this entity from most other chronic T-cell leukemias.

CHRONIC MYELOID LEUKEMIAS

This section will focus on those subtypes of chronic myeloid leukemia in which immunophenotyping is of clinical value or biologic interest: Ph-positive chronic myeloid leukemia (CML) and chronic myeloproliferative diseases, which, like Ph-positive CML, can transform into an acute phase (ie, polycythemia vera [PV] and essential thrombocythemia [ET]). This selection is based on the fact that antigen expression patterns contribute crucially to the correct characterization of blast cells during the acute phase of these diseases but have more limited proven clinical relevance during the more mature, chronic part of the disease.

Philadelphia Chromosome-Positive CML

Chronic myeloid leukemia is a multistep disease that is characterized by two biologically very distinct phases, a chronic and a blastic phase, and a mostly clinically defined accelerated phase preceding blastic transformation.[39] The disease originates in the transformation of a pluripotent hematopoietic precursor cell within the CD34-, HLA-DR-positive stem cell pool. It is a clonal disease in that all affected cells contain the Ph, a translocation between the *ABL* gene on chromosome 9 and the *BCR* gene on chromosome 22, which results in the fusion of portions of these genes (chimeric *BCR/ABL* gene). CD34-positive, HLA-DR-negative immature precursor cells have been shown to be enriched in *BCR/ABL* negative progenitors and thus represent the most suitable pool for autologous transplantation in CML.[40] The *BCR/ABL* messenger ribonucleic acid transcript is translated predominantly into a 210-kD novel protein with tyrosine kinase activity, which has been implicated in the pathogenesis of the disease.[41] Inhibition of this *ABL*-specific tyrosine kinase activity has yielded promising clinical results.[42]

The fact that in the *BCR/ABL* fusion gene, sequences are joined that normally are located on different chromosomes forms the basis for molecular monitoring of Ph-positive CML patients by polymerase chain reaction (PCR) analysis. Along the same line, these junctional sequences translate into a sequence of amino acids that are not expressed in normal cells. Thus, antibodies to the aberrant p210-

kD protein in CML should provide a specific tool for recognition of Ph-transformed cells. Although such antibodies have indeed been produced, they have not found use for diagnostic purposes.

Reflecting the multipotent stem cell origin, cytogenetic or molecular evidence for this genetic abnormality can be found during chronic phase in cells of the myelomonocytic, erythroid, and megakaryocytic lineages and a portion of mature B lymphocytes. Whether T lymphocytes from patients with CML contain the *BCR/ABL* rearrangement is still controversial, but the majority of data suggest that they do not belong to the malignant clone. Figure 5–18 illustrates the biphasic biology of Ph-positive CML.

Chronic Phase

Chronic-phase CML is characterized by the premature release of precursor cells from the bone marrow into the circulation. Studies on adhesion molecules have pointed to a defect in integrin function on the surface of primitive CML progenitor cells compared with normal hematopoietic precursors rather than the absence of certain adhesive receptors. Antigen expression patterns on myeloid cells from bone marrow aspirates during chronic phase show only subtle differences to findings in normal bone marrows. The

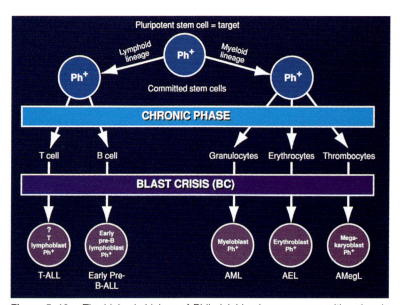

Figure 5–18. The biphasic biology of Philadelphia chromosome-positive chronic myeloid leukemia. T-ALL = T-cell acute lymphoblastic leukemia; early pre-B ALL = CD10-positive precursor B-cell acute lymphoblastic leukemia; AEL = acute erythroleukemia; AMegL = acute megakaryocytic leukemia.

reported appearance of CD33-, CD56-positive myelocytes and metamyelocytes in CML bone marrows is variable, but it has been linked to early detection of relapse after bone marrow transplantation and may thus be of clinical usefulness.[43] In our experience, the most consistent immunophenotypic abnormalities in CML bone marrow are a decrease in lactoferrin-producing cells and a decrease in CD24 expression by myeloid precursor cells, both markers of less than normal maturation. CD34-, HLA-DR-positive blast cells usually remain within the normal range of 1 to 2 percent of total mononuclear cells (Table 5–9).

Blast Crisis

The early detection of increased blast cells in the absence of morphologic and/or clinical evidence of transformation constitutes the immunophenotypic suggestion of accelerated phase and/or beginning blast crisis. Immunophenotypic studies are essential in blast crisis as morphology and cytochemistry are often misleading or inconclusive, respectively. The incidence of lymphoid transformation is around 25 percent, whereas the majority of the cases will develop myeloid blast crisis and a small percentage develop erythroid or megakaryocytic blast crisis. Table 5–9 summarizes antigen expression patterns, which can be used to distinguish various types of blast crisis from chronic-phase or normal bone marrow. Data are based on the literature and our own, in part, unpublished experience.

As in the interpretation of all immunophenotypic analyses, the overlap in antigen expression between normal and leukemic cells must be taken into consideration. For instance, HLA-DR will be seen on nonmalignant monocytes in normal bone marrow and Ph-positive monocytes in chronic-phase bone marrow, as well as on myeloblasts, monocytic blasts, and megakaryoblasts in myeloid blast crisis and on B lymphoblasts in lymphoid blast crisis. Another such example is CD24, a B-lymphoid–associated antigen, which is also expressed by normal myelocytes, metamyelocytes, and granulocytes but not by less mature normal or leukemic myeloid cells. As mentioned before, decreased CD24 expression by otherwise normal-appearing myelocytes and metamyelocytes serves as an indicator of chronic-phase CML.

The most common phenotype in myeloid blast crisis corresponds to that of undifferentiated AML, characterized by low CD65s expression. Although relative monocytosis is an accepted indicator of clinical progression during chronic phase, CD14-positive monocytes or monoblasts rarely dominate during blast crisis. Among lymphoid antigens, CD7 is frequently detected on the myeloid blasts, in the absence of CD2; B-lymphoid–associated antigens are usually lacking. TdT is most commonly detected in a low percentage of myeloblasts, rarely in the entire myeloid population. In addition to selected lymphoid antigen expression by the myeloid blast cells, the simultaneous appearance of distinct myeloid and lymphoid blast populations has also been reported.

The most common phenotype of lymphoid blast crisis is that of early pre-B ALL, characterized by expression of B-lymphoid antigens including CD10 and CD34, as in Ph-positive ALL. Lymphoid blast crisis of CML and Ph-positive ALL may be distinguished molecularly, based on variable breakpoints in the *BCR* gene that lead to distinct BCR/ABL transcripts: b2a2 or b3a2 dominates in CML, whereas e1a2 dominates in ALL. However, these molecular

Table 5–9. IMMUNOPHENOTYPES IN CML BLAST CRISIS COMPARED WITH FINDINGS IN CHRONIC-PHASE OR NORMAL BONE MARROW

Antigen	Normal	CML	M-BC	L-BC	Ery-BC	Mega-BC
Uncommitted antigens						
CD34	1–2%	1–5%	++	++	–	++
HLA-DR	Monos	Monos	++	++	–	++
TdT	1–5%	1–5%	0–15%	++	–	(+)
CD56	–	+-++	+-++	(+)	NA	NA
Myeloid antigens						
MPO	++	++	+-++	–	–	–
CD33/13	++	++	++	0-+	+	+
CD65s	++	++	+	–	–	–
CD11b	++	+	–	–	–	–
LF	++	+	–	–	–	–
Lymphoid antigens						
CD7	–	(+)	+	–	–	+
CD19	–	–	–	++	–	–
CD10	Mature	Mature	–	++	–	–
CD24	++	+	–	++	–	–
Erythroid and megakaryocytic antigens						
H-antigen	–	+	+	–	++	+
CD36	–	–	–	–	++	++
CD41	–	–	–	–	+	++

M-BC = myeloid blast crisis; L-BC = lymphoid blast crisis; Ery-BC = erythroid blast crisis; Mega-BC = megakaryocytic blast crisis; Monos = monocytes; NA = data not available.

rearrangements overlap in that low levels of e1a2 transcripts exist in patients with CML in addition to the CML typical transcript forms, and CML transcripts have been detected in patients with Ph-positive ALL, either alone or in conjunction with e1a2. Terminal deoxynucleotidyl transferase expression is very strong, both in terms of percentage of positive blast cells and fluorescence intensity and biochemical enzyme activity. It should be remembered that CD10 is also expressed by mature myeloid cells so that the finding of some CD10-positive cells in a chronic-phase tissue per se does not always reflect beginning lymphoid blast crisis. Double-staining with myeloid or lymphoid markers of CD10-positive cells will easily settle this issue. As in Ph-positive ALL, presence of CD33 or less often CD13 on the lymphoblasts is not uncommon. Should more than two myeloid antigens be detected, for instance, CD65s in addition to CD33 and CD13, one must consider the possibility of a myeloid transformation. There are two ways to resolve this dilemma. First, seek support for a lymphoid lineage by probing for intracellular CD22 (or CD3), the presence of which would be diagnostic of lymphoid lineage. Second, test for CD117, which, in conjunction with the myeloid antigens, will confirm a myeloid phenotype. In very few cases, multiple lineage overlap is observed, such as CD7 plus limited myeloid antigens in a case of early pre-B ALL.

Not discussed in the table are the rarely reported T-lymphoid blast crises. They often present as extramedullary disease, allowing only for cytochemical testing of tissue sections rather than flow cytometric analysis, which has raised some questions on the reliability of the findings.

The rare erythroid and megakaryocytic blast crises show typical immunophenotypic features of the corresponding acute leukemias. The finding of myeloblast components in addition to erythroblasts or megakaryoblasts is almost universal.

Polycythemia Vera

Immunophenotypic analysis of bone marrow aspirates in PV may demonstrate subtle antigenic abnormalities, such as those seen in chronic-phase CML. Erythroid hyperplasia will be evident from a large number of glycophorin A-staining cells within the mononuclear cell fraction. As in CML, blastic transformation more often presents with a nonlymphoid phenotype, immature myeloid, myelomonocytic, erythroid, or megakaryocytic. Co-expression of myeloid markers with CD7, TdT, and even CD19 has been observed, supporting the concept that PV results from an acquired mutation of a pluripotent hematopoietic stem cell.

The distinction as to whether acute leukemia developing in a patient with PV reflects a natural sequel or a secondary malignancy related to the treatment of the underlying disease is made based on cytogenetic abnormalities rather than immunophenotypic findings.

Essential Thrombocythemia

Leukemic transformation in ET, as in PV, is well recognized, albeit uncommon. Thought to be a clonal stem cell disorder, blast cell phenotypes derived from any of the hematopoietic lineages have been reported to occur in ET blast crisis. Compared with CML or PV, dual myeloid/megakaryocytic or purely megakaryoblastic leukemias are more common in ET.

REFERENCES

1. Paietta E, Andersen J, Wiernik PH. A new approach to analyzing the utility of immunophenotyping for predicting clinical outcome in acute leukemia. Leukemia 1996;10:1–4.
2. Cualing H, Kothari R, Balachander T. Immunophenotypic diagnosis of acute leukemia by using decision tree induction. Lab Invest 1999;79:205–12.
3. Fenaux P, Chastang C, Chevret S, et al. A randomized comparison of all-trans retinoic acid (ATRA) followed by chemotherapy and ATRA plus chemotherapy and the role of maintenance therapy in newly diagnosed acute promyelocytic leukemia. Blood 1999;94:1192–200.
4. Campana D, Coustan-Smith E. Detection of minimal residual disease in acute leukemia by flow cytometry. Cytometry 1999;38:139–52.
5. Weir EG, Cowan K, LeBeau P, Borowitz MJ. A limited antibody panel can distinguish B-precursor acute lymphoblastic leukemia from normal B precursors with four color flow cytometry: implications for residual disease detection. Leukemia 1999;13:558–67.
6. Kishimoto T, Kikutani H, von dem Borne AEG, et al. Leucocyte typing VI. New York: Garland; 1997.

7. Bene MC, Castoldi G, Knapp W, et al. Proposals for the immunological classification of acute leukemias. Leukemia 1995;9:1783–6.

8. Paietta E, Racevskis J, Neuberg D, et al. Expression of CD25 (interleukin-2 receptor α chain) in adult acute lymphoblastic leukemia predicts for the presence of BCR/ABL fusion transcripts: results of a preliminary laboratory analysis of ECOG/MRC Intergroup Study E2993. Leukemia 1997;11:1887–90.

9. Paietta E, Racevskis J, Bennett JM, et al. Differential expression of terminal transferase (TdT) in acute lymphocytic leukemia expressing myeloid antigens and TdT positive acute myeloid leukemia as compared to myeloid antigen negative acute lymphocytic leukemia. Br J Haematol 1993;84:416–22.

10. Paietta E, Neuberg D, Richards S, et al., and the Eastern Cooperative Oncology Group. Rare adult acute lymphocytic leukemia with CD56 expression in the ECOG experience shows unexpected phenotypic and genotypic heterogeneity. Am J Hematol 2001; 66:189–96.

11. Hurwitz CA, Raimondi SC, Head D, et al. Distinctive immunophenotypic features of t(8;21)(q22;q22) acute myeloblastic leukemia in children. Blood 1992;80:3182–8.

12. Tallman MS, Hakimian D, Shaw JM, et al. Granulocytic sarcoma is associated with the 8;21 translocation in acute myeloid leukemia. J Clin Oncol 1993;11:690–7.

13. Baer MR, Stewart CC, Lawrence D, et al. Expression of the neural cell adhesion molecule CD56 is associated with short remission duration and survival in acute myeloid leukemia with t(8;21)(q22;q22). Blood 1997;90:1643–8.

14. Byrd JC, Dodge RK, Carroll A, et al. Patients with t(8;21)(q22;q22) and acute myeloid leukemia have superior failure-free and overall survival when repetitive cycles of high-dose cytarabine are administered. J Clin Oncol 1999;17:3767–75.

15. Paietta E, Andersen J, Yunis J, et al. Acute myeloid leukemia expressing the leucocyte integrin CD11b— a new leukemic syndrome with poor prognosis: result of an ECOG database analysis. Br J Haematol 1998;100:265–72.

16. Melnick A, Licht JD. Deconstructing a disease: RARα, its fusion partners, and their roles in the pathogenesis of acute promyelocytic leukemia. Blood 1999;93:3167–215.

17. Paietta E, Andersen J, Gallagher R, et al. The immunophenotype of acute promyelocytic leukemia (APL): an ECOG study. Leukemia 1994;8:1108–12.

18. Murray CK, Estey E, Paietta E, et al. CD56 expression in acute promyelocytic leukemia (APL): a possible indicator of poor treatment outcome? J Clin Oncol 1999;17:293–7.

19. Scott AA, Head DR, Kopecky KJ, et al. HLA-DR⁻, CD33⁺, CD56⁺, CD16⁻ myeloid/natural killer cell acute leukemia: a previously unrecognized form of acute leukemia potentially misdiagnosed as French-American-British acute myeloid leukemia-M3. Blood 1994;84:244–55.

20. Paietta E. Immunobiology of acute leukemia. In: Wiernik PH, Canellos GP, Dutcher JP, Kyle RA, editors. Neoplastic diseases of the blood. 3rd ed. New York: Churchill Livingstone; 1996. p. 211–47.

21. Adriaansen HJ, te Boekhorst PAW, Hagemeijer AM, et al. Acute myeloid leukemia M4 with bone marrow eosinophilia (M4Eo) and inv(16)(p13q22) exhibits a specific immunophenotype with CD2 expression. Blood 1993;81:3043–51.

22. Paietta E, Racevskis J, Bennett JM, et al. Biologic heterogeneity in Philadelphia chromosome-positive acute leukemia with myeloid morphology: the Eastern Cooperative Oncology Group experience. Leukemia 1998;12:1881–5.

23. Agis H, Beil WJ, Bankl HC, et al. Mast cell-lineage versus basophil lineage involvement in myeloproliferative and myelodysplastic syndromes: diagnostic role of cell-immunophenotyping. Leuk Lymphoma 1996;22:187–204.

24. Harris NL, Jaffe ES, Stein H, et al. A revised European-American classification of lymphoid neoplasms: a proposal from the International Lymphoma Study Group. Blood 1994;84:1361–92.

25. Tbakhi A, Edinger M, Myles J, et al. Flow cytometric immunophenotyping of non-Hodgkin's lymphomas and related disorders. Cytometry 1996;25:113–24.

26. Harris NL, Jaffe ES, Armitage JO, Shipp M. Lymphoma classification: from R.E.A.L. to W.H.O. and beyond. Principles Pract Oncol 1999;13:1–14.

27. Kroft SH, Finn WG, Peterson LC. The pathology of the chronic lymphoid leukemias. Blood Rev 1995;9: 234–50.

28. Eisterer W, Hilbe W, Stauder R, et al. An aggressive subtype of B-CLL is characterized by strong CD44 expression and lack of CD11c. Br J Haematol 1996;93:661–9.

29. Bell PB, Rooney N, Bosanquet AG. CD79a detected by ZL7.4 separates chronic lymphocytic leukemia from mantle cell lymphoma in the leukemic phase. Cytometry 1999;38:102–5.

30. Damle RN, Wasil T, Fais F, et al. Ig V gene mutation status and CD38 expression as novel prognostic indicators in chronic lymphocytic leukemia. Blood 1999;94:1840–7.

31. Hamblin TJ, Davis Z, Gardiner A, et al. Unmutated Ig V_H genes are associated with a more aggressive form of chronic lymphocytic leukemia. Blood 1999;94:1848–54.

32. Hamblin TJ, Orchard JA, Gardiner A, et al. Immunoglobulin V genes and CD38 expression in CLL. Blood 2000;95:2455.

33. Pettitt AR, Zuzel M, Cawley JC. Hairy-cell leukemia: biology and management. Br J Haematol 1999;106: 2–8.

34. Mulligan SP, Travade P, Matutes E, et al. B-ly-7, a monoclonal antibody reactive with hairy cell leukemia, also defines an activation antigen on normal CD8$^+$ T cells. Blood 1990;76:959–64.

35. Garcia-Sanz R, Orfão A, González M, et al. Primary plasma cell leukemia: clinical, immunophenotypic, DNA ploidy, and cytogenetic characteristics. Blood 1999;93:1032–7.

36. Hoyer JD, Ross CW, Li C-Y, et al. True T-cell chronic lymphocytic leukemia: a morphologic and immunophenotypic study of 25 cases. Blood 1995;86:1163–9.

37. Jaffe ES. Classification of natural killer (NK) cell and NK-like T-cell malignancies. Blood 1996;87: 1207–10.

38. Oshimi K. Lymphoproliferative disorders of natural killer cells. Int J Hematol 1996;63:279–90.

39. Thijsen SFT, Schuurhuis GJ, van Oostveen JW, Ossenkoppele GJ. Chronic myeloid leukemia from basics to bedside. Leukemia 1999;13:1646–74.

40. Delforge M, Boogaerts MA, McGlave PB, Verfaillie CM. BCR/ABL$^-$CD34$^+$HLA-DR$^-$ progenitor cells in early chronic phase, but not in more advanced phases, of chronic myelogenous leukemia are polyclonal. Blood 1999;93:284–92.

41. Deininger MWN, Vieira S, Mendiola R, et al. BCR-ABL tyrosine kinase activity regulates the expression of multiple genes implicated in the pathogenesis of chronic myeloid leukemia. Cancer Res 2000;60:2049–55.

42. Druker BJ, Lydon NB. Lessons learned from the development of an Abl tyrosine kinase inhibitor for chronic myelogenous leukemia. J Clin Invest 2000;105:3–7.

43. Lanza F, Bi S, Castoldi G, Goldman JM. Abnormal expression of N-CAM (CD56) adhesion molecule on myeloid and progenitor cells from chronic myeloid leukemia. Leukemia 1993;7:1570–5.

6

Cytogenetic Alterations and Related Molecular Consequences in Adult Leukemia

ELISABETH PAIETTA, PhD

PETER R. PAPENHAUSEN, PhD, FACMG

Cytogenetic analysis in human leukemias began approximately 40 years ago with the majority of the presently known nonrandom chromosome aberrations being discovered by the 1980s. Subsequently, molecular genetic studies were emphasized that have led to the cloning and the characterization of genes involved in the most common recurrent chromosomal abnormalities. Many of these genes were previously unknown. Their pathogenetic effects result from either gene loss or inactivation, deregulated expression of genes in the wrong cell type or at an inappropriate stage of hematopoietic differentiation, gene amplification, or structural alterations and the generation of novel genes. Multivariate analyses have provided convincing evidence that cytogenetic testing provides independent prognostic information in both the acute and the chronic leukemias.

CONVENTIONAL CYTOGENETIC PROCEDURE

Conventional cytogenetics rely on the staining of metaphase cells and therefore depend on dividing neoplastic cells. Anticoagulated bone marrow aspirates are preferred over peripheral blood samples because neoplastic cells are often sparse in the circulation and because leukemic cells in the bone marrow tend to have a higher mitotic rate than in the peripheral blood. Appropriate specimens may also consist of tissue from extramedullary sites of leukemia such as granulocytic sarcomas and effu-sions or lymph node biopsies in lymphomas. The presence of normal, actively proliferating cells, such as marrow erythroid precursor cells, may occasionally overwhelm mitoses from a small number of neoplastic cells. For the same reason, mitogens that stimulate normal lymphocytes are avoided in cytogenetic cultures of malignant cells except for the B-cell mitogen stimulation of small B-lymphocytic leukemia/lymphoma cells. If there is any question as to whether an abnormal karyotype is acquired or congenital, normal lymphocytes from peripheral blood are purposely stimulated with a predominantly T-cell mitogen to determine the constitutional karyotype of a patient.

Rapid transport to the cytogenetic laboratory under the most physiologic conditions (eg, protection from temperature extremes; low-volume bone marrow aspirates should be protected from heparin toxicity) is a prerequisite of successful analysis. Cells are usually cultured for 24 hours prior to the preparation of metaphase spreads, which are arrested by short-term colchicine incubation. Cells are analyzed microscopically. As a general rule, a 20-metaphase analysis constitutes a complete study. This rule does not apply when diagnostic cytogenetic aberrations can be demonstrated in two or more cells, thus constituting an abnormal clone (eg, t[8;21] or t[9;22] or monosomy 7) in a low mitotic sample.

Any deviation from the normal 46-chromosome count is termed aneuploidy. If a cell has 46 chromosomes with structural aberrations, it is termed pseudodiploid. More than 46 chromosomes represents hyperdiploidy, whereas fewer than 46 chromosomes is hypodiploidy. Structural aberrations may affect the long arm of a chromosome (q) or its short arm (p).

CYTOGENETIC ABERRATIONS

There are two major classes of cytogenetic aberrations: those that result in the visible loss or gain of chromosomal material and those that result in a balanced exchange without apparent loss or gain of deoxyribonucleic acid (DNA). Chromosomal loss may be characterized as partial (deletion, del) or complete loss of a chromosome (monosomy). Gains may refer to portions of chromosomes (eg, duplications) or whole chromosomes (trisomy, tetrasomy). Unidentified abnormal chromosomes are labeled as markers (mar). Balanced alterations involve the reciprocal exchange of genetic material either between two or more chromosomes (translocations, t) or between various portions of one chromosome (inversions, inv).

PRIMARY AND SECONDARY CHROMOSOMAL ABNORMALITIES

To date, between 150 and 160 chromosome anomalies have been nonrandomly associated with hematologic disorders. Because they are often found as the sole cytogenetic abnormality, they are termed primary abnormalities. Secondary chromosomal aberrations (not to be confused with typical cytogenetic abnormalities occurring in secondary malignancies) develop in addition to the primary abnormalities and reflect clonal karyotypic evolution. Most secondary changes are monosomies, trisomies, deletions, or isochromosomes. The latter are mirror-image duplications of one chromosome arm with consequent loss of the other arm. Secondary cytogenetic changes are more frequent in acute lymphoblastic leukemia (ALL) than in acute myeloid leukemia (AML) and not only differ with the primary abnormality but may be unique to the hematologic cell type. There are several specific secondary cytogenetic abnormalities that are associated with certain primary abnormalities, such as the loss of one sex chromosome and del(9)(q12q22) in t(8;21) AML or trisomy 22 in inv(16) AML. Trisomy 12 and

t(14;19) in prolymphocytic B-cell leukemia is another example. Others occur as secondary abnormalities in more than one leukemia subtype, such as trisomy 8 or monosomy 7. The prognostic implications of secondary changes in the acute leukemias have not yet been entirely established and will be discussed in the context of individual abnormalities. Additional cytogenetic abnormalities may be seen at the time of relapse or in resistant disease after chemotherapy and therefore can be viewed as conferring survival advantage for the leukemic cells. In chronic myeloid leukemia (CML), clonal evolution is generally considered to be a sign of clinical progression or transformation to blast crisis.

MOLECULAR CONSEQUENCES OF CYTOGENETIC ABERRATIONS

The loss of pivotal DNA sequences involving, for instance, tumor suppressor genes is implicated as the pathogenetic consequence of chromosomal deletions and monosomies. Increased gene dosage due to numeric chromosome gain underlies the leukemogenic role of trisomies and hyperdiploidy in general. The critical genes in numeric chromosome alterations are largely undefined. There is recent evidence that an extra copy of a chromosome that appears normal under the microscope may carry submicroscopic genetic changes, such as the tandem duplication of the *MLL* gene at band 11q23 seen in cases of trisomy 11.

Chromosome translocations can have two distinct effects at the molecular level (Figure 6–1). In the first type, the translocation disrupts an untranslated region of a regulatory gene and places it under the control of the promoter of a very active gene. This allows the production of a normal protein, albeit regulated inappropriately, in the leukemic cells, whereas the same protein may be undetectable in normal counterpart cells. The paradigm for this kind of translocation is that occurring in lymphoid malignancies. During the normal recombination of the variable (V), diverse (D), and junctional (J) regions of the immunoglobulin (Ig) or T-cell receptor (TCR) genes, errors may be made by the recombinase enzyme systems. Such errors result in the translocation of developmentally regulated tran-

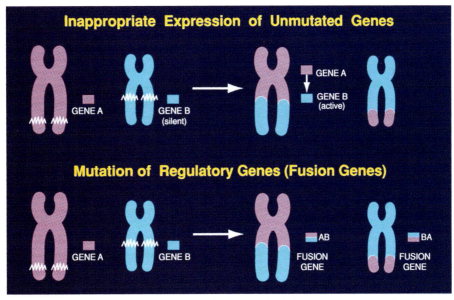

Figure 6–1.   Mechanisms of leukemogenesis as a result of chromosome translocations.

scription factor genes into the vicinity of highly active gene promoters. In the case of lymphoid cells, this results in juxtaposition of putative or known oncogenes to the Ig or TCR gene promoter loci. In the classic example, the (8;14)(q24;q32) translocation in mature B-lineage acute lymphocytic leukemia (Burkitt's-like ALL) places the *c-MYC* gene from chromosome 8 close to and under the control of the very active Ig heavy-chain gene pro-

moter on chromosome 14. The MYC protein interacts with several other transcription factors involved in growth response so that its inappropriate activation will result in uncontrolled cellular proliferation. Additional examples of gene activation by chromosomal translocation are listed in Table 6–1.

In the second type of translocation, fusion of two genes is the mechanism of leukemogenesis (see Figure 6–1). Critical genes located at the breakpoints of

Disease	Translocation	Genes Involved	Transforming Gene (Product)
B-ALL	t(**8**;14)(**q24**;q32)	*c-MYC*/IgH locus	Transcription factor
	t(2;**8**)(p12;**q24**)	*c-MYC*/Igκ locus	- " -
	t(**8**;22)(**q24**;q11)	*c-MYC*/Igλ locus	- " -
T-ALL	t(**8**;14)(**q24**;q11)	*c-MYC*/TCRα-δ locus	- " -
	t(**1**;14)(**p32**;q11)	*TAL-1**/TCRα-δ locus	- " -
	t(**10**;14)(**q24**;q11)	*HOX-11*/TCRα-δ locus	- " -
	t(**11**;14)(**p15**;q11)	*RBTN1*/TCRα-δ locus	- " -
	t(**11**;14)(**p13**;q11)	*RBTN2*/TCRα-δ locus	- " -
	t(7;**19**)(q35;**p13**)	*LYL1*/TCRβ locus	- " -
	t(7;**9**)(q35;**p13**)	*TAL-2*/TCRβ locus	- " -
	t(7;**10**)(q35;**q24**)	*HOX-11*/TCRβ locus	Transcription factor
	t(7;**11**)(q35;**p13**)	*RBTN2*/TCRβ locus	- " -
B-CLL	t(14;**19**)(q32;**q13.1**)	*BCL-3*/IgH locus	Protein-protein interaction
	t(**11**;14)(**q13**;q32)	*BCL-1*/IgH locus	Cell-cycle control
	t(14;**18**)(q32;**q21**)	*BCL-2*/IgH locus	Apoptosis
T-CLL	t(7;**14**)(q35;**q32**)	*TCL1*/TCRβ locus	Oncogene
	t(**14**;14)(q11;**q32**)	*TCL1*/TCRα-δ locus	Oncogene
Early B-ALL	t(5;14)(**q31**;q32)	*IL-3*/IgH locus	Proliferation, eosinophilia

Table 6–1. GENE ACTIVATION THROUGH CHROMOSOME TRANSLOCATION

B-ALL = mature B-lineage ALL; T-ALL = T-lineage ALL; B-CLL = B-cell chronic lymphocytic leukemia; T-CLL = T-cell chronic lymphocytic leukemia; early B-ALL = CD10-positive early pre-B acute lymphocytic leukemia; IgH = immunoglobulin heavy chain; Igκ and Igλ = immunoglobulin light chains; TCR = T-cell receptor; HOX = homeobox-containing genes. *TAL-1 is also termed *SCL* or *TCL-5* gene. The transforming gene and its chromosome location are bolded.

Fusion Genes

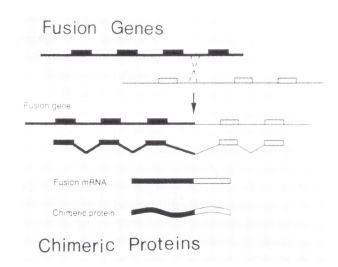

Figure 6–2. The creation of fusion genes and chimeric proteins.

each involved chromosome are disrupted, and portions of these genes are exchanged between the two chromosomes. The creation of fusion genes is schematized in Figure 6–2. When interchromosomal recombinations occur within introns of the genes involved, fusion genes are created that are transcribed into fusion messenger ribonucleic acid (mRNA) transcripts that encode new chimeric proteins. Each translocation will result in the formation of two functional chimeric genes, one on each partner chromosome. In most cases, only one of the hybrid genes is considered a candidate for the transforming gene, based on the gene sequences involved and the in vitro activities of the gene product. However, the reciprocal gene may be transcriptionally active as well. The novel chimeric proteins have properties that differ from those of the wild-type, unaltered proteins and are therefore suspected to be involved in the pathogenesis of these leukemias. Several examples exist for translocations resulting in fusion genes in leukemias, and representatives of these are summarized in Table 6–2. For some of the genes, common alternative or previously used designations have been listed in the legend. The products of most of the genes participating in these translocations have been characterized in terms of their phys-

Table 6–2. CREATION OF NOVEL FUSION GENES THROUGH CHROMOSOME TRANSLOCATIONS			
Disease	**Translocation**	**Fusion Genes**	**Gene Location**
Pre–pre-B ALL (M+)	t(4;11)(q21;q23)	MLL/AF4*	Chr. 4:AF4 and Chr. 11:MLL
Pre–pre-B ALL	t(17;19)(q22;p13)	E2A/HLF	Chr. 17:HLF and Chr. 19:E2A
Early pre-B ALL	t(9;22)(q34;q11)	BCR/ABL	Chr. 9:ABL and Chr. 22:BCR
Pre-B ALL	t(1;19)(q23;p13)	E2A/PBX1	Chr. 1:PBX1 and Chr. 19:E2A
Early pre-B ALL (M+)	t(12;21)(p13;q22)	TEL/AML1	Chr. 12:TEL and Chr. 21:AML1
T-ALL	t(X;11)(q13;q23)	MLL/AFX1	Chr. X:AFX1 and Chr. 11:MLL
AML (CD19+CD56+)	t(8;21)(q22;q22)	AML1/ETO	Chr. 8:ETO and Chr.21:AML1
AML eo	inv (16)(p13q22) or t(16;16)(p13;q22)	CBFβ/MYH11†	Chr. 16p:MYH11 and Chr.16q:CBFβ
APL	t(15;17)(q22;q21)	PML/RARα	Chr. 15:PML and Chr. 17:RARα
APL	t(11;17)(q23;q21)	PLZF/RARα	Chr. 11:PLZF and Chr. 17:RARα
APL	t(5;17)(q35;q21)	NPM/RARα	Chr. 5:NPM and Chr. 17:RARα
AML basophilia	t(6;9)(p23;q34)	DEK/CAN	Chr. 6:DEK and Chr. 9:CAN
AMML erythrophagocytosis	t(8;16)(p11;p13)	MOZ/CBP	Chr. 8:MOZ and Chr. 16:CBP
MPD, AML	t(8;9)(p12;q33)	FGFR1/CEP110	Chr. 8:FGFR1 and Chr. 9:CEP110
Primary/secondary AML	t(11;19)(q23;p13)	MLL/ENL‡	Chr. 11:MLL and Chr. 19:ENL
	t(9;11)(p22;q23)	MLL/AF9	Chr. 9:AF9 and Chr. 11:MLL
	t(11;16)(q23;p13)	MLL/CBP	Chr. 11:MLL and Chr. 16:CBP
	t(6;11)(q27;q23)	MLL/AF6	Chr. 6:AF6 and Chr. 11:MLL
AML, AMegL	t(3;3)(q21;q26) or inv (3)(q21q26)	EVI1	Chr. 3
AML, MDS	t(3;5)(q25;q34)	NPM/MLF1	Chr. 3:MLF1 and Chr. 5:NPM
CML	t(9;22)(q34;q11)	BCR/ABL	Chr. 9:ABL and Chr. 22:BCR
CML-BC	t(3;21)(q26;q22)	AML1/MDS1/EVI1	Chr. 3:MDS1/EVI1 and Chr. 21:AML1
CML, AML, MDS	t(16;21)(p11;q22)	ERG/TLS	Chr. 16:TLS and Chr .21:ERG
CMML	t(5;12)(q33;p13)	TEL/PDGFRβ	Chr. 5:PDGFRβ and Chr. 12:TEL

ALL = acute lymphoid leukemia; AML = acute myeloid leukemia; AML eo = AML with eosinophilia; APL = acute promyelocytic leukemia; AMML = acute myelo-monocytic leukemia; CML-BC = blast crisis of chronic myeloid leukemia; CMML = chronic myelomonocytic leukemia; M+ = positive for selected myeloid antigens.
* The MLL gene is also termed ALL1 or HRX.
† The MYH11 gene is also termed SMMHC.
‡ Different genes located on the same chromosome band may be fused with MLL in the t (11;19).

iologic function. Hypotheses regarding the transforming activity of the respective fusion gene products are based on those normal functional properties. However, the molecular mechanisms of leukemogenesis by fusion proteins remain largely unclear.

Many of the partnering genes in chromosomal translocations have been identified and found to encode cellular factors vital to the fine balance between cell proliferation and differentiation that guarantees regulated hematopoiesis. These are frequently transcription factors, proteins that bind to specific DNA sequences and thereby act as positive or negative regulators of mRNA transcription from responder genes. Transcription factors are grouped according to their DNA-domain binding motif (eg, transcription factors with basic helix-loop-helix motifs such as c-myc and E2A; proteins with helix-turn-helix motifs encoded by homeobox-containing genes, which are major players in the control of cel-

lular differentiation: the zinc finger LIM family such as Rbtn1/Ttg1 and Rbtn2/Ttg2; or transcription factors with runt DNA binding-domain such as the AML1 protein). Other genes involved in gene fusion may code for cytokines or their receptors, which convey growth regulatory signals from the cell membrane to the nucleus. Others are tumor suppressor genes, the products of which normally regulate cell proliferation by limiting passage of cells through the cell cycle. Finally, there are genes involved in programmed cell death or apoptosis.

Aberrant gene expression may result from gene overexpression due to the presence of multiple copies of the same gene. Such gene amplifications present cytogenetically as homogeneous staining regions (HSRs) (Figure 6–3), abnormally banded regions, or as double-minute chromosomes (dmin), the latter being acentric chromosomal fragments that contain amplified DNA sequences.

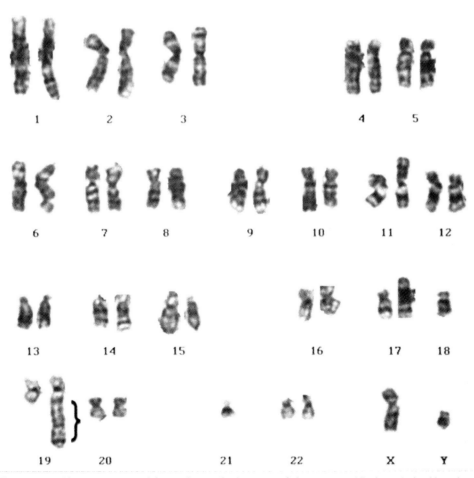

Figure 6–3. Homogeneous staining region on the long arm of chromosome 19, characterized by a long chromosomal segment that does not band (original magnification ×1,600; G banding).

MOLECULAR CYTOGENETICS

In cases in which conventional karyotyping fails to detect chromosomal defects by using banded chromosome spreads, alternative techniques may reveal the presence of cytogenetic abnormalities or gene alterations commonly associated with them. These include molecular cytogenetics in the form of fluorescent in situ hybridization (FISH) and the polymerase chain reaction (PCR), which, although plagued by their own limitations, have circumvented some technical problems associated with routine cytogenetic analysis and have tremendously increased the sensitivity level for detection of genetic defects.

Fluorescent In Situ Hybridization

The FISH technique involves the hybridization of single-stranded DNA probes to homologous single-stranded sequences in chromosomes of metaphase or interphase cells. Various types of FISH probes are available, such as whole-chromosome-specific, centromere-specific, gene-specific, or translocation-specific probes. Figure 6–4 demonstrates the principle of the FISH technique. The molecular probes are fluorescently tagged either directly or by various "sandwich" methods and are detected with a fluorescent microscope. In this way, genetic alterations can be detected at the single cell level, in a dividing (metaphase FISH) or a nondividing cell (interphase FISH), and correlated with morphology and immunophenotypic features of that cell. Fluorescent in situ hybridization is particularly advantageous in patients with acute leukemia in clinical remission. In this situation, cells carrying a patient's diagnostic cytogenetic aberration can be readily enumerated by counting fluorescent signals or hybrid (merged) signals when using translocation-specific probes. The major limitation of the FISH technique is that only those aberrations that are targeted by the probes used will be detected. Fluorescent in situ hybridization is therefore not recommended for establishing an aberrant karyotype at the time of diagnosis, unless the clinical presentation is suggestive of a specific cytogenetic abnormality (eg, abnormal eosinophilia suggesting inv [16]). Although excellent for monitoring the t(9;22) in CML, for instance, when monitoring disappearance of the translocation under interferon therapy, FISH will not detect the various cytogenetic abnormalities associated with evolution of blast crisis.

Polymerase Chain Reaction Technique

Polymerase chain reaction is a method for amplifying selected regions of DNA in vitro through repeated cycles of DNA synthesis, denaturation, and hybridiza-

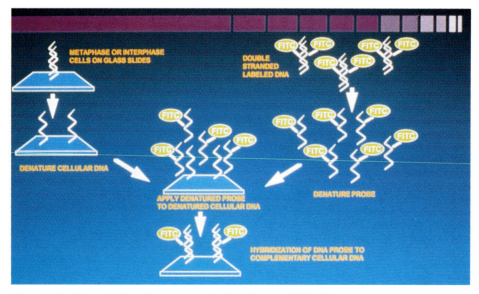

Figure 6–4.   The principle of fluorescent in situ hybridization (FISH). This methodology generally consists of denaturing the DNA in the interphase or metaphase cell and the DNA probe to produce single-stranded DNA. This is followed by a period of competitive hybridization and a wash to remove nonannealed probe. Binding of the fluorochrome-labeled probes is visualized under a fluorescent microscope.

tion. Because the reaction products accumulate exponentially, the concentration of target DNA theoretically doubles with every reaction cycle. Thus, after 20 cycles, the concentration of target DNA may exceed the concentration of nonamplified starting DNA by a factor of over 1 million, thereby, theoretically, allowing the detection of 1 malignant cell among 1 million nonmalignant cells. The high sensitivity of PCR is also its most serious problem since 1 contaminating molecule among 1 million others will result in a false-positive signal. The recent development of LightCycler real-time PCR may have resolved the problem of quantification of PCR products and therefore the quantification of residual disease.

Minimal Residual Disease Detection

To use PCR analysis, the gene sequences to be amplified must be known. This technique is therefore applicable to the detection of translocations for which the partnering genes have been cloned. Standardized PCR analyses of fusion gene transcripts have been developed for the detection of minimal residual disease in many leukemias.[1,2] Recently, molecular abnormalities diagnostic of certain leukemia subtypes have been detected in normal healthy tissues by most sensitive (nested) PCR assays (eg, transcripts from t[4;11], t[14;18], t[9;22], t[8;14] translocations and *MLL* tandem duplications). This has raised two questions: (1) whether results from nested PCR are always indicative of minimal residual disease and (2) whether these fusion transcripts require additional leukemogenic events for progression to clinically recognized malignancy. At least for *MLL* fusion transcripts, it has been suggested that those found in normal bone marrow and blood differ in their composition from those found in leukemic cells. The conclusion to be drawn from these findings is that nested PCR results should be interpreted in the context of additional laboratory and clinical information.

Cryptic Cytogenetic Abnormalities

Polymerase chain reaction analysis has detected gene rearrangements derived from well-characterized chromosome translocations in cells with a normal karyotype. For instance, the incidence of *MLL/AF4* fusion transcripts or *MLL* rearrangements

and duplications arising from other chromosome 11 abnormalities is much higher in leukemias than suggested by conventional cytogenetics. The finding of such cryptic cytogenetic abnormalities may affect prognosis. The *TEL/AML1* fusion gene, which is the most common nonrandom genetic aberration in childhood B-lineage ALL and is occasionally found in adult ALL, is created by a cryptic (12;21) translocation. In children, the presence of this fusion gene defines a subgroup of patients with better than average prognosis. Because of their potential prognostic implications, cryptic translocations are an important target of laboratory analyses. Evidence that genetic lesions may be missed by conventional cytogenetics makes it difficult to assign normal karyotypes to a particular cytogenetic risk group. The fact that most studies demonstrate that patients with a normal karyotype have an intermediate prognosis speaks in favor of the concept that this group may be comprised of a variety of undetected genetic defects.

HOW DO CYTOGENETICS CONTRIBUTE TO LEUKEMIA DIAGNOSIS?

Certain characteristic chromosome abnormalities are lineage specific. For instance, translocations involving Ig or TCR gene loci are typically found in acute or chronic lymphoid malignancies. Other karyotypes are diagnostic of a particular leukemia subtype, such as inv(16), t(8;21), and t(15;17), which are each associated with characteristic morphologic and immunophenotypic features. The (9;22) translocation, termed the Philadelphia (Ph) chromosome, is detected in CML but also in a subgroup of patients with acute lymphoid leukemia, however, with disparate breakpoints in one of the involved genes, the *BCR* gene. Among translocations that create novel fusion genes, one of the partner genes in the fusion process can affect the leukemia phenotype. For instance, t(11;19) with fusion of the *ELL/MEN* gene at 19p13.1 to *MLL* on 11q23 is exclusively found in AML, whereas the same translocation involving the *ENL* gene at 19p13.3 is found in AML and ALL with equal frequency. Finally, there are anomalies that are not subtype restricted. This applies predominantly to chromosome deletions and additions such as loss of chromosome 7 or deletion of the long arm of chromosome 5. Such unbalanced cytogenetic aberrations are associated with particular patient demographics and clinical histories. Several excellent reviews of cytogenetic abnormalities in hematologic malignancies are available to further the reader's understanding.[3–10]

ACUTE LEUKEMIAS

Acute Lymphocytic Leukemia

At least 60 percent of patients with ALL have cytogenetic abnormalities at the microscopic level. The percentage of genetically abnormal patients may be much higher when one considers cryptic translocations, such as t(12;21), which, at least in children, have dramatically increased the prevalence rate of nonrandom genetic lesions. The most common structural chromosome aberrations in ALL are listed in Tables 6–1 and 6–2.

Translocations Involving Antigen Receptor Loci

The majority of structural abnormalities in ALL fall into the category that leads to gene activation through translocation of a regulatory gene, a potential oncogene, into a lymphoid antigen receptor locus.[11,12] Depending on whether Ig or TCR gene loci are involved, the leukemic cells display a B- or T-lymphoid phenotype, respectively. The relevant gene loci are 14q32 for Ig heavy chain, 2p12 for Ig kappa light chain, and 22q11 for Ig lambda light chain and for TCR loci, 7q35 for TCRβ, 14q11 for TCRα/δ, and 7p14 for TCRγ.

The karyotype characteristic of mature B-ALL results in activation of the *C-MYC* oncogene through juxtaposition with Ig heavy- or light-chain loci, **t(8;14)(q24;q32)** (Figure 6–5), **t(2;8)(p12;q24)**, and **t(8;22)(q24;q11)**. A role for inappropriate *C-MYC* expression in neoplastic B-cell proliferation is suggested from experiments in transgenic mice expressing *C-MYC* under the control of Ig heavy-chain enhancer sequences. These mice develop aggressive clonal B-cell malignancies. However, a few cases with mature B-ALL lacking any of these translocations have been described, suggesting that this phenotype may develop through other genetic mechanisms as well. Patients with mature B-ALL tend to have a poorer prognosis than other ALL patients. They also have an increased incidence of central nervous system involvement and extramedullary disease, factors that may contribute to a poorer outcome.

Abnormal expression of *C-MYC* under the control of the TCRα/δ locus in t(8;14)(q24;q11) is associated with T-cell neoplasms, again emphasizing that inappropriate production of *C-MYC* encoded protein is the cause of uncontrolled cellular proliferation. Although T-lineage ALLs overall do better than B-lineage ALL patients, the small **t(8;14)(q24;q11)** subgroup may have a worse prognosis.

Several different proto-oncogenes are activated by translocations in T-ALL, resulting from aberrant recombinase activity, some of which are listed in Table 6–1. The most common one is the stem cell leukemia (*SCL*) or *TAL-1* gene, which is aberrantly expressed after translocation from 1p32-33 into the TCRα/δ or TCRβ locus.[13] The prototype translocation with *SCL* activation is the **t(1;14)(p32;q11)**, occurring in approximately 3 percent of T-ALL. Most patients with *SCL* dysregulation have one or both TCRδ genes deleted and express a CD3-positive TCRα/β-positive phenotype. Although translocations involving the *SCL/TAL-1* gene are cytogenetically detected in only a small number of patients, the *SCL/TAL-1* gene appears activated through other mechanisms in almost 25 percent of patients with T-ALL. The SCL/TAL-1 protein is a transcription factor that was found to be essential for normal hematopoiesis. Its overexpression in transgenic mice, however, induced T-cell malignancies. At least in pediatric studies, the prognosis of patients with SCL/TAL-1 expression is indistinguishable from that of patients without it. *RBTN1* and *RBTN2* genes constitute a distinct family of proto-oncogenes that are activated by tumor-specific translocations in T-ALL (eg, t[11;14][p15;q11]).[14] Their thymic expression in transgenic mice induces T-cell tumors. Interactions between *RBTN1* and *RBTN2* encoded LIM motif transcription factors and the basic helix-loop-helix proteins encoded by *SCL/TAL-1* or by the related *TAL-2* and *LYL1* genes suggest a common leukemogenic pathway in T-ALL harboring genetic alterations that lead to expression of these gene products.

Of interest mostly because of its clinical presentation is **t(5;14)(q31;q32)** in immature B-lineage ALL. This translocation joins the interleukin-3 (IL-3) gene to the Ig heavy-chain gene. It is hypothesized that the peripheral blood eosinophilia associated with this disease may be the result of IL-3 gene activation. In fact, serum IL-3 levels have been found to correlate with disease activity.

Translocations Leading to the Creation of Fusion Genes

Table 6–2 summarizes the most common translocations in ALL that create novel fusion genes.

The **t(4;11)(q21;q23)** is found in < 5 percent of adults with ALL (Figure 6–6). It is associated with a pre–pre-B, CD10-negative immunophenotype that is further characterized by expression of CD15, often in the absence of other myeloid antigens. Occasionally, the same translocation is seen in more mature B-lineage ALL and T-ALL, as well as de novo undifferentiated AML. Among the rare cases of sec-

ondary ALL, t(4;11) is observed disproportionately often when compared with its low incidence in de novo ALL. There is a strong correlation between secondary ALL with t(4;11) and previous treatment with cytostatic drugs targeting DNA topoisomerase II. The 11q23 translocation breakpoints have been identified as cleavage sites for this enzyme. The *MLL (ALL-1, HRX)* gene at 11q23, encoding a transcription factor with homology to the drosophila trithorax gene product, is fused to the *AF4 (FEL)* gene from chromosome 4q21. Although transcripts from both derivative chromosomes have been amplified in leukemic cell lines, the reciprocal *AF4/MLL* gene product has not been found in untreated patients, making the *MLL/AF4* on der(11) the likely leukemogenic fusion product. In adult pre–pre-B ALL patients without cytogenetic evidence of t(4;11), *MLL/AF4* fusion transcripts have been detected by PCR assays. It remains to be established

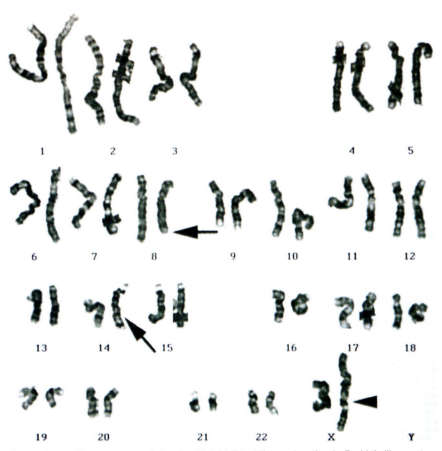

Figure 6–5. Karyotype containing the (8;14)(q24;q32) translocation in Burkitt's-like, mature B-ALL. Arrows point at breaksites on the two involved chromosomes. In this case, an extra copy of 7q (common in lymphoid malignancies) is found on an X chromosome (*arrowhead*) (original magnification ×1,600; G banding).

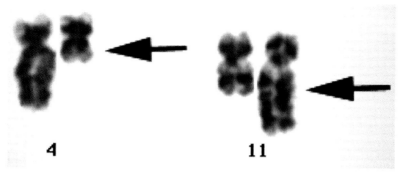

Figure 6–6. Partial karyotype demonstrating the (4;11)(q21;q23) translocation. Arrows refer to breaksites (original magnification ×3,200; G banding).

whether patients carrying cryptic *MLL* translocations share the poor prognostic features of patients with positive cytogenetics. Aside from t(4;11), other 11q23 translocations are recurring abnormalities in both ALL and AML,[15,16] such as **t(1;11)(p32;q23)**, **t(9;11)(p22;q23)**, and **(11;19)(q23;p13)**. Translocation **(X;11)(q13;q23)** is restricted to T-ALL.

Whereas most reports describe t **(1;19)(q23;p13)** (Figure 6–7) predominantly in pediatric pre-B ALL, we have observed this translocation in 20 percent of adult pre-B ALL cases, reflecting an incidence rate almost identical to that in children with this disease subtype. Molecularly, this translocation juxtaposes the *E2A* gene with the *PBX1* gene. E2A proteins function as transcriptional activators, which are essential for normal B-cell development.[17] The translocation creates an *E2A/PBX1* fusion gene on the der(19) chromosome. Cases of t(1;19) ALL without detection of *E2A/PBX1* fusion transcripts have been described, suggesting that this translocation is molecularly heterogeneous. Clinically, t(1;19)

ALL is associated with known risk factors, such as high white count at diagnosis and central nervous system disease, which require intensified treatment approaches. The other chromosomal translocation involving the *E2A* gene, the **t(17;19)(q21;p13)**, is present in < 1 percent of pediatric ALL, mostly of the pre–pre-B phenotype. The same region of the *E2A* gene is fused to the *HLF* (hepatic leukemic factor) gene as is fused to the *PBX1* gene in t(1;19). Like *PBX1*, the *HLF* gene encodes a transcription factor, and the chimeric E2A-PBX1 protein product is implied in the leukemogenic process.

The **(9;22)(q34;q11)** translocation (Figure 6–8), which leads to formation of the Ph chromosome, occurs in at least 25 percent of patients with ALL. The incidence is higher in older patients. It is also the hallmark of CML. The translocation results in the fusion of parts of the *ABL* gene from chromosome 9 with sequences of the *BCR* gene on chromosome 22 creating the *BCR/ABL* fusion gene, which is proposed as the pathogenic molecular event in this disease. The

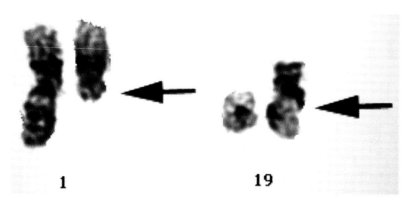

Figure 6–7. Partial karyotype demonstrating the (1;19)(q23;p13) translocation. Arrows refer to breaksites. This anomaly may present as a balanced translocation, as seen here, or as an unbalanced derivative 19 (original magnification ×3,200; G banding).

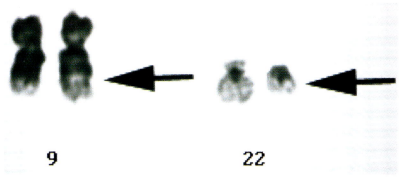

Figure 6–8. Partial karyotype demonstrating the (9;22)(q34;q11) translocation. Arrows refer to breaksites (original magnification ×3,200; G banding).

reciprocal *ABL/BCR* gene fusion product on the derivative chromosome 9 does not appear to be pathogenetically significant (schematized in Figure 6–9). The breakpoint in the *BCR* gene in most cases of Ph-positive ALL differs from that in CML so that gene products of distinct sizes are created. In CML, the *BCR/ABL* mRNA transcript processed from the resulting fusion gene contains *BCR* exon b2 or b3 fused to *ABL* exon a2 (b2a2, b3a2) and is translated into a fusion protein with an approximate molecular mass of 210 kDa. About two-thirds of ALL cases have breakpoints that result in the fusion of *BCR* exon e1 to *ABL* exon a2 (e1a2 junction). In this case, the resulting chimeric mRNA is translated into a smaller 190-kDa fusion protein. In general, this allows the distinction between Ph-positive ALL and lymphoid blast crisis of CML by PCR using primers designed to amplify junction sequences characteristic of each type of gene rearrangement. Figure 6–10 demonstrates the differ-

entially sized PCR products amplified from patients with CML and ALL using these primers. However, in a significant portion of Ph-positive ALL cases without a history suggestive of antecedent CML, CML-typical *BCR/ABL* transcripts alone or in conjunction with ALL-typical transcripts have been detected. Philadelphia chromosome-positive patients usually present with early pre-B ALL immunophenotype, are positive for CD34 and selective myeloid antigens, and express CD25, the alpha-chain of the IL-2 receptor.[18] In most clinical trials, they have an inferior outcome. Whether distinct molecular features add to the prognostic impact of this cytogenetic abnormality is currently unknown. Additional chromosome abnormalities in Ph-positive patients may affect long-term treatment results.[19,20] Molecular testing of ALL patients with normal karyotype and particularly those with insufficient metaphases is recommended. In the Eastern Cooperative Oncology Group (Paietta E, unpublished

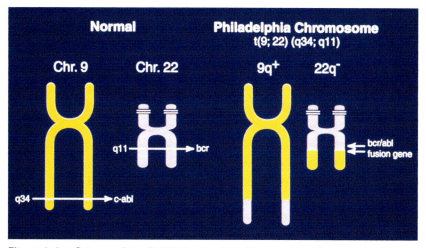

Figure 6–9. Schema of the (9;22) translocation with arrows pointing at breaksites and the resulting *BCR/ABL* fusion site on the 22q- derivative.

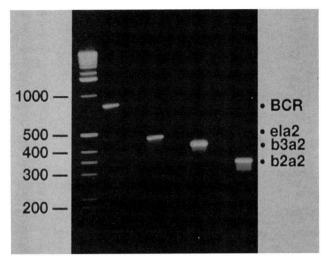

Figure 6–10. Polymerase chain reaction products obtained using primer pairs designed to amplify the three common *BCR/ABL* fusion gene products (e1a2, b3a, b2a2) and normal *BCR* RNA (control for RNA integrity and successful cDNA reverse transcription).

The cryptic **(12;21)(p13;q22)** translocation that results in the *TEL/AML1* fusion gene is found in approximately 25 percent of childhood ALL. Data on adult ALL are limited but suggest a much lower incidence (approximately 3%). The TEL protein is a member of the Ets family of transcription factors.[22] The other target in this translocation is the *AML1 (CBFA2)* gene, a member of the family of core binding factor (CBF) genes. *AML1* represents one of three CBFα subunits that, together with a common CBFβ subunit, comprise functional transcription factors. Both *AML1* and *CBFβ* are involved in several translocations associated with AML. Core binding factor oncoproteins, such as the *TEL/AML1* fusion product, modulate endogenous CBF activities, which may be relevant to transformation. In childhood ALL, the presence of the *TEL/AML1* fusion gene is related to in vitro sensitivity for L-asparaginase.[23]

data) experience of > 300 patients, approximately 2 percent of patients with molecular *BCR/ABL* transcripts are cytogenetically negative for t(9;22). An even higher incidence has been reported by others in a smaller group of patients.[21]

Numeric Chromosome Changes

In terms of numeric changes, hyperdiploidy of > 50 chromosomes is much more common in ALL (5 to

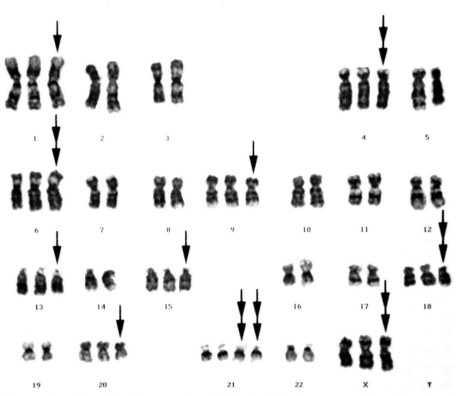

Figure 6–11. Hyperdiploidy in a case of ALL. Gain of certain chromosomes is found to be invariant (*double arrows*). Single arrows designate variable chromosome gain particular to this case (original magnification ×1,600; G banding).

15% of cases) than in AML and is associated with a favorable prognosis (Figure 6–11).[24] Hypodiploidy and near-haploid clones are rare and have a poorer outcome. Other numeric changes are rare in adult ALL. Loss of genetic material from the long arm of chromosome 6, del(6)(q13-15q23) or del (6)(q21), is seen as a secondary alteration in about 10 percent of patients with ALL and also in other lymphoid neoplasms, such as chronic lymphocytic leukemia (CLL) and various lymphomas. Deletions of chromosome 9p, predominantly 9p21-22, are lymphoid lineage specific but not specific for a particular subtype. However, a large percentage of patients with del(9p) or translocations involving 9p present with a T-cell phenotype and certain clinical features, such as a mediastinal mass. The deletions often include the entire interferon gene cluster, the methylthioadenosine phosphorylase gene, and the putative p16[INK4a] (*CDKN2/MTS1*) tumor suppressor gene.

Table 6–3. SELECTED RECURRENT CHROMOSOMAL ABERRATIONS IN AML		
Category	**Critical Genes**	**Disease Subtype**
CBF leukemias		
t(8;21)(q22;q22)	*ETO/AML1*	CD19+ CD56+ AML/M2, M1, M0
t(16;21)(p11;q22)	*MTG16/AML1*	AML/M2, M4, M7
inv(16)(p13q22)	*CBFβ/MYH11*	CD2+ AMML/M4/eosinophilia
t(16;16)(p13;q22)		
t(3;21)(q26;q22)	*MDS1/EVI1/AML1*	MDS, t-AML, CML-BC
CBP and p300 leukemias		
t(8;16)(p11;p13)	*MOZ/CBP*	M4/M5
t(11;16)(q23;p13)	*MLL/CBP*	t-AML, MDS
t(11;22)(q23;q13)	*MLL/p300*	AML
MLL leukemias		
t(1;11)(q21;q23)	*AF1q/MLL*	AMOL/M5
t(6;11)(q27;q23)	*AF6/MLL*	AMML, AMOL/M4, M5
t(9;11)(p22;q23)	*AF9/MLL* or del(11)(q23)	AMOL/M5,few ALL or MDS
t(10;11)(p13;q23)	*AF10/MLL*	AMML, AMOL/M4, M5
t(11;19)(q23;p13.1)	*ELL/MEN/MLL*	AML
t(11;19)(q23;p13.3)	*ENL/MLL*	AML, ALL
t(11;17)(q23;q21)	*MLL/AF17*	AMML, AMOL/M4, M5
+11	Duplicate *MLL*	AML
Fusion genes involving RARα		
t(5;17)(p23;q11-12)	*NPM/RARα*	APL/M3
t(15;17)(q22;q21)	*PML/RARα*	APL/M3
t(11;17)(q23;q21)	*PLZF/RARα*	APL/M3
t(11;17)(q13;q21)	*NuMA/RARα*	APL/M3
Other translocations		
t(6;9)(p23;q34)	*DEK/CAN*	AML/basophilia/M2, M4
t(3;5)(q21;q31)	*MLF1/NPM*	Erythroleukemia/M6
t(3;3)(q21;q26)	*RibophorinI-EVII*	MDS, AMegL
inv(3)(q21q26)		
t(9;22)(q34;q11)	*BCR/ABL*	AML, t-AML
Numeric changes		
del(5)(q13q33)/-5	?	MDS, AML, t-AML
del(7)(q22q34)/-7	?	MDS, AML, t-AML
del(12)(p12)	?	AML, t-AML, MDS, ALL
del(17)(p11-12)	?	AML, t-AML, MDS
del(20)(q11q13)	?	AML, PV, ET, myelofibrosis
dup (1q)	?	AML, PV, ET, myelofibrosis
+4	?	AML/M0
+6	?	AML, MDS
+8	?	AML, PV
+13	?	AML
+19	?	AML, MDS
+21	?	AML, MDS

MDS = myelodysplasia; AML = acute myeloid leukemia; AMML = acute myelomonocytic leukemia; AMOL = acute monocytic leukemia; t-AML = treatment-related AML; APL = acute promyelocytic leukemia; AMegL = acute megakaryocytic leukemia; PV = polycythemia vera; ET = essential thrombocythemia; M1–M5 refer to FAB classifications.

Table 6–4. CYTOGENETIC RISK GROUPS IN DE NOVO AML	
Risk Group	**Cytogenetic Abnormalities**
Favorable	Inv(16)/t(16;16)/del(16q); t(15;17) with and without additional abnormalities; t(8;21) without del(9q) or complex abnormalities
Intermediate	Normal; del(9q), t/del(11q23), del(12p), +6, +8, +21, +22, -Y, some del (7q)
Unfavorable	del(5q)/-5; del(7q)/-7; abn(3q), t(6;9), t(8;16), del(20q), del(17p), +13, complex karyotype (≥ 3 unrelated cytogenetic abnormalities); ring chromosomes, double-minutes, HSRs and other signs of gene amplification

HSR = homogeneous staining region.

Acute Myeloid Leukemia, Myelodysplasia, Polycythemia Vera, and Essential Thrombocythemia

Table 6–3 summarizes the most frequent recurrent chromosomal aberrations in AML, with emphasis on primary anomalies. The table indicates whether there is overlap between primary AML and other hematologic disorders, such as myelodysplasia (MDS), myeloproliferative disorders (MPDs), or treatment-related AML (t-AML). Whenever possible, translocations are grouped according to shared critical genes since this may suggest shared mechanisms of leukemogenesis. Table 6–4 defines risk groups in de novo AML based on cytogenetic abnormalities.

Core Binding Factor Leukemias

Core binding factors participate in the formation of fusion genes in a variety of AML subtypes.[25,26] They are heterodimeric transcription factors containing a common CBFβ subunit and one of three CBFα sub-units. Core binding factor-α corresponds to AML1, the DNA binding domain of which is fused to the *ETO* gene, also known as *MTG8*, on chromosome 8 in the **(8;21)(q22;q22)** translocation (Figure 6–12). The AML1-ETO chimeric product has profound deleterious effects on normal hematopoietic differentiation: it induces proliferation and increases the self-renewal capacity of transfected cells. A recent paradigm suggests the involvement of AML1-ETO in the disruption of chromatin remodeling.[27] Leukemic cells bearing this translocation frequently have a distinct immunophenotype with the expression of the B-cell antigen CD19 along with the neural cell adhesion molecule CD56 on CD34-positive myeloblasts. Although most patients show differentiated FAB M2 morphology with Auer rods, very undifferentiated phenotypes have been reported as well. Patients have consistently higher rates of complete remission than patients with other cytogenetic abnormalities (except inv[16] or t[15;17]) and have superior event-free and overall survival when treated with high-dose cytosine arabinoside in some studies. Leukocytosis at diagnosis is associated with poor survival in these patients. Several secondary cytogenetic abnormalities occur in t(8;21) cells, predominantly the loss of one sex chromosome, del(9)(q13q22) and trisomy 8. To date, only an additional deletion at 9q has been shown to impair survival. *AML1-ETO* fusion may be detected in AML without t(8;21) but with other chromosome 8 abnormalities. In addition to the common t(8;21), *AML1* rearrangements have been detected with several other gene fusion partners (eg, on 17q11 and 1p36 in t-AML). The *AML1* gene may be amplified in situ, which appears as a cytogenetically unidentifiable HSR. In the molecularly related **(16;21)(p11;q22)** translocation, *AML1* is fused to the *ETO* homologous

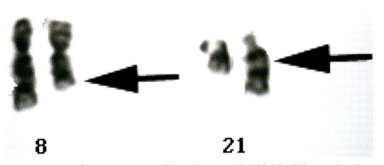

8   **21**

Figure 6–12. Partial karyotype illustrating the (8;21)(q22;q22) translocation. Arrows refer to breaksites (original magnification ×3,200; G banding).

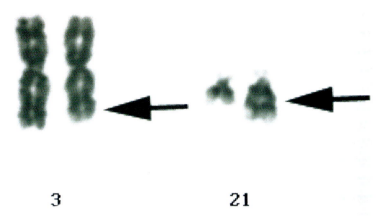

3   **21**

Figure 6–13. Partial karyotype illustrating the (3;21)(q26;q22) translocation. Arrows refer to breaksites (original magnification ×3,200; G banding).

MTG16 gene. Although rare, patients demonstrate variable morphologic characteristics and appear to experience short survival. The **(3;21)(q26;q22)** translocation is detected in myelodysplasia, AML, and t-AML or in the myeloid blast crisis of CML (Figure 6–13).

Inv(16)(p13q22) and the less common **t(16;16)(p13;q22)** involve the CBFβ subunit. Figure 6–14 illustrates a schema for the formation of the inv(16) aberration and its detection by FISH using a breakaway probe. The subtle chromosomal changes seen in association with this inversion are shown in Figure 6–15. The fusion product of the CBFβ and the *MYH11* or *SMMHC* gene (smooth muscle myosin heavy chain) interferes with CBF activities and several other physiologic processes.[28] These leukemias present frequently (85%) with French-American-British (FAB) M4 morphology and abnormal eosinophilia and have an excellent prognosis. The incidence of the subtle inv(16) may be underesti-

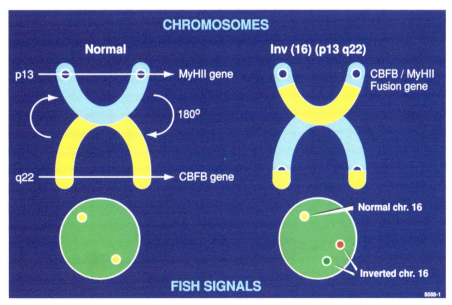

Figure 6–14. Schema of the inv(16)(p13q22). Color coding illustrates the exchange of chromosomal material between the long and short arms of the same chromosome 16 during the inversion. The presumed pathogenetic *CBF*β*-MYH11* fusion gene is created at 16p13. The illustrations underneath represent the results of FISH analysis. Some probes, as in the bicolor inv(16) cocktail illustrated here, are designed to give an overlapping color signal in the normal state (yellow) and to separate into distinct colors when rearranged (red and green). This results in very low background and is ideal for estimates of residual disease.

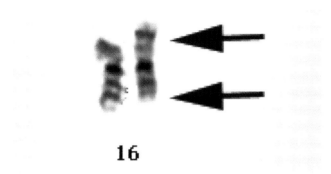

Figure 6–15. Partial karyotype demonstrating the subtle chromosomal changes in inv(16). Arrows point to breaksites on the short and long arms of the same chromosome (original magnification ×3,200; G banding).

mated using standard cytogenetics as compared with PCR. Trisomy 22 in AML with eosinophilia is strongly associated with inv(16), which may be detected at the molecular level even when the inversion is not found. Inv(16) in secondary AML, albeit uncommon, has been observed in patients exposed to topoisomerase II targeting drugs or taxanes. Similar to de novo inv(16) patients, secondary cases seem to benefit from high-dose cytosine arabinoside.

Core Binding Protein and p300 Leukemias

Core binding protein (CBP), the binding protein of the cyclic adenosine monophosphate response element-binding protein, and p300 are critical co-factors for a variety of transcription factors involved in the control of hematopoietic cell differentiation.[29] One class of transcription factors regulated by CBP and p300 is E2A proteins, which have been discussed because of their involvement in t(1;19) of pre-B ALL. Another leukemogenic factor controlled by

p300 is AML1, introduced above. Three leukemia-associated translocations involve CBP or p300 themselves, **t(8;16)(p11;p13)**, **t(11;16)(q23;p13)**, and **t(11;22)(q23;q13)**. In the (8;16) translocation (Figure 6–16), a CBP-derived domain is fused to the MOZ acetyltransferase domain. Transcriptional gene activation is typically associated with acetylation of DNA-associated proteins. The relevance of histone acetylation and deacetylation for gene transcription is further exemplified in leukemias with translocations involving the retinoic acid receptor-α gene (see section on RARα rearrangements). Both the t(11;16) and the t(11;22) fuse the *MLL* gene to **CBP** and *p300*, respectively. Patients with t(11;16) usually have treatment-related leukemias.

Leukemias with MLL Rearrangements, Duplication, or Deletion

In various reciprocal translocations associated with ALL or AML, the *MLL (ALL-1, HRX)* gene located at chromosome 11 band q23 is fused to several different partner genes.[15,16] Each 11q23 abnormality gives rise to a specific fusion gene and, presumably, an oncogenic fusion protein. Interstitial deletions and tandem duplications of *MLL* have also been reported in del(11) (q23) without an apparent partner chromosome and trisomy 11, respectively. The most common fusion partners for *MLL* are *AF4* in t(4;11), which occurs predominantly in ALL, and *AF9* in t(9;11), which is found predominantly in AML. The majority of AML cases present with myelomonocytic or monocytic features. Leukemias arising after treatment for a primary malignancy show a high prevalence of *MLL* rearrangements.

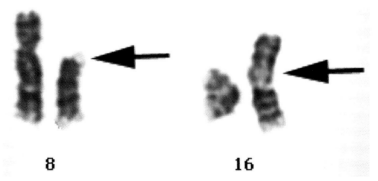

Figure 6–16. Partial karyotype illustrating the (8;16)(p11;p13) translocation. Arrows refer to breaksites (original magnification ×3,200; G banding).

Most of these leukemias develop following treatment with topoisomerase II inhibitors, such as epipodophyllotoxins. The breakpoint cluster region of *MLL* contains sequences with homology to topoisomerase II consensus binding sites, which may explain this association. Typically, secondary AML with *MLL* rearrangements develops with short latency, within a few months or years after treatment. This is in contrast with secondary leukemias bearing aberrations of chromosomes 5 and 7, which develop many years after treatment with alkylating agents or radiation. *MLL/AF4* and *MLL* partial tan-

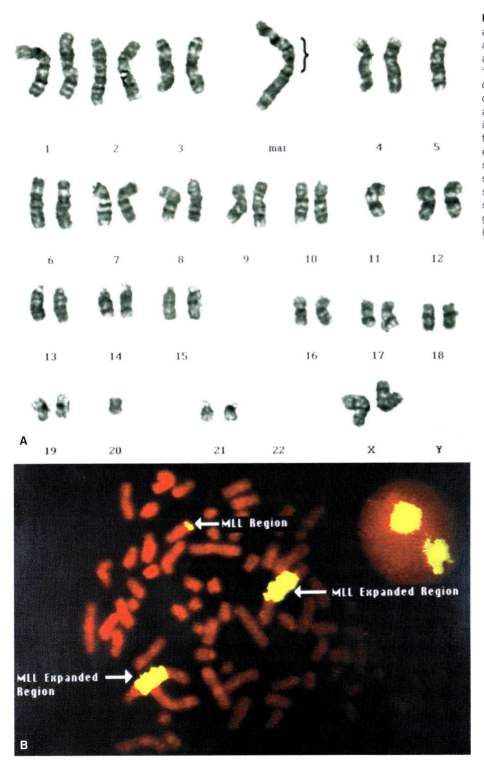

Figure 6–17. *A*, The cytogenetic appearance of a cryptic *MLL* gene amplification. In this case, *MLL* is amplified at the site of the gene "bridging" a 5;11 dicentric marker chromosome (mar) (original magnification ×1,600) G banding. *B*, *MLL* amplification was confirmed by FISH in a near tetraploid clone obtained from this patient. Two dicentrics with expanded *MLL* region (yellow) are seen in the metaphase (chromosomes visible) and interphase cells shown. In the metaphase cell, the small *MLL* signal represents the *MLL* gene on a normal chromosome 11 (original magnification ×1,000).

dem duplication transcripts can be detected in patients with normal karyotypes. Except in AML patients with t(9;11), *MLL* rearrangements or amplifications appear to be indicators of poor survival. An example of cryptic *MLL* gene amplification is demonstrated in Figure 6–17.

Leukemias Involving RARα

The majority of cases with acute promyelocytic leukemia (APL)/FAB M3 are associated with the reciprocal **(15;17)(q22;q21)** translocation (Figure 6–18), which disrupts the *PML* (promyelocytic leukemia) gene on chromosome 15 and the *RARα* gene on chromosome 17.[30] Fluorescent in situ hybridization is helpful in detecting this translocation at the time of minimal residual disease and in nondividing granulocytes after maturation-inducing therapy with all-*trans* retinoic acid (ATRA) (Figure 6–19). The other gene rearrangements found in APL all involve the fusion of *RARα* to one of three other genes, the promyelocytic leukemia zinc finger (*PLZF*) on 11q23, nucleophosmin (*NPM*) on 5p23, or the nuclear matrix-associated (*NuMA*) gene on 11q13. Occasionally, t(15;17) may be found in leukemias with morphology other than M3. In such cases, characteristic immunophenotypic features will support the APL diagnosis. Additional cytogenetic abnormalities do not appear to alter the favorable prognosis of APL. Depending on the breakpoint in the *PML* gene, three distinct types of *PML/RARα* fusion transcripts are formed: the short form (S), the long form (L), and variable isoforms (V), with the V form being the rarest. Although the three isoforms do not seem to alter prognosis, they demonstrate some biologic and clinical differences. Leukemic

promyelocytes containing the S form more often express the T-cell antigen CD2 and the natural killer cell marker CD56 and have a higher incidence of microgranular morphology (M3v) and of additional cytogenetic abnormalities. Both S- and V-form patients tend to present with higher white blood cell counts than those with the L form.

Acute promyelocytic leukemia with the classic t(15;17) shows exquisite sensitivity to ATRA. Although *RARα* is disrupted in an identical place in all of these translocations, patients with the *PLZF/RARα* fusion gene are resistant to the retinoid when given alone. Expression of the PML/RARα fusion protein leads to significant alterations in nuclear architecture, which can be normalized by treating APL cells with ATRA or arsenic compounds. RARα fusion proteins seem to act in a dominant negative fashion, reducing the transcriptional activity of unmutated RARα. Speculations regarding the mechanism of action of ATRA in APL are multiple. It appears that at physiologic levels of ATRA, the fusion receptors do not activate (rather repress) transcription of critical genes for myeloid differentiation. Retinoic acid receptor is pivotal in the regulation of chromatin structure through a balance of histone acetylation and deacetylation.[27] Abnormal histone deacetylation has been observed in APL cells. At physiologic ATRA concentrations, RARα fusion products maintain retinoic acid-responsive genes in a repressed deacetylated state by binding to a nuclear co-repressor molecule. Pharmacologic ATRA levels are necessary to induce conformational changes of RARα and the release of the co-repressor complex. The availability of histone deacetylase inhibitors for the clinic may be exploitable as another targeted therapeutic approach in APL in the future.

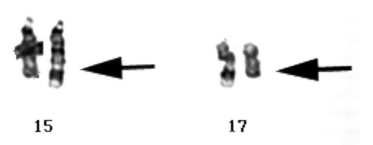

15   **17**

Figure 6–18. Partial karyotype demonstrating the (15;17)(q22;q21) translocation. Arrows point at breaksites (original magnification ×3,200; G banding).

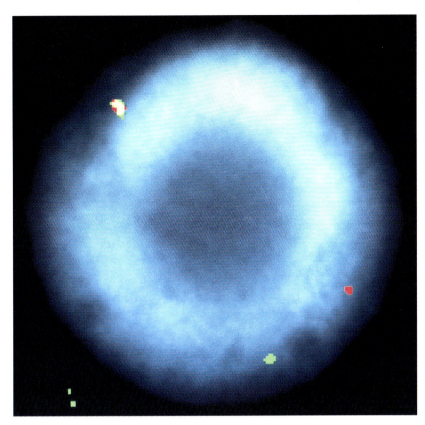

Figure 6–19. Bicolor FISH analysis of APL targets the derivative 15. The gene-specific probe for PML is red, the one for RARα is green and distal to the breaksite. If the (15;17) translocation is present, the labeled probes merge at the PML locus to give the yellow hybrid signal. During the translocation, the reciprocal derivative 17 usually does not receive sufficient red fluorescence from the translocated PML gene segment to be detected (original magnification ×1,000).

In a small percentage of t-AML, APL with t(15;17) has been reported, often following chemotherapy regimens including etoposide. Although topoisomerase II cleavage sites have not been detected within the second RARα intron, the location of the breakpoint in t(15;17), the proposed effect of RARα on chromatin structure may predispose for the development of etoposide-related APL. Reports in the literature on secondary APL include several patients with breast cancer who developed the leukemia after only having had surgery. It is intriguing in this respect that allele losses in the region 17q12-21 have been observed in families with high rates of breast and ovarian cancer and have been shown to involve *BRCA1*, the breast and ovarian cancer susceptibility gene.

NPM, one of the alternate fusion sites for *RARα*, is also involved in other hematologic malignancies, the **t(3;5)(q25;q34)** seen in acute erythroleukemia (AEL)/FAB M6 and MDS and in the t(2;5)(p23;q35) of Ki-1-positive anaplastic lymphomas. Another alternate fusion protein, the chromatin-associated NuMA, regulates mitotic spindle organization and interphase nuclear matrix functions.

Other Structural Chromosome Changes in AML

The **(6;9)(p23;q34)** translocation is a relatively rare abnormality (Figure 6–20). Patients are typically younger than the average, have variable morphology, preceding MDS, present with basophilia, and have an unfavorable prognosis. The break on 9q34 occurs in the *CAN* gene, downstream from the *c-ABL* gene, which is situated in the same chromosome band, and results in the formation of chimeric *DEK/CAN* gene transcripts. The physiologic significance of the *DEK* and *CAN* genes is yet to be elucidated.

Myeloid neoplasms involving abnormalities of the long arm of chromosome 3, **inv(3)(q21q26)**, **t(3;3)(q21;q26)**, and other related aberrations are characterized by disturbed thrombopoiesis. Monosomy 7 or del(7q) are frequent concurrent abnormalities in this karyotype (Figure 6–21). Outcome is generally poor whether these rearrangements are associated with MDS, AML, t-AML, or acute megakaryocytic leukemia (AMegL). Despite the dysplastic megakaryocytopoiesis, the gene encoding thrombopoietin, localized at 3q27-28, is not involved. In the 3q21q26 syndrome, the genes

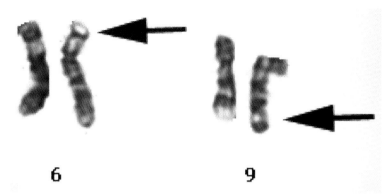

Figure 6–20. Partial karyotype demonstrating the (6;9)(p23;q34) translocation. Arrows point at breaksites (original magnification ×3,200; G-Banding).

involved are the *Ribophorin I* gene at 3q21 and the *EVI1* gene at 3q26. EVI1 is a transcription factor normally not expressed in hematopoietic cells, which may be activated under the control of *Ribophorin I* enhancer elements. The **(3;6)(q21;p21)** translocation in AML combines abnormal thrombopoiesis related to 3q21 with basophilia, possibly associated with the del(6p) reminiscent of t(6;9). Other frequent changes in AMegL in adults are trisomy 21, mono-

somy 5 or 7 or deletion (7q), trisomy 8, and trisomy 19. The **t(1;22)(p13;q13)** is restricted to AMegL/FAB M7 of childhood.

The *FGFR1* gene, which encodes a tyrosine kinase receptor for members of the fibroblast growth factor family, is located at chromosome 8 band p12. This gene is disrupted in several translocations, which result in chimeric proteins with putative oncogenic properties. The **t(8;9)(p12;q33),**

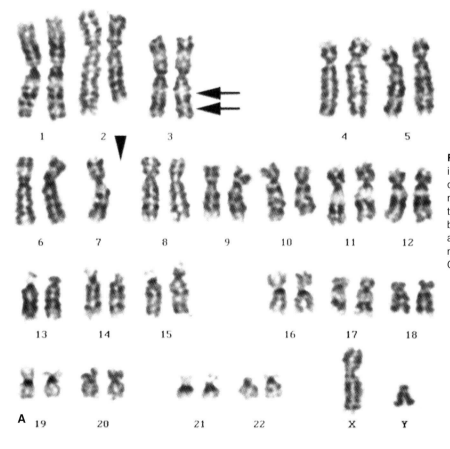

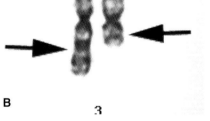

Figure 6–21. *A,* A full karyotype with inv(3)(q21q26) plus monosomy 7, a frequent concomitant alteration (original magnification ×1,600). *B,* A partial karyotype of t(3;3)(q21;q26) with arrows pointing at breaksites. Double arrows indicate inv(3); arrowhead indicates missing second chromosome (7) (original magnification ×3,200; G banding).

which fuses the *FGFR1* gene with the *CEP110* gene, is associated with stem cell MPD. Myeloproliferative disorder is characterized by B- or T-cell lymphoblastic leukemia/lymphoma, myeloid hyperplasia, and peripheral blood eosinophilia, which often progresses to AML.

De novo AML with the Ph chromosome translocation **(9;22)(q34;q11)**, for which a myeloid phenotype was confirmed by immunophenotyping, is rare (< 1%).[31] Additional chromosomal abnormalities include monosomy 7 or 5 and del(5q), all genetic aberrations of multipotent stem cells. The appearance of the Ph chromosome, together with inv(16), may be secondary to or preceding inv(16). Breakpoints in the *BCR/ABL* fusion are heterogeneous. Clonal evolution with acquisition of cytogenetically detected t(9;22) or of *BCR/ABL* transcripts at a late stage of AML is a well-documented phenomenon, particularly in patients with primary t(8;21) or -7.

Deletions or Numeric Changes in AML

Monosomy or interstitial deletions of chromosomes 5, 7, and 17 are typical of patients with MDS, t-AML, or poor prognostic AML.[32,33] Long arm loss of chromosomes 5 and 7 or of chromosome 5 and the short arm of chromosome 17 frequently occur within a single clone, often with numerous additional cytogenetic changes present. It has been hypothesized that loss of a putative tumor suppressor gene from del(5)(q31) may predispose cells to transformation when acquiring a mutation in the *p53* gene during deletion of the short arm of chromosome 17. Many cases with 17p loss are therapy related, either t-MDS or t-AML, appearing after treatment of certain lymphoid neoplasms with alkylating agents or as progression in polycythemia vera (PV) or essential thrombocythemia (ET). The 17p deletion may result from unbalanced translocations involving 17p, monosomy 17, :(17q), or del(17p).

The 5q- syndrome in refractory (macrocytic) anemia is a distinct disease entity with a favorable prognosis (Figure 6–22). Del(5q) in acute leukemia is not restricted to myeloid neoplasms but in rare cases can also be seen in ALL, commonly with expression of myeloid antigens. In AML FAB M1 and M2, it rarely appears as the sole anomaly. In these cases, there is a presumptive submicroscopic

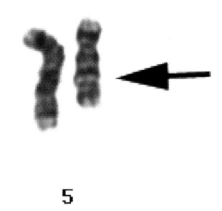

5

Figure 6–22. Partial karyotype of a deletion of the long arm of chromosome 5. The putative tumor suppressor gene is located at 5q31 from minimal deletion studies. Arrow points at breaksite region.

transformation-related additional change. It is often part of a complex karyotype in other AML subtypes, in AML developing after MPDs (such as PV or ET), and particularly in t-AML. It may occasionally be seen in ALL. As mentioned above, the critical deleted gene segment common to all disorders with del(5q) appears to be a putative tumor suppressor gene at 5q31 rather than one of the many other genes concentrated within this chromosome band that are relevant to hematopoiesis (IL-3, IL-4, IL-5, IL-9, granulocyte-macrophage colony-stimulating factor, colony-stimulating factor-1 receptor, etc.).

Partial or complete monosomy 7 is seen in a variety of hematologic malignancies, involving all cell lineages. This suggests that it reflects a genetic defect at a pluripotent stem cell level. The der(1;7) (q10;p10), common in MDS with high transformation rate to AML, results in trisomy 1q and monosomy 7q. Among secondary leukemias following treatment of hematologic and nonhematologic malignancies with alkylating agents or radiation, loss of chromosome 7 is the most common numeric abnormality. Familial MDS and AML with monosomy 7 have been reported. Most deletions in 7q- appear to be interstitial, and there is considerable variety in proximal and distal breakpoints, suggesting that more than one gene may be of importance. The minimal deleted segment appears to be 7q31-32 (Figure 6–23). For -5/5q-, -7/7q-, and 17p- in treatment-related disease, a long interval between initial treatment and outbreak of secondary leukemia is typical (between 2 and 8 years in most studies).

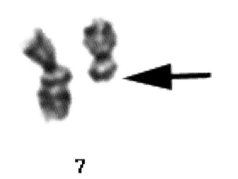

7

Figure 6–23. Partial karyotype of a deletion of the long arm of chromosome 7. Arrow points at breaksite. A putative tumor suppressor gene is located at 7q31-32 (original magnification ×3,200; G banding).

Abnormalities of the short arm of chromosome 12 are found in about 5 percent of AML patients and may also be found in evolved lymphoid disease (Figure 6–24). These leukemias typically develop after MDS or chemotherapy treatment. Aberrations are variable and include translocations, deletions, dicentrics, insertions, and additions with heterogeneous breakpoints on the chromosome. This is by far the most common site for dicentric formation with concomitant loss of regions containing putative tumor suppressor genes.

Deletion of the long arm of chromosome 20 occurs in MDS, MPDs, and AML. Whether del (20q) in MDS is associated with a high rate of transformation to acute leukemia is controversial. The deletion appears to affect a progenitor cell for both the myeloid and B-cell lineages, although cases in lymphoid disease are very rare. It is the most common cytogenetic abnormality in PV and is also found in other MPDs, such as ET and myelofibrosis.

Duplication or partial trisomy of the long arm of chromosome 1 is associated with a disease dis-

12

Figure 6–24. Partial karyotype demonstrating a deletion of the short arm of chromosome 12. Arrow points at breaksite (original magnification ×3,200; G banding).

tribution similar to that of del(20q). It is generally part of a complex karyotype that spans most forms of neoplasia, predominantly myeloma, PV, MDS, AML, and ALL. Distally placed extra 1q segments can "jump" occasionally from chromosome to chromosome in the same patient. Tandem duplications or triplications consistently amplify 1q23 to 1q32.

Trisomy 8 can be found as the sole cytogenetic abnormality in ALL, although infrequently (Figure 6–25). It is the most frequent cytogenetic abnormality in AML and t-AML, occurring in virtually all FAB classes either as primary anomaly or in a complex karyotype. As a secondary change, it most often accompanies the t(15;17) in APL. Tetrasomies and pentasomies of chromosome 8 are preferentially found in monocytic leukemias as a potential clonal evolution secondary to 11q23 aberrations.

Trisomy 13 as the sole cytogenetic abnormality is found in < 1 percent of de novo adult acute leukemia, predominantly of immature myeloid phenotype with lymphoid, often T-cell, antigen expression. The anomaly is associated with a low remission rate and short survival.

Trisomy 4 occurs as single karyotypic anomaly in primary and secondary AML, predominantly of M2, M4, and M0 morphology. In AML, an association with double-minute chromosomes (dmin), markers of gene amplification, has been described.

Trisomy 21 is a common trisomy in patients with AML and MDS in adults. It rarely presents as the primary cytogenetic change. It occurs frequently in addition to -5, -7, +8, t(15;17), inv(16), and t(8;21). Whereas constitutional trisomy 21 in Down syndrome patients is commonly associated with acute megakaryocytic leukemia, this leukemia subtype is uncommon with acquired trisomy 21.

Multiple isodicentric chromosome 21s (duplicate copies of chromosome 21 consisting of two centromeres and two long arms) may be observed in some patients with AML. Because these alterations have a natural mitotic instability, they can rapidly evolve to large copy numbers, as shown in Figure 6–26.

Secondary Leukemias

The occurrence of specific cytogenetic aberrations in secondary leukemias has been discussed in the various previous sections. Aside from karyotypes, which are highly characteristic of secondary leukemias, such as -5/5q-, -7/7q-, and karyotypes with *MLL* gene rearrangements, favorable cytogenetics may be observed as well, such as t(8;21), inv(16), and t(15;17). It appears that treatment response is related to karyotype rather than disease state in that response rates with such favorable cytogenetics in secondary leukemias are identical to those seen in de novo leukemias.[32–35]

CHRONIC LEUKEMIAS

Chronic Lymphoid Leukemias of B-Cell Type

B-Cell Chronic Lymphocytic/Prolymphocytic Leukemia

With the use of B-cell mitogens, more than half of patients with B-CLL demonstrate cytogenetic

abnormalities.[36,37] The most common finding by standard technique is trisomy 12 (Figure 6–27), followed by deletions of the long arm of chromosomes 13, 6, and 11 and additions to 14q32. Interphase cytogenetics by FISH have revealed that deletions of 13q are most common, followed by del(11q), +12, and deletions of 17p. Presumably, some clones do not respond to B-cell mitogens. Interphase FISH analysis in B-CLL patients with normal cytogenetics may be clinically indicated since cytogenetic risk groups have been identified. Patients with trisomy 12 have poorer survival than patients with normal karyotype or with 13q14 aberrations. Inferior prognosis with imminent disease progression is associated with deletions at 11q. Putative transforming genetic events occurring in the most frequent structural anomalies may involve *BCL1* in the 11q deletion, the retinoblastoma tumor suppressor gene in the 13q deletion, and *p53* in the 17p deletion. The (14;18)(q32;q21) translocation is primarily associated with *BCL2* activation and follicular lymphoma,

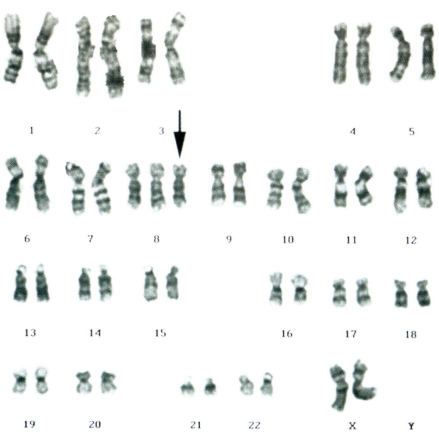

Figure 6–25. Full karyotype with trisomy 8. The arrow points at the extra chromosome (original magnification ×1,600; G banding).

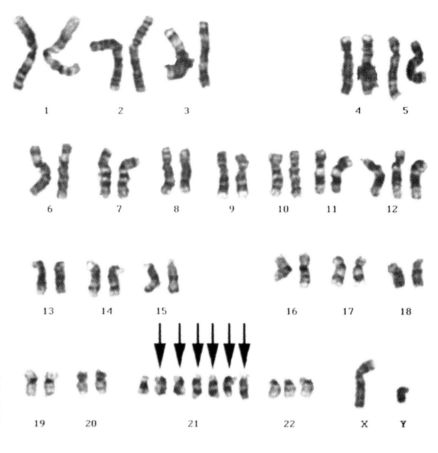

Figure 6–26. Dicentric duplications of chromosome 21 have a natural mitotic instability that results in rapid evolution to increased copy number (*arrow*) (original magnification ×1,600; G banding).

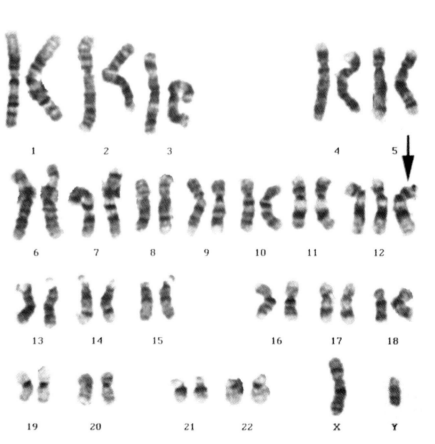

Figure 6–27. Trisomy 12 as a sole anomaly occurs virtually exclusively in B-CLL. The arrow points at the extra chromosome (original magnification ×1,600; G banding).

but it is also common in B-CLL. Atypical, CD5-negative B-CLL shows similar cytogenetic changes as classic B-CLL but with a higher incidence of complex karyotypes. Mantle cell lymphoma may present with a lymphocytosis that, in the absence of immunophenotyping, may be confused with B-CLL. The demonstration of t(11;14)(q13;q32), characteristic of mantle cell lymphoma, will facilitate the diagnosis in such cases.

B-PLL demonstrates frequent deletions at 11q23 and 13q14. With disease progression, clonal evolution is seen in a minority of cases. The (14;19)(q32;q13.1) translocation, which involves the *BCL3* gene on 19q13.1, is a hallmark of B-PLL and is often accompanied by trisomy 12, as in the case shown in Figure 6–28.

Hairy Cell Leukemia

Most cytogenetic studies have not demonstrated a consistent karyotypic abnormality in hairy cell leukemia (HCL). Two-thirds of cases contain clonal abnormalities, often involving chromosomes 1, 2, 5, 6, 11, 19, and 20.[38] Alterations of chromosome 5 are present in approximately 40 percent of patients, most commonly as trisomy 5, pericentric inversions or interstitial deletions involving band 5q13. Trisomy 5, del(2q) or inv(2), and del(1)(q42) distinguish karyotypes in HCL from those of other chronic lymphoid leukemias.

Plasma Cell Leukemia

Cytogenetic analyses in plasma cell leukemia (PCL) usually yield more evaluable metaphases than in multiple myeloma (MM) due to a higher proliferative rate in the former. Most patients have highly complex karyotypes. Many specific cytogenetic abnormalities in PCL are similar to those found in MM, such as recurrent translocations involving 14q32, structural aberrations of chromosome 1 (short or long arm), and monosomy 13 or deletion of 13q.[39] Monosomies 7 and 16 are found more frequently in PCL than MM. On the other hand, trisomies or tetrasomies of chromosomes 3, 5, 6, 9, 11, 15, 17, and 19 are uncommon in PCL, although frequent in MM.

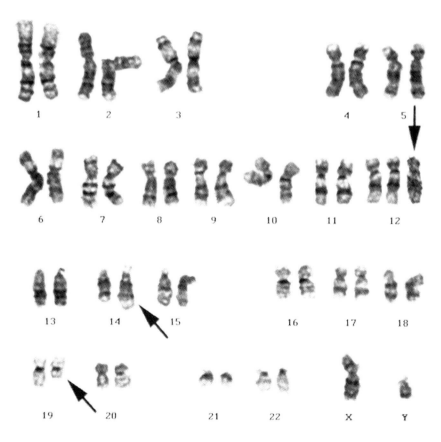

Figure 6–28. Full karyotype with t(14;19) (q32;q13.1) (breakpoints are indicated by arrows) and trisomy 12 (arrow points at extra chromosome) (original magnification ×1,600; G banding).

Chronic Lymphoid Leukemias of T-Cell Type

T-Cell Chronic Lymphocytic/Prolymphocytic Leukemia

T-cell chronic lymphocytic leukemia and T-PLL typically show abnormalities at (14)(q11q32.1) or, to a far lesser extent, Xq28,[40] with overexpression of two homologous genes, *TCL1* and *MTCP1*, respectively. Paracentric inversion of the long arm of chromosome 14, involving bands 14q11 and 14q32, is prominent. 14q11 includes the TCR α/δ locus. 14q32 contains the Ig heavy-chain locus and is commonly involved in genetic changes of B-lymphoid neoplasms; however, the breakpoints in this chromosome region in T-PLL are distant from the Ig heavy-chain gene and instead involve the *TCL1* gene. Trisomy 8q is often seen as a secondary cytogenetic change. Abnormalities involving the long or the short arm of chromosome 6, monosomy 13, or proximal long arm 13 deletions are other karyotypic findings.

Adult T-Cell Leukemia

Adult T-cell leukemia associated with human T-cell leukemia virus-1 infection, like T-CLL/T-PLL, presents with structural abnormalities involving 14q32 and 14q11 or deletions of the long arm of chromosome 6 (6q21). Trisomy 7 or partial trisomy 7q is a recurrent numeric aberration possibly associated with aggressive disease, as are complex karyotypes.[41]

Chronic Myeloid Leukemia

The majority of patients with clinical CML (approximately 90 to 95%) present with the (9;22)(q34;q22) Ph chromosome translocation leading to the formation of the *BCR/ABL* fusion gene (see Figure 6–8). Occasionally (5% of cases), the fusion gene is the result of a complex translocation in which other chromosomes participate in the Ph chromosome formation (complex Ph chromosome). In variant Ph translocations involving a terminal segment of a third chromosome, *BCR/ABL* fusion may be detected in

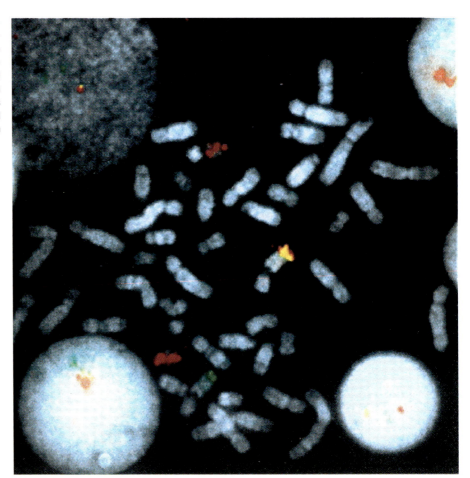

Figure 6–29. Silent Philadelphia chromosome detected by FISH. A submicroscopic insertion of the *BCR* gene into the *ABL* gene produces a classic single yellow fusion signal. The remaining normal ABL gene is represented by the green signal. One of the two red BCR signals appears reduced due to the interstitial gene deletion (original magnification ×1,000).

the absence of cytogenetically apparent involvement of 9q34. With the exception of chromosome Y, all other chromosomes have been involved in variant Ph chromosome translocations. In 2 to 3 percent of CML cases with normal-appearing chromosomes 9 and 22, FISH analysis using DNA probes for specific *BCR* and *ABL* sequences detect submicroscopic non-reciprocal insertions of either a portion of the *BCR* gene into *ABL* (Figure 6–29) or of a portion of the *ABL* gene into *BCR*. This is termed a silent Ph chromosome. In the remaining Ph-negative cases, molecular analysis can frequently identify classic or variant *BCR/ABL* transcripts. This leaves a small group of apparently truly Ph-negative CML patients, which may represent a distinct disease entity.

In t(9;22), a break occurs in the *ABL* gene on chromosome 9 and within the *BCR* gene on chromosome 22. The reciprocal exchange of two segments results in a chromosome 22 with a shortened long arm (22q, the actual Ph chromosome), which carries the *BCR/ABL* fusion gene, and the translocation derivative of chromosome 9 (9q+), which carries the reciprocal *ABL/BCR* fusion gene. In almost all CML patients, the break on chromosome 22 occurs within a segment called the major breakpoint cluster region (M-bcr), and M-bcr exon 2 (b2) or exon 3 (b3) is fused to ABL exon 2 (a2). Few CML patients and the majority of Ph-positive ALL patients show a break within the first intron of the *BCR* gene, in the minor breakpoint cluster region (m-bcr), so that the first exon of *BCR* (e1) is fused to *ABL* a2. Transcripts transcribed from the b2a2 (e13a2) or b3a2 (e14a2) junction trans-

late into a 210-kD fusion protein (p210), whereas the e1a2 junction gives rise to the smaller, 190-kD fusion protein (p190). Low-level transcription of e1a2 mRNA has been detected in most cases of classic CML in addition to b2a2 or b3a2 types. Dominant e1a2 transcription has been reported in cases of chronic myelomonocytic leukemia and MDS, suggesting that these patients may define specific subgroups of CML. Variant *BCR/ABL* fusion genes have been described in a small number of CML patients, such as the c3a2 (e19a2) transcript form in neutrophilic and classic CML in which the break occurs between exons e19 and e20 of the *BCR* gene (originally named exons c3 and c4). This fusion mRNA is translated into a 230-kD protein. Other novel *BCR/ABL* fusion genes reported are *e6a2, e1a3, b2a3,* and *b3a3,* although, theoretically, several additional in-frame fusions between the two genes are possible.[42]

Both *BCR* and *ABL* domains contribute to the oncogenic activity of BCR-ABL proteins. To date, breakpoint localization in the *BCR* and *ABL* genes was not found to correlate with clinical outcome. Polymerase chain reaction with primers designed to detect the major *BCR/ABL* fusion transcripts along with most of the rare variant forms is used to assess the response of patients to therapeutic interventions. Positive PCR results must be interpreted knowing that *BCR/ABL* fusion gene transcripts have been detected in leukocytes of normal individuals.

The acquisition of additional cytogenetic abnormalities during clinically persistent chronic phase is usually indicative of disease progression. Clonal kary-

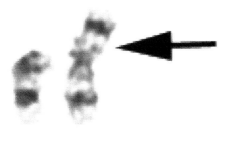

17

Figure 6–30. Isochromosome 17q, as indicated by the arrow in this partial karyotype, is a mirror-image duplication of the long arm of chromosome 17 with a consequent loss of the short arm (original magnification ×3,200; G banding).

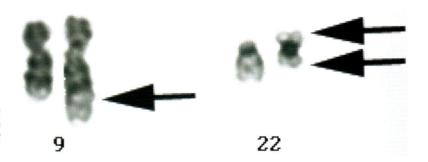

Figure 6–31. Partial karyotype demonstrating the classic derivative (9) of the t(9;22) plus a duplication of the derivative 22 in the form of an isoderivative 22 (original magnification ×3,200; G banding).

otypic evolution occurs in approximately 80 percent of patients who progress to blast crisis. Most frequent additional karyotypic aberrations include trisomy 8, trisomy 19, monosomy 7, a second Ph chromosome, and isochromosome 17q, i(17q) (Figure 6–30). The second Ph chromosome is usually a duplicate of the original translocation derivative but may also appear as an isoderivative 22 (Figure 6–31). In FISH analysis, the extra Ph chromosome can be seen as a third fusion signal (Figure 6–32, bottom). Structural or numeric abnormalities resulting in gain of 7q or loss of 9p are more frequent in lymphoid than in myeloid blast crisis, whereas -7, del(7q), +8, +19, and i(17q) are more common in myeloid transformation. Blast crisis without additional cytogenetic derangements usually demonstrates a lymphoid phenotype.

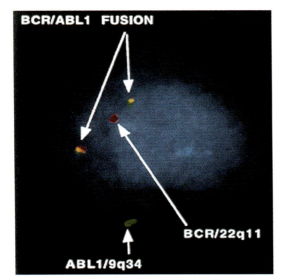

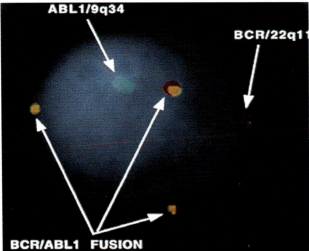

Figure 6–32. Fluorescent in situ hybridization analysis demonstrating a single Ph chromosome that produces the classic *BCR/ABL* and reciprocal *ABL/BCR* yellow fusion signals in the top panel. The bottom panel shows an extra Ph chromosome reflected by a third fusion signal (original magnification ×500).

REFERENCES

1. Cross NCP, Melo JV, Feng L, Goldman JM. An optimized multiplex polymerase chain reaction (PCR) for detection of BCR-ABL fusion mRNAs in hematological disorders. Leukemia 1994;8:186–9.
2. van Dongen JJM, Macintyre EA, Gabert JA, et al. Standardized RT-PCR analysis of fusion gene transcripts from chromosome aberrations in acute leukemia for detection of minimal residual disease. Leukemia 1999;13:1901–28.
3. Clare N, Hansen K. Cytogenetics in the diagnosis of hematologic malignancies. Diagn Hematol 1994;8: 785–807.
4. Harris NL, Jaffe ES, Stein H, et al. A revised European-American classification of lymphoid neoplasms: a proposal from the International Lymphoma Study Group. Blood 1994;84:1361–92.
5. Kroft SH, Finn WG, Peterson LC. The pathology of the chronic lymphoid leukemias. Blood Rev 1995;9: 234–50.
6. Sandberg AA, Chen Z. Cytogenetics of acute leukemia. In: Wiernik PH, Canellos GP, Dutcher JP, Kyle RA, editors. Neoplastic diseases of the blood. 3rd ed. New York: Churchill Livingstone: 1996. p. 249–67.
7. Papenhausen PR, Moscinski LC, Binnie CG. Cytoge-

netic and molecular evaluation in myelodyplastic syndrome and in acute and chronic leukemia. Cancer Control 1997;4:389–98.

8. Donner LR. Cytogenetics of lymphomas: a brief review of its theoretical and practical significance. Cancer Genet Cytogenet 1997;94:20–6.

9. Willman CL. Molecular evaluation of acute myeloid leukemias. Semin Hematol 1999;36:390–400.

10. Dewald GW, Stupca P. 154 chromosome abnormalities in hematologic malignancies. Leuk Res 2000;24:487–9.

11. Boehm T, Rabbitts TH. A chromosomal basis of lymphoid malignancy in man. Eur J Biochem 1989; 185:1–17.

12. Faderl S, Kantarjian HM, Talpaz M, Estrov Z. Clinical significance of cytogenetic abnormalities in adult acute lymphoblastic leukemia. Blood 1998;91: 3995–4019.

13. Begley CG, Green AR. The SCL gene: from case report to critical hematopoietic regulator. Blood 1999;93:2760–70.

14. Wadman I, Li J, Bash RO, et al. Specific in vivo association between the bHLH and LIM proteins implicated in human T cell leukemia. EMBO J 1994;13:4831–9.

15. Rubnitz JE, Behm FG, Downing JR. 11q23 rearrangements in acute leukemia. Leukemia 1996;10:74–82.

16. DiMartino JF, Cleary ML. MLL rearrangements in hematological malignancies: lessons from clinical and biological studies. Br J Haematol 1999;106:614–26.

17. Hunger SP. Chromosomal translocations involving the E2A gene in acute lymphoblastic leukemia: clinical features and molecular pathogenesis. Blood 1996;87:1211–24.

18. Paietta E, Racevskis J, Neuberg D, et al. Expression of CD25 (interleukin-2 receptor α chain) in adult acute lymphoblastic leukemia predicts for the presence of BCR/ABL fusion transcripts: results of a preliminary laboratory analysis of ECOG/MRC Intergroup Study E2993. Leukemia 1997;11:1887–90.

19. Preti HA, O'Brien S, Giralt S, et al. Philadelphia-chromosome-positive adult acute lymphocytic leukemia: characteristics, treatment results, and prognosis in 41 patients. Am J Med 1994;97:60–5.

20. Rieder H, Ludwig W-D, Gassmann W, et al. Prognostic significance of additional chromosome abnormalities in adult patients with Philadelphia chromosome positive acute lymphoblastic leukemia. Br J Haematol 1996;95:678–91.

21. Preudhomme C, Fenaux P, Laï JL, et al. Philadelphia negative, BCR-ABL positive adult acute lymphoblastic leukemia (ALL) in 2 of 39 patients with combined cytogenetic and molecular analysis. Leukemia 1993;7:1054–7.

22. Rubnitz JE, Pui C-H, Downing JR. The role of TEL fusion genes in pediatric leukemias. Leukemia 1999;13:6–13.

23. Ramakers-van Woerden NL, Pieters R, Loonen AH, et al. TEL/AML1 gene fusion is related to in vitro drug sensitivity for L-asparaginase in childhood acute lymphoblastic leukemia. Blood 2000;96:1094–9.

24. Ito C, Kumagai M, Manabe A, et al. Hyperdiploid acute lymphoblastic leukemia with 51 to 65 chromosomes: a distinct biological entity with a marked propensity to undergo apoptosis. Blood 1999;93:315–20.

25. Friedman A. Leukemogenesis by CBF oncoproteins. Leukemia 1999;13:1932–42.

26. Downing JR. The AML1-ETO chimeric transcription factor in acute myeloid leukemia: biology and clinical significance. Br J Haematol 1999;106:296–308.

27. Redner RL, Wang J, Liu JM. Chromatin remodeling and leukemia: new therapeutic paradigms. Blood 1999;94:417–28.

28. Lutterbach B, Hou Y, Durst KL, Hiebert SW. The inv(16) encodes an acute myeloid leukemia 1 transcriptional corepressor. Proc Natl Acad Sci U S A 1999;96:12822–7.

29. Blobel GA. CREB-binding protein and p300: molecular integrators of hematopoietic transcription. Blood 2000;95:745–55.

30. Melnick A, Licht J. Deconstructing a disease: RARα, its fusion partners, and their roles in the pathogenesis of acute promyelocytic leukemia. Blood 1999;93:3167–215.

31. Paietta E, Racevskis J, Bennett JM, et al. Biologic heterogeneity in Philadelphia chromosome-positive acute leukemia with myeloid morphology: the Eastern Cooperative Oncology Group experience. Leukemia 1998;12:1881–5.

32. Johansson B, Mertens F, Mitelman F. Secondary chromosomal abnormalities in acute leukemias. Leukemia 1994;8:953–62.

33. Pedersen-Bjergaard J, Pedersen M, Roulston D, Philip P. Different genetic pathways in leukemogenesis for patients presenting with therapy-related myelodysplasia and therapy-related acute myeloid leukemia. Blood 1995;86:3542–52.

34. Quesnel B, Kantarjian H, Pedersen-Bjergaard J, et al. Therapy-related acute myeloid leukemia with t(8;21), inv(16), and t(8;16): a report on 25 cases and review of the literature. J Clin Oncol 1993;11: 2370–9.

35. Groupe Français de Cytogénétique Hématologique (GFCH). Acute leukemia treated with intensive chemotherapy in patients with a history of previous chemo- and/or radiotherapy: prognostic significance of karyotype and preceding myelodysplastic syndrome. Leukemia 1994;8:87–91.

36. Dierlamm J, Michaux L, Criel A, et al. Genetic abnormalities in chronic lymphocytic leukemia and their clinical and prognostic implications. Cancer Genet Cytogenet 1997;94:27–35.

37. Crossen PE. Genes and chromosomes in chronic B-cell leukemia. Cancer Genet Cytogenet 1997;94:44–51.

38. Haglund U, Juliusson G, Stellan B, Gahrton G. Hairy cell leukemia is characterized by clonal chromosome abnormalities clustered to specific regions. Blood 1994;83:2637–45.

39. Garcia-Sanz R, Orfão A, González M, et al. Primary plasma cell leukemia: clinical, immunophenotypic, DNA ploidy, and cytogenetic characteristics. Blood 1999;93:1032–7.

40. Hoyer JD, Ross CW, Li C-Y, et al. True T-cell chronic lymphocytic leukemia: a morphologic and immunophenotypic study of 25 cases. Blood 1995;86:1163–9.

41. Kamada N, Sakurai , Miyamoto K, et al. Chromosome abnormalities in adult T-cell leukemia/lymphoma: a karyotype review committee report. Cancer Res 1992;52:1481–93.

42. Melo JV. The diversity of BCR-ABL fusion proteins and their relationship to leukemia phenotype. Blood 1996;88:2375–84.

Treatment of Adult Acute Leukemia

MIR YOUSUF ALI, MD
MARTIN S. TALLMAN, MD

ACUTE LYMPHOBLASTIC LUEKEMIA

Although the treatment of adults with acute lymphoblastic leukemia (ALL) is not as successful as that of children, significant progress has been made with the intensification of chemotherapy and the adoption of strategies that parallel those so successful in children.[1] One important reason for the difference in outcome of adults and children with ALL is the higher incidence in adults of unfavorable prognostic factors such as the presence of the Philadelphia (Ph) chromosome.[2] The treatment of adult ALL is generally divided into several phases: (1) induction, (2) consolidation-intensification, (3) central nervous system (CNS) prophylaxis, and (4) maintenance therapy. Bone marrow transplantation (BMT) in first remission may be considered a fifth phase or undertaken in lieu of maintenance. However, the role of BMT in the treatment of adults with ALL is less established than in AML. Clinical and cytogenetic factors that predict for the achievement of complete remission (CR) and remission duration have been well described (Table 7–1) and are useful in identifying the best therapy for a given subgroup[3–10] (Figures 7–1 and 7–2). Furthermore, new prognostic factors such as the loss of retinoblastoma (*Rb*) expression and overexpression of *p53* have recently been described and are together associated with a poor outcome.[11] The *TEL-AML1* fusion gene resulting from the t(12;21)(p13;q22) translocation occurs in approximately 25 percent of patients with precursor B-lineage childhood ALL and has a favorable prognosis.[12] This molecular abnormality occurs

less commonly in adults with ALL (approximately 3% of patients), but its prognostic importance in adults is unknown.[13] This may be attributable to high sensitivity of the leukemic lymphoblasts to L-asparaginase.[14] Major efforts are under way to improve the ability to detect minimal residual disease (MRD) in order to classify patients based on risk of relapse to better direct therapy.

Induction

Remission induction therapy in adult ALL generally includes a combination of vincristine (VCR) and corticosteroids, usually prednisone. Historically, with this combination, 40 to 60 percent of patients achieve a CR, but the median duration of remission was only approximately 3 to 7 months.[15,16] Anthracyclines were subsequently incorporated in induction regimens with a significant improvement in the response rates of 70 to 85 percent. Cancer and Leukemia Group B (CALGB) conducted a randomized trial evaluating the addition of daunorubicin (DNR) to VCR, prednisone, and L-asparaginase and observed a CR in 38 of 46 patients (83%) in the group that received daunorubicin compared to 25 of

Table 7–1. MAJOR PROGNOSTIC FEATURES IN ADULT ACUTE LYMPHOBLASTIC LEUKEMIA

Age < 60 years
WBC < 30,000/µL
T-cell phenotype
Hyperdiploidy
Mediastinal mass (usually T-ALL)
Absence of t(9;22) or t(4;11) or t(8;14)

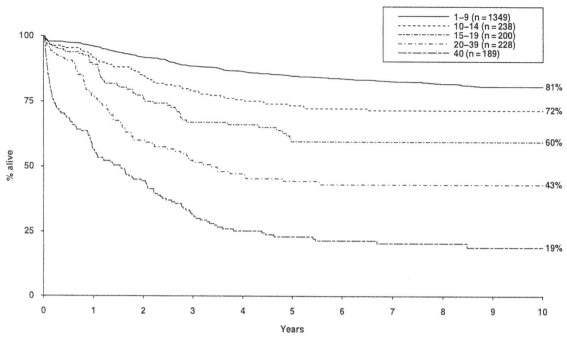

Figure 7–1.   Overall survival by age in MRC protocols UK ALL X and Xa. (From Chessells JM, Hall E, Prentice HG, et al. The impact of age on outcome in lymphoblastic leukemia: MRC UK ALL X and Xa compared: a report from the MRC and Pediatric and Adult Working Parties. Leukemia 1998;12:463–73.)

53 patients (47%) in the control arm (p = .003).[17] This triple-drug regimen of DNR, VCR, and prednisone is now standard remission induction therapy in adult ALL. Induction regimens using VCR, corticosteroids, and anthracyclines routinely yield CR rates that range from 65 to 85 percent, and the induc-

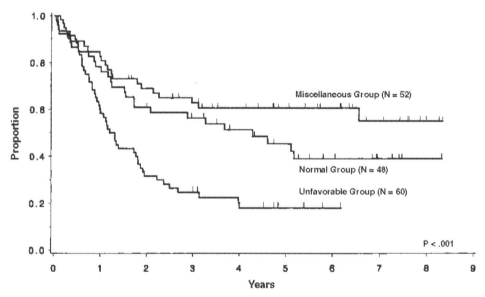

Figure 7–2.   Disease-free survival of patients < age 60 treated on intensive treatment protocols by CALGB by cytogenetic risk group. Miscellaneous risk group includes +21, del (9p) or t(9p), del(12p) t(14q11-11q13), t(14q32) other than t(18;14) and del(6q), hyperdiploid karyotypes (> 50 chromosomes but without any structural abnormalities); unfavorable risk group includes t(9;22), +8, t(4;11), and –7. (Reprinted with permission from Wetzler M, Dodge RK, Mrozek K, et al. Prospective karyotype analysis in adult acute lymphoblastic leukemia: the Cancer and Leukemia Group B experience. Blood 1999;93:3983–93. ©American Society of Hematology.)

tion mortality rates range from 5 to 20 percent (Table 7–2).[18–30] Daunorubicin and doxorubicin are the commonly used anthracyclines, with similar response rates.[4] Mitoxantrone has been shown to produce comparable responses to daunorubicin.[31] In some studies, anthracyclines have been replaced with methotrexate (MTX) and asparaginase, with equivalent CR rates and long-term disease-free survival (DFS) with the potential for decreased cardiotoxicity.[32] Induction therapy with high-dose cytarabine in combination with mitoxantrone, but without VCR-prednisone, has recently been shown to be an effective alternative means of inducing CR in adults with ALL.[33] The addition of L-asparaginase has not been shown to improve CR rate but may have a beneficial impact on long-term outcome in adults.[34] L-Asparaginase was routinely incorporated into treatment programs in adult ALL based on benefits in the therapy of childhood ALL, which led to improved CR rates compared to VCR and prednisone in relapsed patients and in long-term outcome when given to patients in CR.[35,36]

T-Cell Acute Lymphoblastic Leukemia

The addition of cyclophosphamide and cytarabine to VCR-anthracycline-steroid regimens generally has not been associated with an improvement in CR rate or overall prognosis except in the T-cell ALL, where there appears to be an improvement in the CR rates, DFS, and overall survival (OS) with incorporation of these agents.[31,37–40] Cytarabine at lower doses with thioguanine and DNR when added to VCR and prednisone resulted in a CR rate of 91 percent with a median duration of response of 15 months.[37] The addition of cyclophosphamide alone to conventional induction conferred a benefit in outcome for patients with T-cell ALL.[6,28]

Mature B-Cell ALL
(French-American-British Classification L3)

Mature B-cell ALL comprises only approximately 5 percent of adult ALL, but identification of this group at the time of diagnosis is important because these patients benefit from chemotherapy strategies

Author	No. Pts	Induction	Consolidation	Maintenance	CR (%)	DFS (%)	OS (%)
Table 7–2. OUTCOME OF INTENSIVE CHEMOTHERAPY FOR ADULT ALL							
Hoelzer, 1988[4]	368	VCR, pred, dauno, L-asp	CTX, cytarabine, 6-MP, MTX; dex, VCR, Adria, 6-TG	6-MP, MTX	74	37, 5 yr	39, 5 yr
Hussein, 1989[20]	168	VCR, pred, Adria, CTX	Cytarabine, MTX, 6-TG, VCR, pred, L-asp, CTX	VCR, pred, Adria, 6-MP, MTX, actino-D, CTX, BCNU	68	30, 5 yr	~28, 5 yr
Linker, 1991[24]	109	VCR, pred, dauno, L-asp	VCR, pred, dauno, L-asp, teniposide, cytarabine, MTX	MTX, 6-MP	88	42, 10 yr	35, 10 yr
Bouchiex, 1994[5]	572	VCR, pred, CTX, dauno or zorubicin	Dauno or zorubicin cytarabine, L-asp	VCR, pred, dauno, or BCNU, CTX, 6-MP, MTX, actino-D	74[†] 81[‡]	34[†], 3 yr 52[‡], 3 yr	NA[†] NA[‡]
Durrant, 1997[30]	618	VCR, pred, dauno, L-asp	Cytarabine, etoposide, dauno, 6-TG	None	88	28, 5 yr	34, 5 yr
Ludwig, 1998[54]	47	VCR, pred, dauno, L-asp, MTX	CTX, cytarabine, 6-MP, MTX; pred, VCR, dauno, MTX, cytarabine, dex; CTX, cytarabine, 6-TG, MTX, Dex; HiDAC, MTX; HiDMTX, L-asp; teniposide, cytarabine	6-MP, MTX	73	53, 5 yr	~42, 5 yr
Rowe, 1999[69]	920	VCR, pred, dauno, L-asp	CTX, cytarabine, 6-MP, MTX; high-dose MTX, L-asp; etoposide	VCR, pred, MTX, 6-MP, IFN	89	NA	NA

*Patients randomized to early or late consolidation (intensification), both or neither; [†]B-cell phenotype; [‡]T-cell phenotype; [§]Pre-pre–B-cell ALL.
[5] Includes patients with t(94;11) and/or molecular evidence of MLL-AF-4 fusion transcripts.
VCR = vincristine; pred = prednisone; Adria = Adriamycin; L-asp = L-asparaginase; 6-TG = 6-thioguanine; dauno = daunorubicin; actino-D = actinomycin D; MTX = methotrexate; 6-MP = 6-mercaptopurine; CTX = Cytoxan (cyclophosphamide); BCNU = carmustine; dex = dexamethasone, HiDAC = high-dose cytarabine; HiDMTX = high-dose methotrexate; IFN = interferon; NA = not available.

that differ from the treatment for the other groups of ALL. Current strategies for adult B-cell ALL have followed those for the treatment of pediatric patients with B-cell ALL/Burkitt's lymphoma. In children with mature B-cell ALL, cyclophosphamide with high-dose MTX and cytarabine with or without VCR and doxorubicin together with prophylactic intrathecal (IT) chemotherapy using MTX and/or cytarabine has resulted in a marked improvement in the response rates in children.[41,42] A similar approach has been applied in the treatment of adults with B-cell ALL, and CR rates of 70 to 80 percent have been achieved, with DFS approaching 50 percent.[43–46] Due to the high incidence of CNS involvement in this subtype of ALL,[47] strategies emphasize treatment and prophylaxis of this site.[47–50] High-dose MTX and cytarabine penetrate the blood–brain barrier. Their use along with IT methotrexate and/or cytarabine is effective in reducing CNS relapse, frequently observed in mature B-cell ALL. Central nervous system radiation has also been given with methotrexate with an increased incidence of neurotoxicity. Intensive short-term treatment strategies have led to an overall DFS of 50 percent. Relapses usually occur within the first year of therapy.

Role of Growth Factors in the Induction Phase of Treatment.

Death from infections is the major cause of induction failure in adult ALL. Cancer and Leukemia Group B recently concluded a multi-institution, randomized, blinded, placebo-controlled trial using granulocyte colony-stimulating factor (G-CSF) in the induction phase of therapy in adult ALL patients.[51] The median time to recover neutrophils $\geq$ 1,000/μL during the remission induction course was 16 days in the G-CSF arm compared with 22 days in the placebo arm (p = .001). Similarly, the duration of hospitalization was a median of 22 days versus 28 days (p = .02). However there were no differences noted in the duration of fevers in both groups. In the subset of patients over the age of 60 years, a reduction in the number of deaths during induction and a consequent improvement in the CR rates were noted (81% versus 55%; p = .10). After a median follow-up of 4.7 years, there was no difference in either the DFS or OS between the two groups. Other studies have also demonstrated a decrease in the duration of

neutropenia along with a reduction of about 50 percent in the incidence of nonviral infections in patients given growth factors during the induction phase of treatment with the ability to complete therapy earlier with fewer delays in treatment.[52]

Consolidation-Intensification Therapy

Several agents have been used in consolidation-intensification regimens to eradicate MRD, including high doses of cyclophosphamide, asparaginase, cytosine arabinoside, MTX, and etoposide/teniposide with or without an anthracycline (see Table 7–2).[6,20,21,24–28,37–40] Linker and colleagues, using an alternating combination of noncross-reacting drugs in the consolidation phase of the therapy, noted a 42 $\pm$ 6 percent probability of remaining in continued CR with a median follow-up of 77 months.[24] The main complication seen in the consolidation phase of therapy was profound myelosuppression with neutropenic fever requiring antibiotics, seen in about 40 percent of the patients, with three treatment-related deaths. Randomized trials have suggested a benefit from such cyclic intensive postremission therapy. In a large cooperative group trial conducted by the CALGB, 197 patients were treated with a five-drug induction regimen followed by multiagent consolidation, late intensification, CNS prophylaxis, and maintenance, which led to a median survival of 36 months with estimates of the proportion surviving at 3 years of 69 percent for patients < 30 years and 39 percent of those 30 to 59 years of age, and only 17 percent for patients 60 years of age and older (Figure 7–3).[6]

Other studies have evaluated the benefit of consolidation-intensification in the treatment of adult ALL. The European Organization for Research and Treatment of Cancer (EORTC) randomized patients to receive 3-month consolidation with MTX, cytarabine, and thioguanine versus maintenance after induction therapy and found no differences in the DFS.[53] Ludwig and colleagues reported 57 adults with pro-B ALL (previously null cell ALL) given intensive consolidation.[54] Twenty-two patients had leukemic cells with t(4;11) (q21;q23) abnormality and/or *MLL/AF-4* gene rearrangements, and six had other structural abnormalities, including two patients with t(9;22) (q34;q11). Patients were enrolled in two consecutive German multicenter trials. The second trial (study 04/89) included more intensive postremission therapy. Although the CR rate was the same (approximately 75%), the percentage of patients remaining in continuous CR at 5 years was significantly higher among patients receiving the more intensive regimen (10 versus 52%; median 420 days versus median not reached, p = .04). The improved results may be attributable to the intensification of postremission therapy with the addition of high-dose cytarabine and mitoxantrone or the inclusion of allogeneic transplantation in first CR. Cancer and Leukemia Group B carried out a randomized trial of intensification treatment in adults aged 15 to 79 years.[55] Daunorubicin, prednisone, VCR, IT MTX, and asparaginase produced a CR rate of 63 percent. One hundred fifty-one patients were randomly assigned to receive treatment as follows: 74 received intensive cytarabine and DNR and 77 received cycles of mercaptopurine (6-MP) and MTX, followed by 6-MP, MTX, VCR, and prednisone for 3 years in all. Intensification produced major myelosuppression but did not improve remission duration (median, 21 months). No advantage in CR duration or OS was observed from

intensive treatment with DNR and cytarabine following induction of CR. These studies have several limitations, including limited duration of the consolidation-intensification treatment; lack of substantial increase in intensity of the experimental arm than the standard arm; and absence in the consolidation-intensification arm with doses of drugs most effective in improving the outcome in pediatric ALL studies such as high-dose MTX and 6-MP, high-dose cytarabine with cyclophosphamide, and higher doses of asparaginase. However, intensive consolidation has become routine practice in virtually all adult ALL protocols.

Incorporation of high-dose cytarabine into the consolidation-intensification phase has yielded variable results. Patients with T-cell ALL or a high blast count at the time of presentation appear to have an improvement in the remission duration with the incorporation of high-dose cytarabine. In a German multi-institution study, Hoelzer and colleagues reported a 4-year continuous CR rate of 43 percent in a group of 81 high-risk patients intensified with mitoxantrone and high-dose cytarabine compared to 23 percent for 31 patients who were not intensified.[26] The differences could well be explained by differences in the mean age between the two groups, with more older patients in the nonintensified arm.

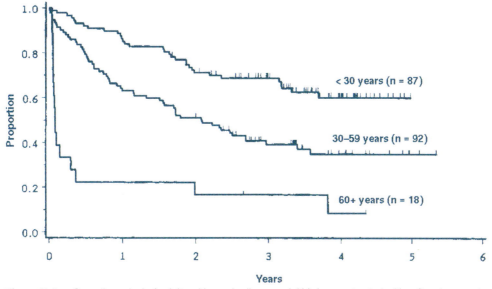

Figure 7–3. Overall survival of adults with newly diagnosed ALL by age treated with a five-drug remission induction regimen with intensive consolidation on CALGB protocol 8811. (Reprinted with permission from Larson RA, Dodge RK, Burns CP, et al. A five-drug remission induction regimen with intensive consolidation for adults with acute lymphoblastic leukemia: Cancer and Leukemia Group B study 8811. Blood 1995;85:2025–37.©American Society of Hematology.)

The Eastern Cooperative Oncology Group (ECOG) using high-dose cytarabine intensification without 6-MP and MTX maintenance showed no improvement in the cure rates.[56]

CNS Prophylaxis. Central nervous system prophylaxis is an important part of the treatment of ALL, since the CNS is a common sanctuary site for leukemic cells. Central nervous system disease is present in approximately 6 percent of adults at diagnosis.[50,57] Prophylactic therapy for prevention of CNS relapse includes IT MTX, cytosine arabinoside, corticosteroids, or a combination of these agents. Prophylactic CNS treatment usually involves cranial irradiation up to 2,400 cGy, with or without IT therapy. Irradiation of the spinal cord can be very myelosuppressive and is generally not done as prophylaxis. Although these strategies have significantly reduced the incidence of CNS relapse, they have been associated with neurotoxicity (demyelination, neurologic changes), particularly when combined with irradiation and IT therapies. Consolidation regimens including high-dose cytarabine and MTX, which cross the blood–brain barrier, may also decrease the risk of CNS leukemia. The combination of high doses of chemotherapy, IT therapy, and cranial irradiation has reduced the relapse rate in the CNS to < 5 percent.[58] Factors associated with a higher rate of CNS relapse include mature B- or T-cell phenotype, high serum lactate dehydrogenase (LDH) levels, a high index of leukemic cell proliferation, very high white blood cell count (WBC) (> 100,000/μL), thrombocytopenia, hepatomegaly, and splenomegaly. These factors may be useful in the development of risk-oriented CNS prophylaxis. Among patients with none of these risk factors, the incidence of CNS leukemia at 1 year was about 5 percent, compared with more than 50 percent in patients with a high LDH and a high proliferative index.

Investigators at The University of Texas M.D. Anderson Cancer Center analyzed the incidence of CNS leukemia after initiation of therapy in patients treated on four consecutive trials for adult ALL, including different CNS prophylactic modalities.[58] The treatment groups included (1) a chemotherapy regimen preceding the VCR-Adriamycin-dexamethasone (VAD) regimen, with no CNS prophylaxis; (2) the VAD regimen with prophylaxis using high-dose systemic chemotherapy; (3) the modified VAD program with high-dose systemic chemotherapy to all patients and IT chemotherapy for high-risk patients after achieving CR; and (4) the hyper-CVAD (cyclophosphamide, vincristine, Adriamycin, dexamethasone) program with early high-dose systemic and IT chemotherapy commencing with induction to all patients, with more IT injections administered to the high-risk group for CNS relapse compared with the low-risk group. A total of 391 patients were included, 73 of whom were treated with pre-VAD, 112 with VAD, 114 with modified VAD, and 92 with hyper-CVAD. The overall CNS relapse rates were 31, 18, 17, and 3 percent, respectively, for the four groups (p < .001). For the high-risk group for CNS relapse, they were 42, 26, 20, and 2 percent, respectively (p < .001). The differences in CNS relapse rates in the low-risk group were not statistically significant. At 3 years, the overall CNS leukemia event-free rates were 48, 76, and 98 percent, respectively (p < .001). In the high-risk group, the CNS event-free rates were 38, 66, 75, and 98 percent, respectively (p < .001); however, there was no difference in the low-risk group. The conclusions from this analysis include the following: (1) high-dose systemic chemotherapy is a useful prophylactic measure, (2) early IT chemotherapy is necessary to reduce the incidence of CNS leukemia overall and in the high-risk group, and (3) a risk-oriented approach is useful to determine the intensity of CNS prophylaxis.

Patients with CNS involvement at the time of presentation may benefit from more aggressive therapy with early high-dose systemic therapy such as cytarabine capable of penetrating the blood–brain barrier. Intracranial radiation may be indicated in patients who have elevated intracranial pressure, indicated by papilledema and headaches with meningeal enhancement on a magnetic resonance imaging scan, or have neurologic signs or symptoms, especially those with cranial nerve root involvement who may benefit from selective irradiation to the base of the skull. One of the proposed schedules for IT therapy includes IT MTX alternating with IT cytarabine twice weekly until the cerebrospinal fluid clears and then weekly for 1 month and once a month thereafter for 2 years. Patients often need an Omaya reservoir placed to carry out this intensive schedule to avoid repeated lumbar punctures, which can result in arachnoiditis and fibrosis.

Maintenance Phase. Methotrexate and 6-MP are the two agents most commonly used for maintenance therapy in children and have been routinely used in adults with ALL.[59,60] However, the most effective regimen has not been determined. Maintenance with oral 6-MP and MTX has been used in various trials in adult ALL in varying schedules. The duration of maintenance therapy required is also unknown but is routinely approximately 2 years or longer.[61,62]

Several studies have omitted maintenance from the therapy altogether. Cancer and Leukemia Group B omitted maintenance after induction and consolidation for a duration of 7 to 9 months and reported a median CR duration of 10 months. Similarly low median duration of CR was also observed in two Eastern Cooperative Oncology Group (ECOG) trials that omitted maintenance after a total duration of consolidation of 8 to 12 months with MTX, asparaginase, cyclophosphamide, Adriamycin, VCR, and prednisone. In these studies, the DFS rates at 2 to 3 years were low (18 and 21%, respectively).

Maintenance therapy with 6-MP and MTX is not required in all patients with ALL. Disease-free survival of 40 to 60 percent has been seen in patients with mature B-cell ALL who are treated with dose-intensive therapy for 3 to 8 months. Patients with Ph-positive ALL do not appear to benefit from the maintenance therapy with 6-MP and MTX. The optimal maintenance therapy for this group of patients is yet to be determined since these patients have relatively high relapse rates with conventional chemotherapy.

An analysis of the associations of individual drug schedules and total doses with overall prognosis in different studies suggests the need for 6-MP and MTX maintenance. Pharmacologic studies have shown significant associations between prognosis and both 6-MP dose delivery and plasma levels, as well as intracellular MTX levels. This suggests that further studies of maintenance schedules may be one area to pursue to improve prognosis.

Philadelphia Chromosome-Positive ALL. Patients with Ph-positive ALL have an extremely poor prognosis with any chemotherapy.[63–67] Investigators at

the M.D. Anderson Cancer Center recently reported the outcome of 38 patients between 1980 and 1991 treated with VAD or with intensive chemotherapy similar to that used for patients with AML.[59] Beginning in 1992, 29 other Ph-positive patients were treated with an intensified chemotherapy (hyper-CVAD).[68] Although the CR rate with the hyper-CVAD program was higher compared to the pre-hyper-CVAD regimens (90 versus 55%, p = .002); the median survival was not different (66 versus 45 weeks, p > .5) (Figure 7–4). However, patients with hyperdiploid Ph-positive ALL treated with hyper-CVAD had a longer CR duration and DFS compared to patients with hypo- and pseudohypodiploid karyotypes (59 versus 42 and 31 weeks, p = .02 and 104, respectively). Nevertheless, there are few, if any, long-term survivors among patients treated with chemotherapy, and such patients must be encouraged to pursue an aggressive strategy of either matched related or unrelated allogeneic transplant.

Prognosis with Contemporary Approaches

In one of the most recent relatively large series published of contemporary intensive chemotherapy for adult ALL, CALGB reported that among 197 patients with a median age of 32 years, treated with cyclophosphamide, DNR, VCR, prednisone, and L-asparaginase, the CR rate was 85 percent.[6] The induction death rate was 9 percent, and only 7 percent had refractory disease. The OS of all 197 patients at 3 years is 50 percent (Figure 7–5). An important difference was seen in OS at 3 years according to age (69% for patients < 30 years old compared with 39% for patients ages 30 to 59 years compared with 17% for those ≥ 60 years of age) (see Figure 7–2 and Table 7–2). Of note, among a small group of patients with no unfavorable prognostic factors, the estimated probability of OS at 5 years was 100 percent (95% confidence interval 77 to 100%). An international trial conducted by the Medical Research Council (MRC) and ECOG for newly diagnosed patients (Table 7–3) has been reported in preliminary form and includes among the largest number of patients treated uniformly.[69] Among 920 patients entered to date at a median age of 29, the CR rate is 89 percent, and the induction death rate is 4.5

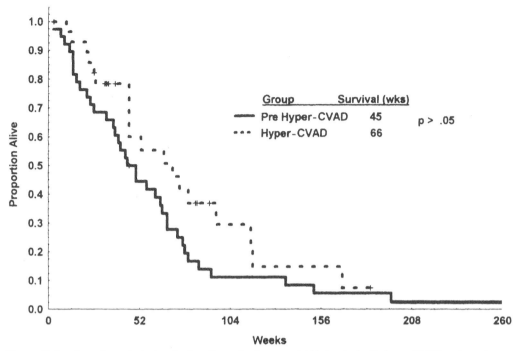

Figure 7–4. Overall survival of patients with newly diagnosed ALL treated with hyper-CVAD and pre-hyper-CVAD chemotherapy. (From Kantarjian HM, O'Brien S, Beran M, et al. Leuk Lymphoma 2000;36:63–73.)

percent. The long-term outcome results await final analysis of the trial. The outcome for older adults (≥ 55 years) with ALL is particularly poor.[70] Although the CR rate is the same as younger adults (approximately 85%) in a series of 40 patients,

Delannoy and colleagues reported a 2-year leukemia-free survival (LFS) of 16 percent.[70] Bassan and colleagues reported a CR rate of approximately 60 percent among 22 older adults with ALL but a 2-year probability of continuous CR of only 13 percent.[71]

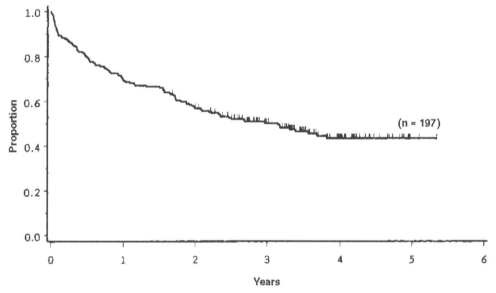

Figure 7–5. Overall survival for 197 patients with newly diagnosed ALL treated with a five-drug induction regimen (cyclophosphamide, daunorubicin, vincristine, prednisone, and L-asparaginase) and intensive multi-agent consolidation, central nervous system prophylaxis, late intensification and maintenance chemotherapy on CALGB protocol 8811. (Reprinted with permission from Larson RA, Dodge RK, Burns CP, et al. A five-drug remission induction regimen with intensive consolidation for adult with acute lymphoblastic leukemia: Cancer and Leukemia Group B study 8811. Blood 1995;85:2025–37. ©American Society of Hematology.)

Table 7–3. TREATMENT FOR ADULT ALL: ECOG PROTOCOL E2993/MRC UKALL XII	

Induction

Phase I (weeks 1 through 4)

Daunorubicin	60 mg/m² IV push days 1, 8, 15, 22
Vincristine	1.4 mg/m² IV push days 1, 8, 15, 22 (maximum 2 mg per dose)
Prednisone	60 4 mg/m² PO qd days 1–28
L-Asparaginase	10,000 units/m² IM or IV in 100 mL D5W over 30 min qd days 17–28
Methotrexate	12.5 mg IT day 15 only, unless patient received treatment for CNS leukemia as per Section 5.213

If CNS leukemia is present at diagnosis, methotrexate IT or via an Omaya reservoir is given weekly until blasts are not present in spinal fluid. Twenty-four cGy cranial irradiation and 12 Gy to the spinal cord are administered concurrent with Phase II.

Phase II (weeks through 8) (should be postponed until the total WBC exceeds 3 × 10⁹/L)

Cyclophosphamide	650 mg/m² IV in 250 cc normal saline for 30 min days 1, 5, and 29
Cytarabine	75 mg/m² IV in 100 cc D5W for 30 min days 1–4, 8–11, 15–18, 22–25
6-Mercaptopurine	60 mg/m² PO qd days 1–28
Methotrexate	12.5 mg IT days 1, 8, 15, 22 (unless patient was treated for occult disease during Phase I)

Intensification* (weeks 12 through 16) (begins 4 weeks from day 28 of induction Phase II; this again can be postponed until the white count exceeds 3 x 10⁹/L)

High-dose methotrexate	3 g/m² IV in NS 500 mL over 2 hours days 1, 8, 22
L-Asparaginase	10,000 IU/m² IV in 100 mL D5W × 30 min days 2, 9, 23
Leucovorin rescue	10 mg/m² IV in 50 mL D5W q 6 hours × 4 doses beginning 22–24 hours after completion of MTX; then 10 mg/m² PO q 6 hours × 72 hours

Allogeneic/MUD BMT or Autologous BMT†

Perform harvest (from marrow, from peripheral blood, or from both) within 4–7 weeks from start of intensification. Postpone harvest until marrow cellularity on biopsy ≥ 20%

Day –6 to day –4	Fractionated TBI total dose; for 1,320 cGy; for males only: 400-cGy testicular boost
Day –3	Etoposide 60 mg/kg IV
Day 0	Allogeneic/MUD or autologous marrow infusion
Day 0	GM-CSF 250 µg/m² daily subcutaneous until ANC ≥ 1,000/µL on 3 consecutive days
Day +30	Interferon-α 3 MU SC 3 × per week for Ph-positive patients to continue for 15 months; must be postponed until WBC > 3.0 × 10⁹/L and platelets > 100 × 10⁹/L

CNS prophylaxis for patients randomized to conventional and consolidation without occult disease (see Section 5.311)

Conventional Consolidation/Maintenance‡ (begins after intensification when WBC > 3.0 × 10⁹/L and platelets > 100 × 10⁹/L)

Cycle I consolidation

Cytarabine	75 mg/m² UV in 500 cc D5W over 30 min, days 1–5
Etoposide	100 mg/m² IV in 500 mL NS over 1 hour days 1–5
Vincristine	1.4 mg/m² IV push days 1, 8, 15, 22 (maximum 2 mg/dose)
Dexamethasone	10 mg/m² PO days 1–28

Cycle II consolidation (beginning 4 weeks from day 1 of first cycle or when WBC > 3.0 × 10⁹/L, except cycle IV, which will begin 2 months from day 1 following cycle III or when WBC > 3.0 × 10⁹/L)

Cytarabine	75 mg/m² IV in 500 cc D5W over 30 min days 1–5
Etoposide	100 mg/m² IV in 500 cc normal saline over 60 min days 1–5

Cycle III consolidation (begin 4 weeks from day 1 of cycle II or when WBC > 3.0 × 10⁹/L)

Daunorubicin	25 mg/m² IV push days 1, 8, 15, 22
Cyclophosphamide	650 mg/m² IV in 250 cc normal saline over 30 min day 29
Cytarabine	75 mg/m² IV 100 cc D5W over 30 min days 31–34, 38–41
6-Thioguanine	60 mg/m² PO days 29–42

Cycle IV consolidation (identical to cycle II but will begin 8 weeks from day 1 following cycle III, or when WBC > 3.0 × 10⁹/L)

Cytarabine	75 mg/m² IV in 500 cc D5W over 30 min days 1–5
Etoposide	100 mg/m² IV in 500 cc normal saline over 60 min days 1–5

Maintenance therapy (to continue for 2¹/₂ years from start of intensification)

Vincristine	1.4 mg/m² IV every 3 months (maximum 2 mg/dose) with prednisone
Prednisone	60 mg/m² PO × 5 days every 3 months with vincristine
6-Mercaptopurine	75 mg/m² PO/day
Methotrexate	20 mg/m² PO or IV once per week for 2¹/₂ years
Interferon-α	For Ph-positive randomized patients; 3 MU SC 3 × per week to continue for 15 months; must be postponed until WBC > 3 × 10⁹/L and platelets > 100 × 10⁹/L

Bone Marrow Transplantation

Allogeneic Bone Marrow Transplantation

Allogeneic BMT in Patients with Standard-Risk ALL in First Remission. Allogeneic BMT is an effective therapy for patients with ALL, although the role has been less established than in AML (Table 7–4).[29,69,72–84] The timing of transplantation in adults with standard risk is controversial because prognostic factors guide risk-adapted therapy.

Horowitz and colleagues conducted a retrospective analysis of patients who received intensive consolidation and maintenance with the Berlin-Frankfurt-Munster (BFM) regimen compared with patients undergoing allogeneic BMT in first remission in the International Bone Marrow Transplant Registry (IBMTR).[83] After accounting for age and lead-time bias to BMT, the 5-year LFS rate was 44 percent in patients who underwent allogeneic BMT compared with 38 percent in patients treated with maintenance and consolidation chemotherapy (not statistically significant). The major cause of treatment failure in the chemotherapy group was leukemia relapse (cumulative risk at 5 years 59%), with a 4 percent probability of treatment-related deaths, whereas the probabilities in the BMT group were 26 and 39 percent, respectively. The investigators were not able to identify any subgroup of patients who benefited from BMT.

In a prospective study conducted in France, patients between the ages of 15 and 40 years in first remission with a human leukocyte antigen (HLA)-identical sibling assigned to undergo allogeneic BMT had an estimated 3-year DFS of 43 percent; those under the age of 50 years and without a donor randomized to undergo an autologous BMT or receive maintenance chemotherapy had a 3-year DFS rate of 39 and 32 percent, respectively (not statistically significant).[84] Patients over the age of 50 years receiving maintenance chemotherapy had a significantly shorter 3-year DFS rate of only 24 percent. In the update of this trial, the 5-year DFS rates were 45 percent for the allogeneic BMT group and 31 percent for the control group, which combined the autologous BMT and chemotherapy groups (p = .1). Patients at high risk (ie, Ph-positive ALL, null or undifferentiated ALL, age older than 35 years, WBC count over 30.0×10^9/L, or time to CR longer than 4 weeks) who received allogeneic BMT had a 5-year DFS of 39 percent compared with 14 percent for patients who received other therapies (p = .01). For patients at standard risk, the 5-year DFS rates were 48 percent in the allogeneic BMT group and 43 percent in the nonallogeneic BMT group (no significant difference). The International ALL trial conducted by the MRC and ECOG has reported an EFS of 58 percent at 3 years for 173 patients undergoing HLA-matched allogeneic transplantation in first CR.[69] The EFS at 3 years for patients who were Ph-negative is 63 percent, 71 percent for standard-risk patients, and 57 percent for high-risk patients (excluding those with the Ph chromosome). The OS at 3 years is 60 percent, 75 percent for standard-risk patients, and 58 percent for high-risk patients (excluding those with

Table 7–4. RESULTS OF ALLOGENEIC BONE MARROW TRANSPLANTATION IN ADULT ALL IN FIRST CR						
Study	N	Risk	DFS/LFS (%)	RR (%)	TRM (%)	Median Follow-up (mo)
Blume, 1987[74]	39	Standard, high*	63	16	26	18
Doney, 1987[75]	46	Standard	28; 5 yr	41	38	50
Vernant, 1988[76]	27	Standard, high	59; 6 yr	11	15	56
Chao, 1991[77]	53	High	61; 5 yr	10	35	66
Fiere, 1993[29]	122	Standard	43; 3 yr	36	20	22
Sutton, 1993[80]	184	Standard	50; 6 yr	31	27.6	82
Sebban, 1994[81]	75	Standard	48; 5 yr	17	11	NA
	41	High	39; 5 yr	44	24	NA
Attal, 1995[82]	43	Standard†	68; 3 yr	31	12	27
Deconinck, 1997[84]	42	High‡	40; 7 yr	NA	38	66
Rowe, 1999[69]	173	Standard, high	63; 3 yr	NA	21	NA

*Thirty-one of 39 patients had one (n = 23) or more (n = 8) high-risk features; †3 patients had the Philadelphia chromosome; ‡10 patients had the Philadelphia chromosome.
NA = not available.

the Ph chromosome). In a retrospective study conducted by the IBMTR comparing the outcome of patients with ALL in first CR undergoing either chemotherapy treatment alone or HLA-matched allogeneic BMT, the LFS at 5 years was significantly worse with chemotherapy than with transplants in patients ≤ 30 years old (30 versus 53%, p = .02) but not in patients older than 30 years (26 versus 30%, p = .70) (Figures 7–6 and 7–7).[85]

Allogeneic BMT in Patients with High-Risk ALL Including Philadelphia Chromosome-Positive ALL.
Attempts have been made to improve the survival in patients with Ph-positive ALL with allogeneic BMT.[84–91] Barrett and colleagues reported an overall relapse-free survival at 2 years of 31 percent in 67 patients with Ph-positive ALL after allogeneic BMT.[87] Subset analysis revealed a 2-year LFS of 38 percent in patients transplanted in first remission, 41 percent for patients transplanted after first relapse, and 25 percent for patients failing to achieve remissions at the time of transplant. Kroger and colleagues noted an estimated LFS of 46 percent at 3 years and 34 percent at 5 years for patients with Ph-positive ALL after an allogeneic BMT in first remission.[90] Patients below the age of 30 were found to have a better estimated OS at 3 years of 61 versus 11 percent (p < .001). The treatment-related

mortality was 25 percent, mainly from infections and graft-vs-host disease (GVHD). These results were a marked improvement when compared with the less than 10 percent cure rates with conventional chemotherapy seen in this population of patients. Deconinck and colleagues reported an OS of 45 ± 9 percent with a median follow-up of 66 months in a group of 42 patients with high-risk ALL who underwent an allogeneic BMT when performed in the first remission.[84] Preliminary results from the International ALL trial from the MRC and ECOG reported the results of the treatment of 138 Ph-positive patients.[91] The 3-year OS for patients undergoing matched related donor transplantation in first CR was 38 percent compared with 0 percent for those receiving only chemotherapy and no transplant. Given the extremely poor prognosis for patients with Ph-positive ALL, every effort should be made to have such patients undergo a transplant, preferably a matched allogeneic transplant or a matched unrelated donor transplant.

Transplantation for Patients with Relapsed or Refractory ALL.
Adults with ALL refractory to primary induction chemotherapy or who relapse following a first remission have a very poor prognosis. Although remission can be induced in 40 to 70 percent of cases with salvage chemotherapy, these usu-

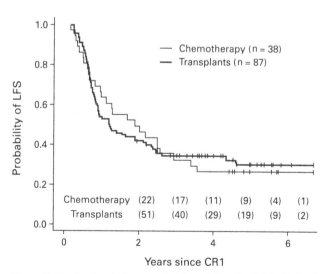

Figure 7–6. Leukemia-free survival for adults with ALL in first CR age ≤ 30 years. (From Oh H, Gale RP, Zhang M-J, et al. Chemotherapy vs HLA-identical sibling bone marrow transplants for adults with acute lymphoblastic leukemia in first remission. Bone Marrow Transplant 1998;22:253–7.)

Figure 7–7. Leukemia-free survival for adults with ALL in first CR age > 30 years. (From Oh H, Gale RP, Zhang M-J, et al. Chemotherapy vs HLA-identical sibling bone marrow transplants for adults with acute lymphoblastic leukemia in first remission. Bone Marrow Transplant 1998;22:253–7.)

ally are short-lived, with less than 5 percent of the patients being alive at 2 years from the start of salvage chemotherapy. Both allogeneic and autologous stem cell transplantation have been used in this setting. Martino and colleagues reported the results of patients with primary refractory or relapsed ALL who underwent autologous or allogeneic transplantation after salvage chemotherapy.[92] The CR rate with salvage chemotherapy was 78 percent. Of the 19 patients assigned to autologous stem cell transplantation, 10 did not undergo transplantation (9 due to early relapse and 1 due to a fungal infection). Eight of the nine patients receiving autologous stem cell transplantation relapsed 2 to 30 months post-transplant. All 10 patients assigned to allogeneic stem cell transplantation received the assigned treatment. There were four transplant-related deaths, and the remaining six patients were alive with a disease-free interval between 9.7 and 92.6 months. In an intent-to-treat analysis, the mean OS from CR for those assigned to autologous stem cell transplantation and allogeneic stem cell transplantation was 11.3 months and 60.1 months, respectively (p < .01). This study emphasizes the difficulty in carrying out transplantation among adults with refractory or relapsed ALL. In addition, autologous stem cell transplantation appears to offer little benefit in this setting, and allogeneic stem cell transplantation from a related or unrelated donor should be considered after achieving a CR with salvage chemotherapy.

Autologous and Matched Unrelated Donor Transplantation in ALL

Autologous BMT using cells harvested in CR and cryopreserved can be used as a source of stem cells after high-dose chemotherapy. However, the value of autologous BMT for adults with ALL in first remission is undetermined.

Fiere and colleagues conducted a randomized trial between autologous BMT and maintenance chemotherapy after consolidation therapy and reported that both autologous BMT and maintenance chemotherapy produced comparable 3-year DFS rates (39 ± 5% versus 32 ± 5%) and OS durations (49 ± 5% versus 42 ± 5%).[29] Patients who relapsed late, after 36 months, were observed in the chemotherapy arm. This study did not demonstrate a survival benefit of autologous BMT compared to maintenance chemotherapy in patients with ALL who received consolidation therapy. A large series evaluated 6 years of consecutive autologous transplants for ALL at the University of Minnesota and the Dana-Farber Cancer Institute compared with matched unrelated donor (MUD) transplants.[93] Most of the transplants were performed in early first or second remission. In adults over 18 years in second CR, DFS for MUD transplantation was significantly better than that seen with autologous BMT (42 ± 22% versus 0%; p < .006). The transplant-related mortality was significantly higher in the MUD-BMT group compared with the autologous BMT group (48 ± 24% versus 8 ± 11%). Evidence of the role of graft-versus-leukemia (GVL) effect in the reduction of the relapse was evident by the fact that risk of relapse beyond day 100 after transplantation was significantly higher in the autologous BMT group compared with the MUD group (85 ± 17% versus 26% ± 24%; p = .001). Improvements in the purging procedures (monoclonal antibodies), BMT preparative regimens (more selective anti-ALL agents), or therapy following BMT for residual disease such as adoptive immunotherapy, antibody-based approaches, or interferon may improve the outcome. The identification and quantification of MRD in harvested cells prior to autologous stem cell transplantation by polymerase chain reaction (PCR) to detect immunoglobulin gene rearrangements may be highly predictive of relapse (Figure 7–8).[94]

Matched unrelated donor transplantation has substantial limitations compared with matched sibling allogeneic transplantation. These include delays in donor identification, increased toxicity, particularly related to GVHD, and graft rejection. However, a potential advantage includes a decreased risk of relapse, presumably related to GVL effect. Unrelated donor BMT may be appropriate to consider in high-risk or relapsed patients with no available sibling donor, particularly for patients with Ph-positive ALL.

Minimal Residual Disease

The development of immunologic and molecular techniques to detect residual disease in ALL is important to distinguish patients with different risks of relapse. These techniques include flow cytometric sorting and immunophenotyping, clonogenic assays, and detection of leukemia-specific deoxyribonucleic acid (DNA) or ribonucleic acid (RNA) sequences by Southern blot or PCR.[95] The presence of residual clonal cells using these techniques may predict the risk of relapse and OS in patients who have attained a morphologic remission.[96,97] During induction chemotherapy, there is a three- to four-log reduction in the number of leukemic cells, but even after a CR is achieved, residual disease can be detected.[98] In some patients, an increase in leukemic cells can be demonstrated by PCR months before it becomes clinically evident. One approach for detecting MRD is to identify the rearrangement of immunoglobulin (Ig) or T-cell receptor (TCR) genes.[98] The clonal nature of ALL is manifested by a specific and unique rearrangement of these genes in all malignant cells, whereas normal cells have a germline configuration. Amplification of such a leukemia-specific marker by PCR can identify one leukemic cell among 1 million normal cells. The principle of this technique is based on amplifying and identifying the specific rearrangement that occurs during the differentiation of B and T cells in the Ig heavy chain (the hypervariable sequence known as the complementary determinant region III) and the TCR, respectively.

Knechtli and colleagues, using a PCR-based MRD analysis, examined the remission specimens of 64 patients receiving allogeneic BMT.[97] The specimens were collected 6 to 81 days (median 23 days) prior to transplantation. Samples were rated high-level positive (sensitivity 10^{-2} to 10^{-3}), low-level positive (sensitivity 10^{-3} to 10^{-5}), or negative. The 2-year EFS rates for these groups were 0, 36, and 73 percent, respectively ($p < .001$). The major limitation of this technique is that because the specific rearrangement is unique for each clone, specific probes must be generated for each patient. The Seattle Marrow Transplant Team evaluated the presence of *bcr-abl* fusion messenger RNA (mRNA) transcript by PCR after allogeneic transplantation.[98] The relative risk of relapse after transplant associated with a positive PCR assay compared with a negative assay was 5.7 (95% confidence interval 1.2 to 2.6, $p \leq .05$) Furthermore, patients expressing the p[190]

bcr-abl mRNA relapse more frequently than those expressing p[210] *bcr-abl* mRNA (7 of 10 patients versus 1 of 8, $p = .02$, log rank). Zetterquist and colleagues have reported that the presence of mixed chimerism as detected by analysis of immunoglobulin heavy-chain and TCR gene rearrangement in patients who have undergone allogeneic stem cell transplantation predicts relapse.[99] Mizuta and colleagues have shown that detection of MRD by PCR amplification of a region of the immunoglobulin gene in harvested cells predicts relapse after autologous transplantation.[94] An alternative approach is the blast-colony assay, described by Estrov and colleagues.[100] With this assay, in vitro growth of lymphoblastic colonies during CR was observed in patients who later experienced relapse. The presence of disease as detected by this method is not always associated with relapse, and a threshold for prediction of adverse outcome has not been established. Verhagen and colleagues have shown that probes can be used to develop patient-specific, real-time PCR assays to accurately detect almost all IgH gene rearrangements.[101,102] Metaphase fluorescent in situ hybridization to detect chromosomal trisomy and/or translocation was used in 25 patients with ALL in CR.[103] Low numbers of abnormal cells (0.05% to < 1%) may disappear in subsequent tests. However, the presence of > 1 percent in any sample preceded relapse after chemotherapy or translocation.

Treatment of Relapsed and Refractory Disease

Treatment for patients with relapsed and refractory ALL is unsatisfactory. A variety of salvage chemotherapy regimens have been identified including high-dose cytarabine with or without L-asparaginase,[104] mitoxantrone,[104–109] and amsacrine.[110] Kantarjian and colleagues have reported very encouraging results with hyper-CVAD (cyclophosphamide, VCR, Adriamycin, dexamethasone) high-dose MTX, and cytarabine all followed by POMP (prednisone, VCR, MTX, and 6-MP) maintenance in newly diagnosed patients.[111] This has become a popular salvage regimen.

Biologic agents have been explored in this setting including interferon[112] and interleukin-4.[113] B43-

Genistein is a CD19 receptor-directed tyrosine kinase inhibitor that has been tested in refractory B-lineage ALL.[114] Among 15 patients treated in a phase I dose escalating trial, 2 patients who had failed marrow transplantation and were in second or greater relapse achieved a bone marrow remission by day 28. Preliminary studies testing the Abl tyrosine kinase inhibitor STI-571 in patients with Ph-positive ALL have been encouraging with respect to the achievement of CR.[115]

Coagulopathy Associated with L-Asparaginase

L-Asparaginase has become routinely administered to patients with ALL.[116–118] It is associated with several important toxicities including liver disease and a life-threatening coagulopathy that includes both hemorrhage and thrombosis.[119–126] The drug depletes proteins including antithrombin III, plasminogen, and fibrin. Daily evaluation of fibrinogen levels, prothrombin time, and D-dimer during the first 10 days of induction to determine if disseminate intravascular coagulation is present and to maintain the platelet count $\geq$ 20,000/μL and the fibrinogen level $\geq$ 100 mg/dL with fresh frozen plasma and cryoprecipitation has been suggested.[125]

Prognosis

Individual prognostic factors for response to therapy and for survival have been well recognized in adult ALL. Multivariate analyses in different studies have identified several consistent independent patient and disease-associated poor-prognosis features for survival. These include older age, elevated leukocyte count, specific karyotype abnormalities, or delay (more than 4 or 6 weeks) in achieving a CR. Depending on these characteristics, patients can be categorized as having standard-risk ALL (about 25 to 30% of patients), with an expected long-term survival above 50 percent, or high-risk ALL (70 to 75% of patients), with an expected long-term survival below 30 percent. Future studies will apply risk-oriented approaches such that patients with high-risk ALL will receive experimental or novel treatment strategies (allogeneic BMT, autologous BMT, dose intensification, and new agents).

ACUTE MYELOID LEUKEMIA

The treatment of acute myeloid leukemia (AML) generally involves the administration of cytotoxic chemotherapy to eradicate the malignant cells, which permits restoration of normal hematopoiesis by normal residual stem cells. Approximately 50 to 75 percent of adults with AML achieve complete remission (CR) with an anthracycline and cytarabine.[127–130] However, the majority of patients eventually relapse because of regrowth of residual leukemic cells. Therefore, the long-term disease-free survival (DFS) is only 20 to 30 percent of patients who achieve a first CR, despite intensive consolidation chemotherapy. In an Eastern Cooperative Oncology Group (ECOG) analysis of the outcome of more than 1,400 patients with previously untreated AML entered on five successive clinical treatment trials in which daunorubicin and cytarabine were given for induction and successive trials included increasingly intensive postremission therapy, 62 percent of patients achieved CR, but 76 percent have relapsed or died.[131,132] The overall survival (OS) for all patients at 5 years is only 15 percent. The 5-year OS rate ranged between 9 and 33 percent for patients less than age 55 years and 6 to 15 percent for patients age 55 years and older (Figure 7–9). Among patients younger than age 55 years, both the DFS and OS increased with more intensive postremission strategies. The Cancer and Leukemia Group B (CALGB) has shown that the administration of multiple courses of very intensive consolidation with high-dose cytarabine (3 g/m²

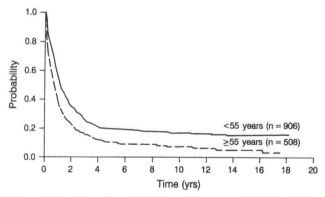

Figure 7–9. Overall survival from diagnosis of 1,414 patients treated on 5 ECOG clinical trials conducted between 1976 and 1994 for patients with previously untreated AML. All protocols included daunorubicin and cytarabine for induction with increasingly intensive postremission therapy. (From Bennett JM, Young ML, Andersen JW, et al. Long-term survival in acute myeloid leukemia: the Eastern Cooperative Oncology Group experience. Cancer 1997;80:2205–9.)

dose) consolidation has resulted in a 4-year continuous CR rate of 44 percent for patients younger than age 61 years (Figure 7–10).[133]

These and other studies have clearly demonstrated that the outcome for adults with AML depends not only on the age of the patient but also on the intensity of postremission therapy and on the biologic characteristics of the disease, including karyotype and expression of the multidrug-resistant (mdr) phenotype. The French-American-British (FAB) classification has been widely adopted since its initial description in 1976 and allows for the uniformity of diagnosis of morphologic subtypes of AML.[134,135] It remains useful but does not by itself account for all subtypes since the recognition of biologic subtypes is based on cytogenetics, immunophenotyping, and molecular genetics. Advances in these areas have led to a new proposed World Heath Organization classification that attempts to correlate morphology, cytochemistry, immunophenotype, karyotype, and molecular genetics with clinical features (Table 7–5).[136] Improvements in outcome have occurred primarily because of better supportive care, increased intensity of postremission chemotherapy, the development of bone marrow (stem cell) transplantation, and in acute promyelocytic leukemia, where the specific genetic abnormality is targeted with the vitamin A derivative all-*trans* retinoic acid (ATRA). Baudard and colleagues have demonstrated an improvement in CR rate and

Table 7–5. PROPOSED WORLD HEALTH ORGANIZATION CLASSIFICATION OF ACUTE MYELOID LEUKEMIA
AML with specific cytogenetic defects
AML with features of t(8;21)
AML with features of inv(16)
Promyelocytic leukemia with t(15;17)
Promyelocytic leukemia with t(v;17)
AML with t(6;9)
AML with trilineage dysplasia (dysplasia involving > 50% of all cell lineages)
Classify using subgroups (M0–M7)
AML without defining cytogenetic defects or dysplasia
AML M1–M6
Myeloid sarcoma
Acute panmyelosis with myelofibrosis
AML arising in a previously myelodysplastic syndrome
Therapy-related AML
Alkylating agent related
Topoisomerase II inhibitor related

5-year OS in younger patients treated over a 16-year period (Figure 7–11).[137]

Standard Induction Chemotherapy

The treatment of patients with AML can be divided into two phases, remission induction and postremission therapy. During the past 30 years, a series of successive studies has led to an induction regimen that has become routinely used. Approximately 30 to 40 percent of patients achieve CR with either cytarabine or daunorubicin given as a single agent.[138–140] Complete remission is generally achieved in more

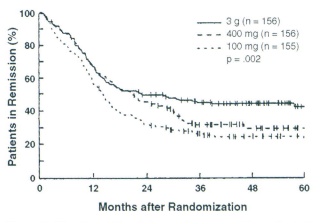

Figure 7–10. Probability of disease-free survival for patients 60 years old or younger according to dose of cytarabine given as postremission therapy (doses were to be 400 mg/m² or 3 g/m² twice daily on days 1, 3, and 5 for 4 courses). (From Mayer RJ, Davis RB, Schiffer CA, et al. For the Cancer and Leukemia Group B: intensive postremission chemotherapy in adults with acute myeloid leukemia. N Engl J Med 1994;331:896–903.)

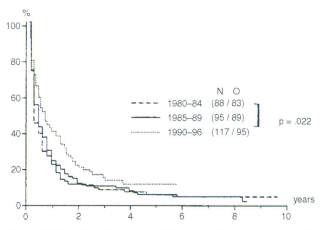

Figure 7–11. Overall survival of 784 consecutively treated patients less than age 60 years treated at a single institution by year of diagnosis between 1980 and 1995. (From Baudard M, Beauchamp-Nicoud A, Delmer A, et al. Has the prognosis of adult patients with acute myeloid leukemia improved over years? A single institution experience of > 784 consective patients over a 16-year period. Leukemia 1999;13:1481–90.)

than 50 percent of patients when these agents are combined. The CALGB established that 3 days of daunorubicin and 7 days of cytarabine are associated with a better outcome than 2 days and 5 days, respectively, and that 10 days of cytarabine did not improve outcome compared with 7.[129,141] Daunorubicin at a dose of 30 mg/m^2 is inferior compared with 45 mg/m^2 in patients less than age 60 years and less toxic than Adriamycin 30 mg/m^2.[128] Finally, 100 mg/m^2 of cytarabine is equally as effective as 200 mg/m^2.[142] Therefore, the most common contemporary induction chemotherapy is daunorubicin 45 mg/m^2/d intravenously (IV) for 3 days and cytarabine 100 mg/m^2 by continuous IV infusion for 7 days. Since this combination regimen was established, a number of studies have explored strategies to improve the CR rate, including alternative anthracyclines, the addition of agents such as etoposide, or adding high-dose cytarabine (HiDAC).[143]

Anthracyclines in Induction

The anthracyclines include daunorubicin, doxorubicin, mitoxantrone (a synthetic deoxyribonucleic acid [DNA] intercalator based on the anthracenedione structure and considered as an anthracycline analog), aclarubicin, and the synthetic agent 4-demethoxydaunorubicin or idarubicin. Idarubicin may have advantages as an induction agent because of higher lipid solubility; increased cellular uptake; induction of more DNA single-strand breaks; its conversion to an alcoholic derivative; 13-hydroxyidarubicin, an active metabolite with a prolonged plasma half-life; greater toxicity of AML blast cells; and less dependency on P-glycoprotein efflux.[144–147]

Four prospective randomized trials have compared idarubicin to daunorubicin and provide some evidence that idarubicin may be superior, particularly in young adults (Table 7–6).[148–151] In three of the studies, idarubicin was associated with a statistically significantly higher CR rate, particularly in younger patients, compared with daunorubicin; was more effective in eradicating leukemia after one course; and was associated with a lower incidence of resistant leukemia. The study by Mandelli and colleagues for the Gruppo Italiano Malattie Ematologiche Maligne dell'Adulto (GIMEMA) was the only trial that did not show a higher CR rate with idarubicin.[151] This trial

included patients with an antecedent myelodysplastic syndrome, a population of patients excluded by Berman and colleagues.[148] Although patients with an antecedent myelodysplastic syndrome were eligible in the studies by Wiernik and Vogler,[149,150] only a small percentage of such patients were included. The study by Mandelli and colleagues was designed for patients older than 55 years, whereas the studies by Wiernik and Vogler did not restrict the upper age limit. The CR rate with idarubicin was not lower among patients with hyperleukocytosis in the studies by Berman and Wiernik and colleagues[148,149] but was among patients treated with daunorubicin. One of the difficulties in comparing long-term advantages of idarubicin to daunorubicin is that postremission therapy varied between studies. Nevertheless, one can conclude that higher CR rates have been achieved with idarubicin in younger patients, and idarubicin may be beneficial in patients presenting with hyperleukocytosis. In these studies, idarubicin at either 12 or 13 mg/m^2 was compared with daunorubicin at a dose of 45 mg/m^2. Therefore, it is not clear that any observed improvement represents an inherent biologic advantage of a particular drug rather than biologic dose equivalence. There has not been a prospective randomized trial comparing daunorubicin at a dose of 45 mg/m^2 with either 60 mg/m^2 or 70 mg/m^2. In a retrospective analysis, Usui and colleagues reported that the optimal dose of daunorubicin in induction was approximately 280 mg/m^2 (40 mg/m^2 for 7 days), which is greater than the doses routinely administered of 40 to 60 mg/m^2 for 3 days.[152] Furthermore, it is not clear that OS with idarubicin is superior to that achieved with daunorubicin since two studies showed an advantage and two

Table 7–6. RANDOMIZED TRIALS COMPARING IDARUBICIN TO DAUNORUBICIN IN INDUCTION IN AML			
Study	Anthracycline	No. Pts	% CR
Berman[148]	IDA	60	80
	DNR	60	58
Wiernik[149]	IDA	97	70
	DNR	111	59
Vogler[150]	IDA	105	71
	DNR	113	58
Mandelli[151]	IDA	124	40
	DNR	125	39

CR = complete remission; IDA = idarubicin; DNR = daunorubicin.

did not. A meta-analysis by the AML Collaborative Group reported similar early induction failure rates (20% for idarubicin versus 18% for daunorubicin; p = .4) but fewer late (after day 40) induction failures with idarubicin (62 versus 53%; p = .002).[153] Among patients achieving CR, fewer patients assigned to idarubicin relapsed (p = .008), but somewhat more died in CR, resulting in a nonsignificant benefit in DFS (p = .07). Overall survival was better with idarubicin (13 versus 9% alive at 5 years; p = .03).

Mitoxantrone is associated with a relatively steep dose-response in clonogenic assays of leukemia cells and has a favorable extramedullary toxicity profile.[154] Mitoxantrone[155–157] and aclarubicin,[158] a class III anthracycline whose uptake and outward transport is largely unaffected in multidrug-resistant cell lines, may also offer advantages. Mitoxantrone appears at least as effective and aclarubicin more effective than daunorubicin in younger patients with respect to CR rate but not OS, and both may be associated with less resistant leukemia. Amsacrine, a DNA intercalator distinct from anthracyclines, was compared with daunorubicin 50 mg/m^2, given with cytarabine, and 6-thioguanine (6-TG) was associated with a higher CR rate (70 versus 54%; p = .03), more frequent achievement of CR with only one cycle (48 versus 28%, p = .03), and improved OS (p = .01).[159]

Several other studies have addressed the dose and choice of anthracyclines, specifically in older patients. Buchner and colleagues compared daunorubicin 30 mg/m^2 with 60 mg/m^2 during induction in patients older than age 60 followed by consolidation and monthly maintenance for 3 years.[160] The CR rate was higher among patients receiving the higher dose (52 versus 45%; p = .026), and the CR rate was higher after one cycle (38 versus 20%; p = .001). Survival was significantly improved only among patients older than age 65 years (14 versus 5%; p = .002). A trial that included a small number of patients by Feldman and colleagues compared high-dose mitoxantrone at 80 mg/m^2 for 5 days.[161] Complete remission was achieved in 57 percent of patients with the high-dose mitoxantrone compared with 43 percent with standard dose. However, the median time to relapse was 6 months, and there was no statistically significant difference between the two groups and no difference in toxicity.

The ECOG completed a prospective randomized trial of daunorubicin versus idarubicin versus mitoxantrone as the anthracycline given together with cytarabine in 350 evaluable patients older than 55 years.[162] The study was also designed to compare the CR rates with and without granulocyte-macrophage colony-stimulating factor (GM-CSF) priming to recruit leukemia cells into the cell cycle. A preliminary analysis shows that the CR rates achieved with the three different anthracyclines did not differ. There was a trend toward a decreased induction mortality rate on the mitoxantrone arm. In the European Organization for the Research and Treatment of Cancer (EORTC)-HOVON collaborative trial, patients 60 years of age and older were randomized to receive either daunorubicin 30 mg/m^2 for 3 days or mitoxantrone 8 mg/m^2 for 3 days plus cytarabine 100 mg/m^2 by continuous infusion for 7 days.[163] There was a modestly higher CR rate with mitoxantrone (46.6%) compared with daunorubicin (38.0%) (p = .067), likely related to a reduced probability of resistant leukemia (47 versus 32%; p = .001) since the induction mortality was somewhat higher with mitoxantrone (21 versus 15%). However, among patients who achieved CR, there was no difference in either DFS or OS. Another prospective trial conducted as a collaboration between the EORTC and GIMEMA prospectively evaluated daunorubicin and mitoxantrone given with cytarabine and etoposide in younger adults.[164] Patients then received cytarabine 500 mg/m^2 every 12 hours for 6 days with the same induction intercalating agent. There was no difference in CR rate or in induction mortality, DFS, or OS between the three induction arms. Therefore, there is no evidence that one anthracycline is better than another for induction in older adults. Whether one agent is better in younger adults is less clear.

Randomized Trials of Cytarabine Dose in Induction

Cytarabine is one of the most active single drugs for the treatment of AML. Modifications in both the dose and duration of cytarabine have been evaluated. In a prospective randomized trial conducted at the University of California-Los Angeles, intermediate-dose cytarabine at 500 mg/m^2 given with daunorubicin 60 mg/m^2 gave similar results to 200 mg/m^2 with respect to both CR rates (71 and 74%, respectively) and DFS.[165] Patients receiving the higher dose of cytarabine did have a higher CR rate after one course of induction, but this was not statistically significant.

Since a number of studies have shown that HiDAC is effective treatment for patients with relapsed and refractory leukemia, several trials have tested the benefits of HiDAC in induction. Three prospective randomized trials have directly compared HiDAC with standard induction while using the same postremission therapy in both arms (Table 7–7). The Australian Leukemia Study Group (ALSG) compared HiDAC 3 g/m^2 every 12 hours for 8 days on alternate days plus daunorubicin 50 mg/m^2 and etoposide to conventional induction with etoposide.[166] The Southwest Oncology Group (SWOG) compared cytarabine 2 g/m^2 every 12 hours for 6 days plus daunorubicin 45 mg/m^2 to conventional induction.[167] Neither trial showed a higher CR rate with HiDAC compared with standard induction, but the higher-dose regimen was associated with increased hematologic and extramedullary toxicity, including nausea, emesis, and ophthalmologic toxicity. In one of these studies, patients randomized to HiDAC had increased cerebellar toxicity. Both studies showed a longer DFS, but not OS, among patients receiving the high-dose regimen. However, these studies do not provide information as to whether HiDAC must be given in induction or would yield similar outcome results if HiDAC was given as consolidation.

Randomized Trials of Additional Drugs During Induction

The ALSG previously compared standard-dose cytarabine plus daunorubicin (7 + 3) to 7 + 3 plus etoposide 75 mg/m^2/d for 7 days (7 + 3 + 7) followed by consolidation with the same agents over a shorter time, 5 + 2 versus 5 + 2 + 5.[168] Patients then received maintenance with cytarabine and 6-TG for 2 years. Although there was a significantly longer DFS on the etoposide arm, OS was not longer. Updated results reveal that the median OS was not significantly improved on 7 + 3 + 7 compared with 7 + 3 (13 versus 9 months; p = .24).[169] The 5- and 10-year survival rates for 7 + 3 + 7 were 19 and 16 percent,

respectively, compared with 16 and 12 percent, respectively, for 7 + 3. However, the OS among patients less than age 55 was significantly longer on the 7 + 3 + 7 arm (p = .04) with a 5- and 10-year OS of 25 and 25 percent, respectively, and 17 and 14 percent for 7 + 3. Older patients experienced significantly more toxicity and no benefit in outcome. Therefore, in younger patients, intensified induction appears to improve CR duration and OS without necessarily improving the CR rate.

Updated results of the HiDAC + 3 + 7 versus 7 + 3 + 7 trial show that the median remission duration was 46 months for HiDAC + 3 + 7 and 12 months for 7 + 3 + 7 (p = .0007).[169] The DFS among patients achieving CR at 5 years was 48 percent with the HiDAC arm compared with 25 percent on the 7 + 3 + 7 arm, and there were no relapses on either arm beyond 54 months. The difference in OS between the two arms approached statistical significance (p = .053). These data suggest that intensified induction, as administered here, may improve outcome.

The potential advantage of adding etoposide in induction was also tested by the Medical Research Council (MRC) in the United Kingdom in the AML10 trial.[170] More than 1,800 patients age 55 years and younger were randomized to either 7 + 3 (daunorubicin 50 mg/m^2) + 6-TG or 7 + 3 (daunorubicin 50 mg/m^2) + etoposide 100 mg/m^2/d for 5 days. All patients achieving CR received two cycles of consolidation. Induction mortality was somewhat higher on the etoposide arm (9 versus 6%; p = .06). The CR rates between the two arms did not differ. Similarly, there were no differences in either DFS (42 at 6 years for 7 + 3 and 43% for 7 + 3 + 5) or OS (40 for both groups). This trial further suggests that the addition of etoposide to standard anthracycline-

Table 7–7. RANDOMIZED STUDIES OF HIDAC (H) VERSUS STANDARD-DOSE CYTARABINE (S) IN INDUCTION IN AML

Author	N		CR (%)		DFS (5-Yr) (%)		OS (5-Yr) (%)	
	S	H	S	H	S	H	S	H
Schiller[165]	51	50	71	74	20	28	25	37
Bishop[166]	152	149	74	71	23	41	25	31
Weick[167]	493	172	58	55	21	33	22	32

HiDAC = high-dose cytosine arabinoside; CR = complete remission; DFS = disease-free survival; OS = overall survival.

cytarabine induction is not associated with improved outcome, although the results may be confounded by the potential contribution of 6-TG.

Randomized Trials of Sequential Standard-Dose Cytarabine Followed by High-Dose Cytarabine in Induction

Investigators at Tufts-New England Medical Center administered HiDAC on days 8, 9, and 10 of induction to exploit potential recruitment into the cell cycle and to avoid administering an entire second cycle of induction for patients with residual leukemia after a first cycle.[171] Complete remission was achieved in 89 percent of patients, and essentially all patients achieved CR after one cycle of chemotherapy. Both ECOG and SWOG have completed phase II studies testing this strategy. No difference was observed in the CR rate among patients given the intensified induction compared with standard induction in either trial.[172,173] The German AML Cooperative Group randomized newly diagnosed patients to either two courses of standard-dose cytarabine with daunorubicin and 6-TG or one course of the same chemotherapy followed by HiDAC with mitoxantrone on day 21 regardless of the marrow findings.[174] There were no differences in the CR rates (65% in the standard dose versus 71% on the HiDAC arm; p = NS) or in the induction death rate (18 versus 14%; p = NS) or the RFS at 5 years (29 versus 35%; p = NS). However, high-risk patients (> 40% residual blasts on the D16 marrow, unfavorable kary-

otype, and elevated lactate dehydrogenase) had a higher CR rate (65 versus 49%; p = .004), a superior EFS at 5 years (17 versus 12%, p = .012), and median OS at 5 years (13 versus 8 months; p = .009).

Hematopoietic Growth Factors During Induction

Hematopoietic growth factors have been shown to shorten the period of neutropenia after induction therapy in AML. Most prospective clinical trials have been conducted in older patients where the risk of death from marrow aplasia justified the concern for leukemia cell stimulation. Many prospective randomized trials have been carried out, but with different designs, patient ages, and induction regimens (Table 7–8).[175–186] In the ECOG trial, patients between ages 55 and 70 received daunorubicin 60 mg/m^2 plus cytarabine 100 mg/m^2 for 7 days.[176] The CR rate was better for the GM-CSF arm (60%) compared with the placebo arm (44%) (p = .08), and median times were significantly shorter on the GM-CSF arm. Furthermore, infectious toxicity was significantly reduced on the GM-CSF arm (p = .015). In an intent-to-treat analysis considering all randomized patients, the median survival was significantly longer for patients receiving GM-CSF (10.6 versus 4.8 months). This difference was attributable to increased early mortality in the placebo group. The design of the CALGB trial reported by Stone and colleagues differed in that patients received GM-CSF or placebo on day 8 (versus day 11 in the

					CR (%)	Median Days ANC to 1,000/μL
Author	No. Pts	Growth Factor	Start Day	Marrow Aplasia	Growth Factor	Control
Rowe[176]	117	GM-CSF	11	Yes	60/44	12/18
Dombret[177]	173	G-CSF	8	No	70/47*	21/27*
Heil[178]	521	G-CSF	8	No	69/68	20/25
Godwin[179]	234	G-CSF	11	Yes	42/49	3–4 days
Stone[180]	379	GM-CSF	8	No	52/54	15/17
Zittoun[181]	53	GM-CSF	8	No	48/77*	Not different
Löwenberg[181]	316	GM-CSF	1–8	No	63/61	26/31*
Link[183]	187	G-CSF	9	No	60/43*	12/18*
Goldstone[184]	800	G-CSF	8	No	72/75	15/20
Witz[185]	209	GM-CSF	1	No	63/61	22/26*

Table 7–8. RANDOMIZED TRIALS OF GROWTH FACTOR AFTER INDUCTION THERAPY IN AML

GM-CSF = granulocyte-macrophage colony-stimulating factor; G-CSF = granulocyte colony-stimulating factor.
Adapted from Rowe JM, Liesveld JL. Hematopoietic growth factors in acute leukemia. Leukemia 1997;11:328–41.
*p ≤ .05.

ECOG study) immediately after completion of induction therapy, irrespective of whether marrow aplasia had been achieved.[180] Furthermore, 30 percent of patients discontinued the study drug in either arm because of perceived toxicity. There was no difference in CR rates among patients assigned to GM-CSF (51%) versus placebo (54%) (p = .61). The incidence of both severe and lethal infection did not differ between the two groups. The incidence of regrowth of leukemia also did not differ. The median duration of neutropenia was only minimally shorter among patients receiving GM-CSF (15 versus 17 days; p = .02). Although all studies demonstrated a shorter period of myelosuppression, such an effect did not translate to a clinically meaningful benefit in all trials. In the French study, the CR rate was increased, but survival was not prolonged.[177] Neither of the studies conducted by the CALGB or SWOG showed that a shorter period of myelosuppression resulted in improvement in either CR rate or OS.

Although growth factors shorten the period of neutropenia following induction chemotherapy and in several studies significantly reduced morbidity, the CR rate and OS are generally not improved. Importantly, growth factors appear safe and do not appear to be an associated risk of leukemic cell stimulation.

Postremission Therapy

A variety of approaches have been explored to prevent relapse. Such strategies have included low-dose maintenance therapy, intensive consolidation therapy, or high-dose chemotherapy or chemoradiotherapy with either allogeneic or autologous bone marrow or stem cell transplantation.

Maintenance Therapy

A prospective randomized trial conducted by the ECOG suggested that maintenance therapy with 6-TG plus cytarabine 60 mg/m^2 once a week for 2 years offered a benefit in remission duration compared to no maintenance treatment (median remission duration of 8.1 versus 4.1 months (p = .003), although no significant survival difference was identified.[187] Buchner and colleagues recently analyzed long-term follow-up data and observed a benefit to monthly maintenance for 3 years (5-year DFS 23 versus

6%).[188] In a EORTC-HOVON trial, 76 patients ($\geq$ 61 years of age) achieving CR were randomized to no further therapy and 75 patients to eight cycles of low-dose cytarabine (10 mg/m^2 subcutaneously) every 12 hours for 12 days every 6 weeks following consolidation with the same agents used induction.[163] An advantage DFS was observed among patients receiving maintenance low-dose cytarabine (median DFS 20 versus 7% and 5-year DFS 13 versus 7%; p = .006), but OS was not different (5-year OS 18 versus 15%, p = .29). The AML9 study, conducted by the MRC in the United Kingdom, randomized patients in CR to maintenance treatment for 1 year with eight courses of cytarabine 70 mg/m^2 subcutaneously every 12 hours and 6-TG 100 mg/m^2 orally every 12 hours for 5 days per month followed by four courses of COAP (cyclophosphamide, vincristine, cytarabine, and prednisone) or observation.[189] Such therapy delayed but did not prevent relapse with no improvement in the OS at 5 years. Therefore, contemporary studies employing various maintenance regimens consistently show a benefit in DFS but not OS.

Intensive Consolidation Chemotherapy

Retrospective analyses of cooperative group studies[5,6] have suggested that increasing the intensity of postremission therapy is beneficial. Several studies have prospectively evaluated the role of intensive postremission consolidation with HiDAC. The CALGB randomly assigned 596 patients in CR to receive four courses of cytarabine at one of three doses: 100 mg/m^2/d by continuous IV infusion for 5 days, 400 mg/m^2/d by continuous IV infusion for 5 days, and 3 g/m^2 as a 3-hour IV infusion twice daily on days 1, 3, and 5 (see Figure 7–10).[133] High rates of central nervous system toxicity were observed in patients older than 60 years randomized to the high-dose regimen. Randomization was subsequently limited to patients 60 years of age or younger. Disease-free survival was 21 percent in the 100-mg group, 25 percent in the 400-mg group, and 39 percent in the 3-g group. The results were most significant in patients with favorable cytogenetics. This trial demonstrated a dose-response effect for cytarabine in patients undergoing postremission therapy. Although the HiDAC regimen used in this trial has become widely adopted, it must be noted that after the four courses of cytarabine, all patients received four monthly cycles of cytarabine 100 mg/m^2 every 12 hours for 5 days by subcutaneous injection and daunorubicin 45 mg/m^2 IV infusion on day 1. Remissions achieved in this trial were quite durable, with few relapses after 20 months. (In an ECOG trial, patients without HLA-matched siblings were randomized to 2 years of continuous outpatient maintenance therapy with cytarabine and 6-TG or a single course of intensive consolidation with cytarabine 3 g/m^2 IV every 12 hours for 12 doses followed by amsacrine 100 mg/m^2 per day IV for 3 days.[190]) The event-free survival at 4 years was 27 percent for the intensive consolidation arm and 16 percent for the maintenance arm (p = .068). This difference was statistically significant in patients younger than 60 years of age. The Swiss Group for Clinical Cancer Research (SAKK) randomized younger patients to one course of consolidation with either high-dose cytarabine at 3 g/m^2 twice daily for 6 days or standard-dose cytarabine 100 mg/m^2 by continuous IV infusion for 7 days each with daunorubicin 45 mg/m^2 for 3 days after two cycles of induction, which included daunorubicin 45 mg/m^2 IV for 3 days plus cytarabine 100 mg/m^2 by continuous IV infusion for 7 days and then M-amsacrine 120 mg/m^2 IV daily for 5 days plus etoposide 80 mg/m^2 daily for 5 days as a continuous IV infusion.[191] Among the 112 patients in CR, the estimated DFS at 4 years was 25 ± 6 percent for standard-dose cytarabine consolidation compared with 37 ± 6 percent for high-dose cytarabine. The median OS was also better (24.6 versus 32.6 months; p = .07) These data suggest that a single course of intensive consolidation with high-dose cytarabine leads to as good an outcome as multiple courses of intensive putatively noncross-resistant chemotherapy.[192,193]

The number of courses of HiDAC required for optimal postremission therapy is uncertain. The Finnish Leukemia Group randomized patients less than age 65 years in CR after two courses of induction to either four additional consolidation courses after two courses of HiDAC-containing consolidation or observation.[194] No benefit was observed for patients randomized to the longer consolidation program, suggesting that early intensive consolidation is likely the most important influence on outcome rather than the total number of cycles (Figure 7–12).

Allogeneic Bone Marrow (Stem Cell) Transplantation

Allogeneic bone marrow or stem cell transplantation has become an effective strategy for patients with AML in first CR (Table 7–9).[195–210] Reinfusion of hematopoietic stem cells from an HLA-matched sibling donor following myeloablative chemotherapy or chemoradiotherapy takes advantage of both the antileukemic effects of the preparative regimen and of graft-versus-leukemia effect against potential residual leukemic cells, contributed by the reinfused stem cells. Approximately 50 to 60 percent of younger patients in first CR appear to be cured since the risk of relapse is generally less than 20 percent. However, transplant-related mortality (within the first 100 days post-transplant) remains approximately 20 to 25 percent related to graft-versus-host disease (GVHD), cytomegalovirus infections, and fungal infections and has diminished the benefits in outcome afforded by the reduction in relapse rate. New techniques such as T-cell depletion[203,211–213] and nonmyeloablative transplantation[214–216] may diminish the incidence of GVHD and other toxicities and improve outcome. Importantly, the same cytogenetic abnormalities that confer a poor prognosis with intensive consolidation chemotherapy also confer a relatively poor prognosis after allogeneic transplantation.[210,217] Allogeneic stem

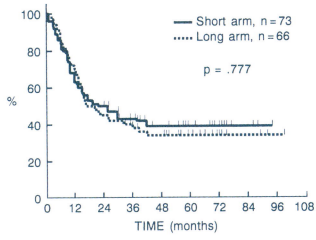

Figure 7–12. Projected relapse-free survival of patients randomized to a short arm (two cycles of high-dose cytarabine containing consolidation chemotherapy followed by two induction cycles) or a long arm (six cycles of consolidation). (From Elonen E, Almqvist A, Hanninen A, et al. Comparison between four and eight cycles of intensive chemotherapy in adult acute myeloid leukemia: a randomized trial of the Finnish Leukemia Group. Leukemia 1998;1041–8.)

Table 7–9. ALLOGENEIC BONE MARROW (STEM CELL) TRANSPLANTATION FOR AML IN FIRST CR					
Author	No. Pts	TRM (%)	RR (%)	DFS (%)	OS (%)
Champlin,[197] 1985	23	43	40	60*, 4 yr	40
Forman,[202] 1987	69[†]	30	16	51, 4 yr	NA
Clift,[312] 1987	231	25	25	46, 5 yr	48, 5 yr
Appelbaum,[200] 1988	33	36	15	48, 5 yr	48, 5 yr
McGlave,[198] 1988	73	7	9	62, 7 yr	NA
Geller,[201] 1989[‡]	49	49	8	45, 3 yr	46
Schiller,[204] 1992	28	32	32	48, 5 yr	45, 5 yr
Young,[203] 1992[§]	31	42	13	45, 3 yr	45, 3 yr
Fagioli,[205] 1994	91	26	29	NA	53, 5 yr
Keating,[207] 1996	169	22	23	60, 3 yr	NA
Labar,[208] 1996	46	18	12	71, 7 yr	NA
Mehta,[206] 1996	85	33[‖]	25[‖]	48, 10 yr	NA
Reiffers,[209] 1996	36	12	24	67, 3 yr	65, 3 yr
Ferrant,[210], 1995[#]	346	NA	22	57, 3 yr	59, 3 yr
Soiffer,[211] 1997[§]	14	16	25	63, 4 yr	71, 4 yr

* Freedom from relapse; [†]includes 20 patients ages 1–19 years; [‡]includes 27 patients who received low-dose cyclophosphamide ± methylprednisone or intramuscular cyclosporine as graft-versus-host disease prophylaxis; [§]T-cell depletion; [‖]at 10 years; only two relapses beyond 2 years; [#]results for standard-risk patients. NA = not available.

cell transplantation may be an effective initial strategy for patients with secondary AML.[218] A retrospective analysis from the International Bone Marrow Transplant Registry suggests no advantage to any dose of consolidation chemotherapy for patients with AML undergoing allogeneic transplant in first CR once CR is achieved with a standard induction program (Figure 7–13).[219] In addition, Cahn and colleagues, on behalf

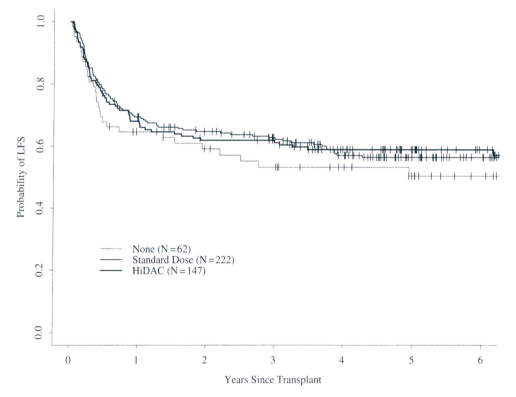

Figure 7–13.   Retrospective analysis of leukemia-free survival for patients with AML in first CR following induction given either no consolidation chemotherapy, standard-dose cytarabine consolidation, or high-dose cytarabine consolidation. (Reprinted with permission from Tallman MS, Rowlings PA, Milone G, et al. Effect of postremission chemotherapy prior to HLA-identical sibling transplantation for acute myelogenous leukemia in first complete remission. Blood 2000;96:1254–8. ©American Society of Hematology.)

of the European Cooperative Group for Blood and Marrow Transplantation (EBMT), also failed to observe any difference in outcome with any dose of cytarabine consolidation prior to allogeneic stem cell transplantation.[220] Allogeneic stem cell transplantation also appears to be a better approach than either chemotherapy or autologous stem cell transplantation for patients with AML in second CR.[221,222]

An important issue concerns the inherent practical difficulty in carrying out allogeneic transplantation. Such a strategy is frequently only completed in approximately 60 percent of intended cases[223] and in less than 10 percent of all patients with newly diagnosed AML treated at a single center.[224]

Autologous Stem Cell Transplantation

Autologous stem cell transplantation is an alternative approach for patients who lack a suitable HLA-matched allogeneic donor (Table 7–10).[193,225–242] One advantage is that this strategy is not limited by donor availability since every patient can serve as his or her own donor. However, a potential disadvantage is that there is no graft-versus-leukemia effect, which appears to be an important component contributing to the curative potential of allogeneic transplantation. In the aggregate experience, the OS rate is approximately 45 to 55 percent. The treatment-related mortality rates associated with autologous transplantation in most recent studies are very low or zero.[172,236,239,240] A number of trials have tested the benefits of purging to eradicate the leukemic cells, but no prospective comparative trial has been conducted.[226,237] The major limitation of autologous stem cell transplantation is leukemic relapse attributable to residual disease, contamination of the reinfused cells, and the absence of a putative graft-versus-leukemia effect. Whether autologous stem cell transplantation provides an advantage compared to intensive consolidation chemotherapy has not been definitively established.

Comparative Benefit of Intensive Postremission Chemotherapy, Allogeneic Bone Marrow Transplantation, and Autologous Bone Marrow Transplantation for AML in First Remission

Several studies have compared the benefits of intensive consolidation with HiDAC, autologous bone marrow (or stem cell) transplantation, and allogeneic bone marrow transplantation. Autologous stem cell transplantation permits escalation of chemotherapy doses but is limited by the lack of putative graft-versus-leukemia effect associated with allogeneic transplantation. Furthermore, there is a theoretical risk of infusion of occult residual leukemic cells. Allogeneic transplantation provides the best antileukemic potential but is consistently

Table 7–10. AUTOLOGOUS BONE MARROW (STEM CELL) TRANSPLANTATION FOR AML IN FIRST CR					
Author	No. Pts	TRM (%)	RR (%)	DFS (%)	OS (%)
Gorin,[227] 1986	60	NA	NA	67, 2 yr	45, 2 yr
Löwenberg,[242] 1990	32	9	53	35, 3 yr	33, 3 yr
Gorin,[228] 1991	671*	NA	41	48, 7 yr	NA
Gulati,[229] 1992	15	0	27	72, 4 yr	NA
Cassileth,[230] 1993	39	6	33	54, 3 yr	NA
Linker,[231] 1993	58	3	22	76, 3 yr	NA
Sanz,[232] 1993	24	13	60	35, 2.5 yr	~53, 2.5 yr
Sierra,[233] 1993	24	4	48	48, 3 yr	NA
Laporte,[234] 1994	64	18	25	58, 8 yr	NA
Cahn,[235] 1995	111	28	52	34, 4 yr	35, 4 yr
Cahn,[235] 1995	786	14	50	43, 4 yr	48, 4 yr
Miggiano,[236] 1996	51	0	24	71, 5 yr	77, 5 yr
Stein,[237] 1996	60	8	44	49, 2 yr	NA
Schiller,[238] 1997	59	33	54	42, 3 yr	47, 3 yr
Gondo,[239] 1997	42	0	21	79, 3 yr	NA
Martin,[240] 1998	35	0	47	52, 4 yr	52, 4 yr
Visani,[241] 1999	44	NA	52	~45, 4 yr	NA

*Six percent of patients received purged marrow; †all patients received purged marrow.
NA = not applicable.

associated with a higher risk of treatment-related mortality than the other two strategies. All of these studies have been assigned younger patients with an HLA-matched donor to allogeneic transplantation and randomize other patients to either consolidation chemotherapy or autologous transplantation or between the latter two strategies (Table 7–11).[193,243–245] The earliest study carried out as a collaboration between the EORTC and GIMEMA assigned 168 patients in first CR to allogeneic transplantation and randomized 126 patients to a second cycle of consolidation with cytarabine 2 g/m² every 12 hours days 1 to 4 plus daunorubicin 45 mg/m² days 5 to 7 and 128 patients to autologous transplantation with cyclophosphamide/total body irradiation as the preparative regimen.[243] Only 74 percent of patients randomized to autologous transplantation actually completed the treatment because of early relapse and toxicity. Nevertheless, the DFS at 4 years, by an intent-to-treat analysis, was approximately 50 percent. This outcome is not different than that achieved among patients undergoing allogeneic transplantation who had a DFS of 55 percent at 4 years. These results were significantly better than that observed among patients receiving consolidation (30%). However, the OS at 4 years for all three treatment groups was similar (59% allogeneic, 56% autologous, 46% consolidation). Whereas relapse was more frequent among patients randomized to autologous transplantation, treatment-related mortality was higher among those assigned allogeneic transplantation. Despite a similar trial design, different observations were made in the ECOG/SWOG/CALGB Intergroup trial.[244] The DFS associated with allogeneic transplantation was not significantly

longer (43% at 4 years) than that associated with autologous transplantation (34%) or consolidation with HiDAC (34%). However, OS following HiDAC was longer than that after autologous or allogeneic transplantation. This finding likely relates to the opportunity to undergo transplantation at relapse following consolidation (Figure 7–14). In the study by the GOELAM, there was no difference in the 4-year DFS or OS between patients randomized to autologous transplantation and those randomized to consolidation.[245] The trial conducted by the MRC was unique because it demonstrated that autologous transplantation following three cycles of consolidation (two similar to induction and one including cytarabine 1 g/m² every 12 hours for 3 days) reduced the risk of relapse, and a statistical effect was seen on OS (Figure 7–15).[193] There has never been a randomized study of allogeneic transplantation among patients with an HLA-compatible sibling.

Several limitations of these studies are present. First, a substantial proportion of patients randomized to autologous transplantation fail to complete the assigned treatment. Second, although allogeneic transplantation offers the potential for graft-versus-leukemia effect and is associated with the lowest risk of relapse, higher treatment-related mortality, compared to autologous transplantation and consolida-

Table 7–11. PROSPECTIVE RANDOMIZED TRIALS OF CONSOLIDATION CHEMOTHERAPY VERSUS BMT IN AML			
	DFS/OS—4 Year (%)		
Author	Consolidation	Autologous BMT	Assigned Allogeneic BMT
Zittoun,[243] 1995	30/46	48/56	55/59
Cassileth,[244] 1998	34/52	34/43	43/46
Harousseau,[245] 1997	43/59	48/52	49/55
Burnett,[193] 1998	40/57*	54/45	—

*7 years.

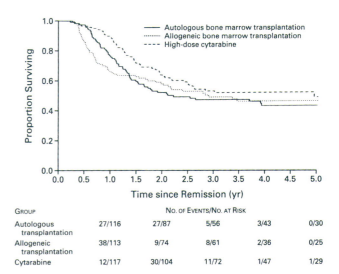

Group	No. of Events/No. at Risk				
Autologous transplantation	27/116	27/87	5/56	3/43	0/30
Allogeneic transplantation	38/113	9/74	8/61	2/36	0/25
Cytarabine	12/117	30/104	11/72	1/47	1/29

Figure 7–14. Overall survival of patients with AML according to type of postremission therapy, HLA-matched allogeneic bone marrow transplantation, autologous stem cell transplantation, or high-dose cytarabine consolidation chemotherapy. (From Cassileth PA, Harrington DP, Appelbaum FR, et al. Chemotherapy compared with autologous or allogeneic bone marrow transplantation in the management of acute myeloid leukemia in first remission. N Engl J Med 1998;339:1649–56.)

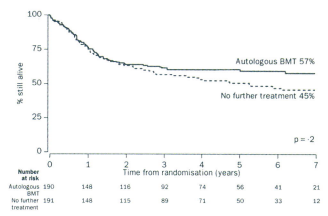

Figure 7–15. Overall survival for patients with AML randomized to either autologous stem cell transplantation or no further therapy, following three cycles of consolidation after successful induction. (From Burnett AK, Goldstone AH, Stevens RM, et al. Randomized comparison of addition of autologous bone marrow transplantation to intensive chemotherapy for acute myeloid leukaemia in first remission: results of MRC AML 10 Trial. Lancet 1998;351:700–8.)

tion chemotherapy, diminishes the impact of the greater antileukemic potential and, therefore, a benefit in OS is not observed. Third, it is likely that the mortality rate associated with both autologous and allogeneic transplantation will likely continue to decrease as the techniques of transplantation improve, such as the introduction of autologous peripheral blood stem cell transplantation and improvements in T-cell depletion techniques for allogeneic transplantation.[203,211–213] In addition, placental cord blood transplantation from both related and unrelated donors offers the immediate availability of stem cells for reconstitution, lowers the risk of infectious disease transmission, and offers the potential of a lower incidence of GVHD.[246–249] Transplantation with nonmyeloablative purine analog containing preparative regimens appears to permit satisfactory engraftment with potentially less toxicity and may expand the population of patients who can benefit.[214–216] New treatments for GVHD such as thalidomide may further decrease morbidity and mortality.[250] The use of peripheral blood allogeneic stem cells for allogeneic transplantation will require further study to determine if blood-derived stem cells are the preferred source for hematopoietic reconstitution.[251–254] Furthermore, recent studies suggest that the outcome for allogeneic transplantation in patients older than age 40 may not be less favorable than in younger patients.[255] There are also constantly chang-

ing improvements in all three postremission strategies including consolidation chemotherapy, which all make frequent re-evaluation of the benefits and hazards of each approach important.[133,256]

Treatment for Acute Promyelocytic Luekemia

Acute promyelocytic leukemia (APL) deserves separate consideration because it is treated differently from all other subtypes of AML and has become the most curable. Since the first report in 1988,[257] a number of phase II trials have confirmed the effectiveness of the vitamin A derivative ATRA as differentiation therapy in patients with APL.[258–269] Two prospective randomized trials have compared ATRA, with or without chemotherapy, to chemotherapy alone for induction (Table 7–12).[268,269] Following CR, patients in both trials received two cycles of consolidation (7 + 3 then intermediate-dose cytarabine + daunorubicin in the APL91 trial and 7 + 3 then HiDAC + daunorubicin in the North American Intergroup trial). In the latter trial, patients in CR after two cycles of consolidation were randomized to either 1 year of daily maintenance ATRA or observation. In both trials, the CR rates on both arms were not statistically different. However, event-free survival, DFS, and OS were markedly improved with ATRA such that approximately 70 percent of patients remain disease free at 4 years. This benefit was attributable to a decrease in the relapse rate with ATRA. In the North American Intergroup trial, patients induced with standard induction chemotherapy and maintained with ATRA had an outcome identical to those patients who received ATRA during induction. Patients who were assigned to receive ATRA for both induction and consolidation had the most favorable outcome (Figure 7–16). The most serious and life-threatening complication of differentiation therapy with ATRA is the retinoic acid syndrome, a cardiorespiratory distress syndrome manifested by interstitial pulmonary infiltrates, pleural or pericardial effusions, hypoxemia, and episodic hypotension with otherwise unexplained weight gain.[270,271] The syndrome has been associated with rapid development of hyperleukocytosis in many but not all patients, which can be observed with ATRA induction.[268,269] However, the syndrome may

Table 7–12. PROSPECTIVE TRIALS OF ATRA IN APL					
Trial	No. Pts	Induction	% CR	% ED	% DFS/EFS
Randomized					
APL91 (Europe)[268]	54	ATRA (+ chemo)	97	9	79
	47	Chemo	81	8	50
APL93 (Europe)[273]	109	ATRA → chemo	95	8	75
	99	ATRA + chemo	94	7	86
North American Intergroup[271]	172	ATRA	72	11	67
	174	Chemo	69	14	32
UK MRC (England)[274]	119	ATRA (5d) → chemo	70	23	59
	120	ATRA + chemo	87	12	78
Nonrandomized					
GIMEMA (Italy)[265]	535	ATRA + chemo	93	7	78/65
JALSG (Japan)[267]	196	ATRA ± chemo	88	9	62/54
PETHEMA (Spain)[266]	100	ATRA + chemo	87	11	Too early

develop in patients with relatively low white blood cell counts (WBCs).[271,272] The syndrome typically resolves quickly with early administration of corticosteriods (dexamethasone 10 mg bid for at least 3 days) at the earliest sign or symptom. The pathophysiology of the syndrome involves interstitial infiltration of the lung parenchyma with maturing myeloid cells rather than leukostasis with vascular obstruction (Figure 7–17). The APL93 trial provides compelling evidence that administering concurrent ATRA plus chemotherapy reduces the relapse rate compared with sequential ATRA for induction followed by chemotherapy.[273] This was observed even among patients presenting with a relatively low WBC. Therefore, the standard induction strategy for APL now includes ATRA plus chemotherapy for all patients. The MRC randomized patients to either a short course of ATRA (5 days) in an effort to reduce the coagulopathy but avoid the retinoic acid syndrome with chemotherapy or concomitant ATRA plus chemotherapy until CR and found that the latter strategy was associated with an improved outcome.[274] Although the best chemotherapy regimen to include in induction is not established, recent studies indicate that anthracycline alone during induction is sufficient.[265,266] The best consolidation regimen has not been established; however, it appears that all patients should receive at least two cycles of consolidation with either anthracycline + cytarabine as in the APL91 trial, anthracycline + cytarabine followed by HiDAC as in the North American Intergroup Trial, or intermediate-dose cytarabine + idarubicin and then

mitoxantrone + etoposide + cytarabine + 6-TG as in the GIMEMA trial. The precise role of maintenance therapy with ATRA continues to evolve. The North American Intergroup Trial and the APL93 trial both suggest a beneficial role. Lo Coco and colleagues have suggested a benefit to treating patients with chemotherapy in molecular relapse (defined as the

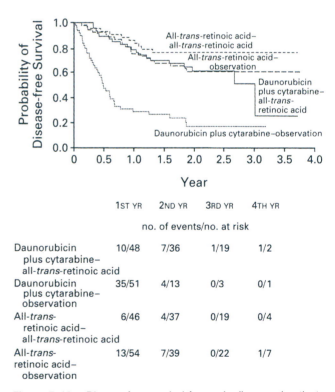

Figure 7–16. Disease-free survival for newly diagnosed patients with APL assigned to either chemotherapy or ATRA for induction and either ATRA maintenance or observation on North American Intergroup Protocol 0129. (From Tallman MS, Andersen JW, Schiffer CA, et al. All-trans retinoic acid in acute promyelocytic leukemia. N Engl J Med 1997;337:1021–8.)

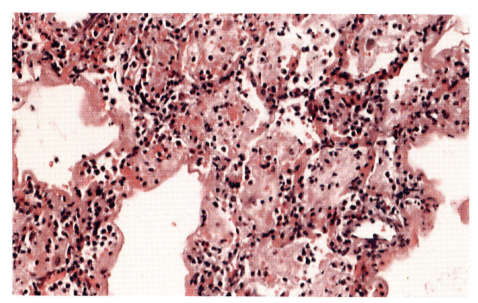

Figure 7–17. Photomicrograph of lung parenchyma from a patient with the retinoic acid syndrome showing infiltration of the parenchyma with mature myeloid cells. (Reprinted with permission from Tallman MS, Andersen JW, Schiffer CA, et al. Clinical description of 44 patients with acute promyelocytic leukemia who developed the retinoic acid syndrome. Blood 2000;95:90–5. ©American Society of Hematology.)

reappearance of reverse transcriptase-polymerase chain reaction positivity for the *PML-RARα* fusion transcript on two successive marrow samples obtained during postconsolidation serial monitoring) rather than at the time of hematologic relapse (Figure 7–18).[275] Patients who relapse after ATRA-containing induction followed by intensive consolidation can be reinduced with ATRA followed by intensive consolidation and then autologous stem cell transplantation.[276] Such a strategy results in a 3-year DFS rate of 77 percent (Figure 7–19).

A new approach for patients who relapse after ATRA or those who demonstrate resistance to ATRA

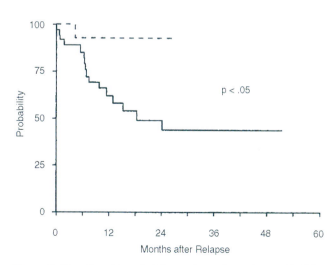

Figure 7–18. Overall survival from relapse for patients with APL treated at the time of molecular relapse compared to the time of hematologic relapse (historic control population). (Reprinted with permission from Lo Coco F, Diverio D, Avvisati G, et al. Therapy of molecular relapse in acute promyelocytic leukemia. Blood 1999;94:2225–9. ©American Society of Hematology.)

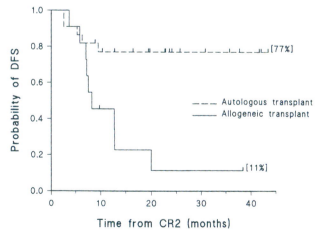

Figure 7–19. Kaplan-Meier plots of DFS following autologous and allogeneic stem cell transplant for patients with acute promyelocytic leukemia in second CR following induction with ATRA followed by intensive consolidation chemotherapy. (From Thomas X, Dombret H, Cordonnier C, et al. Treatment of relapsing acute promyelocytic leukemia by all-*trans* retinoic acid therapy followed by timed sequential chemotherapy and stem cell transplantation. APL Study Group. Acute promyelocytic leukemia. Leukemia 2000;14:1006–13.)

Table 7–13. PHASE II TRIALS OF ARSENIC TRIOXIDE IN APL		
Trial	N	CR (%)
Previously treated	42	52
Harbin[277]	47	85
Shanghai[280]	12	92
U.S. multicenter[281]	40	85
Previously untreated	30	73
Harbin[277]	11	73

is arsenic trioxide, which has recently been shown to be very effective in this setting (Table 7–13).[277–281] In a multicenter phase II trial conducted in the United States, 85 percent of patients achieved CR.[281] Furthermore, 75 percent of patients had no evidence of residual disease by molecular studies after two cycles (25 days each) of treatment. The mechanisms of action appear to be down-regulation of *Bcl-2* expression at the mRNA and protein levels with degradation of *PML-RARα* fusion protein and activation of caspaces[282–285] treatment of older adults.

Suggested Strategies for Primary Therapy of AML for Patients Not Participating in a Clinical Trial

For patients ≤ 55 years of age, standard induction includes either daunorubicin or idarubicin and cytarabine. Hematopoietic growth factors may be administered safely following induction. If an HLA-compatible sibling is available, allogeneic BMT, either immediately after induction or after a single cycle of intensive postremission therapy, which may include cytarabine either 3 g/m² every 12 hours for 6 days or 3 g/m² twice daily on days 1, 3, and 5, can be considered. If no HLA-compatible sibling is available, postremission therapy is given with one cycle of cytarabine as above with an autologous stem cell transplant using peripheral blood-derived stem cells or four cycles of cytarabine if an autologous stem cell transplant is not to be carried out.

For patients > 55 to 65 years of age, induction with either daunorubicin, idarubicin, or mitoxantrone and cytarabine is given followed by consolidation with cytarabine 1.5 g/m² every 12 hours for 6 days for one to two cycles. Autologous stem cell transplantation may be considered if concurrent medical problems do not preclude such an approach. For patients older than 69, the dose of postremission cytarabine may be reduced to 1.5 g/m² for six doses.

Specific karyotype abnormalities may influence therapeutic decisions. For example, patients with favorable karyotypes may fare particularly well with a standard induction regimen of daunorubicin plus standard-dose cytarabine followed by intensive consolidation (Figure 7–20).[256,286,287] or transplant.[210,217,288] The outcome of patients with unfavorable karyotypes is poor with intensive cytarabine consolidation. The use of high-dose cytarabine with daunorubicin in induction does not appear to increase the CR rate among patients with unfavorable karyotype abnormalities such as monosomy 7, inv(3), or t(6;9).[289] Therefore, allogeneic transplan-

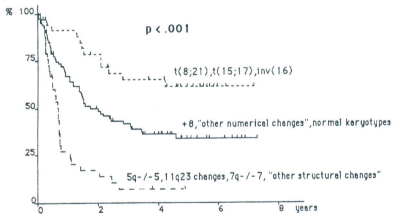

Figure 7–20. Probabilities of continuous CR of previously untreated patients with AML according to chromosomal groups. (From Dastague N, Payen C, Lafage-Pochitaloff M, et al. Prognostic significance of karyotype in de novo adult acute myeloid leukemia. The BGMT group. Leukemia 1995;9:1491–8.)

tation should be strongly considered. However, it is difficult to be definitive about such strategies since controversies exist.

Treatment of Patients with Persistent Disease After a First Course of Induction

The best treatment for patients with persistent disease following an anthracycline-cytarabine–based induction regimen has not been determined. There are data that suggest that the administration of high-dose cytarabine leads to a higher CR rate compared with a second cycle of induction chemotherapy with standard-dose cytarabine.[290] Nevertheless, the DFS at 5 years may be less if a second cycle of chemotherapy is required to achieve CR. Among patients who do attain a CR with a second induction regimen, allogeneic transplantation is the most important factor predictive of long-term EFS and OS.[291]

Treatment of Patients with Relapsed or Refractory AML

The outcome for patients with relapsed AML is dependent on the duration of first remission, and the only patients with any chance for long-term survival[292,293] appear to be those whose first CR duration was greater than 6 months (Figure 7–21).[292] The second CR rate varies from 22 to 68 percent, depending on the duration of first CR and initial cytogenetic finding.[294–301] A variety of reinduction regimens have been evaluated including amsacrine plus etoposide,[294] high-dose cytarabine-containing programs,[296–300] regimens testing modulation of multidrug resistance,[302–306] and novel agents such as topotecan[307,308] and biologic approaches such as interleukin-2.[309–311] Finally, several studies have shown that either allogeneic or autologous stem cell transplantation for patients in either first relapse, second remission, or with refractory disease may result in a cure for some patients.[312–317] Matched unrelated donor transplantation is still associated with a high transplant-related mortality rate but also may provide long-term survival for some patients.[318–322] Mylotarg® is an immunoconjugate that includes an anti-CD33 antibody linked to the potent cytotoxic agent calicheamicin (Figure 7–22).[323,324] This agent induces remission in 30 percent of patients in first

relapse with a first CR duration of at least 6 months.[324] Such remissions may permit further intensive treatment, such as stem cell transplantation.

CHRONIC LYMPHOCYTIC LEUKEMIA

The treatment of patients with chronic lymphocytic leukemia (CLL) has evolved rapidly during the last decade. A variety of new therapeutic strategies including purine nucleoside analogs, monoclonal antibodies, and stem cell transplantation are now available. However, whether they will replace traditional alkylating agent-based chemotherapy has not been determined.

Patients with early-stage disease and some patients with an indolent or smoldering form of CLL have an overall survival rate that approaches that of the normal population of the same age.[325,326] Therefore, many patients with CLL often require no therapy at the time of diagnosis and can be observed. Most investigators agree on the need to treat patients with advanced-stage CLL (Rai stages 3–4, Binet stages B and C) and to observe patients with earlier stages of disease for progression or appearance of disease-related symptoms requiring treatment since the clinical course may be variable.[327] Factors that predict for less favorable prognosis include clinical stage, older age, short lymphocyte doubling time, diffuse pattern of involvement in the bone marrow, and cytogenetic abnormalities.[325,328–332] Recently, a cohort of patients with 11q deletions have been

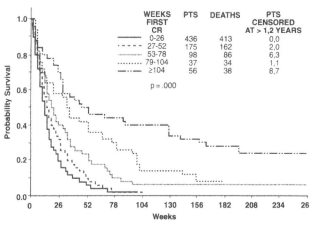

Figure 7–21. Probability of survival for patients with relapsed or primary refractory AML treated between 1980 and 1995. (From Estey E. Treatment of refractory AML. Leukemia 1996;10:932–6.)

- **hP67.6 - humanized anti-CD33 antibody**
- **Blue - linker**
- **Red - calicheamicin**

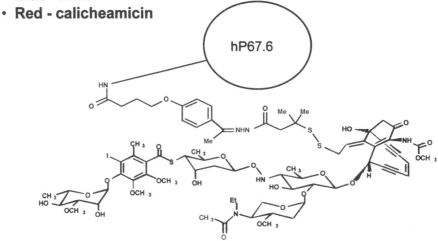

Figure 7–22. Structure of Mylotarg®, an anti-CD33-calicheamicin immunoconjugate.

identified and such patients have extensive nodal involvement and a poor prognosis (Figure 7–23).[333–335] Randomized trials have confirmed that treatment of patients with early-stage disease with alkylating agents does not improve survival and, in fact, may have a deleterious effect on outcome.[335–337] Criteria for initiation of therapy generally include

(1) worsening constitutional symptoms attributable to the disease; (2) progressive or symptomatic lymphadenopathy or hepatosplenomegaly, hypersplenism, or organ dysfunction; (3) a short doubling time of the peripheral blood lymphocyte count; (4) recurrent infections; and (5) immune-mediated complications such as warm-antibody–mediated autoimmune hemolytic anemia or autoimmune thrombocytopenia (Table 7–14).[338,339]

The response criteria for patients with CLL have been recently revised (see Table 7–14).[339] A complete remission (CR) requires absence of all evidence of disease for at least 2 months, including all adenopathy and hepatosplenomegaly determined by examination and radiographic techniques, absence of constitutional symptoms, a normal complete blood count, and a bone marrow aspirate and biopsy of the lymphocytes representing the nucleated cells without lymphoid nodules. A partial remission (PR) classification has been established to identify therapeutic agents with biologic effects.

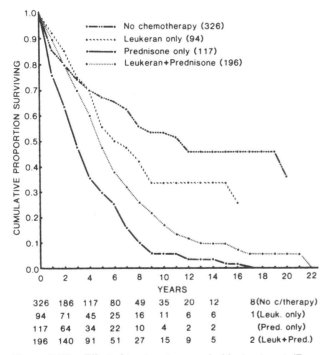

Figure 7–23. Effect of treatment on survival by treatment. (From Skinnider LF, Tan L, Schmidt J, Armitage G. Chronic lymphocytic leukemia. A review of 745 cases and assessment of clinical staging. Cancer 1982;50:2951–5.)

Conventional Treatment

Historically, the most common initial treatment regimen in CLL has been chlorambucil alone or a combination of chlorambucil and prednisone, which produces response rates of 38 to 75 percent.[340–343] This variability appears to be due to differences in the precise response criteria used and in the drug doses administered. Corticosteriods are routinely used in combination with alkylating agents since these drugs are themselves lymphocytolytic. In addition, corticosteroids may also be used alone to treat autoimmune hemolytic anemia or autoimmune thrombocytopenia associated with CLL. For example, prednisone may be given if the only indication for treatment is either autoimmune hemolytic anemia or autoimmune thrombocytopenia. Alternatively, if the underlying disease requires treatment, it is routine to administer chlorambucil either on a daily basis with a relatively low dose of, for example, 0.07 mg/kg/d or on an intermittent basis with a larger dose of 0.7 mg/kg every 3 to 4 weeks or 30 mg/kg every 2 weeks. However, it is not clear that one schedule, either continuous or intermittent administration, is superior.[343] The dose-limiting toxicity of all schedules of alkylating agents is myelosuppression. There is no improvement in survival

with the addition of prednisone to chlorambucil.[18] Cyclophosphamide is an alternative alkylating agent that can also be administered on a daily basis at 50 to 150 mg/d orally or intermittently 1,000 to 2,000 mg every 2 to 4 weeks orally. It has been suggested that cyclophosphamide may have a less suppressive effect on the platelet count. Therefore, in patients with thrombocytopenia attributable to bone marrow infiltration rather than immune mediated, this may be the preferred alkylating agent. The combination of cyclophosphamide, vincristine, and prednisone (CVP) has also been associated with response rates between 33 and 72 percent.[342–344] As with other single alkylating agent administration such as chlorambucil, different cyclophosphamide doses and schedules, patient characteristics, and less strict response criteria may contribute to the wide variation in response rates reported. Importantly, randomized trials have shown

Table 7–14. COMPARISON OF NATIONAL CANCER INSTITUTE WORKING GROUP AND IWCLL GUIDELINES FOR CLL

Variable	NCI	IWCLL
Diagnosis		
Lymphocytes ($\times 10^9$/L)	> 5; ≥ 1 B-cell marker (CD19, CD20, CD23) + CD5	≥ 10 + B-phenotype or bone marrow involved < 10 + both of above
Atypical cells (%) (eg, prolymphocytes)	< 55	Not stated
Duration of lymphocytes	None required	Not stated
Bone marrow lymphocytes (%)	≥ 30	> 30
Staging	Modified Rai, correlate with Binet active disease (details in document)	IWCLL
Eligibility for trials		A: lymphs > 50 x 10^9/L doubling time < 12 mo diffuse marrow B, C: all patients
Response criteria		
Complete remission		
Physical examination	Normal	Normal
Symptoms	None	None
Lymphocytes ($\times 10^9$/L)	≤ 4	< 4
Neutrophils ($\times 10^9$/L)	≥ 1.5	> 1.5
Platelets ($\times 10^9$/L)	> 100	> 100
Hemoglobin (g/dL)	> 11 (untransfused)	Not stated
Bone marrow lymphocytes (%)	< 30; no nodules	Normal, allowing nodules or focal infiltrates
Partial remission		
Physical examination (nodes and/or liver, spleen) plus ≥ 1 of	≥ 50% decrease	Downshift in stage
neutrophils ($\times 10^9$/L),	≥ 1.5	
platelets ($\times 10^9$/L),	> 100	
hemoglobin (g/dL)	> 11 or 50% improvement	
Duration of complete or partial remission	≥ 2 mo	Not stated
Progressive disease		Upshift in stage
Physical examination (nodes, liver, spleen)	≥ 50% increase or new	
Circulating lymphocytes	≥ 50% increase	
Other	Richter's syndrome	
Stable disease	All others	No change

From Cheson BD, Bennett JM, Grever MR, et al. National Cancer Institute-sponsored working group guidelines for chronic lymphocytic leukemia: revised guidelines for diagnosis and treatment. Blood 1996;87:4990–7.

that the outcome with CVP is not improved compared with that with chlorambucil and prednisone.[344–346]

Attempts to intensify chemotherapy approaches have been made by adding a variety of antileukemic agents to alkylating agent plus corticosteroid-based regimens. Several studies have tested the potential benefits of adding doxorubicin (Adriamycin). Higher response rates but no improvement in overall survival have been observed among patients treated with an Adriamycin-based regimen such as cyclophosphamide, Adriamycin, vincristine, and prednisone (CHOP) compared with chlorambucil plus prednisone.[347–350] Other combination regimens in CLL include the M2 program (vincristine, prednisone, cyclophosphamide, melphalan, and carmustine)[351] and doxorubicin, vincristine, and cytosine arabinoside (POACH).[352] These regimens have yielded slightly higher CR rates but are more toxic and not clearly superior to chlorambucil plus prednisone. Therefore, the most common initial treatment for patients with CLL continues to be an alkylating agent, most often chlorambucil, with or without prednisone. However, the clinical development of new agents such as the purine analogs, with novel mechanisms of action, has renewed interest in changing this approach.

New Drugs

Purine Analogs

Fludarabine. Fludarabine (9-β-D arabinofuranosyl 2-fluoroadenine monophosphate) is a fluorinated purine analog with remarkable activity in CLL (Table 7–15).[353–362] This agent is resistant to the action of adenosine deaminase.[363,364] The phosphorylated form of the drug accumulates intracellularity and inhibits deoxyribonucleic acid (DNA), ribonucleic acid (RNA), and protein synthesis.[365–368] Among other enzymes, the triphosphate drug 2-fluoroadenosine arabinoside triphosphate inhibits DNA polymerase and ribonucleotide reductase and competes with

			Response		
Reference	**No. Patients**	**Prior Therapy**	**Complete %**	**Partial %**	**None %**
Fludarabine					
Grever	21	21	1 (15) 4	3 (14)	17 (81)
Keating	78	78	26 (74) 33	15 (19)	33 (42)
Keating	35	0	4 (20) 11	2 (6)	7 (20)
Hiddemann	20	20	0	7 (35)	9 (45)
Puccio	42	42	0	22 (52)	20 (48)
Bergmann	18	18	1 (6)	12 (67)	6 (33)
Spriano	27	23	1 (25) 4	9 (39)	13 (57)
Spriano	4	0		3 (75)	0
Sorenson	703	703	21 (3)	205 (29)	476 (68)
2-Chlorodeoxyadenosine					
Saven	90	90	4 (4)	40 (44)	54 (60)
Juliusson	18	18	7 (39)	5 (28)	6 (33)
Betticher	11	11	3 (27)	5 (45)	6 (33)
Tallman	26	26	0	8 (31)	18 (69)
Tallman					
Saven	20	0	5 (25)	12 (60)	3 (15)
Juliusson	17	0	4 (41) 23	5 (29)	5 (29)
Delannoy	19	0	9 (47)	5 (26)	5 (26)
Robak	33	0	12 (36)	13 (39)	8 (24)
Robak	10	10	1 (10)	4 (40)	5 (50)
Deoxycoformycin					
Grever	20	27	1 (4)	4 (14)	23 (92)
Dillman	26	26	1 (4)	3 (12)	22 (85)
Dillman	26	26	0	7 (27)	19 (73)
Ho	13	0	0	6 (46)	7 (54)
Deardon	17	17	0	6 (25) 35	11 (65)

Adapted from Tallman MS, Hakimian D. The purine nucleoside analogs: emerging roles in indolent lymphoproliferative disorders. Blood 1995;86:2463–74.

deoxyadenosine triphosphate (dATP) required by DNA polymerase.[364,369-371]

In the first large study of fludarabine in patients with advanced CLL, fludarabine was administered intravenously at a dose of 25 to 30 mg/m² for 5 days every 3 to 4 weeks to previously treated patients.[357] Complete response was seen in 13 percent of patients and PR in 28 percent. The term nodular partial remission has been used to describe the bone marrow in patients whose only evidence of disease was persistence of lymphoid nodules.[348] In this trial, nodular PR was observed in 16 percent of patients. The response to fludarabine and survival both correlate with the stage of disease, extent of prior therapy, and the degree of sensitivity to prior alkylating agent exposure (Figure 7–24).[358,362]

Fludarabine has been used alone or in combination with prednisone in both treated and untreated patients, producing high response rates compared with the experience with conventional regimens.[357] Lower response rates were observed in patients with advanced CLL, older patients, and patients who had previously undergone therapy. The addition of oral prednisone, 30 mg/m² for 5 days, to fludarabine did not improve results and was associated with increased morbidity due to the occasional occurrence of unusual, often opportunistic infections, such as *Pneumocystis carinii* pneumonia or listeriosis.[372]

O'Brien and colleagues have explored maintenance therapy with interferon after remission induction with fludarabine and observed no benefit.[373]

Fludarabine has been prospectively compared with chlorambucil in a large randomized intergroup trial.[374] Although the CR rate was higher with fludarabine, no improvement in overall survival was present. Fludarabine has also been compared with cyclophosphamide, Adriamycin, and prednisone in a prospective randomized trial.[375] A higher response rate was observed for fludarabine in both treated and untreated patients, although the difference was statistically significant only in the untreated patients. Among untreated patients, remission duration and survival did not differ between the two treatment groups. However, among untreated patients, fludarabine was associated with significantly longer remissions with a trend toward longer survival (Figure 7–25). Finally, the French Cooperative Group has reported preliminary results of a randomized comparison of fludarabine; cyclophosphamide, Adriamycin (50 mg/m² day 1), and prednisone (CAP); and cyclophosphamide, vincristine, Adriamycin (25 mg/m² day 1), and prednisone (CHOP).[376] Lower response rates and increased risk of death among the patients randomized to CAP have resulted in early closure of that arm. In a follow-up report, there was no difference in overall survival between the three

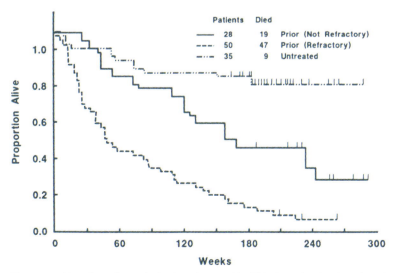

Figure 7–24. Overall survival of patients with CLL by prior treatment and response status. (Reprinted with permission from Keating MJ, O'Brien S, Kantarjian H, et al. Long-term follow-up of patients with chronic lymphocytic leukemia treated with fludarabine as a single agent. Blood 1993;81:2878–84. ©American Society of Hematology.)

treatments, despite the fact that the rate of hematologic remission was higher among the patients randomized to fludarabine (41 versus 30% for CHOP; p = .006; 15% with CAP; p = .0001).[377]

Several investigators have attempted to combine fludarabine with alkylating agents given the potential for synergy.[378–385] In one trial, which included a small number of patients, Weiss and colleagues identified a dose of fludarabine of 15 mg/m^2/d for 5 days as the maximal tolerated dose when given with chlorambucil 20 mg/m^2.[380] The Southwest Oncology Group (SWOG) also conducted a phase I trial of the same combination and concluded that these agents could be safely combined at the following doses: chlorambucil 15 mg/m^2 on day 1 and fludarabine 20 mg/m^2/d for 5 days.[381] The dose-limiting toxicity was thrombocytopenia. Fludarabine has been combined with cyclophosphamide and appears very promising.[383–385] Investigators at Johns Hopkins University treated 21 patients with previously untreated CLL at a dose of cyclophosphamide 600 mg/m^2 day 1 and fludarabine 20 mg/m^2 days 1 to 5.[383] Ten patients achieved CR and 10 PR. Three patients developed either acute immune hemolytic anemia or thrombocytopenia. The German CLL Study Group treated patients with advanced CLL (Binet stages B and C) with fludarabine 30 mg/m^2/d IV and cyclophosphamide 250 mg/m^2/d IV days 1 to 3 every 28 days for 6 cycles.[385] Among 25 evaluable patients, 3 CRs and 19 PRs were observed, for an overall response rate of 88 percent. No patients experienced a grade 3 or 4 infection. Hemolytic anemia following fludarabine in patients with CLL is uncommon but well recognized, and may be severe and fatal. Weiss and colleagues have reported a mortality rate of 29 percent attributable to complications of hemolytic anemia associated with fludarabine.[386]

2-Chlorodeoxyadenosine. 2-Chlorodeoxyadenosine (2-CdA), like fludarabine, does not inhibit adenosine deaminase (ADA) but is resistant to the enzyme. This agent is phosphorylated by deoxycytidine kinase, resulting in the intracellular accumulation of 2-CdA triphosphate, which inhibits ribonucleotide reductase.[387] An initial phase I trial established the safety of this drug in lymphoproliferative disorders.[388] Following an initial pilot trial of 18

patients with advanced CLL that showed favorable results,[389] investigators at Scripps Clinic conducted a larger trial in which 2-CdA was given to 90 patients with relapsed and refractory CLL and resulted in CR and PR rates of 4 and 40 percent, respectively.[390] A number of subsequent studies have confirmed the activity of 2-CdA in previously treated patients.[391–396] In the aggregate experience, the CR rates are approximately 5 to 40 percent and PR rates are 20 to 45 percent. Significantly higher CR and PR rates have been seen in previously untreated patients.[396–401] Robak and colleagues recently reported a large series of 194 patients with previously untreated CLL.[400] The CR rate was 45.4 percent, and the overall response rate was 82.5 percent among patients with stage I and II disease. The CR rate was 54.5 percent compared with 34.1 percent

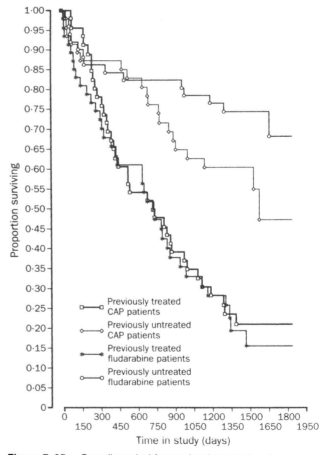

Figure 7–25. Overall survival for previously treated and untreated patients with either fludarabine or CAP (cyclophosphamide, Adriamycin, prednisone). (From The French Cooperative Group on CLL. Multicentre prospective randomized trial of fludarabine versus cyclophosphamide, doxorubicin and prednisone (CAP) for treatment of advanced stage chronic lymphocytic leukemia. Lancet 1996;347: 1432–8.)

for patients with stage II and III disease (p = .0002). The median survival from the beginning of treatment with 2-CdA was significantly shorter among previously treated patients (16.3 months) compared with previously untreated patients (19.4 months) (p < .0001) (Figures 7–26 and 7–27). Similar to fludarabine, 2-CdA has also been associated with autoimmune hemolytic anemia.[402] However, the most prominent toxicities have been myelosuppression, primarily thrombocytopenia, and infections. Patients previously treated with fludarabine who are no longer responsive have only a 20 percent response rate to 2-CdA.[403] Betticher and colleagues have suggested that a lower dose of 0.5 mg/kg per cycle as a subcutaneous injection may be associated with fewer infections with preservation of the antitumor activity in lymphomas.[404]

Pentostatin. Intravenous pentostatin (2'-deoxycoformycin) directly inhibits ADA and is a third purine analog studied in CLL.[405,406] However, the overall response rate of 26 percent has been modest, and this analog appears less effective than either fludarabine or 2-CdA as a single agent.[406–409] Lack of response to purine analogs has been correlated with p53 gene deletion.[410]

Monoclonal Antibodies. Two monoclonal antibodies, IDEC-C2B8 (anti-CD20)[411–413] and CAMPATH-1H (humanized anti-CD52),[414–418] have been recently tested in patients with CLL. Preliminary studies suggest modest response rates with Rituxan® (rituximab). However, among 29 patients with relapsed or refractory CLL treated with CAMPATH-1H, 11 patients (38%) achieved a PR and 1 (4%) achieved CR.[414] Chronic lymphocytic leukemia cells were rapidly eliminated from the blood in 28 of the 29 patients (97%), and CR in the bone marrow was achieved in 36 percent of patients. Keating and colleagues reported among 92 evaluable patients with refractory CLL that the overall response rate was 33 percent, with 2 percent CR, 31 percent partial response, and 59 percent stable disease.[418] Patients with bulky disease responded the least well. The projected time to progress for responders is at 9+ months. These preliminary data suggest that CAMPATH-1H may be most effective for peripheral circulating leukemic cells.

Biologic Agents

Interferon-α yields a low response rate in previously treated patients, but 50 percent of patients

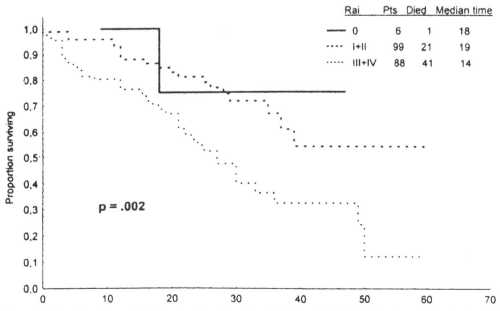

Figure 7–26. Overall survival of previously untreated patients treated with 2-chlorodeoxyadenosine by Rai stage. (From Robak T, Blonski JZ, Kasznicki M, et al. Cladribine with or without prednisone in the treatment of previously treated and untreated B-cell chronic lymphocytic leukemia—updated results of the multicentre study of 378 patients. Br J Haematol 2000;108:357–68.)

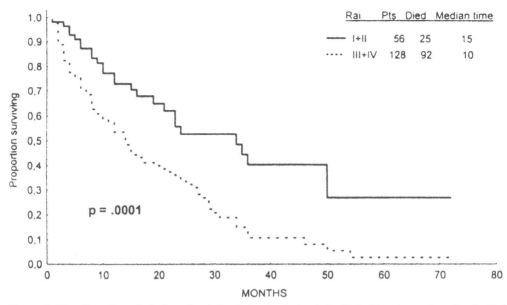

Figure 7–27. Overall survival of previously treated patients treated with 2-chlorodeoxyadenosine by Rai stage. (From Robak T, Blonski JZ, Kasznicki M, et al. Cladribine with or without prednisone in the treatment of previously treated and untreated B-cell chronic lymphocytic leukemia—updated results of the multicentre study of 378 patients. Br J Haematol 2000;108:357–68.)

with previously untreated stage A CLL show a greater than 50 percent reduction in their absolute lymphocyte counts.[419–422]

Other cytokines investigated in CLL have included interleukins (IL-2, IL-4) and tumor necrosis factor.[423] Hematopoietic growth factors such as granulocyte colony-stimulating factor (G-CSF) and granulocyte-macrophage colony-stimulating factor (GM-CSF) may ameliorate chemotherapy or disease-induced neutropenia.

Stem Cell Transplantation

It is only recently that high-dose chemotherapy has been applied to patients with CLL because the majority of patients are older adults. However, the techniques of transplantation such as improved supportive care, better graft-versus-host disease (GVHD) prophylaxis, the use of peripheral blood-derived hematopoietic stem cells for reconstitution, and post-transplant hematopoietic recovery have made this approach feasible in this population.[424–435]

Michallet and colleagues for the European Group for Blood and Marrow Transplantation and the International Bone Marrow Transplant Registry carried out a retrospective analysis of 54 patients (median age 41 years, range 21 to 58) undergoing human leukocyte antigen (HLA)-identical sibling bone marrow transplantation (BMT) between 1984 and 1992.[432] The majority of patients had advanced disease (3 patients had Rai stage 0 disease, 10 stage 1, 10 stage 2, 7 stage 3, and 22 stage 4). Thirty-eight patients (70%) achieved CR, and 24 (44%) remain alive at a median of 27 months (range 5 to 80 months) after transplantation with a 3-year probability of overall survival of 46 percent.

Stem cell transplantation for patients with CLL remains investigational (Table 7–16). In a review of 26 evaluable patients who underwent allogeneic BMT, 11 remain alive and disease free at 5 to 48 months, with a projected 4-year overall survival of 40 percent. In general, studies show engraftment in 90 percent of patients, acute GVHD in approximately 30 percent, and chronic GVHD in approximately 40 percent of patients. Three-year survival rates are approximately 45 percent. Autologous BMT in select patients with CLL is currently under investigation. Recent trials have shown that patients transplanted with marrow cells rendered negative for the *bcl-2* rearrangement at the molecular level (by polymerase chain reaction) have prolonged disease-free survival.[431] Prolonged persistence of minimal residual disease may be identical and may correlate with the tumor burden prior to transplantation.[433] Allogeneic transplantation can induce durable remission in patients with CLL who are refractory not only to alkylating agents but also to fludarabine.[434] A recent report of 23 patients with B-cell CLL undergoing allogeneic transplantation between 1988 and 1997 (14 with chemorefractory disease, 20 matched related, and 3 matched unrelated) demonstrated that the only favorable prognostic factor for failure-free survival and overall survival was the use of cyclophosphamidc/total body irradiation preparative regimen rather than a preparative regimen of cyclophosphamide/etoposide/total body irradiation (Figure 7–28).[429] The incidence of grade II to IV GVHD was 54 percent. Fourteen patients are alive and disease free at a median of 26 months (range 9 to 115 months), including 2 patients who received matched unrelated transplants. The obligatory immunosuppressive consequences of allogeneic transplantation combined with the underlying inherent immune suppression related to the disease have resulted in a high incidence of infectious complications.[436]

Other Novel Agents with Antileukemic Effects In Vitro

Theophylline

The methylxanthine derivative theophylline has been shown to induce apoptosis in CLL cells.[437–439] The mechanism of action is believed to be inhibition of intracellular cyclic adenosine monophosphate degradation. Furthermore, theophylline appears to synergize with alkylating agents in the induction of apoptosis.[440,442] Clinical trials are under way to determine if this agent is effective, particularly in early-stage disease.

Depsipeptide

Depsipeptide has marked, in vitro, rapid, selective cytotoxicity against human CLL cells.[441–443] Preliminary data suggest that this agent induces cell-cycle arrest at the G0 to G1 stage of the cell cycle, possibly by inhibition of the ras transduction pathway and down-regulation of c-myc messenger ribonucleic

Table 7–16. RESULTS OF BMT IN CHRONIC LYMPHOCYTIC LEUKEMIA

Reference	No. Patients	Conditioning Regimen	Median Age (Yr)	Types of Transplants	Status at Transplant	Toxic Deaths	No. Patients Alive in CR (Duration in Mo)
Rabinowe,[425] 1993	20	Cy/TBI	40	8 allo	7 MRD, 1 CR	1	7 (11–18+)
			45	12 auto	10 MRD, 2 CR	0	4 (13–31+)
Khouri,[426] 1994	22	Cy/TBI	42	10 allo	Relapse 4	1	9 (2–36+)[†]
			59	11 auto	(2–29+)		
				1 syn			
Bartlett-Pandite,[427] 1994	45	Cy/TBI	45	13 allo[‖]	45 chemotherapy	2	8 (1–52+)
				32 auto[#]		3	26
Michallet,[432] 1996	54	Cy/TBI	41	Allo[‖]	7 response	1	24 (5–80+)
					19 stable	30	
					21 progressive		
Sutton,[428] 1998	20	Cy/TBI	55	20 auto	20 chemosensitive[‡‡]	2	6 (median 36)
Schey,[435] 1999	10	Cy/TBI	51	10 auto	6 untreated	0	7 (22)
					4 previously treated[§§]		
Pavletic,[429] 2000	23[**]	Cy/TBI or Cy/VP16/TBI	46	46 allo	14 chemorefractory	9	14 (9–115)
Dreger,[430] 2000	37	Cy/TBI	49	37 auto	14 chemonaive	0	NA

Cy = cyclophosphamide; TBI = total body irradiation; MRD = minimal residual disease; CR = complete remission; allo = allogeneic; auto = autologous; syn = syngeneic.
*Seven patients had marrow treated with anti-CD19 monoclonal antibodies and immunomagnetic separation.
†Two patients in near-complete remission.
‡Marrow purged with multiple anti–B-cell monoclonal antibodies.
§Nineteen patients received one additional drug.
‖T-cell depletion with anti-CD6 monoclonal antibodies.
#Bone marrow purged with multiple anti–B-cell monoclonal antibodies.
**Includes three patients receiving matched unrelated donor transplants.
††MD status (< 10% marrow involvement, < 2 cm lymph nodes, and no organomegaly).
‡‡10 CR after chemotherapy, 5 PR and 5 NR.
§§Patients received fludarabine as cytoreductive treatment prior to transplant.

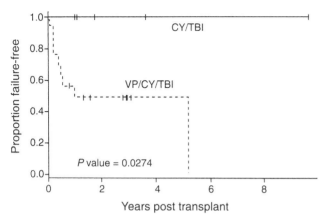

Figure 7–28. Failure-free survival of 6 B-cell patients after allogeneic stem cell transplantation with a preparative regimen of cyclophosphamide and total body irradiation (TBI) compared with 16 patients who received etoposide, cyclophosphamide, and TBI. (From Pavletic ZS, Arrowsmith ER, Bierman PJ, et al. Outcome of allogeneic stem cell transplantation for B-cell chronic lymphocytic leukemia. Bone Marrow Transplant 2000;25:717–22.)

acid.[441–444] In addition, this agent also decreases the *bcl-2:bax* ratio and p27 expression.[444]

Protein Kinase Inhibitors

Flavopiridol and 7-hydroxystaurosporine are protein kinase inhibitors. Flavopiridol is a semisynthetic molecule that is a flavone derivative of the alkaloid rohitukine.[445] 7-Hydroxystaurosporine (UCN-01) is a derivative of the protein kinase inhibitor staurosporine.[446] Both agents induce apoptosis of B-cell CLL cells possibly by down-regulating a variety of antiapoptotic proteins MCI-1, X-linked inhibitor of apoptosis (XIAP), and BAG-1 in all samples tested and Bcl-2 in approximately one half of samples.[447] Future clinical studies will determine if these agents are clinically useful.

Summary

Chronic lymphocytic leukemia remains a generally indolent and incurable disease. A number of new approaches have been developed, many of which have been tested clinically. New agents such as the purine analogs and monoclonal antibodies have excellent antileukemic efficacy and can induce both morphologic and molecular remissions. However, it is not clear that such advances translate into improved survival for patients and may have long-term conse-

quences. Therefore, alkylating agents, with or without prednisone, remain the initial treatment of choice for most patients not participating in a clinical trial. Evaluating new strategies earlier in the natural history of the disease may improve survival and justify a change in the conventional therapies.

CHRONIC MYELOGENOUS LEUKEMIA

Major progress has been made both in understanding the molecular pathogenesis of chronic myeloid leukemia (CML) and in the therapy. The t(9;22) translocation results in the formation of the Philadelphia (Ph) chromosome and a Bcr/Abl fusion protein, and this process provides a proliferative advantage for the leukemia cells. Historically, treatment has included drugs such as busulfan and hydroxyurea, which suppress leukocytosis and thrombocytosis and control splenomegaly. Whereas interferon-α can eradicate the Ph chromosome containing malignant cells, allogeneic stem cell transplantation has the potential to cure approximately 60 percent of all patients. Most recently, the oral tyrosine kinase inhibitor STI-571 has been shown to induce complete hematologic remission in every patient in the chronic phase with minimal toxicity but also to eradicate the leukemic cells in a significant proportion of patients in less than 6 months. These exciting advances have required a re-evaluation of therapeutic strategies.

Therapy of Patients in the Chronic Phase

Conventional Therapy and Other Chemotherapeutic Approaches

Historically, therapy for chronic myelogenous leukemia (CML) in the chronic phase has consisted of busulfan (Myleran) or hydroxyurea (Hydrea). Busulfan allows long periods of hematologic control and is inexpensive and therefore attractive when socioeconomic issues are important or in patients for whom follow-up is erratic. However, busulfan is associated with lung, marrow, and heart fibrosis and can cause an Addison's-like disease in 10 percent of patients. Prolonged myelosuppression may be observed. The dose of busulfan is usually 0.1 mg/kg/d until the white blood cell (WBC) counts decrease by 50 percent, and then the dose is reduced by 50 percent. Therapy is discontinued when the WBC count drops below 20,000/μL and is restarted when it increases above 50,000/μL.

Hydroxyurea has a lower toxicity profile than busulfan but is associated with shorter control of the peripheral blood counts. It is usually given at a dose of 40 mg/kg/d and is reduced by 50 percent when the WBC count drops below 20,000/μL. The dose is then adjusted individually to keep the WBC count at 5 to 10,000/μL. In a pilot phase II trial of higher doses, hydroxyurea (2 g/m^2/d) was given until the absolute neutrophil count reached < 1,000/μL.[448] At least 25 percent of Ph-negative cells were observed, with one patient achieving a complete cytogenetic remission. However, the responses were transient.

A large randomized study from Germany prospectively compared hydroxyurea with busulfan in patients with chronic-phase CML.[449] Patients treated with hydroxyurea had a longer median duration of the chronic phase (47 versus 37 months; p = .04) and a longer overall survival (58 versus 45 months; p = .008) than those treated with busulfan. The toxicity profile was more favorable for hydroxyurea. Improvements in the peripheral blood counts were not accompanied by a significant reduction in the percentage of cells bearing the Ph chromosome. These agents are successful in controlling the peripheral blood counts. However, they do little in maintaining patients in chronic phase and preventing them from transforming into the accelerated phase or blast crisis.

Anagrelide. Anagrelide belongs to the imidazole (2,1-b) quinazolin-2-1 series of compounds. This agent reduces megakaryocyte size and ploidy and is very effective in the control of thrombocytosis.[450,451] Anagrelide is given at a starting dose of 0.5 mg orally two to four times a day. The daily dose is then increased gradually to control the platelet count. The dose should not excel 10 mg/d.

Other chemotherapeutic agents such as 6-mercaptopurine (Purinethol), melphalan (Alkeran), thioguanine, and thiotepa have been used less frequently, sometimes in combination with busulfan. In one small study, continuous-infusion low-dose cytarabine at 15 to 30 mg/m^2/d was used with patients achieving a good hematologic response and cytogenic remissions.[452]

Homoharringtonine. Homoharringtonine is a plant alkaloid from the *Cephalotaxus fortuneii* tree, found in the Fugian province of China. This agent acts by blocking peptide bone formation following binding of the aminoacyl-transfer ribonucleic acid bonding to the ribosome. Investigators at The University of Texas M.D. Anderson Cancer Center performed a phase II study of homoharringtonine in 71 patients with CML who were either refractory to interferon (IFN) or were in late chronic phase (more than 1 year from diagnosis) and reported a 72 percent complete hematologic remission (CHR) rate of 72 percent and a cytogenetic response rate of 30 percent, which included a complete or major cytogenetic response of 22 percent.[453] Among 93 patients in early chronic phase (less than 1 year from diagnosis) treated with homoharringtonine, the complete hematologic rate was 92 percent and the cytogenetic response rate was 68 percent.[454] Studies combining homoharringtonine with low-dose cytarabine in patients who had failed IFN therapy have led to cytogenetic responses.[455,456] Toxicities have included diarrhea, headaches, cardiovascular toxicity, drug fever, fatigue, nausea, and vomiting, all usually in less than 10 percent of patients.

Interferon in the Treatment of CML in Chronic Phase

In the early 1980s, IFN-α was introduced into the therapy for CML following observations of in vitro inhibition of myeloid colony formation when normal or CML progenitors were cultured in its presence.[457] The first report in humans used partially pure IFN-α to treat 51 patients in chronic phase.[458,459] A CHR was achieved in 71 percent. However, more importantly, cytogenetic responses (ie, suppression of the Ph-positive clone) were observed in 39 percent of patients.[457] Recombinant human IFN-α soon became available and had similar results to those achieved with natural IFN-α. At the M.D. Anderson Cancer Center, 274 patients were treated with IFN-α 5 million units/m^2/d.[460] Eighty percent of the patients achieved a CHR with cytogenetic responses seen in

58 percent (major 38%, complete 26%), and the median survival was 89 percent. Good-risk patients had a major cytogenic response in 50 percent of patients, and the median survival was 102 months. Several other trials have shown a CHR varying from 80 percent to 22 percent with a major cytogenic response varying between 20 and 0 percent depending on the dose of the IFN used.[461–463]

Various investigators have used different criteria to assess responses to treatment, making comparisons difficult. The M.D. Anderson Cancer Center's criteria for response to therapy are presented in Table 7–17.

There appears to be a dose-response effect with IFN-α in CML in chronic phase. Lower-dose schedules are associated with inferior results compared with higher-dose schedules. In a study from Italy, patients in chronic-phase CML were randomized to receive 2 M units/m² three times a week (tiw) or 5 M units/m² three times a week with CHR rates of 24 versus 47 percent (p = .06), respectively.[15] Moreover, it was observed that patients who failed to respond to lower doses responded when given higher doses of IFN-α. Higher responses were observed when patients were treated with a daily schedule.[461] The dose used in most studies that have yielded a significant response is 5 M units/m²/d.

Patient Characteristics Affect Response Rates to Interferon

Patients with a poor performance status, presence of symptoms at diagnosis, splenomegaly, anemia, leukocytosis, high percentage of circulating blasts, peripheral nucleated red blood cells, and bone marrow basophilia are associated with a low likelihood of achieving a major cytogenic response to IFN. Similarly, the stage of the disease at the time of presentation is a major determinant of response. Patients in early chronic phase within 1 year of diagnosis have the best response. Kantarjian and colleagues found that patients in early chronic phase had a CHR of 60 to 80 percent with a major cytogenic response of 20 to 30 percent compared with a CHR rate of 50 to 60 percent and major cytogenic response of < 10 percent when patients were treated in late chronic phase. The CHRs in the accelerated phase and blast crisis were 30 to 40 percent and 20 to 30 percent, respectively, with none of the patients achieving a major cytogenic response.[460]

Comparisons of Interferon to Conventional Chemotherapy

In view of phase II data that showed that IFN-α was effective in inducing CHR and major cytogenic remission in patients with CML, several phase III studies were undertaken to compare IFN-α to chemotherapy.

The Italian Cooperative Group on Chronic Myeloid Leukemia compared IFN-α with conventional chemotherapy (hydroxyurea or busulfan) in patients with chronic-phase CML and showed a cytogenetic response (defined as > 33% of metaphases negative for Ph-chromosome) of 30 percent in the IFN-α group compared with 5 percent in the conventional chemotherapy group (p < .001). Figure 7–29 shows the overall survival for patients assigned to IFN-α who were alive and in chronic phase after 8 months (landmark analysis).[463] The time to progression from the chronic phase to an accelerated or blast phase was longer in the IFN group than in the chemotherapy group (median > 72 versus 45 months; p < .001) (Figure 7–30), as was survival (median 72 versus 52 months; 6-year survival 50 versus 29%; p = .002 for both comparisons) (Figure 7–31). Treatment was discontinued in 16 percent of patients in the IFN arm due to side effects.

In a randomized multicenter study from Germany, the benefits of IFN versus busulfan or hydroxyurea on survival of Ph-positive CML were examined. A total of 513 Ph-positive patients were randomized as follows: 133 for IFN, 186 for busul-

Table 7–17. RESPONSE CRITERIA FOR TREATMENT OF CHRONIC-PHASE CML		
Response	Category	Criteria
Hematologic remission	Complete	Normalization of WBC counts to < 9,000/μL with normal differential
	Partial	Decrease in WBC count to ≤ 50% of pretreatment level and to < 20,000/μL or normalization of WBC with persistent splenomegaly or immature peripheral cells
Cytogenetic responses	Complete	No evidence of Ph-positive cells
	Partial	1 to 34% of metaphases Ph-positive
	Minor	35 to 95% of metaphases Ph-positive
	None	Persistence of Ph chromosomes in all analyzable cells.

*Major cytogenetic response includes complete and partial responses.

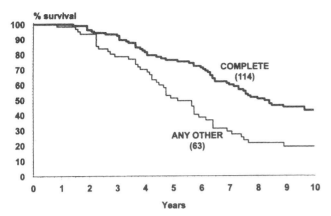

Figure 7–29. Overall survival of patients with CML in chronic phase assigned to interferon-α who were alive and in chronic phase after 8 months (landmark analysis). (Reprinted with permission from The Italian Cooperative Study Group on Chronic Myeloid Leukemia. Long-term follow-up of the Italian trial of interferon-alpha versus conventional chemotherapy in chronic myeloid leukemia. Blood 1998;92:1541–8. ©American Society of Hematology.)

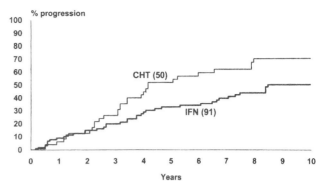

Figure 7–30. Time to prognosis to accelerated or blast phase for CML patients in the chronic phase assigned to either interferon-α or chemotherapy with hydroxyurea or busulfan (10 patients). (Reprinted with permission from The Italian Cooperative Study Group on Chronic Myeloid Leukemia. Long-term follow-up of the Italian trial of interferon-alpha versus conventional chemotherapy in chronic myeloid leukemia. Blood 1998;92:1541–8. ©American Society of Hematology.)

fan, and 194 for hydroxyurea. Interferon-treated patients have a significant survival advantage over busulfan-treated (p − .008) but not over hydroxyurea-treated patients (p = .44).[464] The longer survival was attributable to slower progression to blast crisis. The median survival of IFN-treated patients is 5.5 years (5-year survival 59%; 95% confidence interval [CI], 48 to 70%), of busulfan-treated patients is 3.8 years (5-year survival 32%; CI 24 to 40%), and of hydroxyurea-treated patients is 4.7 years (5-year survival 44%; CI 36 to 53%). Cytogenetic IFN responders had no significant survival advantage over nonresponders (p = .2). The lack of survival advantage among the IFN patients compared with the hydroxyurea group can be explained by a lower actual dose of IFN-α delivered in this study (2×10^6 units/m²/d) with fewer major cytogenetic responses and the fact that some patients may not have been in chronic phase at the time of therapy.

A third study conducted by the Medical Research Council (MRC) showed a survival advantage for IFN-α compared to chemotherapy.[465]

Significance of Cytogenetic Response with Interferon-α

The cytogenic responses observed with IFN-α are durable in more than 50 percent of patients, and the durability is greater in patients who achieve a com-

plete or major cytogenetic response.[461] In patients treated with IFN, achievements of a CHR at 3 months, a cytogenic response at 12 months, and a major cytogenic response at 24 months are associated with a better outcome. In a multivariate analysis, achieving a major cytogenetic response (< 35% Ph-positive cells) with IFN-α (5×10^6 units/m²/d or the maximally tolerated lower dose) in patients with chronic-phase CML was associated with an improved survival (p < .001).

Combination Therapy Using Interferon-α

Interferon has been combined with different agents in an attempt to improve the response in patients with

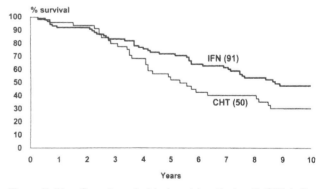

Figure 7–31. Overall survival for low-risk patients with CML in the chronic phase assigned to either interferon-α or chemotherapy with hydroxyurea or busulfan (10 patients). (Reprinted with permission from The Italian Cooperative Study Group on Chronic Myeloid Leukemia. Long-term follow-up of the Italian trial of interferon-alpha versus conventional chemotherapy in chronic myeloid leukemia. Blood 1998;92:1541–8. ©American Society of Hematology.)

chronic-phase CML. Cytarabine has been shown to have in vivo suppression of CML cells, with in vivo responses as a single agent in low doses.[466,467] In a phase II study at the M.D. Anderson Cancer Center, 142 patients with Ph-positive early chronic-phase CML received subcutaneous injections of IFN-α 5×10^6 units/m²/d and cytosine arabinoside 10 mg/d.[468] A CHR was achieved in 92 percent of patients. A cytogenetic response was seen in 74 percent; it was major in 50 percent (Ph-positive < 35%) and complete in 31 percent (Ph-positive 0%). In another study from the French Cooperative Group, patients were randomized to either IFN-α with hydroxyurea (n = 361) or IFN-α, hydroxyurea with cytarabine (20 mg/m²/d for 10 days monthly) (n = 360) and found a significant improvement in the survival in the IFN-cytarabine-hydroxyurea arm compared with the IFN-α-hydroxyurea arm (5-year rates 70 versus 60%; p = .02).[469] The cytarabine group was also found to have a significantly higher rate of CHR at 6 months (66 versus 55%; p < .01) and higher cytogenetic responses at 1 year (overall 61 versus 50%; major 41 versus 24%; p < .001). A similar benefit was also seen in the Italian trial, which compared IFN-α with cytarabine (n = 275) versus IFN-α alone (n = 265).[470] Survival was superior in the combination arm but significantly so only in the low-risk group (p = .01). These investigators also noted an improvement in the cytogenetic response rate in the combination arm at 12 months (41 versus 34%; major 17 versus 9%; p < .01).

Interferon has safely been combined with hydroxyurea in an effort to achieve a faster hematologic response and reduce the toxicity associated with IFN-α by using lower doses of interferon. The Benelux CML Study Group conducted a randomized study comparing hydroxyurea with the combination of hydroxyurea with low-dose IFN (3×10^6 units five times a week).[471] Although the hematologic and cytogenetic responses in the IFN group were higher than in the control group, the duration of chronic phase from randomization was not statistically different with 53 and 44 months in the IFN and control groups, respectively. The cytogenetic response rates for the IFN arm were 9 percent complete and 7 percent partial responders. No advantage for survival calculated from diagnosis was seen for the IFN group (median

64 months) compared with the control group (median, 68 months). However, there was a definite survival benefit in the IFN group that attained a major cytogenetic response. This study strengthens the observation that higher doses of IFN-α are associated with an increased likelihood of obtaining a major cytogenetic response that, in turn, is associated with an improvement in overall survival.

The use of IFN-α as a maintenance drug following the induction of intensive chemotherapy does not improve the survival rate or the durability of cytogenetic responses over those achieved with IFN-α alone.[472] In a pilot study, 32 patients with Ph-positive CML were treated with intensive chemotherapy induction followed by IFN-α maintenance. Intensive chemotherapy consisted of three cycles of daunorubicin 120 mg/m² on day 1, cytarabine 80 mg/m² daily for 10 days, vincristine 2 mg on day 1, and prednisone 100 mg daily for 5 days (DOAP). Maintenance therapy with IFN-α at a dose of 3×10^6 to 5×10^6 units/m²/d was adjusted according to counts and toxicity. The outcome of patients was compared with a matched historic population of 64 patients treated with IFN-α alone. Overall, 60 percent of patients had a cytogenetic response (partial or complete) with induction chemotherapy, but only eight (25%) had a sustained cytogenetic response with IFN-α maintenance. After a median follow-up of 67 months, the 6-year survival rate of the 32 patients was 58 percent, compared with 36 percent for the matched historic group (p = .084). The durable cytogenetic responses were 25 percent and 19 percent, respectively (p = .48). It has been suggested that response to IFN-α correlated with specific human leukocyte antigen (HLA) phenotype.[473]

Side Effects of Interferon-α

Side effects of IFN-α include fludarabine-like symptoms such as myalgias, arthralgias, fever, and headaches; neurologic toxicity including depression and memory loss; and autoimmune phenomena such as autoimmune hemolytic anemia or thrombocytopenia, Raynaud's phenomena, hypothyroidism, and systemic lupus erythematosus. Approximately 20 percent of patients developed neutralization antibodies and became resistant to therapy with IFN-α.

Allogeneic Bone Marrow (Stem Cell) Transplantation in CML

Allogeneic bone marrow transplantation (BMT) has been a major advance resulting in cure of CML. Several studies have reported long-term survival of 50 to 75 percent and a disease-free survival of 30 to 70 percent in patients with chronic-phase CML after allogeneic BMT.[474–482]

The Italian Cooperative Group on CML reported their experience with 258 patients prospectively registered to receive allogeneic BMT or conventional therapy with hydroxyurea or busulfan.[483] Nineteen percent of the patients (50/258) received an allogeneic BMT and 43 percent were in the BMT group versus 25 percent in the non-BMT group (p = .24). However, in the subgroup age < 30 years, the difference was statistically significant (65% versus 35%; p = .03).

The International Bone Marrow Transplant (IBMT) Registry and the German CML Study Group published the data comparing patients treated with non–T-cell–depleted BMT in chronic phase (584 patients reported to the IBMT Registry) with a group of patients treated on a randomized trial of the German CML Study Group (n = 196).[484] The non-BMT group received hydroxyurea (n = 121) or IFN-α (n = 75). The median age for the transplant group was 35 versus 41 years in the non-BMT group (p = .001). The 7-year survival was 58 percent with transplant versus 32 percent (p = .001) in the nontransplant group (42% with IFN and 22% with hydroxyurea). The survival advantage was greater in patients who had intermediate- or high-risk prognostic factors and those transplanted within 1 year of diagnosis.

The outcome of allogeneic transplantation in CML depends on a host of different factors. Younger patients have a better outcome with allogeneic transplantation due to a lower rate of transplant-related complications compared with the risk of relapse. The cutoff age for allogeneic transplantation is controversial. Gale and colleagues noted a relative risk of death of 1.4 in the group that was transplanted after age 35 years.[484] Other studies have also shown a decline in the long-term survival after age 30 years.[474–482] With improvement of supportive care and proper selection of patients, transplants have become safer for older patients.[485] The risk of transplant-related mortality and morbidity should be taken into consideration before recommending allogeneic transplants to the patients in chronic phase of CML.

The stage of disease at the time of transplantation is another important factor. The long-term survival rates after BMT are better when performed in the chronic (50 to 60%) compared with the accelerated phase (15 to 40%), with the worst outcome when performed in blast crisis (< 15%).[474–478] This is mainly due to the high rate of relapse and substantial risk of transplant-related morbidity. Patients who undergo transplantation in the accelerated phase solely on the basis of chromosomal analysis (ie, double Ph chromosome, trisomy 8, or isochrome 17) have a better outcome than patients transplanted in the accelerated phase by hematologic or bone marrow morphologic criteria.[486] There is much debate as to the best timing for transplantation in the chronic phase of CML. Biggs and colleagues noted a survival rate of 70 percent in the group of patients with chronic-phase CML who were transplanted within 1 year of the disease compared with 40 percent in those transplanted beyond 1 year.[478] A similar benefit on long-term survival (8-year survival probabilities) was also noted by the European Group for Bone Marrow Transplantation (69 versus 49%; p = .01 univariate analysis; not significant on multivariate analysis).[489] The data from the IBMT Registry also showed an improved survival with transplantation in early chronic phase.[476] The Seattle Group noted no significant difference in the outcome in the group transplanted between 1 and 2 years from diagnosis compared with greater than 1 year but noted a critical drop in survival rates beyond 2 years from diagnosis.[488,489]

Patients who were treated with busulfan were found to have a poorer outcome,[478] whereas prior exposure to IFN-α did not adversely affect the overall survival, incidence of graft-versus-host disease (GVHD), and time for hematologic recovery.[476]

Early studies of allogeneic transplantation in CML used conditioning regimens containing total body irradiation (TBI) and cyclophosphamide. These resulted in an increase in the risk of death due to causes other than relapse.[474,475,477] Busulfan has been substituted for TBI with an outcome that is comparable.[478] In a prospective randomized trial comparing the conditioning regimens of cyclophosphamide and TBI with cyclophosphamide and busulphan, the Seattle Marrow Transplant Team noted no significant differences in the 3-year probabilities of survival (0.80 for both), relapse (0.13 for both), and event-free survival (cyclophosphamide-TBI, 0.68; busulfan-cyclophosphamide, 0.71) in the speed of engraftment or incidence of veno-occlusive disease of the liver.[490] There was significantly more acute GVHD disease in the cyclophosphamide-TBI group. Fever days, positive blood cultures, hospitalizations, major elevation in creatinine, and inpatient hospital days were significantly more common in the cyclophosphamide-TBI group than in the busulfan-cyclophosphamide group.[490] Other preparative regimens have also shown similar results.[491]

The incidence and severity of GVHD can be reduced by T-cell depletion of the donor bone marrow prior to transplantation. Although this, in fact, reduces the incidence and severity of GVHD, it also can lead to an increase in the incidence of graft failures and a higher rate of relapse.[492,493]

Salvage Therapy After Bone Marrow Transplantation

Several approaches have been adopted in an attempt to treat patients who have relapsed after allogeneic transplantation for CML.

A second transplantation has been attempted in patients who relapse after one allogeneic BMT with some success.[494] Performance status at the time of second transplantation and the time to relapse after the first transplant affect the outcome. Patients who relapse within 6 months from transplantation have a poor outlook.

Interferon-α has been frequently employed in the treatment of relapse after an allogeneic BMT.[495–498] Patients in cytogenic relapse have a better response than those in hematologic relapse (58% cytogenetic response with 43% complete response versus 46% cytogenetic response with 28% complete response). Patients who have received a non–T-cell–depleted marrow have a higher response to IFN than patients with a lower tumor burden.[496] The median time to attain complete cytogenetic remission with IFN is about 7.5 months, and responses are durable in most patients.

Donor lymphocyte infusion (DLI) is the most effective salvage therapy for relapse after transplantation for CML. The cytogenetic response and CHR rates range from 60 to 80 percent with 3-year disease-free survival rates between 30 and 90 percent.[499–507] Among 30 patients treated with DLI, the Kaplan-Meier estimates of molecular remission at 2 years after DLI for patients treated in early (cytogenetic or molecular) relapse was 86.6 percent, whereas for patients in late (hematologic) relapse, it was 47.3 percent.[507] The risks with DLI include myelosuppression and severe GVHD, which results in significant morbidity and mortality.

Interferon has been combined with DLI in the treatment of relapsed CML after allogeneic transplantation. Polymerase chain reaction (PCR) showed a complete cytogenetic response in six of eight patients in chronic phase at the time of treatment, whereas the three patients who were in accelerated phase after relapse failed to respond. Van Rhee and colleagues have shown that lymphocytes from sibling and matched unrelated donors are associated with equal efficacy.[506]

Matched Unrelated Donor Transplantation in Chronic Myelogenous Leukemia

Only a small fraction of patients with CML had a matched related donor for allogeneic transplantation. This has led to a heightened interest in matched unrelated donor (MUD) transplantation for such patients.[508–514] The National Bone Marrow Transplant Program published results of MUD transplantation in CML in 1993.[508] The program found an actuarial incidence of hematologic relapse at 2 years of 11 percent with a 2-year disease-free survival of 45 ± 21 percent in patients transplanted within 1 year of diagnosis in chronic phase compared with 36 ± 11 percent for patients in chronic phase transplanted beyond 1 year. The incidence of grade II and IV acute GVHD was 54 ± 10 percent and chronic GVHD was 52 ± 10 percent. A lower incidence of both grade II and IV acute GVHD (p = .0003) and extensive chronic GVHD (p = .01) was associated with the use of T-cell–depleted marrow.

With improvement in the molecular testing of HLAs and a better control of GVHD, the incidence of morbidity and mortality with MUD transplantation can be significantly reduced. The Seattle Marrow

Transplant Team reported an estimated 5-year survival of 74 percent in patients under the age of 50 years after a MUD transplantation within 1 year of diagnosis of chronic-phase CML.[514] The incidence of grade II and IV GVHD was 35 percent, and the estimated 5-year risk of relapse was 10 percent. The rate of graft failure was 10 percent.

In an updated analysis of MUD transplantation from the National Marrow Donor Program, the overall survival among good-risk patients was very dependent on the age of the patient.[512] The overall survival for patients age less than 20 years was similar to that among patients between ages 20 and 35 (63.2 and 67.2%, respectively) but less for patients older than 35 years (47%) (Figure 7–32).

Until experience with MUD transplantation has matured, this procedure should be reserved for patients who are young (< 45 to 50 years), in chronic phase of the disease, and have a fully matched donor available. In addition, transplantation should be carried out within the first year of diagnosis.

Given the theoretical possibility of impairment of engraftment or unfavorable influence on relapse rate or outcome with exposure to IFN prior to transplantation, this issue has been addressed in several studies. There is some evidence that the administration of IFN-α prior to MUD transplantation has a deleterious effect on outcome if given within 3 to 6 months of transplantation.[513] However, this has not been uniformly demonstrated for patients receiving matched related transplants. A retrospective analysis by Hehlmann and colleagues suggested that the outcome of allogeneic transplantation, both related and unrelated, is not compromised if IFN is discontinued within 3 months of transplant.[515] Beelen and colleagues reported that prolonged (> 12 months) exposure to IFN-α prior to transplantation resulted in an increased incidence of graft failure (non-HLA–matched donors) and fatal infections, which led to increased treatment-related mortality and overall survival.[516] Two studies analyzing outcome in patients receiving HLA-identical transplants did not report an adverse effect on outcome with prior IFN exposure.[517,518] In the study by Tomas and colleagues, IFN was discontinued a median of 60 days (range 9 to 270) prior to transplantation.[518]

Autologous Bone Marrow/Peripheral Blood Stem Cell Transplantation

Patients with CML have early progenitor cells that do not have the t(9,22) (*bcr/abl* gene).[519] These stem cells are responsible for normal hematopoiesis to exist alongside the predominantly malignant CML clone. Leukapheresis allows collection of the normal early progenitor cells during early recovery from intensive chemotherapy. Cells harvested in this fashion have a lower risk of contamination with *bcr/abl*-positive cell.[520,521] With these facts in mind, autografting was attempted in patients with chronic-phase CML.[522–531] Although there is some degree of suppression of the Ph-positive cell in 40 to 70 percent of patients, this is usually transient, and the disease eventually returned. It is not clear if there is prolongation in survival after autografting. Boiron and colleagues for the European Bone Marrow Transplant Group reported that for 41 patients not responding to IFN, the overall survival at 2 and 4 years was 84 and 51 percent, respectively.[529]

Several techniques have been developed to in vitro purge the marrow to reduce the contamination of Ph-positive cells. These include long-term bone

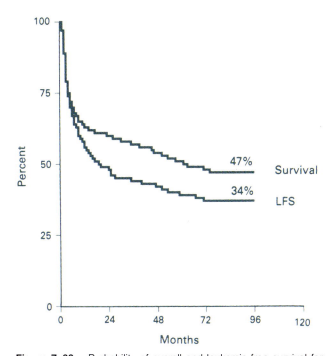

Figure 7–32. Probability of overall and leukemia-free survival for patients undergoing bone marrow transplantation in first chronic phase (n = 947). (From Gratwohl A, Hermans J, Niederwieser D, et al. Bone marrow transplantation for chronic myeloid leukemia long-term results. Bone Marrow Transplant 1993;12:509–16.)

marrow culture that can select Ph-negative cells, manipulations with cyclophosphamide derivative, IFNs, antisense oligodeoxynucleotides to c-myb or bcr/abl tyrosine kinase inhibitors, and other immunologic approaches.[532–544] The ideal purging technique is still unknown and is an area of active research.

Decitabine

Decitabine is a hypomethylating deoxycytidine nucleoside analogue that has been tested in chronic myeloid leukemia both in chronic phase and in blast crisis.[544,545] In blast crisis, the overall response rate is approximately 25 percent.[544] The most important toxicity is prolonged myelosuppression, with a median time to granulocyte recovery of 48 days and a recovery of platelets to 30,000/μL of 31 days.

Tyrosine Kinase Inhibitors

STI-571 is an inhibitor of the protein tyrosine kinase associated with bcr/abl, the platelet-derived growth factor receptor, and c-kit.[546,547] This agent shows selectively for the abl protein tyrosine kinase in vitro and in vivo and specifically inhibits proliferation of bcr/abl-expressing cells.[548] In a phase I trial for patients failing IFN-α, 54 patients receive daily oral STI-571 at 10 different doses, and 23 (96%) of 24 patients receiving at least 300 mg/d for 4 weeks achieved CHR.[549] Furthermore, remission was achieved in 3 weeks, and all patients were sustained

for up to 8 months. Within 2 months of treatment, 33 percent of patients had attained a cytogenetic remission by fluorescent in situ hybridization (FISH) complete cytogenetic remission with 300 mg or more of STI-571 within 2 months of initiating therapy. Grade 2 myelosuppression was observed in 5 of 24 patients, and grade 3 was observed in 2 of 24 patients treated with 300 mg or more.

STI-571 has also been tested in patients with CML in blast crisis and bcr/abl-positive acute lymphoblastic leukemia or lymphoid blast crisis.[550] Twenty-two patients (12 with myeloid blast crisis and 10 with ALL or lymphoid blast crisis) were treated with STI-571. Eleven of 15 patients who completed at least 28 days of therapy responded with at least 50 percent reduction of blood or bone marrow blasts. Four patients (one with CML lymphoid blast crisis, one with CML myeloid blast crisis, and two with ALL) achieved the complete disappearance of leukemia from the marrow and peripheral blood for at least 28 days. Phase II studies including larger numbers of patients with chronic-phase CML, blast crisis, and bcr/abl-positive ALL are ongoing. Preliminary studies have also suggested that combining STI-571 with other antineoplastic agents may be useful.[551] Additional ongoing trials include a phase I trial of STI-571 plus low-dose cytarabine; phase II trials in patients in chronic phase, accelerated phase, and blast crisis who have failed IFN; and a phase III prospective randomized trial for previously untreated patients in first chronic phase. The precise role of

Table 7–18. ALLOGENEIC BONE MARROW (STEM CELL) TRANSPLANTATION FOR CML IN FIRST CHRONIC PHASE

Author	No. Pts	TRM (%)	DFS (%)	OS (%)
Speck,[474] 1984	39	31	93, 3 yr	63, 3 yr
Thomas,[475] 1986	67	34	49, 3 yr	~50, 3 yr
Goldman,[476] 1988	405	40	46, 4 yr*	55, 4 yr
Clift,[477] 1991†	57 (12.0 Gy)	27	58, 4 yr	60, 4 yr
	59 (15.75 Gy)		66, 4 yr	66, 4 yr
Biggs,[478] 1992	62	34	NA	58, 3 yr
Wagner,[479] 1992	79	42‡	54§	52, 4.5 yr
Gratwohl,[480] 1993	947	42‖	34#	47, 8 yr
Savage,[482] 1997	205	37**	NA	58, 5 yr
Hehlmann,[515] 1999	104	35	NA	57, 5 yr

*Leukemia-free survival.
†Randomized trial of 12.0 and 15.75 Gy total body irradiation each with cyclophosphamide.
‡Includes 4 patients whose cause of death is listed as other.
§Event-free survival for patients < age 30.
‖At 5 years leukemia-free survival at 8 years.
**Includes 28 patients in accelerated phase, 10 in blast phase.
NA = not available.

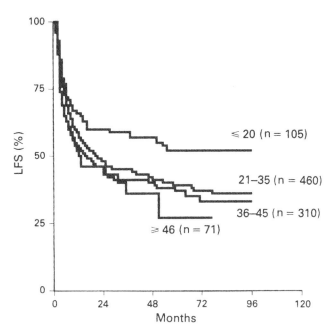

Figure 7–33. Overall survival in good risk patients with CML in chronic phase undergoing matched unrelated donor transplantation by age. (Reprinted with permission from McGlave PB, Shu XO, Wen U, et al. Unrelated donor marrow transplantation for chronic myelogenous leukemia. 9 years' experience of the National Marrow Program. Blood 2000;95:2219–25. ©American Society of Hematology.)

STI-571 in the treatment of patients with CML is rapidly evolving. Studies have recently demonstrated that *bcr/abl*-positive cells can develop resistance to STI-571 by overexpression of *bcr/abl* and possibly other mechanisms.[552]

Treatment of Advanced-Stage CML

The treatment of patients with CML in the accelerated phase or blast crisis remains formidable. Patients with an early accelerated phase undergo allogeneic transplantation and have a reasonably favorable outcome. However the allogeneic transplantation is carried out in the blast crisis, only approximately 18 percent of patients fare well.[474] Generally, it is routine practice to attempt to eradicate the leukemic cells prior to definitive procedures such as BMT. Various chemotherapeutic strategies have been attempted.[551,553–557] Kouides and Rowe have shown an overall response rate (complete plus partial response) of 69 percent (9 of 3 patients) with achievement of a second chronic phase in 54 percent (7 of 13 patients) with an intensified induction regimen of daunorubicin 70 mg/m²/d on days 1 to 3 plus

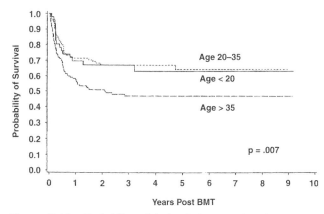

Figure 7–34. Probability of leukemia-free survival for patients undergoing bone marrow transplantation in first chronic phase by age. (From Gratwohl A, Hermans J, Niederwieser D, et al. Bone marrow transplantation for chronic myeloid leukemia long-term results. Bone Marrow Transplant 1993;12:509–16.)

cytarabine 200 mg/m²/d by continuous infusion on days 1 to 9.[554] Kantarjian and colleagues tested high-dose cytarabine at 1.5 g/m²/d over 24 hours for 4 days with daunorubicin at 120 mg/m² intravenously in 48 patients in accelerated phase or blast crisis and reported that 29 percent (14 of 48 patients) achieved a CHR and +5 percent (7 patients) achieved a second chronic phase.[553] Montefusco and colleagues investigated the addition of etoposide 100 mg/m²/d and carboplatin 150 mg/m²/d every 12 hours on days 1 to 3 and 8 to 10.[556] Eleven of 17 patients (65%) achieved complete remission, and 7 of the 11 responding

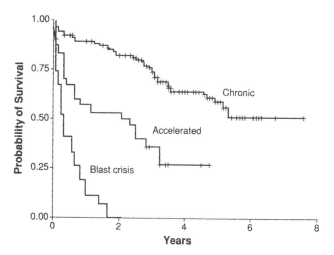

Figure 7–35. Overall survival for 198 patients with CML undergoing autologous stem cell transplantation for chronic (n = 141) or accelerated phase (n = 27). (Reprinted with permission from Bhatia R, Verfaillie CM, Miller JS, McGlave PB. Autologous transplantation therapy for chronic myelogenous leukemia. Blood 1997;89:2623–34. ©American Society of Hematology.)

Table 7–19. THERAPY OF CML BLAST CRISIS

Author	No. Pts	Regimen	CHR (%)	TRM (%)	Remission Duration (Mo)	Overall Survival (Mo)
Kantarjian,[553] 1992	24	Daunorubicin 120 mg/m* Cytarabine 1.5 g Solu-Medrol 100 mg	33	25	1–18	
Kouides,[554] 1995	14	Daunorubicin 70 mg/m* Cytarabine 200 mg/m*	69[†]	29	1.6–7.8	NA
Lipton,[555] 1996	14	Mitoxantron 12 mg/m* Cytarabine 1.5 mg/m* Vincristine 1 mg/m* Solu-Medrol 40 mg/m*	64	21	1–5	7–14
Montefusco,[556] 1997	17	Etoposide 100 mg/m* Cytarabine 500 mg/m* Carboplatin 150 mg/m*	65	27	7+–16+	7+–38+
Dann,[557] 1998	17	Cladribine 15 mg/m*	47[†]	26	.26–16.2[‡]	
Druker,[548] 1999	15[§]	STI-571	73[‖]			

NA = not applicable.
*Nontransplanted parent.
[†]Complete plus partial remission.
[‡]Time-to-treatment failure.
[§]Ten myeloid blast crisis patients.
[‖]Response defined as 50% or greater decrease in the percentage of peripheral or bone marrow blasts. Four patients achieved complete disappearance of the leukemia from the marrow and peripheral blood including one lymphoid blast crisis, one myeloid blast crisis, and two patients with ALL.

patients (64%) achieved a cytogenetic response with conversion to all Ph-negative metaphases. Cladribine was tested in 19 patients in blast crisis at doses of 16 to 20 mg/m^2/d for 5 days.[557] The complete remission plus partial remission rate was 47 percent.

Summary and Recommended Treatment Strategies

Allogeneic transplantation remains the only proven curative treatment for patients with CML. Therefore, for younger patients with a suitable HLA-matched donor, transplantation can be considered the treatment of choice. The age above which the toxicities and mortality rate increase to make this approach too toxic to recommend as initial therapy has not been definitively established; however, most investigators would consider ages 45 to 55 years as the upper age limit. For older patients and those without a suitable donor, IFN, with or without low-dose cytarabine, is considered the best initial strategy. An alternative for younger patients is a matched unrelated transplant. Following transplantation, serial PCR and cytogenetic studies are done. If the PCR becomes positive less than 12 months after transplant, the PCR can be followed. If relapse occurs within 12 months after transplant, IFN or DLI is considered. If the PCR becomes

positive or cytogenetic or morphologic relapse occurs after 12 months from transplant, IFN-α or DLI is considered. If after 12 months from transplant, the PCR becomes positive, the best approach is not known. One can consider DLI or IFN-α. For patients who responded well to IFN-α by achieving a major cytogenetic response (greater than or at least 65% reduction in Ph-positive cells), one can consider stopping the IFN-α after a period of time, such as 3 to 5 years. If there is less than a major cytogenetic response, low-dose cytarabine can be added. The role of STI-571 is under active investigation. A clinical trial randomizing untreated patients to either STI-571 or IFN-α plus low-dose cytarabine is under way.

REFERENCES

1. Pui C-H, Evans WE. Acute lymphoblastic leukemia. N Engl J Med 1998;339:605–15.
2. Chessels JM, Hall E, Prentice HG, et al. The impact of age on outcome in lymphoblastic leukemia: MRC UK ALL X and Xa compared: a report from the MRC and Pediatric and Adult Working Parties. Leukemia 1998;12:463–73.
3. Maccarini M, Carbelli G, Amadori S, et al. Adolescent and adult acute lymphoblastic leukemia: prognostic features and outcome of therapy. A study of 293 patients. Blood 1982;60:677–84.
4. Hoelzer D, Thiel E, Loffler H, et al. Prognostic factors

in a multicentre study for treatment of acute lymphoblastic leukemia in adults. Blood 1988;71:123–31.

5. Boucheix C, David B, Sebban C, et al. Immunophenotype of adult acute lymphoblastic leukemia, clinical parameters, and outcome: an analysis of a prospective trial including 562 tested patients (LALA87). Blood 1994;84:1603–12.

6. Larson RA, Dodge RK, Burns CP, et al. A five-drug remission induction regimen with intensive consolidation for adults with acute lymphoblastic leukemia: Cancer and Leukemia Group B study 8811. Blood 1995;85:2025–37.

7. The Group Francois de Cytogenetique Hematologique. Cytogenetic abnormalities in adult acute lymphoblastic leukemia: correlations with hematologic findings and outcome. A collaborative study of the Groupe Francais de Cytogenetique Hematologique. Blood 1996;87:3135–42.

8. Gaynor J, Chapman D, Little C, et al. A cause-specific hazard rate analysis of prognostic factors among 199 adults with acute lymphoblastic leukemia: the Memorial Hospital experience since 1969. J Clin Oncol 1988;6:1014–30.

9. Czuczman MS, Dodge RK, Stewart CC, et al. Value of immunophenotype in intensively treated adult acute lymphoblastic leukemia: Cancer and Leukemia Group B study 8364. Blood 1999;93:3931–9.

10. Wetzler M, Dodge RK, Mrozek K, et al. Prospective karyotype analysis in adult acute lymphoblastic leukemia: the Cancer and Leukemia Group B experience. Blood 1999;93:3983–93.

11. Tsai T, Davalath S, Rankin C, et al. Tumor suppressor gene alteration in adult acute lymphoblastic leukemia (ALL). Analysis of retinoblastoma (Rb) and p53 gene expression in lymphoblasts of patients with de novo, relapsed, or refractory ALL treated in Southwest Oncology Group studies. Leukemia 1996;10:1901–10.

12. Rubnitz JE, Downing JR, Pui GH, et al. TEL gene rearrangement in acute lymphoblastic leukemia: a new genetic marker with prognostic significance. J Clin Oncol 1997;15:1150–7.

13. Aguilar RCT, Sohal J, Rhee FV, et al. TEL/AML1 fusion in acute lymphoblastic leukaemia of adults. Br J Haematol 1996;95:673–7.

14. Woerden NLR, Pieters R, Loonen AH, et al. TEL/AML1 gene fusion is related to in vitro drug sensitivity for L-asparaginase in childhood acute lymphoblastic leukemia. Blood 2000;96:1094–9.

15. Amadori S, Montuoro A, Meloni G, et al. Combination chemotherapy for acute lymphoblastic leukemia in adults: results of a retrospective study in 82 patients. Am J Hematol 1980;8:175–83.

16. Hess CE, Zirkle IW. Results of induction therapy with vincristine and prednisone alone in adult acute lymphoblastic leukemia: report of 43 patients and review of the literature. Am J Hematol 1982;13:63–71.

17. Gottlieb AJ, Weinberg V, Ellison RR, et al. Efficacy of daunorubicin in the therapy of adult acute lymphocytic leukemia: a prospective randomized trial by Cancer and Leukemia Group B. Blood 1984;64:267–74.

18. Schauer P, Arlin ZA, Mertelsmann R, et al. Treatment of acute lymphoblastic leukemia in adults: results of the L-10 and L-10M protocols. J Clin Oncol 1983;1:462–70.

19. Barnett MJ, Greaves MF, Amess JAL, et al. Treatment of acute lymphoblastic leukemia in adults. Br J Haematol 1986;64:455–68.

20. Hussein KK, Dahlberg S, Head D, et al. Treatment of acute lymphoblastic leukemia in adults using intensive induction, consolidation, and maintenance chemotherapy. A Southwest Oncology Group Study. Blood 1989;73:57–63.

21. Radford JE, Burns CP, Jones MP, et al. Adult acute lymphoblastic leukemia: results of the Iowa HOP-L Protocol. J Clin Oncol 1989;7:58–66.

22. Mandelli F, Annino L, Rotoli B, et al. The GIMEMA ALL 0183 trial: analysis of 10-year follow-up. GIMEMA Cooperative Group, Italy. Br J Haematol 1996;92:665–72.

23. Kantarjian HM, Walters RS, Keating MJ, et al. Results of the vincristine, doxorubicin, and dexamethasone regimen in adults with standard- and high-risk acute lymphoblastic leukemia. J Clin Oncol 1990;8:994–1004.

24. Linker CA, Levitt LJ, O'Donnell M, et al. Treatment of adult acute lymphoblastic leukemia with intensive cyclic chemotherapy: a follow-up report. Blood 1991;78:2814–22.

25. Finnish Leukemia Group. Long-term survival in acute lymphoblastic leukemia in adults. A prospective study of 51 patients. Eur J Haematol 1992;48:75–82.

26. Hoelzer D, Thiel E, Loffler M, et al. The German multicentre trials for treatment of acute lymphoblastic leukemia in adults. Leukemia 1992;6:175–7.

27. Hoelzer D, Thiel E, Ludwig WD, et al. Follow-up of the first two successive German multicentre trials for adult ALL (01/81 and 02/84). German Adult ALL Study Group. Leukemia 1993;7:S130–4.

28. Schiffer CA, Larson RA, Bloomfield CD, for the CALGB. Cancer and Leukemia Group B (CALGB) studies in adult acute lymphoblastic leukemia. Leukemia 1992;6:171–4.

29. Fiere D, Lapage E, Sebban C, et al. Adult acute lymphoblastic leukemia: a multicentre randomized trial testing bone marrow transplantation as post remission therapy. J Clin Oncol 1993;11:1990–2001.

30. Durrant IJ, Prentice HG, Richards SM, et al. Intensification of treatment for adults with acute lym-

phoblastic leukaemia: results of U.K. Medical Research Council randomized trial UKALL XA. Medical Research Council Working Party on Leukaemia in Adults. Br J Haematol 1997;99:84–92.

31. Cuttner J, Mick R, Budman DR, et al. Phase III trial of brief intensive treatment of adult acute lymphocytic leukemia comparing daunorubicin and mitoxantrone: a CALGB study. Leukemia 1991;5:425–31.

32. Wiernik PH, Dutcher JP, Gucalp R, et al. MOAD therapy for acute lymphocytic leukemia [abstract]. Proc Am Soc Clin Oncol 1990;9:205.

33. Weiss M, Maslak P, Feldman E, et al. Cytarabine with high dose mitoxantrone induces rapid remission in adult acute lymphoblastic leukemia without the use of vincristine or prednisone. J Clin Oncol 1996;14: 2480–5.

34. Nagura E, Kimura K, Yamada K, et al. Nation-wide randomized comparative study of doxorubicin, vincristine, and prednisolone combination therapy with and without L-asparaginase for adult acute lymphoblastic leukemia. Cancer Chemother Pharmacol 1994;33:359–65.

35. Sallan S, Hitchcock-Bryan S, Gelber R, et al. Influence of intensive asparaginase in the treatment of childhood non-T-cell acute lymphoblastic leukemia. Cancer Res 1983;43:5601–7.

36. Clavell L, Gelber R, Cohen H, et al. Four agent induction and intensive asparaginase therapy for treatment of childhood acute lymphoblastic leukemia. N Engl J Med 1986;315:657–63.

37. Kasparu H, Sreter L, Holowiiecki I, et al. Intensified induction therapy for ALL in adults: a multicenter trial. Onkologie 1991;14(Suppl 12):80.

38. Cortes J, Kantarjian HM. Acute lymphoblastic leukemia: a comprehensive review with emphasis on biology and therapy. Cancer 1995;76:2393–417.

39. Rohatiner AZS, Bassan R, Battista R, et al. High dose cytosine arabinoside in the initial treatment of adults with acute lymphoblastic leukemia. Br J Cancer 1990;62:454–58.

40. Hoelzer D, Thiel E, Loffler H, et al. Intensified chemotherapy and mediastinal irradiation in adult T-cell acute lymphoblastic leukemia. In: Gale RP, Hoelzer D, editors. Acute lymphoblastic leukemia. New York: Alan R. Liss; 1990. p. 221–9.

41. Sullivan MP, Ramirez I. Curability of Burkitt's lymphoma with high-dose cyclophosphamide high-dose methotrexate therapy and intrathecal chemoprophylaxis. J Clin Oncol 1985;3:627–36.

42. Murphy SB, Bowman WP, Abromowitch M, et al. Results of treatment of advanced-stage Burkitt's lymphoma and B cell (SIg+) acute lymphoblastic leukemia with high-dose fractionated cyclophosphamide and coordinated high-dose methotrexate and cytarabine. J Clin Oncol 1986;4:1732–9.

43. Hoelzer D, Ludwig W-D, Thiel E, et al. Improved outcome in acute lymphoblastic leukemia in adult B-cell acute lymphoblastic leukemia. Blood 1996;87: 495–508.

44. Patte C, Michon J, Frappaz D, et al. Therapy of Burkitt and other B-cell acute lymphoblastic leukemia and lymphoma: experience with LMB protocols of the SFOP (French Pediatric Oncology Society) in children and adults [review]. Baillieres Clin Haematol 1994;7:339–48.

45. Lee EJ, Pettroni GR, Freter CE, et al. Brief duration high intensity chemotherapy for patients with small non-cleaved lymphoma and FAB L-3 acute lymphoblastic leukemia in adults: preliminary results of CALGB 9251 [abstract]. Proc Am Soc Clin Oncol 1997;16:24a.

46. Pees HW, Radke H, Schwamborn J, et al. The BFM protocol for HIV-negative Burkitt's lymphomas and L3 ALL in adult patients. A high chance for cure. Ann Hematol 1992;65:201–5.

47. Gokbuget N, Hoelzer D. Meningeosis leukaemica in adult acute lymphoblastic leukaemia. J Neurooncol 1998;38:167–80.

48. Omura GA, Moffitt S, Vogler WR, et al. Combination chemotherapy of adult acute lymphoblastic leukemia with randomized central nervous system prophylaxis. Blood 1980;55:199–204.

49. Willemze R, Drenthe-Schank AM, van Rossom J, et al. Treatment of acute lymphoblastic leukemia in adolescents and adults. Comparison of two schedules for CNS leukemia prophylaxis. Scand J Hematol 1980;24:421.

50. Kantarjian HM, Walters RS, Smith TL, et al. Identification of risk groups for development of central nervous system leukemia in adults with acute lymphoblastic leukemia. Blood 1988;72:1784–9.

51. Larson RA, Dodge RK, Linker CA, et al. A randomized controlled trial of filgrastim during induction and consolidation chemotherapy for adults with acute lymphoblastic leukemia: CALGB study 9111. Blood 1998;92:1556–64.

52. Ottoman OG, Hoelzer D, Gracien E, et al. Concomitant granulocyte colony-stimulating factor and induction chemotherapy in adult lymphoblastic leukemia: a randomized phase III trial. Blood 1995;86:444–50.

53. Stryckmans P, De Witte TH, Marie JP, et al. Therapy of adult ALL: overview of 2 successive EORTC studies: (ALL-2 & ALL-3). The EORTC Leukemia Cooperative Study Group. Leukemia 1992;6:199 203.

54. Ludwig WD, Reider H, Bartram CR, et al. Immunophenotypic and genotypic features, clinical characteristics, and treatment outcome of adult pro-B acute lymphoblastic leukemia: results of the German multicenter trials GMALL 03/87 and 04/89. Blood 1998;92:1898–909.

55. Ellison RR, Mick R, Cuttner J, et al. The effects of post induction intensification treatment with cytarabine and daunorubicin in adult acute lymphoblastic leukemia: a prospective randomized clinical trial by Cancer and Leukemia Group B. J Clin Oncol 1991; 9:2002–15.

56. Cassileth PA, Anderson JW, Bennett JM, et al. Adult lymphocytic leukemia: the Eastern Cooperative Oncology Group experience. Leukemia 1992;6:178–81.

57. Clarkson B, Ellis S, Little C, et al. Acute lymphoblastic leukemia in adults. Semin Oncol 1985;12:160–79.

58. Cortes J, O'Brien SM, Pierce S, et al. The value of high-dose systemic chemotherapy and intrathecal therapy for central nervous system prophylaxis in different risk groups of adult acute lymphoblastic leukemia. Blood 1995;86:2091–7.

59. Gale RP, Butturini A. Maintenance chemotherapy and cure of childhood acute lymphoblastic leukaemia. Lancet 1991;338:1315–8.

60. Bleyer WA, Sather HN, Nickerson HJ, et al. Monthly pulses of vincristine and prednisone prevent bone marrow and testicular relapse in low-risk childhood acute lymphoblastic leukemia: a report of the CCG-161 study by the Children's Cancer Study Group. J Clin Oncol 1991;9:1012–21.

61. Miller DR, Leikin SL, Albo VC, et al. Three versus five years of maintenance therapy are equivalent in childhood acute lymphoblastic leukemia: a report from the Children's Cancer Study Group. J Clin Oncol 1989;7:316–25.

62. Childhood ALL Secretariat, CTSU, Radcliffe Infirmary, Oxford, UK. Duration and intensity of maintenance chemotherapy in acute lymphoblastic leukaemia: overview of 42 trials involving 12,000 randomized children. Childhood ALL Collaborative Group. Lancet 1996;347:1783–8.

63. Secker-Walker LM, Craig JM, Hawkins JM, Hoffbrand AV. Philadelphia positive acute lymphoblastic leukemia in adults: age distribution, BCR breakpoint and prognostic significance. Leukemia 1991;5:196–9.

64. Gotz G, Weh HJ, Walter TA, et al. Clinical and prognostic significance of the Philadelphia chromosome in adult patients with acute lymphoblastic leukemia. Ann Hematol 1992;64:97–100.

65. Annino L, Ferrari A, Cedrone M, et al. Adult Philadelphia-chromosome-positive acute lymphoblastic leukemia: experience of treatments during a ten-year period. Leukemia 1994;8:664–7.

66. Westbrook CA, Hooberman AL, Spino C, et al. Clinical significance of the BCR-ABL fusion gene in adult acute lymphoblastic leukemia: a Cancer and Leukemia Group B Study (8762). Blood 1992;80: 2983–90.

67. Faderl S, Kantarjian HM, Thomas DA, et al. Outcome of Philadelphia chromosome-positive adult acute lymphoblastic leukemia. Leuk Lymphoma 2000;36: 263–73.

68. Kantarjian HM, O'Brien S, Beran M, et al. Update of the hyper-CVAD program in newly diagnosed adult acute lymphoblastic leukemia (ALL) [abstract]. Blood 1995;80:173a.

69. Rowe JM, Richards S, Wiernik PH, et al. Allogeneic bone marrow transplantation (BMT) for adults with acute lymphoblastic leukemia (ALL) in first complete remission (CR): early results from the International ALL trial (MRC UK ALL/ECOG E2993) [abstract]. Blood 1999;94:732.

70. Delannoy A, Sebban C, Cony-Makhoul P, et al. Age-adapted induction treatment of acute lymphoblastic leukemia in the elderly and assessment of maintenance with interferon combined with chemotherapy. A multicentric prospective study in forty patients. French Group for Treatment of Adult Acute Lymphoblastic Leukemia. Leukemia 1997;11:1429–34.

71. Bassan R, DiBona E, Lerede T, et al. Age-adapted moderate-dose induction and flexible outpatient postremission therapy for elderly patients with acute lymphoblastic leukemia. Leuk Lymphoma 1996;22:295–301.

72. Thomas ED, Sanders JE, Flournoy N, et al. Marrow transplantation for patients with acute lymphoblastic leukemia: a long-term follow-up. Blood 1983;62:1139–41.

73. Weisdorf DJ, Nesbit ME, Ramsay NK, et al. Allogeneic bone marrow transplantation for acute lymphoblastic leukemia in remission: prolonged survival associated with acute graft-versus-host disease. J Clin Oncol 1987;5:1348–55.

74. Blume KG, Forman SJ, Snyder DS, et al. Allogeneic bone marrow transplantation for acute lymphoblastic leukemia during first complete remission. Transplantation 1987;43:389–92.

75. Doney K, Buckner CD, Kopecky KJ, et al. Marrow transplantation for patients with acute lymphoblastic leukemia in first marrow remission. Bone Marrow Transplant 1987;2:355–63.

76. Vernant JP, Marit G, Maraninchi D, et al. Allogeneic bone marrow transplantation in adults with acute lymphoblastic leukemia in first complete remission. J Clin Oncol 1988;6:227–31.

77. Chao NJ, Forman SJ, Schmidt GM, et al. Allogeneic bone marrow transplantation for high-risk acute lymphoblastic leukemia during first complete remission. Blood 1991;78:1923–7.

78. Copelan EA, Biggs JC, Avalos BR, et al. Radiation-free preparation for allogeneic bone marrow transplantation in adults with acute lymphoblastic leukemia. J Clin Oncol 1992;10:237–42.

79. Barrett AJ, Horowitz MM, Gale RP, et al. Marrow transplantation for acute lymphoblastic leukemia:

factors affecting relapse and survival. Blood 1989;74:862–71.

80. Sutton L, Kuentz M, Cordonnier C, et al. Allogeneic bone marrow transplantation for adult acute lymphoblastic leukemia in first complete remission: factors predictive of transplant-related mortality and influence of total body irradiation modalities. Bone Marrow Transplant 1993;12:583–9.

81. Sebban C, Lepage E, Vernant JP, et al. Allogeneic bone marrow transplantation in adult acute lymphoblastic leukemia in first complete remission: a comparative study. J Clin Oncol 1994;12:2580–7.

82. Attal M, Blaise D, Marit G, et al. Consolidation treatment of adult acute lymphoblastic leukemia: a prospective randomized trial comparing allogeneic versus autologous bone marrow transplantation and testing the impact of recombinant interleukin-2 after autologous bone marrow transplantation. Blood 1995;86:1619–28.

83. Horowitz MM, Messerer D, Hoelzer D, et al. Chemotherapy compared with bone marrow transplantation for adults with acute lymphoblastic leukemia in first remission. Ann Intern Med 1991;115:13–8.

84. Deconinck E, Cahn J-Y, Milpied N, et al. Allogeneic bone marrow transplantation for high-risk acute lymphoblastic leukemia in first remission: long-term results for 42 patients conditioned with an intensified regimen (TBI, high-dose Ara-C and melphalan). Bone Marrow Transplant 1997;20:731–5.

85. Oh H, Gale RP, Zhang MJ, et al. Chemotherapy vs HLA-identical sibling bone marrow transplants for adults with acute lymphoblastic leukemia in first remission. Bone Marrow Transplant 1998;22:253–7.

86. Wingard JR, Piantadosi S, Santos GW, et al. Allogeneic bone marrow transplantation for patients with high-risk acute lymphoblastic leukemia. J Clin Oncol 1990;8:820–30.

87. Barrett AJ, Horowitz MM, Ash RC, et al. Bone marrow transplantation for Philadelphia chromosome positive acute lymphoblastic leukemia. Blood 1992;79:3067–70.

88. Miyamura K, Tanimoto M, Morishima Y, et al. Detection of Philadelphia chromosome-positive acute lymphoblastic leukemia by polymerase chain reaction: possible eradication of minimal residual disease by marrow transplantation. Blood 1992;79:1366–70.

89. Keil F, Kalhs P, Haas OA, et al. Relapse of Philadelphia chromosome positive acute lymphoblastic leukaemia after marrow transplantation: sustained molecular remission after early and dose-escalating infusion of donor leucocytes. Br J Haematol 1997;97:161–4.

90. Kroger N, Kruger W, Wacker-Backhaus G, et al. Intensive conditioning regimen in bone marrow transplantation for Philadelphia chromosome positive acute lymphoblastic leukemia. Bone Marrow Transplant 1998;22:1029–33.

91. Goldstone AH, Richards S, Wiernik PH, et al. Philadelphia chromosome positive patients with adult lymphoblastic leukemia (ALL). Early results from the International ALL trial (MRC UK ALL XII/ECOG E2993 [abstract]). Blood 1999;94:3071.

92. Martino R, Bellido M, Brunet S, et al. Allogeneic or autologous stem cell transplantation following salvage chemotherapy for adults with refractory or relapsed acute lymphoblastic leukemia. Bone Marrow Transplant 1998;21:1023–7.

93. Weisdorf DJ, Billett AL, Hannan P, et al. Autologous versus unrelated donor allogeneic marrow transplantation for acute lymphoblastic leukemia. Blood 1997;90:2962–8.

94. Mizuta S, Ito Y, Kohno A, et al. Accurate quantitation of residual tumor burden at bone marrow harvest predicts timing of subsequent relapse in patients with common ALL treated by autologous bone marrow transplantation. Bone Marrow Transplant 1999;24:777–84.

95. Potter MN. The detection of minimal residual disease in acute lymphoblastic leukemia. Blood Rev 1992;6:68–82.

96. Yamada M, Wasserman R, Lange B, et al. Minimal residual disease in childhood B-lineage lymphoblastic leukemia: persistence of leukemic cells during the first 18 months of treatment. N Engl J Med 1990;323:448–55.

97. Knechtli CJC, Goulden NJ, Hancock JP, et al. Minimal residual disease status before allogeneic bone marrow transplantation is an important determinant of successful outcome for children and adolescents with acute lymphoblastic leukemia. Blood 1998;92:4072–9.

98. Radich J, Gehly G, Lee A, et al. Detection of bcr-abl transcripts in Philadelphia chromosome-positive acute lymphoblastic leukemia after marrow transplantation. Blood 1997;89:2602–9.

99. Zetterquist H, Mattsson J, Uzunel M, et al. Mixed chimerism in the B cell lineage is a rapid and sensitive indicator of minimal residual disease in bone marrow transplant recipients with pre-B cell acute lymphoblastic leukemia. Bone Marrow Transplant. 2000;25:843–51.

100. Estrov Z, Grunberger T, Dube ID, et al. Detection of residual acute lymphoblastic leukemia cells in cultures of bone marrow obtained during remission. N Engl J Med. 1986;315:538–42.

101. Pongers-Willemse MJ, Verhagen OJ, Tibbe GJ, et al. Real-time quantitative PCR for the detection of minimal residual disease in acute lymphoblastic leukemia using junctional region specific TaqMan probes. Leukemia 1998;12:2006–14.

102. Verhagen OJHM, Willemze MJ, Breunis WB, et al. Application of germline IGH probes in real-time quantitative PCR for the detection of minimal residual disease in acute lymphoblastic leukemia. Leukemia 2000;14:1426–35.

103. El-Rifai W, Ruutu T, Vettenranta K, et al. Follow-up of residual disease using metaphase-FISH in patients with acute lymphoblastic leukemia in remission. Leukemia 1997;11:633–8.

104. Hoelzer D. High-dose chemotherapy in adult acute lymphoblastic leukemia. Semin Oncol 1991;28:84–9.

105. Hiddemann W, Buchner T, Heil G, et al. Treatment of refractory acute lymphoblastic leukemia in adults with high dose cytosine arabinoside and mitoxantrone (HAM). Leukemia 1990;4:637–40.

106. Rosen PJ, Rankin C, Head DR, et al. A phase II study of high dose ARA-C and mitoxantrone for treatment of relapsed or refractory adult acute lymphoblastic leukemia. Leuk Res 2000;24:183–7.

107. Kantarjian HM, Estey EH, O'Brien S, et al. Intensive chemotherapy with mitoxantrone and high-dose cytosine arabinoside followed by granulocyte-macrophage colony-stimulating factor in the treatment of patients with acute lymphocytic leukemia. Blood 1992;79:876–81.

108. Mazza JJ, Leong T, Rowe JM, et al. Treatment of adult patients with acute lymphocytic leukemia in relapse. Leuk Lymphoma 1996;20:317–9.

109. Milpied N, Gisselbrecht C, Harousseau JL, et al. Successful treatment of adult acute lymphoblastic leukemia after relapse with prednisone, intermediate-dose cytarabine, mitoxantrone, and etoposide (PAME) chemotherapy. Cancer 1990;66:627–31.

110. Arlin ZA, Feldman E, Kempin S, et al. Amsacrine with high-dose cytarabine is highly effective therapy for refractory and relapsed acute lymphoblastic leukemia in adults. Blood 1998;72:433–5.

111. Kantarjian HM, O'Brien S, Keating JM, et al. Update of the hyper-CVAD dose intensive regimen in adult acute lymphocytic leukemia [abstract]. Blood 1998;92:1285.

112. Haas OA, Mor W, Gadner H, Bartram CR. Treatment of Ph-positive acute lymphoblastic leukemia with alpha-interferon. Leukemia 1988;2:555.

113. Okabe M, Kuni-eda Y, Sugiwura T, et al. Inhibitory effect of interleukin-4 on the in vitro growth of Ph1-positive acute lymphoblastic leukemia cells. Blood 1991;78:1574–80.

114. Messinger Y, Chen LL, O'Neil K, et al. Treatment of therapy-refractory B-lineage acute lymphoblastic leukemia with an apoptosis-inducing-CD19-directed tyrosine kinase inhibitor [abstract]. Blood 1999;94:1317.

115. Druker BJ, Kantarjian HM, Sawyers C, et al. Activity of an abl specific tyrosine kinase inhibitor in patients with bcr-abl positive acute myelogenous leukemia in blast crisis [abstract]. Blood 1999;94:3082.

116. Haskell CM, Canellos GP, Leventhal BG, et al. L-Asparaginase: therapeutic and toxic effects in patients with neoplastic disease. N Engl J Med 1969;281:1028–34.

117. Jones B, Holland JF, Glidewell O, et al. Optimal use of L-asparaginase (NSC-109229) in acute lymphocytic leukemia. Med Pediatr Oncol 1977;3:387–400.

118. Nesbit ME, Ertel I, Hammond DG, et al. L-Asparaginase as a single agent in acute lymphoblastic leukemia: survey of studies from Children's Cancer Study Group. Cancer Treat Rep 1981;65:101–7.

119. Priest JR, Ramsay NK, Latchaw RE, et al. Thrombotic and hemorrhagic strokes complicating early therapy for childhood acute lymphoblastic leukemia. Cancer 1980;46:1548–54.

120. Priest JR, Ramsay NK, Steinherz PG, et al. A syndrome of thrombosis and hemorrhage complicating L-asparaginase therapy for childhood acute lymphoblastic leukemia. J Pediatr 1982;100:984–9.

121. Barbui T, Rodeghiero F, Meli S, et al. Fatal pulmonary embolism and antithrombin III deficiency in adult lymphoblastic leukemia during L-asparaginase therapy. Acta Haematol 1983;69:188–91.

122. Legnani C, Palareti G, Pession A, et al. Intravascular coagulation phenomena associated with prevalent fall in fibrinogen and plasminogen during L-asparaginase treatment in leukemic children. Haemostasis 1988;18:179–86.

123. Andrew M, Brooker L, Mitchell L. Acquired antithrombin III deficiency secondary to asparaginase therapy in childhood acute lymphoblastic leukemia. Blood Coagul Fibrinolysis 1994;5:S24–36.

124. Sarris A, Cortes J, Kantarjian H, et al. Disseminated intravascular coagulation in adult acute lymphoblastic leukemia: frequent complications with fibrinogen levels less than 100 mg/dl. Leuk Lymphoma 1996;1:85–92.

125. Alberts SR, Bretscher M, Wiltsie JC, et al. Thrombosis related to the use of L-asparaginase in adults with acute lymphoblastic leukemia: a need to consider coagulation monitoring and clotting factor replacement. Leuk Lymphoma 1999;32:489–96.

126. Bushman JE, Palmieri D, Whinna HC, Church FC. Insight into the mechanism of asparaginase-induced depletion of antithrombin III in treatment of childhood acute lymphoblastic leukemia. Leuk Res 2000;24:559–65.

127. Rai KR, Holland JF, Glidewell OJ, et al. Treatment of acute myelocytic leukemia: A study by Cancer and Leukemia Group B. Blood 1981;58:1203–12.

128. Yates J, Glidewell O, Wiernik P, et al. Cytosine arabinoside with daunorubicin or Adriamycin for therapy of acute myelocytic leukemia: a CALGB study. Blood 1982;60:454–62.

129. Priesler HD, Anderson K, Rai K, et al. The frequency of long-term remission in patients with acute myelogenous leukemia treated with conventional maintenance chemotherapy: a study of 760 patients with a minimum follow-up of 6-years. Br J Haematol 1989;71:189–94.

130. Bandini G, Zuffa E, Rosti G, et al. Long-term outcome of adults with acute myelogenous leukemia: results of a prospective randomized study of chemotherapy with a minimal follow-up of 7 years. Br J Haematol 1991;77:486–90.

131. Rowe JM, Andersen J, Cassileth PA, et al. Clinical trials of adults with acute myelogenous leukemia: experience of the Eastern Cooperative Oncology Group. In: Hiddemann W, Buchner T, Wormann B, et al., editors. Acute leukemia IV: experimental approaches and novel therapies. Berlin: Springer-Verlag; 1994. p. 542.

132. Bennett JM, Young ML, Andersen JW, et al. Long-term survival in acute myeloid leukemia: the Eastern Cooperative Oncology Group experience. Cancer 1997;80:2205–9.

133. Mayer RJ, Davis RB, Schiffer CA, et al. For the Cancer and Leukemia Group B: intensive postremission chemotherapy in adults with acute myeloid leukemia. N Engl J Med 1994;331:896–903.

134. Bennett JM, Catovsky D, Daniel MT, et al. Proposals for the classification of the acute leukemias. Br J Haematol 1976;33:451–8.

135. Bennet JM, Catovsky D, Daniel MT, et al. Proposed revised criteria for the classification of acute myeloid leukemia. A report from the French-American-British Group. Ann Intern Med 1985;103:620–5.

136. Harris NL, Jaffe ES, Diebold J, et al. World Heath Organization classification of neoplastic diseases of the hematopoietic and lymphoid tissues: Report of the Clinical Advisory Committee meeting—Airlie House, Virginia, November 1997. J Clin Oncol 1999;17:3835–49.

137. Baudard M, Beau Champ-Nicoud A, Delmer A, et al. Has the prognosis of adult patients with acute myeloid leukemia improved over years? A single institution experience of > 784 consecutive patients over a 16-year period. Leukemia 1999;13:1481–90.

138. Freireich E. Arabinosyl cytosine: a 20-year update. J Clin Oncol 1987;5:523–4.

139. Coltman CA, Freireich EJ, Pendleton O, et al. Adult acute leukemia studies using cytarabine: early Southwest Oncology Group trials. Med Pediatr Oncol 1982;10:173–83.

140. Weil M, Glidewell OJ, Jacquillat C, et al. Daunorubicin in the therapy of acute granulocytic leukemia. Cancer Res 1973;33:921–8.

141. Preisler H, Davis RB, Kirshner J, et al. Comparison of three remission induction regimens and two postre-mission strategies for the treatment of acute non-lymphocytic leukemia: a Cancer and Leukemia Group B Study. Blood 1987;69:1441–9.

142. Dillman RO, Davis RB, Green MR, et al. A comparative study of two different doses of cytarabine for acute myeloid leukemia: a phase III study of Cancer and Leukemia Group B. Blood 1991;78:2520–6.

143. Rowe JM, Tallman MS. Intensifying induction therapy in acute myeloid leukemia: has a new standard of care emerged? Blood 1997;90:2121–6.

144. Speth PA, Minderman H, Haanen C. Idarubicin vs daunorubicin: preclinical and clinical pharmacokinetic studies. Semin Oncol 1989;16:2–9.

145. Curtis JE, Minden MD, Minkin S, et al. Sensitivities of AML blast stem cells to idarubicin and daunorubicin: a comparison with normal hematopoietic progenitors. Leukemia 1995;9:396–404.

146. Ross D, Tang Y, Comblatt B. Idarubicin (IDA) is less vulnerable to transport-mediated multidrug resistance (MDR) than its metabolite idarubicin (IDA-ol) or daunorubicin [abstract]. Blood 1993;10:1015.

147. Roovers DJ, van Vliet M, Bloem AC, et al. Idarubicin overcomes P-glycoprotein-related multidrug resistance: comparison with doxorubicin and daunorubicin in human multiple myeloma cell lines. Leuk Res 1999;23:539–48.

148. Berman E, Heller G, Santorsa J, et al. Results of a randomized trial comparing idarubicin and cytosine arabinoside with daunorubicin and cytosine arabinoside in adult patients with newly diagnosed acute myelogenous leukemia. Blood 1991;77:1666–74.

149. Wiernik PH, Banks PL, Case DC Jr, et al. Cytarabine plus idarubicin or daunorubicin as induction and consolidation therapy for previously untreated adult patients with acute myeloid leukemia. Blood 1992;79:313–9.

150. Vogler WR, Velez-Garcia E, Weiner RS, et al. A phase III trial comparing idarubicin and daunorubicin in combination with cytarabine in acute myelogenous leukemia: a Southeastern Cancer Study Group study. J Clin Oncol 1992;10:1103–11.

151. Mandelli F, Petti MC, Ardia A, et al. A randomized clinical trial comparing idarubicin and cytarabine to daunorubicin and cytarabine in the treatment of acute non-lymphoid leukaemia. A multicentric study from the Italian Co-operative Group GIMEMA. Eur J Cancer 1991;27:750–5.

152. Usui N, Dohashi N, Kobayashi T, et al. Role of daunorubicin in the induction therapy for adult acute myeloid leukemia. J Clin Oncol 1998;16:2086–92.

153. The AML Collaborative Group. A systematic collaborative overview of randomized trials comparing idarubicin with daunorubicin (or other anthracycline) as induction therapy for acute myeloid leukemia. Br J Haematol 1998;103:100–9.

154. Grant S, Arlin Z, Gewirtz D. Effect of pharmacologically relevant concentrations of mitoxantrone or the in vitro growth of leukemic blast progenitors. Leukemia 1991;5:336–9.

155. Arlin Z, Case DC Jr, Moore J, et al. Randomized multicenter trial of cytosine arabinoside with mitoxantrone or daunorubicin in previously untreated adult patients with acute nonlymphocytic leukemia (ANLL). Leukemia 1990;4:177–83.

156. Wahlin A, Hornsten P, Hedenus M, et al. Mitoxantrone and cytarabine versus daunorubicin and cytarabine in previously untreated patients with acute myeloid leukemia. Cancer Chemother Pharmacol 1991;28: 480–3.

157. Pavlovsky S, Gonzalez-Llaven J, Garcia-Martinez MA, et al. A randomized study of mitoxantrone plus cytarabine versus daunorubicin plus cytarabine in the treatment of previously untreated adult patients with acute nonlymphocytic leukemia. Ann Hematol 1994;60:11–5.

158. Hansen OP, Pedersen-Bjergaard J, Ellegaard J, et al. Aclarubicin plus cytosine arabinoside versus daunorubicin plus cytosine arabinoside in previously untreated patients with acute myeloid leukemia: a Danish national phase III trial. The Danish Society of Hematology Study Group on AML, Denmark. Leukemia 1991;5:510–6.

159. Berman E, Arlin ZA, Gaynor J, et al. Comparative trial of cytarabine and thioguanine in combination with amsacrine or daunorubicin in patients with untreated acute nonlymphocytic leukemia: results of the L-16M protocol. Leukemia 1989;3:115–21.

160. Buchner T, Hiddemann W, Wormann B, et al. Daunorubicin 60 instead of 30 mg/sqm improves response and survival in elderly patients with AML [abstract]. Blood 1997;90:2596.

161. Feldman E, Seiter K, Damon L, et al. A randomized trial of high versus standard-dose mitoxantrone with cytarabine in elderly patients with acute myeloid leukemia. Leukemia 1997;11:485–9.

162. Rowe JM, Neuberg D, Friedenberg W, et al. A phase III study of daunorubicin vs idarubicin vs mitoxantrone for older adult patients (> 55 years) with acute myelogenous leukemia (AML) [abstract]. A study of the Eastern Cooperative Oncology Group (E3993). Blood 1998;92:1284.

163. Löwenberg B, Suciu S, Archimbaud E, et al. Mitoxantrone versus daunorubicin in induction-consolidation chemotherapy—the value of low-dose cytarabine for maintenance of remission, and an assessment of prognostic factors in acute myeloid leukemia in the elderly: final report. European Organization for the Research and Treatment of Cancer and the Dutch-Belgian Hemto-Oncology Cooperative HOVON Group. J Clin Oncol 1998;16:872–81.

164. Zittoun R, Suici S, Dewitte T, et al. Comparison of three intercalating agents in induction and consolidation in acute myelogenous leukemia (AML) followed by autologous or allogeneic transplantation. Preliminary results of the EORTC-GIMEMA AML-10 randomized trial [abstract]. Blood 1999;94:2923.

165. Schiller G, Gajewski J, Nimer S, et al. A randomized study of intermediate-dose cytarabine as intensive induction for acute myelogenous leukemia. Br J Haematol 1992;81:170–7.

166. Bishop JF, Matthews JP, Young GA, et al. A randomized trial of high-dose cytarabine in induction in acute myeloid leukemia. Blood 1996;87:1710–7.

167. Weick JK, Kopecky KJ, Appelbaum DR, et al. A randomized investigation of high-dose versus standard-dose cytosine arabinoside with daunorubicin in patients with previously untreated acute myeloid leukemia: a Southwest Oncology Group Study. Blood 1996;88:2841–51.

168. Bishop JF, Lowenthal RM, Joshua D, et al. Etoposide in acute nonlymphocytic leukemia: Australian Leukemia Study Group. Blood 1990;75:27–32.

169. Bishop JF, Matthews JP, Young GA, et al. Intensified induction chemotherapy with high-dose cytarabine and etoposide for acute myeloid leukemia: a review and updated results from the Australian Leukemia Study Group [review]. Leuk Lymphoma 1998;28: 315–27.

170. Hann IM, Stevens RF, Goldstone AH, et al. Randomized comparison of DAT versus ADE as induction chemotherapy in children and younger adults with acute myeloid leukemia. Results of the Medical Research Council's 10th AML Trial (MRC AML10). Blood 1997;89:2311–8.

171. Mitus AJ, Miller KB, Schenkien DP, et al. Improved survival for patients with an acute myelogenous leukemia. J Clin Oncol 1995;13:560–9.

172. Cassileth PA, Lee SJ, Miller KB, et al. Feasibility study of adding high-dose cytarabine (HDAC) in induction (IND) and in consolidation (CONS) before autologous stem cell transplant (ASCT) in adult acute myeloid leukemia (AML) [abstract]. Blood 1998;92:4559.

173. Petersdorf S, Rankin C, Terebolu H, et al. A phase II study of standard dose daunomycin and cytosine arabinoside (Ara-C) with high-dose Ara-C induction therapy followed by sequential high-dose Ara-C consolidation for adults with previously untreated acute myelogenous leukemia: a Southwest Oncology Group study (SWOG 9500) [abstract]. Proc Am Soc Clin Oncol 1998;17:55.

174. Buchner T, Hiddemann W, Wormann B, et al. Double induction strategy for acute myeloid leukemia: the effect of high-dose cytarabine with mitoxantrone instead of standard-dose cytarabine with daunoru-

bicin and 6-thioguanine: a randomized trial by the German AML Cooperative Group. Blood 1999;93: 4116–24.

175. Buchner T, Hiddemann W, Koenigsmann M, et al. Recombinant human granulocyte-macrophage colony-stimulating factor after chemotherapy in patients with acute myeloid leukemia at higher age or after relapse. Blood 1991;78:1190–7.

176. Rowe JM, Andersen J, Mazza JJ, et al. A randomized placebo-controlled study of granulocyte-macrophage colony stimulating factor in adult patients (> 55–70 years of age) with acute myelogenous leukemia (AML): a study of the Eastern Cooperative Oncology Group (E1490). Blood 1995;86:457–62.

177. Dombret H, Chastang C, Fenaux P, et al. A controlled study of recombinant human granulocyte colony-stimulating factor in elderly patents after treatment for acute myelogenous leukemia. N Engl J Med 1995;332:1678–83.

178. Heil G, Hoelzer D, Sanz MA, et al. A randomized, double-blind, placebo-controlled, phase III study of filgrastim in remission induction and consolidation therapy for adults with de novo acute myeloid leukemia. Blood 1997;90:4710–8.

179. Godwin JR, Kopecky KJ, Head DR, et al. A double-blind placebo-controlled trial of granulocyte colony-stimulating factor in elderly patients with previously untreated acute myeloid leukemia: a Southwest Oncology Group Study (903). Blood 1998;91:3607–15.

180. Stone RM, Berg DT, George SL, et al. for the Cancer and Leukemia Group B. Granulocyte-macrophage colony-stimulating factor after initial chemotherapy for elderly patients with primary acute myelogenous leukemia. N Engl J Med 1995;332:1671–7.

181. Zittoun R, Suciu S, Mandelli F, et al. Granulocyte-macrophage colony-stimulating factor associated with induction treatment of acute myelogenous leukemia. A randomized trial by the European Organization for Research and Treatment of Cancer and Leukemia Cooperative Groups. J Clin Oncol 1996;14:2150–9.

182. Löwenberg B, Suciu S, Archimbaud E, et al. Use of recombinant GM-CSF during and after remission induction chemotherapy in patients aged 61 years and older with acute myeloid leukemia: final report of AML-11, a phase III randomized study of the Leukemia Cooperative Group of the European Organization for the Research and Treatment of Cancer and the Dutch-Belgium Hemato-Oncology Cooperative Group. Blood 1997;90:2952–61.

183. Link H, Wandt H, Schonrock-Nabulski P, et al. G-CSF (Lenograstim) after chemotherapy for acute myeloid leukemia: a placebo controlled trial [abstract]. Blood 1996;88:2654.

184. Goldstone AH, Burnett AK, Milligan DW, et al. Lack of

benefit of G-CSF on complete remission and possible increased relapse risk in AML: an MRC study of 800 patients [abstract]. Blood 1997;90:2595.

185. Witz F, Harousseau JL, Sadoun A, et al. GM-CSF during and after remission induction treatment for elderly patients with acute myeloid leukemia (AML). Hematol Blood Transfus 1997;40:852–6.

186. Schiffer CA. Hematopoietic growth factors as adjuncts to the treatment of acute myeloid leukemia. Blood 1996;88:3675–85.

187. Cassileth PA, Harrington DP, Hines JD, et al. Maintenance chemotherapy prolongs remission duration in adult acute nonlymphocytic leukemia. J Clin Oncol 1988;6:583–7.

188. Buchner T, Hiddemann W, Wormann B, et al. Late events in AML. Data from long-term observation of patients in two trials starting in 1981 and 1985 [abstract]. Blood 1997;90:2247.

189. Rees JKH, Gray RG, Wheatley K. Dose intensification in acute myeloid leukaemia: greater effectiveness at lower cost. Principal report of the Medical Research Council's AML9 Study. Br J Haematol 1996;94: 89–98.

190. Cassileth P, Lynch E, Hines JD, et al. Varying intensity of post-remission therapy in acute myeloid leukemia. Blood 1992;79:1924–30.

191. Fopp M, Fey MF, Bacchi M, et al. Post-remission therapy of adult acute myeloid leukemia: one cycle of high-dose versus standard-dose cytarabine. Ann Oncol 1997;8:251.

192. Tallman MS, Appelbaum FR, Amos D, et al. Evaluation of intensive consolidation therapy for adults with acute nonlymphocytic leukemia using high-dose cytosine arabinoside with asparaginase and amsacrine with etoposide. J Clin Oncol 1987;5:918–26.

193. Burnett AK, Goldstone AH, Stevens RM, et al. Randomized comparison of addition of autologous bone-marrow transplantation to intensive chemotherapy for acute myeloid leukaemia in first remission: results of MRC AML10 trial. Lancet 1998;351: 700–8.

194. Elonen E, Almqvist A, Hanninen A, et al. Comparison between four and eight cycles of intensive chemotherapy in adult acute myeloid leukemia: a randomized trial of the Finnish Leukemia Group. Leukemia 1998;12:1041–8.

195. Thomas ED, Buckner CD, Clift RA, et al. Marrow transplantation for acute nonlymphoblastic leukemia in first remission. N Engl J Med 1979;301:579–99.

196. Appelbaum FR, Dahlberg S, Thomas ED, et al. Bone marrow transplantation or chemotherapy after remission induction for adults with acute nonlymphoblastic leukemia: a prospective comparison. Ann Intern Med 1984;101:581–8.

197. Champlin RE, Ho WG, Gale RP, et al. Treatment of

acute myelogenous leukemia. A prospective controlled trial of bone marrow transplantation versus consolidation chemotherapy. Ann Intern Med 1985;102:285–91.

198. McGlave PB, Haake RJ, Bostrom BC, et al. Allogeneic bone marrow transplantation for acute nonlymphocytic leukemia in first remission. Blood 1988;72:1512–7.

199. Ferrant A, Doyen C, Delannoy A, et al. Allogeneic or autologous bone marrow transplantation in acute nonlymphocytic leukemia in first remission. Bone Marrow Transplant 1991;7:303–9.

200. Appelbaum FR, Fisher LD, Thomas ED. Chemotherapy v marrow transplantation for adults with acute nonlymphocytic leukemia: a five-year follow-up. Blood 1988;72:179–84.

201. Geller RB, Saral R, Piantadosi S, et al. Allogeneic bone marrow transplantation after high-dose busulfan and cyclophosphamide in patients with acute nonlymphocytic leukemia. Blood 1989;73:2209–18.

202. Forman SJ, Krance RA, O'Donnell MR, et al. Bone marrow transplantation for acute nonlymphoblastic leukemia during first complete remission. An analysis of prognostic factors. Transplantation 1987;43:650–3.

203. Young JW, Papadopoulos EB, Cunningham I, et al. T-cell depleted allogeneic bone marrow transplantation in adults with acute nonlymphoblastic leukemia in first remission. Blood 1992;79:3380–7.

204. Schiller GJ, Nimer SD, Territo MC, et al. Bone marrow transplantation versus high-dose cytarabine-based consolidation chemotherapy for acute myelogenous leukemia in first remission. J Clin Oncol 1992;10:41–6.

205. Fagioli F, Bacigalupo A, Frassoni F, et al. Allogeneic bone marrow transplantation for acute myeloid leukemia in first complete remission: the effect of FAB classification and GVHD prophylaxis. Bone Marrow Transplant 1994;13:247–57.

206. Mehta J, Powles R, Treleaven J, et al. Long-term follow-up of patients undergoing allogeneic bone marrow transplantation for acute myeloid leukemia in first complete remission after cyclosphosphamide-total body irradiation and cyclosporine. Bone Marrow Transplant 1996;18:741–6.

207. Keating S, Suciu S, de Witte T, et al. Prognostic factors of patients with acute myeloid leukemia (AML) allografted in first complete remission: an analysis of the EORTC GIMEMA AML 8A Trial. Bone Marrow Transplant 1996;17:993–1001.

208. Labar B, Masszi T, Morabito F, et al. Allogeneic bone marrow transplantation for acute leukemia—IGCI experience. Bone Marrow Transplant 1996;17:1009–12.

209. Reiffers J, Stoppa AM, Attal M, et al. Allogeneic vs autologous stem cell transplantation vs chemotherapy in patients with acute myeloid leukemia in first complete remission: the BGMT 87 Study. Leukemia 1996;10:1874–82.

210. Ferrant A, Doyen C, Delannoy A, et al. Karyotype in acute myeloblastic leukemia: prognostic significance in a prospective study assessing bone marrow transplantation in first remission. Bone Marrow Transplant 1995;15:685–90.

211. Soiffer RJ, Fairclough D, Robertson M, et al. CD6-depleted allogeneic bone marrow transplantation for acute leukemia in first complete remission. Blood 1997;89:3039–47.

212. Papadapoulos EB, Carabasi MH, Castro-Malaspina H, et al. T-cell-depleted allogeneic bone marrow transplantation as postremission therapy for acute myelogenous leukemia: freedom from relapse in the absence of graft-versus-host disease. Blood 1998;91:1083–90.

213. Aversa F, Terenzi A, Carotti A, et al. Improved outcome with T-cell-depleted bone marrow transplantation for acute leukemia. J Clin Oncol 1999;17:1545–50.

214. Giralt S, Estey E, Albitar M, et al. Engraftment of allogeneic hematopoietic progenitor cells with purine analog-containing chemotherapy: harnessing graft-versus-leukemia without myeloablative therapy. Blood 1997;89:4531–6.

215. Slavin S, Nagler A, Naparstek E, et al. Nonmyeloablative stem cell transplantation and cell therapy as an alternative to conventional bone marrow transplantation with lethal cytoreduction for the treatment of malignant and nonmalignant hematologic diseases. Blood 1998;91:756–63.

216. Georges GE, Storb R, Thompson JD, et al. Adoptive immunotherapy in canine mixed chimeras after nonmyeloablative hematopoietic cell transplantation. Blood 2000;95:3262–9.

217. Gale RP, Horowitz MM, Weiner RS, et al. Impact of cytogenetic abnormalities on outcome of bone marrow transplants in acute myelogenous leukemia in first remission. Bone Marrow Transplant 1995;16:203–8.

218. Anderson JE, Gooley TA, Schoch G, et all. Stem cell transplantation for secondary acute myeloid leukemia: evaluation of transplantation as initial therapy or following induction chemotherapy. Blood 1997;89:2578–85.

219. Tallman MS, Rowlings PA, Milone G, et al. Effect of postremission chemotherapy prior to HLA-identical sibling transplantation for acute myelogenous leukemia in first complete remission. Blood 2000;96:1254–8.

220. Cahn Y, Labopin M, Gorin NC. Impact of cytosine arabinoside (Ara-C) dose given at induction or consolidation before allogeneic or autologous stem cell transplantation (SCT) for acute myeloblastic leukemia in first remission [abstract]. Blood 1997;90:1002.

221. Gale RP, Horowitz MM, Rees JKH, et al. Chemotherapy versus transplants for acute myeloid leukemia in second remission. Leukemia 1996;10:13–9.

222. Tomas JF, Gomez-Garcia de Soria V, Lopez-Lorenzo JL, et al. Autologous or allogeneic bone marrow transplantation for acute myeloid leukemia in second complete remission. Importance of duration of first complete remission in final outcome. Bone Marrow Transplant 1996;17:979–84.

223. Berman E, Little C, Gee T, et al. Reasons that patients with acute myelogenous leukemia do not undergo allogeneic bone marrow transplantation. N Engl J Med 1992;326:156–60.

224. Gamberi B, Bandini G, Visani G, et al. Acute myeloid leukemia from diagnosis to bone marrow transplantation: experience from a single center. Bone Marrow Transplant 1994;14:69–72.

225. Rizzoli V, Mangoni L, Carlo-Stella C. Autologous bone marrow transplantation in acute myelogenous leukemia [review]. Leukemia 1992;6:1101–6.

226. Gorin NC. Autologous stem cell transplantation in acute myelocytic leukemia. Blood 1998;92:1073–90.

227. Gorin NC, Herve P, Aegerter P, et al. Autologous bone marrow transplantation for acute leukaemia in remission. Br J Haematol 1986;64:385–95.

228. Gorin NC, Labopin M, Meloni G, et al. Autologous bone marrow transplantation for acute myeloid leukemia in Europe: further evidence of the role of marrow purging by mafosfamide. Leukemia 1991;5:896–904.

229. Gulati S, Acaba L, Yahalom J, et al. Autologous bone marrow transplantation for acute myelogenous leukemia using 4-hydroperoxycyclophosphamide and VP-16 purged bone marrow. Bone Marrow Transplant 1992;10:129–34.

230. Cassileth PA, Andersen J, Lazarus HM, et al. Autologous bone marrow transplant in acute myeloid leukemia in first remission. J Clin Oncol 1993;11:314–9.

231. Linker CA, Ries CA, Damon LE, et al. Autologous bone marrow transplantation for acute myeloid leukemia using busulfan plus etoposide as a preparative regimen. Blood 1993;81:311–8.

232. Sanz MA, de la Rubia J, Sanz GF, et al. Busulfan plus cyclophosphamide followed by autologous blood stem-cell transplantation for patients with acute myeloid leukemia in first complete remission: a report from a single institution. J Clin Oncol 1993; 11:1661–7.

233. Sierra J, Grañena A, Garcia J, et al. Autologous bone marrow transplantation for acute leukemia: results and prognostic factors in 90 consecutive patients. Bone Marrow Transplant 1993;12:517–23.

234. Laporte J, Douay L, Lopez M, et al. One hundred twenty-five adult patients with primary acute leukemia autografted with marrow purged by mafosfamide: a 10-year single institution experience. Blood 1994;84:3810–8.

235. Cahn JY, Labopin M, Mandelli F, et al. Autologous bone marrow transplantation for first remission acute myeloblastic leukemia in patients older than 50 years: a retrospective analysis of the European Bone Marrow Transplant Group. Blood 1995;85:575–9.

236. Miggiano MC, Gherlinzoni F, Rosti G, et al. Autologous bone marrow transplantation in late first complete remission improves outcome in acute myelogenous leukemia. Leukemia 1996;10:402–9.

237. Stein AS, O'Donnell MR, Chai A, et al. In vivo purging with high-dose cytarabine followed by high-dose chemoradiotherapy and reinfusion of unpurged bone marrow for adult acute myelogenous leukemia in first complete remission. J Clin Oncol 1996;14:2206–16.

238. Schiller G, Lee M, Miller T, et al. Transplantation of autologous peripheral blood progenitor cells procured after high-dose cytarabine-based consolidation chemotherapy for adults with acute myelogenous leukemia in first remission. Leukemia 1997; 11:1533–9.

239. Gondo H, Harada M, Miyamoto T, et al. Autologous peripheral blood stem cell transplantation for acute myelogenous leukemia. Bone Marrow Transplant 1997;20:821–6.

240. Martin C, Torres A, Leon A, et al. Autologous peripheral blood stem cell transplantation (PBSCT) mobilized with G-CSF in AML in first complete remission. Role of intensification therapy in outcome. Bone Marrow Transplant 1998;21:375–82.

241. Visani G, Lemoli RM, Tosi P, et al. Use of peripheral blood stem cells for autologous transplantation in acute myeloid leukemia patients allows faster engraftment and equivalent disease-free survival compared with bone marrow cells. Bone Marrow Transplant 1999;24:467–72.

242. Löwenberg B, Verdonck LJ, Dekker AW, et al. Autologous bone marrow transplantation in acute myeloid leukemia in first remission: results of a Dutch prospective study. J Clin Oncol 1990;2:287–94.

243. Zittoun RA, Mandelli F, Willemze R, et al. Autologous or allogeneic bone marrow transplantation compared with intensive chemotherapy in acute myeloid leukemia. N Engl J Med 1995;332:217–23.

244. Cassileth P, Harrington D, Appelbaum FR, et al. Chemotherapy compared with autologous or allogeneic bone marrow transplantation in the management of acute myeloid leukemia in first remission. N Engl J Med 1998;339:1649–56.

245. Harousseau J-L, Cahn JY, Pignon B, et al. Comparison of autologous bone marrow transplantation and intensive chemotherapy as postremission therapy in adult acute myeloid leukemia. Blood 1997;90:2978–86.

246. Wagner JE, Rosenthal J, Sweetman R, et al. Successful transplantation of HLA-matched and HLA-mismatched umbilical cord blood from unrelated

donors: analysis of engraftment and acute graft-versus-host disease. Blood 1996;88:795–802.

247. Gluckman E, Rocha V, Boyer-Chammard A, et al. Outcome of cord-blood transplantation from related and unrelated donors. Eurocord Transplant Group and the European Blood and Marrow Transplantation Group. N Engl J Med 1997;337:373–81.

248. Rubinstein P, Carrier C, Scaradavou A, et al. Outcomes among 562 recipients of placental-blood transplants from unrelated donors. N Engl J Med 1998;339:1565–77.

249. Rocha V, Wagner JE, Sobocinski KA, et al. Graft-versus-host disease in children who have received a cord-blood or bone marrow transplant from an HLA-identical sibling. N Engl J Med 2000;342:1846–54.

250. Parker P, Chao N, Nademanee A, et al. Thalidomide as salvage therapy for chronic graft-versus-host disease. Blood 1995;89:3604–9.

251. Bensinger WI, Clift R, Martin P, et al. Allogeneic peripheral blood stem cell transplantation in patients with advanced hematologic malignancies: a retrospective comparison with marrow transplantation. Blood 1996;88:2794–800.

252. Glass B, Uharek L, Zeis M, et al. Allogeneic peripheral blood progenitor cell transplantation in a murine model: evidence for an improved graft-versus-leukemia effect. Blood 1997;90:1694–700.

253. Brown RA, Adkins D, Khoury H, et al. Long-term follow-up of high-risk allogeneic peripheral-blood stem-cell transplant recipients: graft-versus-host disease and transplant-related mortality. J Clin Oncol 1999;17:806–12.

254. Cornelissen JJ, Fibbe W, Schattenberg AV, et al. A retrospective Dutch study comparing T cell-depleted allogeneic blood stem cell transplantation vs T cell-depleted allogeneic bone marrow transplantation. Bone Marrow Transplant 1998;21(Suppl 3):S66–70.

255. Cahn JY, Labopin M, Schattenberg A, et al. Allogeneic bone marrow transplantation for acute leukemia in patients over the age of 40 years. Acute Leukemia Working Party of the European Group for Bone Marrow Transplantation (EBMT). Leukemia 1997;11:416–9.

256. Byrd JC, Dodge RK, Carroll A, et al. Patients with t(8;21) (q22;q22) and acute myeloid leukemia have superior failure-free and overall survival when repetitive cycles of high-dose cytarabine are administered. J Clin Oncol 1999;17:3767–75.

257. Huang ME, Ye YC, Chen SR, et al. Use of all-trans retinoic acid in the treatment of acute promyelocytic leukemia. Blood 1988;72:567–72.

258. Castaigne S, Chomienne C, Daniel MT, et al. All-trans retinoic acid as a differentiation therapy for acute promyelocytic leukemia. I. Clinical results. Blood 1990;76:1704–9.

259. Warrell RP Jr, Miller WH Jr, Scheinberg DA, et al. Differentiation therapy of acute promyelocytic leukemia with tretinoin (all-trans-retinoic acid). N Engl J Med 1991;324:1385–93.

260. Fenaux P, Castaigne S, Dombret H, et al. All-trans-retinoic acid followed by intensive chemotherapy gives a high complete remission rate and may prolong remissions in newly diagnosed acute promyelocytic leukemia: a pilot study on 26 cases. Blood 1992;80:2176–81.

261. Chen ZX, Xue YQ, Zhang R, et al. A clinical and experimental study on all-trans retinoic acid-treated acute promyelocytic leukemia patients. Blood 1991;78:1413–9.

262. Kanamaru A, Takemoto Y, Tanimoto M, et al. All-trans retinoic acid for the treatment of newly diagnosed acute promyelocytic leukemia. Japan Adult Leukemia Study Group. Blood 1995;85:1202–6.

263. Ohno R, Yoshida H, Fukutani H, et al. Multi-institutional study of all-trans-retinoic acid as a differentiation therapy of refractory acute promyelocytic leukemia. Leukaemia Study Group of the Ministry of Health and Welfare. Leukemia 1993;7:1722–7.

264. Avvisati G, Lo Coco F, Diverio D, et al. AIDA (all-trans retinoic acid + idarubicin) in newly diagnosed acute promyelocytic leukemia: a Gruppo Italiano Malattie Ematologiche Maligne dell'Adulto (GIMEMA) pilot study. Blood 1996;88:1390–8.

265. Mandelli F, Diverio D, Avvisati G, et al. Molecular remission in PML/RARα-positive acute promyelocytic leukemia by combined all-trans retinoic acid and idarubicin (AIDA). Blood 1997;90:1014–21.

266. Sanz MA, Martin G, Rayon C, et al. A modified AIDA protocol with anthracycline-based consolidation results in high antileukemic efficacy and reduced toxicity in newly diagnosed PML/RARalpha-positive acute promyelocytic leukemia. PETHEMA group. Blood 1999;94:3015–21.

267. Asou N, Adachi K, Tamura J, et al. Analysis of prognostic factors in newly diagnosed acute promyelocytic leukemia treated with all-trans-retinoic acid and chemotherapy. Japan Adult Leukemia Study Group. J Clin Oncol 1998;16:78–85.

268. Fenaux P, Le Deley MC, Castaigne S, et al. Effect of all trans-retinoic acid in newly diagnosed acute promyelocytic leukemia. Results of a multicenter randomized trial. European APL 91 Group. Blood 1993;82:3241–9.

269. Tallman MS, Andersen JW, Schiffer CA, et al. All-trans retinoic acid in acute promyelocytic leukemia. N Engl J Med 1997;337:1021–8.

270. De Botton S, Dombret H, Sanz M, et al. Incidence, clinical features, and outcome of all-trans-retinoic acid syndrome in 413 cases of newly diagnosed acute promyelocytic leukemia. Blood 1998;92:2712–8.

271. Tallman MS, Andersen JW, Schiffer CA, et al. Clinical description of 44 patients with acute promyelocytic leukemia who developed the retinoic acid syndrome. Blood 2000;95:90–5.

272. Vahdat L, Maslak P, Miller WH Jr, et al. Early mortality and the retinoic acid syndrome in acute promyelocytic leukemia: impact of leukocytosis, low-dose chemotherapy, PMN/RAR-alpha isoform, and CD13 expression in patients treated with all-trans retinoic acid. Blood 1994;84:3843–9.

273. Fenaux P, Chastang C, Chevret S, et al. A randomized comparison of all trans-retinoic acid (ATRA) followed by chemotherapy and ATRA plus chemotherapy and the role of maintenance therapy in newly diagnosed acute promyelocytic leukemia. The European APL Group. Blood 1999;94:1192–200.

274. Burnett AK, Grimwade D, Solomon E, et al. Presenting white blood cell count and kinetics of molecular remission predict prognosis in acute promyelocytic leukemia treated with all-trans retinoic acid: results of the randomized MRC trial. Blood 1999;93:4131–43.

275. Lo Coco F, Diverio D, Avvisati G, et al. Therapy of molecular relapse in acute promyelocytic leukemia. Blood 1999;94:2225–9.

276. Thomas X, Dombret H, Cordonnier C, et al. Treatment of relapsing acute promyelocytic leukemia by all-trans retinoic acid therapy followed by timed sequential chemotherapy and stem cell transplantation. APL Study Group. Acute promyelocytic leukemia. Leukemia 2000;14:1006–13.

277. Zhang P, Wang SY, Hu XH, et al. Arsenic trioxide treated 72 cases of acute promyelocytic leukemia. Chin J Haematol 1996;17:58–60.

278. Shen Z-X, Chen G-Q, Ni J-H, et al. Use of arsenic trioxide (As2O3) in the treatment of acute promyelocytic leukemia (APL) II. Clinical efficacy and pharmacokinetics in relapsed patients. Blood 1997;89:3354–60.

279. Soignet SL, Maslak P, Wang Z-G, et al. Complete remission after treatment of acute promyelocytic leukemia with arsenic trioxide. N Engl J Med 1998;339:1341–8.

280. Niu C, Yan H, Yu T, et al. Studies on treatment of acute promyelocytic leukemia with arsenic trioxide: remission induction, follow-up, and molecular monitoring in 11 newly diagnosed and 47 relapsed acute promyelocytic leukemia patients. Blood 1999;94:3315–24.

281. Soignet SL, Frankel S, Tallman M, et al. US multicenter trial of arsenic trioxide (AT) in acute promyelocytic leukemia (APL) [abstract]. Blood 1999;94:698a.

282. Chen GQ, Zhu J, Shi XG, et al. In vitro studies on cellular and molecular mechanisms of arsenic trioxide (As2O3) in the treatment of acute promyelocytic leukemia: As2O3 induces NB4 cell apoptosis with downregulation of Bcl-2 expression and modulation of PML-RAR alpha/PML proteins. Blood 1996;8:1052–61.

283. Akao Y, Mizoguchi H, Kojima S, et al. Arsenic induces apoptosis in B-cell leukaemic cell lines in vitro: activation of caspases and down-regulation of Bcl-2 protein. Br J Haematol 1998;102:1055–60.

284. Huang XJ, Wiernik PH, Klein RS, Gallagher RE. Arsenic trioxide induces apoptosis of myeloid leukemia cells by activation of caspases. Med Oncol 1999;16:58–64.

285. Perkins C, Kim CN, Fang G, Bhalla KN. Arsenic induces apoptosis of multidrug-resistant human myeloid leukemia cells that express Bcr-Abl or overexpress MDR, MRP, Bcl-2, or Bcl-x(L). Blood 2000;95:1014–22.

286. Dastugue N, Payen C, Lafage-Pochitaloff M, et al. Prognostic significance of karyotype in de novo adult acute myeloid leukemia. The BGMT group. Leukemia. 1995;9:1491–8.

287. Grimwade D, Walker H, Oliver F, et al. The importance of diagnostic cytogenetics on outcome in AML: analysis of 1,612 patients entered into the MRC AML 10 trial. Blood 1998;92:2322–33.

288. Slovak ML, Kopecky KJ, Cassileth PA, et al. Karyotype analysis predicts outcome of pre- and postremission therapy in adult acute myeloid leukemia (AML). A SWOG/ECOG Intergroup Study [abstract]. Blood 1998;92:2795.

289. Stein AS, O'Donnell MR, Slovak ML, et al. High-dose cytosine arabinoside and daunorubicin induction therapy for adult patients with de novo non M3 acute myelogenous leukemia: impact of cytogenetics on achieving a complete remission. Leukemia 2000;14:1191–6.

290. Anderlin P, Ghadder HM, Smith TL, et al. Factors predicting complete remission and subsequent disease-free survival after a second course of induction therapy in patients with acute myeloid leukemia resistant to the first. Leukemia 1996;964–9.

291. Liso V, Iacopino P, Avvisati G, et al. Outcome of patients with acute myeloid leukemia who failed to respond to a single course of first-line induction therapy: a GIMEMA study of 218 unselected consecutive patients. Leukemia 1996;10:1443–52.

292. Estey E. Treatment of refractory AML [review]. Leukemia 1996;10:932–6.

293. Vignetti V, Orsini E, Petti MC, et al. Probability of long-term disease-free survival for acute myeloid leukemia patients after first relapse: a single-centre experience. Ann Oncol 1996;7:933 8.

294. Tschapp L, von Fliedner VE, Sauter C, et al. Efficacy and clinical cross-resistance of a new combination therapy (AMSA/VP16) in previously treated patients with acute nonlymphocytic leukemia. J Clin Oncol 1986;4:318–24.

295. Keating MJ, Kantarjian HM, Smith TL, et al. Response to salvage therapy and survival after relapse in acute

myelogenous leukemia. J Clin Oncol 1989;7: 1071–80.

296. Hiddemann W, Aul C, Maschmeyer G, et al. High-dose versus intermediate-dose cytosine arabinoside combined with mitoxantrone for the treatment of relapsed and refractory acute myeloid leukemia: results of an age adjusted randomized comparison. Leuk Lymphoma 1993;10:133–7.

297. Kern W, Aul C, Maschmeyer G, et al. Superiority of high-dose over intermediate-dose cytosine arabinoside in the treatment of patients with high-risk acute myeloid leukemia: results of an age-adjusted prospective randomized comparison. Leukemia 1998;12:1049–55.

298. Karanes C, Kopecky KJ, Head DR, et al. A phase III comparison of high-dose ARA-C (HIDAC) versus HIDAC plus mitoxantrone in the treatment of first relapse or refractory acute myeloid leukemia. Southwest Oncology Group Study. Leuk Res 1999; 23:787–94.

299. Kern W, Schoch C, Haferlach T, et al. Multivariate analysis of prognostic factors in patients with refractory and relapsed acute myeloid leukemia undergoing sequential high-dose cytosine arabinoside and mitoxantrone (S-HAM) salvage therapy: relevance of cytogenetic abnormalities. Leukemia 2000;14:226–31.

300. Carella AM, Carlier P, Pungolino E, et al. Idarubicin in combination with intermediate-dose cytarabine and VP-16 in the treatment of refractory or rapidly relapsed patients with acute myeloid leukemia. Leukemia 1993;7:196–9.

301. Lee S, Tallman MS, Oken MM, et al. Duration of second complete remission compared with first complete remission in patients with acute myeloid leukemia. Leukemia (in press).

302. List AF, Spier C, Greer J, et al. Phase I/II trial of cyclosporine as a chemotherapy-resistance modifier in acute leukemia. J Clin Oncol 1993;11:1652–60.

303. Kornblau SM, Estey EH, Madden T, et al. Phase I study of mitoxantrone plus etoposide with multidrug blockade by sdz PSC-833 in relapse or refractory acute myeloid leukemia. J Clin Oncol 1997;15:1796–802.

304. Tallman MS, Lee S, Sikic B, et al. Mitoxantrone, etoposide and cytosine arabinoside plus cyclosporine in patients with relapsed or refractory acute myeloid leukemia: an Eastern Cooperative Oncology Group pilot study. Cancer 1999;85:358–67.

305. Advani R, Saba HI, Tallman MS, et al. Treatment of refractory and relapsed acute myelogenous leukemia with combination chemotherapy plus the multidrug resistance modulator valspodar (PSC 833). Blood 1999;93:787–95.

306. Chauncey TR, Rankin C, Anderson JE, et al. A phase I study of induction chemotherapy for older patients with newly diagnosed acute myeloid leukemia (AML) using mitoxantrone, etoposide, and the MDR modulator PSC-833: a Southwest Oncology Group study 9617. Leuk Res 2000;24:567–74.

307. Kantarjian HM, Beran M, Ellis A, et al. Phase I study of topotecan, a new topoisomerase I inhibitor, in patients with refractory or relapsed acute leukemia. Blood 1993;81:1146–51.

308. Cortes J, Estey EH, Beran M, et al. Cyclophosphamide, Ara-C and topotecan (CAT) for patients with refractory or relapsed acute leukemia. Leuk Lymphoma 2000;36:479–84.

309. Maraninchi D, Blaise D, Viens P, et al. High-dose recombinant interleukin-2 and acute myeloid leukemia in relapse. Blood 1991;78:2182–7.

310. Meloni G, Foa R, Vignetti M, et al. Interleukin-2 may induce prolonged remissions in advanced acute myeloid leukemia. Blood 1994;84:2158–63.

311. Meloni G, Vignetti M, Andrizzi C, et al. Interleukin-2 for the treatment of advanced acute myeloid leukemia patients with limited disease: updated experience with 20 cases. Leuk Lymphoma 1996;21:429–35.

312. Clift RA, Buckner CD, Thomas ED, et al. The treatment of acute nonlymphoblastic leukemia by allogeneic bone marrow transplantation. Bone Marrow Transplant 1987;2:243–58.

313. Schmitz N, Gassmann W, Rister M, et al. Fractionated total body irradiation and high-dose VP-16-213 followed by allogeneic bone marrow transplantation in advanced leukemias. Blood 1988;72:1567–73.

314. Petersen FB, Lynch MHE, Clift RA, et al. Autologous marrow transplantation for patients with acute myeloid leukemia in untreated first relapse or in second complete remission. J Clin Oncol 1993;11: 1353–60.

315. Przepiorka D, Ippoliti C, Khouri I, et al. Allogeneic transplantation for advanced leukemia: improved short-term outcome with blood stem cell grafts and tacrolimus. Transplantation 1996;62:1806–10.

316. Demirer T, Petersen FB, Bensinger WI, et al. Autologous transplantation with peripheral blood stem cells collected after granulocytic colony stimulating factor in patients with acute myelogenous leukemia. Bone Marrow Transplant 1996;18:29–34.

317. Grigg AP, Szer J, Beresford J, et al. Factors affecting the outcome of allogeneic bone marrow transplantation for adults with refractory or relapsed acute leukemia. Br J Haematol 1999;107:409–18.

318. Schiller G, Feig SA, Territo M, et al. Treatment of advanced acute leukaemia with allogeneic bone marrow transplantation from unrelated donors. Br J Haematol 1994;88:72–8.

319. Kernan NA, Bartsch G, Ash RC, et al. Analysis of 462 transplantations from unrelated donors facilitated by the National Marrow Donor Program. N Engl J Med 1993;328:593–602.

320. Beatty PG, Anasetti C, Hansen JA, et al. Marrow transplantation from unrelated donors for treatment of hematologic malignancies: effect of mismatching for one HLA locus. Blood 1993;81:249–53.

321. Sierra J, Storer B, Hansen JA, et al. Transplantation of marrow cells from unrelated donors for treatment of high-risk leukemia: the effect of leukemic burden, donor HLA-matching, and marrow cell dose. Blood 1997;89:4226–35.

322. Kodera Y, Morishima Y, Kato S, et al. Analysis of 500 bone marrow transplants from unrelated donor (UR-BMT) facilitated by the Japan Marrow Donor Program: confirmation of UR-BMT as a standard therapy for patients with leukemia and aplastic anemia. Bone Marrow Transplant 1999;24:995–1003.

323. Sievers EL, Appelbaum FR, Spielberger RT, et al. Selective ablation of acute myeloid leukemia using antibody-targeted chemotherapy: a phase I trial of an anti-CD33 calicheamicin immunoconjugate. Blood 1999;93:3678–84.

324. Sievers EL, Larson RA, Estey E, et al. Preliminary results of the efficacy and safety of CMA-676 in patients with AML in first relapse [abstract]. Proc Am Soc Clin Oncol 1999;18:21.

325. Rai KR, Sawitsky A, Cronkite EP, et al. Clinical staging of chronic lymphocytic leukemia. Blood 1975;46:219–34.

326. Montserrat E, Vinolas N, Reverles JC, et al. Natural history of chronic lymphocytic leukemia on the progression and prognosis of early clinical stages. Nouv Rev Fr Hematol 1988;30:459–61.

327. Rozman C, Bosch F, Montserrat E. Chronic lymphocytic leukemia: a changing natural history? Leukemia 1997;11:775–8.

328. Zwiebel JA, Cheson BD. Chronic lymphocytic leukemia: staging and prognostic factors. Semin Oncol 1998;25:42–59.

329. Montserrat E, Sanchez-Bisoni J, Vinolas N, et al. Lymphocyte doubling time in chronic lymphocytic leukemia: analysis of its prognosis significance. Br J Haematol 1986;62:567–75.

330. Rozman C, Montserrat E, Rodriguez-Fernandez JM, et al. Bone marrow histologic pattern—the best single prognostic parameter in chronic lymphocytic leukemia: a multivariate survival analysis of 329 cases. Blood 1984;64:642–8.

331. Pangalis GA, Boussiotis VA, Kittas C. B-chronic lymphocytic leukemia. Disease progression in 150 untreated stage A and B patients as predicted by bone marrow pattern. Nouv Rev Fr Hematol 1988;30:373–5.

332. Juliusson G, Oscier DG, Fichett M, et al. Prognostic subgroups in B-cell CLL defined by specific chromosomal abnormalities. N Engl J Med 1990;323:720–4.

333. Fegan C, Robinson H, Thompson P, et al. Karyotype evolution in CLL: identification of a new sub-group of patients with deletions of 11q and advanced or progressive disease. Leukemia 1995;9:2003–8.

334. Dohner H, Stilgenbauer S, James MR, et al. 11q deletions identify a new subset of B-cell chronic lymphocytic leukemia characterized by extensive nodal involvement and inferior prognosis. Blood 1997;89: 2516–22.

335. The French Cooperative Group. Effects of chlorambucil and therapeutic decision in initial forms of chronic lymphocytic leukemia (stage A): results of a randomized clinical trial on 612 patients. Blood 1990;75:1414–21.

336. Skinnider LF, Tan L, Schmidt J, Armitage G. Chronic lymphocytic leukemia: a review of 745 cases and assessment of clinical staging. Cancer 1982;50: 2951–5.

337. Bruiatelli M, Jaksic B, Planinc-Peraica A, et al. Treatment of chronic lymphocytic leukemia in early and stable phase of the disease: long-term results of a randomized trial. Eur J Haematol 1995;55:158–63.

338. Cheson BD, Bennett JM, Rai KR, et al. Guidelines for clinical protocols for chronic lymphocytic leukemia. Am J Haematol 1988;29:152–63.

339. Cheson BD, Bennett JM, Grever MR, et al. National Cancer Institute-sponsored working group guidelines for chronic lymphocytic leukemia: revised guidelines for diagnosis and treatment. Blood 1996;87:4990–7.

340. Han T, Ezdinli EZ, Shimaoka K, et al. Chlorambucil vs combined chlorambucil therapy in chronic lymphocytic leukemia. Cancer 1973;31:502–8.

341. Knospe WH, Loeb V, Huguley CM. Biweekly chlorambucil treatment of chronic lymphocytic leukemia. Cancer 1974;33:555–62.

342. Jaksic B, Brugiatelli M. High-dose continuous chlorambucil vs intermittent chlorambucil plus prednisone for treatment of B-CLL-IGCI Cl-1 trial. Nouv Rev Fr Hematol 1988;30:437–42.

343. Sawitsky A, Rai KR, Glidewell O, et al. Comparison of daily versus intermittent chlorambucil and prednisone therapy in the treatment of patients with chronic lymphocytic leukemia. Blood 1977;50:1049–59.

344. Montserrat E, Alcala A, Parody R, et al. Treatment of chronic lymphocytic leukemia in advanced stages. A randomized trial comparing chlorambucil plus prednisone versus cyclophosphamide, vincristine, and prednisone. Cancer 1985;56:2369–75.

345. Catovsky D, Fooks J, Richards S. The UK Medical Research Council CLL trial 1 and 2. Nouv Rev Fr Hematol 1988;30:423–7.

346. The French Cooperative Group on Chronic Lymphocytic Leukemia. A randomized clinical trial of chlorambucil vs COP in stage B chronic lymphocytic leukemia. Blood 1990;75:1422–5.

347. The French Cooperative Group on Chronic Lymphocytic Leukemia. Effectiveness of "CHOP" regimen in advanced untreated chronic lymphocytic leukemia. Lancet 1986;II:1346–9.

348. Hansen MM, Andersen E, Birgens H, et al. CHOP versus chlorambucil plus prednisone in chronic lymphocytic leukemia. Leuk Lymphoma 1991;5:97–100.

349. Kimby E, Mellstedt H. Chlorambucil prednisone versus CHOP in symptomatic chronic lymphocytic leukemia of B-cell type. A randomized trial. Leuk Lymphoma 1991;5:93–6.

350. Spanish Cooperative Group PETHEMA. Treatment of chronic lymphocytic leukemia: a preliminary report of Spanish (PETHEMA) trials. Leuk Lymphoma 1991;5:89–91.

351. Tallman MS, Hakimian D. The purine nucleoside analogs: emerging roles in indolent lymphoproliferative disorders. Blood 1995;86:2463–74.

352. Kempin S, Lee BJ III, Koziner B, et al. Combination chemotherapy of advanced chronic lymphocytic leukemia: the M2 protocol (vincristine, BCNU, cyclophosphamide, melphalan and prednisone). Blood 1982;60:1110–21.

353. Keating MJ, Scouros M, Murphy S, et al. Multiple agent chemotherapy (POACH) in previously treated and untreated patients with chronic lymphocytic leukemia. Leukemia 1988;2:157–64.

354. Grever MR, Kopecky KJ, Coltman CA. Fludarabine monophosphate: a potentially useful agent in chronic lymphocytic leukemia. Nouv Rev Fr Hematol 1988;30:457–9.

355. Keating MJ, Kantarjian H, Talpaz M, et al. Fludarabine: a new agent with major activity against chronic lymphocytic leukemia. Blood 1989;74:19–25.

356. Hiddemann W, Rottmann R, Wormann B, et al. Treatment of advanced chronic lymphocytic leukemia by fludarabine: results of a clinical phase II study. Ann Hematol 1991;63:1–4.

357. Robertson LE, Huh YO, Butler JJ, et al. Response assessment in chronic lymphocytic leukemia after fludarabine plus prednisone: clinical, pathologic, immunophenotype and molecular analysis. Blood 1992;80:29–36.

358. Keating MJ, O'Brien S, Kantarjian H, et al. Long-term follow-up of patients with chronic lymphocytic leukemia treated with fludarabine as a single agent. Blood 1993;81:2878–84.

359. Puccio CA, Mittleman, Lichtman SM, et al. Immunosuppressive effects and clinical response of fludarabine in refractory chronic lymphocytic leukemia. Ann Oncol 1993;4:371–5.

360. Spriano M, Clavio M, Carrara P, et al. Fludarabine in untreated and previously treated B-CLL patients. A report on efficacy and toxicity. Haematologica 1994;79:218–24.

361. Sorensen JM, Vena DA, Fallavollita A, et al. Treatment of refractory chronic lymphocytic leukemia with fludarabine phosphate via the group C, protocol mechanism of the National Cancer Institute: five-year follow-up report. J Clin Oncol 1997;15:458–65.

362 Keating MJ, Smith TL, Lerner S, et al. Prediction of prognosis following fludarabine used as secondary therapy for chronic lymphocytic leukemia. Leuk Lymphoma 2000;37:71–85.

363. Lee WW, Benitz A, Goodman A, et al. Potential anticancer agents LX: synthesis of the B-anomer of 9-(d-arabinofuranosyl)adenosine. J Am Chem Soc 1960;82:2648.

364. Brockman RW, Schabel FM Jr, Montgomery JA. Biologic activity of A-B-D-arabinofuranosyl-2-fluoroadenosine, a metabolically stable analog of 9-β-D-arabinofurosyladenosine. Biochem Pharmacol 1977;26:2193–6.

365. Noker PE, Duncan GF, El Dareer SM, et al. Disposition of 9-β-arabinofuranosyl-2-fluoroadenine 5'-phosphate in mice and dogs. Cancer Treat Rep 1983;67:445–56.

366. Huang P, Chubb S, Plunkett W. Termination of DNA synthesis by 9-beta-D-arabinofuranosyl-2-fluoroadenosine. A mechanism for cytotoxicity. J Biol Chem 1990;265:16617–16625.

367. Catapano CV, Chandler K, Fernandes DJ. Inhibition of primer RNA formation in CCRF-CEM leukemia cells by fludarabine triphosphate. Cancer Res 1991;51:1829–35.

368. Yang S-W, Huang P, Plunkett W, et al. Dual mode of inhibition of purified DNA ligase I from human cells by 9-beta-D-arabinofuranosyl-2-fluoroadenosine triphosphate. J Biol Chem 1992;267:2345–49.

369. Parker WB, Bapat AR, Shen JX, et al. Interaction of 2-halogenated dATP analogs (F, Cl, and Br) with human DNA polymerases, DNA primase, and ribonucleotide reductase. Mol Pharmacol 1988;34:485–91.

370. Plunkett W, Chubb S, Alexander L, et al. Comparison of the toxicity and metabolism of 9-beta-D-arabinofuranosyl-2-fluoroadenine and 9-beta-D-arabinofuranosyladenine in human lymphoblastoid cells. Cancer Res 1980;40:2349–55.

371. White EL, Shaddix SC, Brockman RW, et al. Comparison of the toxicity and metabolism of 9-β-D-arabinofuranosyl-2-fluoroadenine and 9-β-D-arabinofuranosyladenine on target enzymes from mouse tumor cells. Cancer Res 1982;42:2260–4.

372. Anaisse E, Kontoyiannis DP, Kantarjian H, et al. Listerosis in patients with chronic lymphocytic leukemia who were treated with fludarabine and prednisone. Ann Intern Med 1992;117:466–9.

373. O'Brien S, Kantarjian H, Beran M, et al. Interferon maintenance therapy for patients with chronic lymphocytic leukemia in remission after fludarabine therapy. Blood 1995;86:1296–300.

374. Rai K, Peterson B, Elias L, et al. A randomized comparison of fludarabine and chlorambucil for patients with previously untreated chronic lymphocytic leukemia: a CALGB, SWOG, CTG/NCI-C, and ECOG Intergroup study [abstract]. Blood 1996;88:1419.

375. The French Cooperative Group on CLL. Multicentre prospective randomized trial of fludarabine versus cyclophosphamide, doxorubicin and prednisone (CAP) for treatment of advanced stage chronic lymphocytic leukemia. Lancet 1996;347:1432–8.

376. Leporrier M, Chevret S, Cazin B, et al. Randomized comparison of fludarabine, CAP, in 695 previously untreated stage B and C chronic lymphocytic leukemia (CLL). Early stopping of the CAP accrual [abstract]. Blood 1997;90:2357.

377. Leporrier M, Chevret S, Cazin B, et al. Randomized clinical trial comparing two anthracycline-containing regimens (CHOP and CAP) and fludarabine (FDR) in advanced chronic lymphocytic leukemia [abstract]. Blood 1999;94:2682.

378. Koel U, Li L, Nowak B. Fludarabine and cyclophosphamide: synergistic cytotoxicity associated with inhibition of interstrand cross-link removal [abstract]. Proc Am Assoc Cancer Res 1997;38:2.

379. Bellosillo B, Villamor N, Colomer D. In vitro evaluation of fludarabine in combination with cyclophosphamide and/or mitoxantrone in B-cell chronic lymphocytic leukemia. Blood 1999;94:2836–43.

380. Weiss M, Spies T, Berman E, Kempin S. Concomitant administration of chlorambucil limits dose intensity of fludarabine in previously treated patients with chronic lymphocytic leukemia. Leukemia 1994;8:1290–3.

381. Elias L, Stock-Novack D, Head DR, et al. A phase I trial of combination fludarabine monophosphate and chlorambucil in chronic lymphocytic leukemia: a Southwest Oncology Group study. Leukemia 1993;7:361–5.

382. Frewin R, Turner D, Tighe M. Combination therapy with fludarabine and cyclophosphamide as salvage treatment in lymphoproliferative disorders. Br J Haematol 1999;104:612–3.

383. Flinn IW, Byrd JC, Morrison C, et al. Fludarabine and cyclophosphamide: a highly active and well tolerated regimen for patients with previously untreated chronic lymphocytic leukemia [abstract]. Blood 1998;92:424.

384. Morrison VA, Rai KR, Peterson B, et al. The impact of therapy with chlorambucil (C), fludarabine (F) or fludarabine and chlorambucil (F+C) or infections in patients with chronic lymphocytic leukemia (CLL): an Intergroup study (CALGB 9011) [abstract]. Blood 1998;92:2020.

385. Hallek M, Wilhelm M, Emmerich B, et al. Fludarabine plus cyclophosphamide (FC) and dose intensified chlorambucil (DIC) for the treatment of chronic lymphocytic leukemia (CLL): results of two phase II studies (CLL-2 protocol) of the German CLL study group (GCLLSG) [abstract]. Blood 1999;94:1402.

386. Weiss RB, Freiman J, Kweder SL, et al. Hemolytic anemia after fludarabine therapy for chronic lymphocytic leukemia. J Clin Oncol 1998;16:1885–9.

387. Carson DA, Wasson DB, Taetle R, et al. Specific toxicity of 2-chlorodeoxyadenosine toward resting and proliferative human lymphocytes. Blood 1983;62:737–74.

388. Carson DA, Wasson DB, Beutler E. Anti-leukemic and immunosuppressive activity of 2-chloro-2'-deoxyadenosine. Proc Natl Acad Sci U S A 1984;81:2232–6.

389. Piro LD, Carrera CJ, Beutler E, et al. 2-Chlorodeoxyadenosine: an effective new agent for the treatment of chronic lymphocytic leukemia. Blood 1988;72:1069–73.

390. Saven A, Carrera CJ, Carson DA, et al. 2-Chlorodeoxyadenosine treatment for refractory chronic lymphocytic leukemia. Leuk Lymphoma 1991;5:133–8.

391. Juliusson G, Liliemark J. High complete remission rate from 2-chloro-2'-deoxyadenosine in previously treated patients with B-cell chronic lymphocytic leukemia: response predicted by rapid decrease of blood lymphocyte count. J Clin Oncol 1993;11:679–89.

392. Betticher DC, Fey MF, von Rohr A, et al. High incidence of infections after 2-chlorodeoxyadenosine (2-CDA) therapy in patients with malignant lymphomas and chronic and acute leukaemias. Ann Oncol 1994;5:57–64.

393. Tallman MS, Hakimian D, Zanzig C, et al. Cladribine (2-CdA) in the treatment of relapsed and refractory chronic and lymphocytic leukemia. J Clin Oncol 1995;13:983–8.

394. Juliusson G, Liliemark J. Long-term survival following cladribine (2-chlorodeoxyadenosine) therapy in previously treated patients with chronic lymphocytic leukemia. Ann Oncol 1996;7:373–9.

395. Robak T, Blonski JZ, Urbanska-Rys H, et al. 2-Chlorodeoxyadenosine (cladribine) in the treatment of patients with chronic lymphocytic leukemia 55 years old and younger. Leukemia 1999;13:518–23.

396. Robak T, Blasinska-Morawiec M, Blonsici JZ, et al. 2-Chlorodeoxyadenosine (cladribine) in the treatment of elderly patients with B-cell chronic lymphocytic leukemia. Leuk Lymphoma 1999;34:151–7.

397. Saven A, Lemon RH, Kosty M, et al. 2-Chlorodeoxyadenosine in patients with untreated chronic lymphocytic leukemia. J Clin Oncol 1995;13:570–4.

398. Juliusson G, Christiansen I, Hansen MM, et al. Oral cladribine as primary therapy for patients with B-

cell chronic lymphocytic leukemia. J Clin Oncol 1996;14:2160–6.

399. Delannoy A, Martiat P, Gala JL, et al. 2-Chlorodeoxyadenosine (CdA) for patients with previously untreated chronic lymphocytic leukemia (CLL). Leukemia 1995;9:1130–5.

400. Robak T, Blonski JZ, Kasnicki M, et al. Cladribine with or without prednisone in the treatment of previously treated and untreated B-cell chronic lymphocytic leukemia—updated results of the multicentre study of 378 patients. Br J Haematol 2000;108:357–68.

401. Tallman MS, Wollins E, Jain V, et al. Leustatin in the treatment of patients with previously untreated chronic lymphocytic leukemia [abstract]. Blood 1997;90:2574.

402. Chasty RC, Myint H, Oscier DG, et al. Autoimmune haemolysis in patients with B-CLL treated with chlorodeoxyadenosine (CdA). Leuk Lymphoma 1998;29:391–8.

403. O'Brien S, Kantarjian H, Estey E, et al. Lack of effect of 2-chlorodeoxyadenosine therapy in patient with chronic lymphocytic leukemia refractory of fludarabine. N Engl J Med 1994;330:319–22.

404. Betticher DC, von Rohr A, Ratschiller D, et al. Fever infections, but maintained antitumor activity with lower-dose standard-dose cladribine in pretreated low-grade non-Hodgkin's lymphoma. J Clin Oncol 1998;16:850–8.

405. Fox RM, Mann CJ, Kefford RF. Deoxyadenosine toxicity to human peripheral blood lymphocytes: implications for 2-deoxycoformycin as a potential immunosuppressive drug. Cancer Treat Symp 1984;2:33–6.

406. Grever MR, Leiby JM, Kraut EH, et al. Low-dose deoxycoformycin in lymphoid malignancy. J Clin Oncol 1985;3:1196–201.

407. Dillman RO, Mick R, McIntyre OR. Pentostatin in chronic lymphocytic leukemia: a phase II trial of Cancer and Leukemia Group B. J Clin Oncol 1989; 7:433–8.

408. Ho AD, Thaler J, Stryckmans P, et al. Pentostatin in refractory chronic lymphocytic leukemia: a phase II trial of the European Organization for Research and Treatment of Cancer. J Natl Cancer Inst 1990;82: 1416–20.

409. Dearden C, Catovsky D. Deoxycoformycin in the treatment of mature B-cell malignancies. Br J Cancer 1990;62:4–5.

410. Dohner H, Fischer K, Bentz M, et al. p53 gene deletion predicts for poor survival and non-response to therapy with purine analogs in chronic B-cell leukemias. Blood 1995;85:1580–9.

411. Pedersen IM, Jurlander J. The chimeric anti-CD20 antibody Rituxan® can induce MAP-kinase phosphorylation, up-regulation of proapoptotic proteins and

412. Winker U, Schulz HR, Jensen M, et al. Toxicity and efficacy of the antiCD20 antibody Rituxan® in patients with B-CLL chronic lymphocytic leukemia. A phase III study [abstract]. Blood 1999; 94:1396.

413. Murphy TJ, Ling G, Flinn IW, et al. Infusion-related events following Rituxan® therapy in chronic lymphocytic leukemia/small lymphocytic leukemia (CLL/SLL): association with inflammatory cytokines [abstract]. Blood 1999;94:1397.

414 Osterborg A, Fassas AS, Anagnostopoulos A, et al. Humanized CD52 monoclonal antibody campath-1H as first-line treatment in chronic lymphocytic leukemia. Br J Haematol 1996;93:151–3.

415. Osterborg A, Dyer MJS, Bunjes D, et al. Phase II multicenter study of human CD52 antibody in previously treated chronic lymphocytic leukemia. J Clin Oncol 1997;15:1567–74.

416. Bowen AL, Zomas A, Emmett E, et al. Subcutaneous CAMPATH-1H in fludarabine resistant/relapse chronic lymphocytic and B-prolymphocytic leukemia. Br J Haematol 1997;90:617–9.

417. Rai KR, Hoffman M, Janson D. Immunosuppression and opportunistic infections in patients with chronic lymphocytic leukemia following CAMPATH-1H therapy [abstract]. Blood 1995;80:348.

418. Keating MJ, Byrd J, Rai K, et al. Multicenter study of campath-1H in patients with chronic lymphocytic leukemia (B-CLL) refractory to fludarabine [abstract]. Blood 1999;94:3118.

419. Talpaz, M, Rosenblum M, Kurzrock R, et al. Clinical and laboratory changes induced by alpha interferon in chronic lymphocytic leukemia—a pilot study. Am J Hematol 1987;24:341–50.

420 Rozman C, Montserrat E, Vinolas N, et al. Recombinant A$_2$-interferon in the treatment of B-chronic lymphocytic leukemia in early stages. Blood 1988;71:1295–8.

421. Pangalis GA, Griva E. Recombinant alfa-2b-interferon therapy in untreated, stages A and B chronic lymphocytic leukemia. Cancer 1988;61:869–72.

422. Pozzato G, Franzin F, Moretti M, et al. Low-dose "natural" alpha-interferon in B-cell derived chronic lymphocytic leukemia. Hematologica 1992;77:413–7.

423. Kay NE, Oken MM, Mazza JJ, et al. Evidence for tumor reduction in refractory or relapsed B-CLL patients treated with infusional interleukin 2. Nouv Rev Fr Hematol 1988;30:475–8.

424. Michallet M, Corront B, Hollard D, et al. Allogeneic bone marrow transplantation in chronic lymphocytic leukemia: 17 cases. Report from the EBMTG. Bone Marrow Transplant 1991;7:275–9.

425. Rabinowe SN, Soiffer RJ, Gribben JG, et al. Autolo-

gous and allogeneic bone marrow transplantation for poor prognosis patients with B-cell chronic lymphocytic leukemia. Blood 1993;82:1366–76.

426. Khouri IF, Keating MJ, Vriesendorp HM, et al. Autologous and allogeneic bone marrow transplantation for chronic lymphocytic leukemia: preliminary results. J Clin Oncol 1994;12:748–58.

427. Bartlett PF, Soffer R, Gribben JG, et al. Autologous and allogeneic bone marrow transplantation for B-cell CLL: balance between toxicity and efficacy [abstract]. Blood 1994;84:2129.

428. Sutton L, Maloum K, Gonzalez H, et al. Autologous hematopoietic stem cell transplantation as salvage treatment for advanced B-cell chronic lymphocytic leukemia. Leukemia 1998;12:1699–707.

429. Pavletic ZS, Arrowsmith ER, Bierman PJ, et al. Outcome of allogeneic stem cell transplantation for B-cell chronic lymphocytic leukemia. Bone Marrow Transplant 2000;25:717–22.

430. Deger P, Dohner H, Emmerich B, et al. A prospective multicenter study of early autologous stem cell transplantation (ASCT) in CLL (CLL-3 study): first interim analysis [abstract]. Bone Marrow Transplant 2000;25:23.

431. Provan D, Bartlett-Pandite L, Zwicky C, et al. Eradication of polymerase chain reaction detectable chronic lymphocytic leukemia cells is associated with improved outcome after bone marrow transplantation. Blood 1996;88:2228–35.

432. Michallet M, Archimaud E, Bandin G, et al. HLA-identical sibling bone marrow transplantation in younger patients with chronic lymphocytic leukemia. Ann Intern Med 1996;124:311–5.

433. Mattsson J, Uzunel M, Remberger M, et al. Minimal residual disease is common after allogeneic stem cell transplantation in patients with B-cell chronic lymphocytic leukemia and may be controlled by graft-versus-host disease. Leukemia 2000;14:247–54.

434. Khouri I, Przepiorka D, van Besien K, et al. Allogeneic blood or marrow transplantation for chronic lymphocytic leukemia: timing of transplantation and potential effect of fludarabine on acute graft-versus-host disease. Br J Haematol 1997;97:466–73.

435. Schey SA, Absan G, Jones R. Dose intensification and molecular response in patients with chronic lymphocytic leukemia: a phase II single centre study. Bone Marrow Transplant 1999;24:989–93.

436. Zomas A, Mehta J, Powles R, et al. Unusual infections following allogeneic bone marrow transplantation for chronic lymphocytic leukemia. Bone Marrow Transplant 1994;14:799–803.

437. Mentz F, Mossalayi MD, Ouaaz F, et al. Theophylline synergizes with chlorambucil in inducing apoptosis of B-chronic lymphocytic leukemia cells. Blood 1996;88:2172–82.

438. Mentz F, Merle-Beral H, Ouaaz F, Binet JL. Theophylline, a new inducer of apoptosis in B-CLL: role of cyclic nucleotides. Br J Haematol 1995;90:957–9.

439. Mentz F, Merle-Beral H, Dalloul AH. Theophylline-induced B-CLL apoptosis is partly dependent on CD38 expression and endogenous IL-10 production. Leukemia 1999;3:78–84.

440. Binet JL, Mentz F, Leblond V, Merle-Beral H. Synergistic action of alkylating agents and methylxanthine derivatives in the treatment of chronic lymphocytic leukemia. Leukemia 1995;9:2159–64.

441. Ueda H, Nakajima H, Hori Y, et al. FR901228, a novel antitumor bicyclic depsipeptide produced by Chromobacterium violaceum no. 968. I. Taxonomy, fermentation, isolation, physico-chemical and biological properties, and antitumor activity. J Antibiot (Tokyo) 1994;47:301–10.

442 Nakajima H, Kim YB, Terano H, et al. FR901228, a potent antitumor antibiotic, is a novel histone deacetylase inhibitor. Exp Cell Res 1998;241:126–33.

443. Byrd JC, Shinn C, Ravi R, et al. Depsipeptide (FR99228): a novel therapeutic agent with selective, in vitro activity against human B-cell chronic lymphocytic leukemia cells. Blood 1999;94:1401–8.

444. Ueda H, Nakajima H, Hori Y, et al. Action of FR901228, a novel antitumor bicyclic depsipeptide produced by Chromobacterium violaceum no. 968, on Ha-ras transformed NIH3T3 cells. Biosci Biotechnol Biochem 1994;58:1579–83.

445. Arguello F, Alexander M, Sterry JA, et al. Flavopiridol induces apoptosis of normal lymphoid cells, causes immunosuppression, and has potent antitumor activity in vivo against human leukemia and lymphoma xenografts. Blood 1998;91:2482–90.

446. Seynaeve CM, Kazanietz MG, Blumberg PM, et al. Differential inhibition of protein kinase C isozymes by UCN-01, a staurosporine analogue. Mol Pharmacol 1994;45:1207–14.

447. Kitada S, Zapata JM, Andreeff M, Reed JC. Protein kinase inhibitors flavopiridol and 7-hydroxy-staurosporine down-regulate antiapoptosis proteins in B-cell chronic lymphocytic leukemia. Blood 2000;96:393–7.

448. Kolitz JE, Kempin SJ, Schluger A, et al. A phase II pilot trial of high-dose hydroxyurea in chronic myelogenous leukemia. Semin Oncol 1992;19(Suppl 9):27–33.

449. Hehlmann R, Heimpel H, Hasford J, et al. Randomized comparison of busulfan and hydroxyurea in chronic myelogenous leukemia: prolongation of survival by hydroxyurea. Blood 1993;82:398–407.

450. Silverstein MN, Petitt RM, Solberg LA Jr, et al. Anagrelide: a new drug for treating thrombocytosis. N Engl J Med 1988;318:1292–4.

451. Silverstein MN. Anagrelide Study Group. Anagrelide,

a therapy for thrombocythemic states: experience in 577 patients. Am J Med 1992;92:69–76.

452. Robertson MJ, Tantravahi R, Griffin JD, et al. Hematologic remission and cytogenetic improvement after treatment of stable-phase chronic myelogenous leukemia with continuous infusion of low-dose cytarabine. Am J Hematol 1993;43:95–102.

453. O'Brien S, Kantarjian H, Keating M, et al. Homoharringtonine therapy induces responses in patients with chronic myelogenous leukemia in late chronic phase. Blood 1995;86:3322–6.

454 O'Brien S, Kantarjian H, Feldman E, et al. Sequential homoharringtonine (HHT) and interferon (IFN-A) produce high hematologic and cytogenetic response rates in Philadelphia chromosome positive (Ph) chronic myelogenous leukemia (CML) [abstract]. Proc Am Soc Clin Oncol 1995;14:1006.

455. Kantarjian H, O'Brien S, Keating M, et al. Homoharringtonine (HHT) and low-dose cytosine arabinoside (ara-C) combination therapy has significant activity in patients (pts) with late phase Philadelphia chromosome (Ph) positive chronic myelogenous leukemia (CML) [abstract]. Blood 1996;88:578a.

456. Ernst T, Soiffer R, Stone R. Homoharringtonine with low-dose cytarabine combination therapy induces both hematologic and cytogenetic remissions in patients with chronic myelogenous leukemia (CML) [abstract]. Blood 1996;88:578a.

457. Verma DS, Spitzer G, Gutterman JU, et al. Human leukocyte interferon preparation blocks granulopoietic differentiation. Blood 1979;54:1423–7.

458. Talpaz M, Kantarjian HM, McCredie K, et al. Hematologic remission and cytogenetic improvement induced by recombinant human interferon alpha in chronic myelogenous leukemia. N Engl J Med 1986;314:1065–9.

459. Talpaz M, Kantarjian HM, McCredie KB, et al. Clinical investigation of human alpha interferon in chronic myelogenous leukemia. Blood 1987;69:1280–8.

460. Kantarjian H, Smith TL, O'Brien S, et al. Prolonged survival in chronic myelogenous leukemia after cytogenetic response to interferon-alpha therapy. Ann Intern Med 1995;122:254–61.

461. Alimena G, Morra E, Lazzarino M, et al. Interferon alpha 2B as therapy for Ph-positive chronic myelogenous leukemia: a study of 82 patients treated with intermittent or daily administration. Blood 1988;72:642–7.

462. Kantarjian HM, Deisseroth A, Kurzrock R, et al. Chronic myelogenous leukemia: a concise update. Blood 1993;82:691–703.

463. The Italian Cooperative Study Group on Chronic Myeloid Leukemia. Interferon α2a compared with conventional chemotherapy for the treatment of chronic myeloid leukemia. N Engl J Med 1994;330:820–5.

464. Hehlmann R, Heimpel H, Hasford J, et al. Randomized comparison of interferon-alpha with busulfan and hydroxyurea in chronic myelogenous leukemia. The German CML Study Group. Blood 1993;82:398–407.

465. Alan NC, Richards SM, Shepherd PC. UK Medical Research Council randomized, multicentre trial of interferon-alpha n1 for chronic myeloid leukaemia: improved survival irrespective of cytogenetic response. The UK Medical Research Council's Working Parties for Therapeutic Trials in Adult Leukaemia. Lancet 1995;345:1392–7.

466. Sokal JE, Leong SS, Gomez GA. Preferential inhibition by cytarabine of CFR-GM from patients with chronic granulocytic leukemia. Cancer 1987;59:197–202.

467. Robertson MJ, Tantravahi R, Griffin JD, et al. Hematologic remission and cytogenetic improvement after treatment of stable phase chronic myelogenous leukemia with continuous infusion of low-dose cytarabine. Am J Hematol 1993;43:95–102.

468. Kantarjian HM, O'Brien S, Smith TL, et al. Treatment of Philadelphia chromosome-positive early chronic phase chronic myelogenous leukemia with daily doses of interferon alpha and low dose cytarabine. J Clin Oncol 1999;17:284–92.

469. Guilhot F, Chastang C, Michallet C, et al. Interferon alpha 2b combined with cytarabine versus interferon alone in chronic myelogenous leukemia. N Engl J Med 1997;337:223–9.

470. Tura S, on behalf of the Italian Cooperative Study Group on CML. Cytarabine increases karyotypic response in interferon-alpha treated chronic myelogenous leukemia patients: results of a national prospective randomized trial [abstract]. Blood 1998;92:317a.

471. The Benelux CML Study Group. Randomized study on hydroxyurea alone versus hydroxyurea combined with low-dose interferon-alpha 2b for chronic myeloid leukemia. Blood 1998;91:2713–21.

472. Kantarjian HM, Talpaz M, Keating MJ, et al. Intensive chemotherapy induction followed by interferon-alpha maintenance in patients with Philadelphia chromosome-positive chronic myelogenous leukemia. Cancer 1991;68:1201–7.

473. Cortes J, Fayad L, Kantarjian H, et al. Association of HLA phenotype and response to interferon-alpha in patients with chronic myelogenous leukemia. Leukemia 1998;12:455–62.

474. Speck B, Bortin MM, Champlin R, et al. Allogeneic bone marrow transplantation for chronic myelogenous leukemia. Lancet 1984;1:665–8.

475. Thomas ED, Clift RA, Fefer A, et al. Marrow transplantation for the treatment of chronic myelogenous leukemia. Ann Intern Med 1986;104:155–63.

476. Goldman JM, Gale RP, Horowitz MM, et al. Bone marrow transplantation for chronic myelogenous

leukemia in chronic phase. Ann Intern Med 1988;108:806–14.

477. Clift RA, Buckner CD, Appelbaum FR, et al. Allogeneic marrow transplantation in patients with chronic myeloid leukemia in the chronic phase: a randomized trial of two irradiation regimens. Blood 1991;77:1660–5.

478. Biggs JC, Szer J, Crilley P, et al. Treatment of chronic myeloid leukemia with allogeneic bone marrow transplantation after preparation with BuCy2. Blood 1992;80:1352–7.

479. Wagner JE, Zahurak M, Piantadosi S, et al. Bone marrow transplantation of chronic myelogenous leukemia in chronic phase: evaluation of risks and benefits. J Clin Oncol 1992;10:779–89.

480. Gratwohl A, Hermans J, Niederwieser D, et al. Bone marrow transplantation for chronic myeloid leukemia: long-term results. Bone Marrow Transplant 1993;12:509–16.

481. Clift RA, Buckner CD, Thomas ED, et al. Marrow transplantation for chronic myeloid leukemia: a randomized study comparing cyclophosphamide and total body irradiation with busulfan and cyclophosphamide. Blood 1994;84:2036–43.

482. Savage DG, Szydlo RM, Chase A, et al. Bone marrow transplantation for chronic myeloid leukaemia: the effects of differing criteria for defining chronic phase on probabilities of survival and relapse. Br J Haematol 1997;99:30–5.

483. Italian Cooperative Study Group on Chronic Myeloid Leukaemia. Evaluating survival after allogeneic bone marrow transplant for chronic myeloid leukaemia in chronic phase: a comparison of transplant versus no-transplant in a cohort of 258 patients first seen in Italy between 1984 and 1986. Br J Haematol 1993;85:292–9.

484 Gale RP, Hehlmann R, Zhang MJ, et al. Survival with bone marrow transplantation versus hydroxyurea or interferon for chronic myelogenous leukemia. Blood 1998;91:1810–9.

485. Clift RA, Appelbaum FR, Thomas ED. Treatment of chronic myeloid leukemia by marrow transplantation. Blood 1993;82:1954–6.

486 Clift RA, Buckner CD, Thomas ED, et al. Marrow transplantation for patients in accelerated phase of chronic myelocytic leukemia [review]. Blood 1994;84:4368–73.

487. van Rhee F, Szydlo RM, Hermans J, et al. Long term results after allogeneic bone marrow transplantation for chronic myelogenous leukemia in chronic phase: a report from the Chronic Leukemia Working Party of the European Group for Blood and Bone Marrow Transplantation. Bone Marrow Transplant 1997;20:553–60.

488. Clift RA, Storb R. Marrow transplantation for CML:

the Seattle experience. Bone Marrow Transplant 1996;17(Suppl 3):S1–3.

489. Clift RA, Anasetti C. Allografting for chronic myelogenous leukemia. Baillieres Clin Haematol 1997;10:319–36.

490. Clift RA, Buckner CD, Thomas ED, et al. Marrow transplantation for chronic myeloid leukemia: a randomized study comparing cyclophosphamide and total body irradiation with busulfan and cyclophosphamide. Blood 1994;84:2036–43.

491. Snyder DS, Negrin RS, O'Donnell MR, et al. Fractionated total-body irradiation and high-dose etoposide as a preparatory regimen for bone marrow transplantation for 94 patients with chronic myelogenous leukemia in chronic phase. Blood 1994;84:1672–9.

492. Marmont AM, Horowitz MM, Gale RP, et al. T-cell depletion of HLA-identical transplants in leukemia. Blood 1991;78:2120–30.

493 Schattenberg A, De Witte T, Preijers F, et al. Allogeneic bone marrow transplantation for leukemia with marrow grafts depleted of lymphocytes by counterflow centrifugation. Blood 1990;75:1356–63.

494. Mrsic M, Horowitz MM, Atkinson K, et al Second HLA-identical sibling transplants for leukemia recurrence. Bone Marrow Transplant 1992;9:269–75.

495. Higano CS, Chielens D, Raskind W, et al. Use of α-2a-interferon to treat cytogenetic relapse of chronic myeloid leukemia after marrow transplantation. Blood 1997;90:2549–54.

496. Luis Steegmann J, Casado F, Granados E, et al. Treatment of chronic myeloid leukemia relapsing after allogeneic bone marrow transplantation: the case for giving interferon. Blood 1998;91:2617–9.

497. Higano CS, Raskind WH, Singer JW. Use of alpha interferon for the treatment of relapse of chronic myelogenous leukemia in chronic phase after allogeneic bone marrow transplantation. Blood 1992;80:1437–42.

498. Higano C, Raskind W, Singer J. Alpha interferon treatment of cytogenetic-only relapse of chronic myelogenous leukemia after marrow transplantation [abstract]. Proc Am Soc Clin Oncol 1993;12:307.

499. Kolb HJ, Schattenberg A, Goldman JM, et al. Graft vs leukemia effect of donor lymphocyte transfusion in marrow grafted patients. European Group for Blood and Marrow Transplantation Working Party on Chronic Leukemia. Blood 1995;86:2041–50.

500. Hertenstein B, Wiesneth M, Jurgen N, et al. Interferon-α and donor buffy coat transfusions for treatment of relapsed chronic myeloid leukemia after allogeneic bone marrow transplantation. Transplantation 1993;56:1114–8.

501. Bar BM, Schattenberg A, Mensink EJ, et al. Donor leukocyte infusion for chronic myeloid leukemia relapsed after allogeneic bone marrow transplantation. J Clin Oncol 1993;11:513–9.

502. Drobyski WR, Keever CA, Roth MS, et al. Salvage immunotherapy using donor leukocyte infusions as treatment for relapsed chronic myelogenous leukemia after allogeneic bone marrow transplantation: efficacy and toxicity of a defined T-cell dose. Blood 1993;82:2310–8.

503. Porter DL, Roth MS, McGarigle C, et al. Induction of graft-versus-host disease as immunotherapy for relapsed chronic myeloid leukemia. N Engl J Med 1994;330:100–6.

504. Collins RH Jr, Shpilberg O, Drobyski WR, et al. Donor leucocyte infusion in 140 patients with relapsed malignancy after allogeneic transplantation. J Clin Oncol 1997;15:433–44.

505. Kolb HJ, Mittermuller J, Clemm C, et al. Donor leucocyte transfusions for treatment of recurrent chronic myelogenous leukemia in marrow transplanted patients. Blood 1990;76:2462–5.

506. van Rhee F, Savage D, Blackwell J, et al. Adoptive immunotherapy for relapse of chronic myeloid leukemia after allogeneic bone marrow transplant: equal efficacy of lymphocytes from sibling and matched unrelated donors. Bone Marrow Transplant 1998;21:1055–61.

507. Raanani P, Dazzi F, Sohal J, et al. The rate and kinetics of molecular response to donor leucocyte transfusions in chronic myeloid leukaemia patients treated for relapse after allogeneic bone marrow transplantation. Br J Haematol 1999;99:945–50.

508. McGlave P, Bartsch G, Anasetti C, et al. Unrelated donor marrow transplantation therapy for chronic myelogenous leukemia: initial experience of the National Marrow Donor Program. Blood 1993;81:543–50.

509. Marks DI, Cullis JO, Ward KN, et al. Allogeneic bone marrow transplantation for chronic myeloid leukemia using sibling and volunteer unrelated donors. A comparison of complications in the first 2 years. Ann Intern Med 1993;119:207–14.

510. Spencer A, Szydlo RM, Brookes PA, et al. Bone marrow transplantation for chronic myeloid leukemia with volunteer unrelated donors using ex vivo or in vivo T-cell depletion: major prognostic impact of HLA class I identity between donor and recipient. Blood 1995;86:3590–7.

511. Lee SJ, Kuntz KM, Horowitz MM, et al. Unrelated donor bone marrow transplantation for chronic myelogenous leukemia: a decision analysis. Ann Intern Med 1997;127:1080–8.

512. Hansen JA, Gooley TA, Martin PJ, et al. Bone marrow transplantation from unrelated donors for patients with chronic myeloid leukemia. N Engl J Med 1998;338:962–8.

513. Morton AJ, Gooley T, Hansen JA, et al. Association between pretransplant interferon-alpha and outcome after unrelated donor marrow transplantation for chronic myelogenous leukemia in chronic phase. Blood 1998;92:394–401.

514. McGlave PB, Shu YO, Wen W, et al. Unrelated donor marrow transplantation for chronic myelogenous leukemia. 9 years' experience of the National Marrow Program. Blood 2000;95:2219–25.

515. Hehlmann R, Hochhaus A, Kolb HJ, et al. Interferon-alpha before allogeneic bone marrow transplantation in chronic myelogenous leukemia does not affect outcome adversely, provided it is discontinued at least 90 days before the procedure. Blood 1999;94:3668–77.

516. Beelen DW, Graeven U, Elmaagacli AH, et al. Prolonged administration of interferon-alpha in patients with chronic-phase Philadelphia chromosome-positive chronic myelogenous leukemia before allogeneic bone marrow transplantation may adversely affect transplant outcome. Blood 1995;85:2981–90.

517. Giralt SA, Kantarjian HM, Talpaz M, et al. Effect of prior interferon alfa therapy on the outcome of allogeneic bone marrow transplantation for chronic myelogenous leukemia. J Clin Oncol 1993;11:1055–61.

518. Tomas JF, Lopez-Lorenzo JL, Requena MJ, et al. Absence of influence of prior treatment with interferon on the outcome of allogeneic bone marrow transplantation for chronic myeloid leukemia. Bone Marrow Transplant 1998;22:47–51.

519. Leemhuis T, Leibowitz D, Cox G, et al. Identification of BCR/ABL-negative primitive hematopoietic progenitor cells within chronic myeloid leukemia marrow. Blood 1993;81:801–7.

520. Carella AM, Pollicardo N, Pungolino E, et al. Mobilization of cytogenetically "normal" blood progenitor cells by intensive conventional chemotherapy for chronic myeloid and acute lymphoblastic leukemia. Leuk Lymphoma 1993;9:477–83.

521. Kantarjian H, Talpaz M, Hester J, et al. Collection of peripheral blood diploid cells from chronic myelogenous leukemia patients early in the recovery phase from myelosuppression induced by intensive chemotherapy [abstract]. Blood 1994;84:382a.

522. Bhatia R, Verfaillie CM, Miller JS, McGlave PB. Autologous transplantation therapy for chronic myelogenous leukemia [review]. Blood 1997;89:2623–34.

523. Brito-Babapulle F, Bowcock SJ, Marcus RE, et al. Autografting for patients with chronic myeloid leukemia in chronic phase: peripheral blood stem cells may have a finite capacity for maintaining haemopoiesis. Br J Haematol 1989;73:76–81.

524. Kantarjian HM, Talpaz M, LeMaistre CF, et al. Intensive combination chemotherapy and autologous bone marrow transplantation leads to the reappearance of Philadelphia chromosome-negative cells in chronic myelogenous leukemia. Cancer 1991;67:2959–65.

525. Reiffers J, Goldman J, Meloni G, et al. on behalf of the Chronic Leukemia Working Party of the EBMT. Autologous stem cell transplantation in chronic myelogenous leukemia: a retrospective analysis of the European Group for Bone Marrow Transplantation. Bone Marrow Transplant 1994;14:407–10.

526. Talpaz M, Kantarjian H, Khouri I, et al. Diploid cells collected from chronic myelogenous leukemia patients during recovery from conventional dose-induced myelosuppression generate complete cytogenetic remissions after autologous transplantation [abstract]. Blood 1994;84:537a.

527. Reiffers J, Trouette R, Marit G, et al. Autologous blood stem cell transplantation for chronic granulocytic leukaemia in transformation: a report of 47 cases. Br J Haematol 1991;77:339–45.

528. Khouri IF, Kantarjian HM, Talpaz M, et al. High-dose chemotherapy and unpurged autologous stem cell transplantation for chronic myelogenous leukemia: the M.D. Anderson experience [abstract]. Blood 1994;84:537a.

529. Boiron J-M, Cahn J-Y, Meloni G, et al. Chronic myeloid leukemia in first chronic phase not responding to α-interferon: outcome and prognostic factors after autologous transplantation. Bone Marrow Transplant 1999;24:259–64.

530. Khouri IF, Kantarjian HM, Talpaz M, et al. Results with high-dose chemotherapy and unpurged autologous stem cell transplantation in 73 patients with chronic myelogenous leukemia. The MD Anderson experience. Bone Marrow Transplant 1996;17:775–9.

531. Pigneux A, Faberes C, Boiren JM, et al. Autologous stem cell transplantation in chronic myeloid leukaemia: a single center experience. Bone Marrow Transplant 1999;24:265–70.

532. Dunbar CE, Stewart FM. Separating the wheat from the chaff: selection of benign hematopoietic cells in chronic myeloid leukemia. Blood 1992;79:1107–10.

533. Turhan AG, Humphries RK, Eaves CJ, et al. Detection of breakpoint cluster region- negative and nonclonal hematopoiesis in vitro and in vivo after transplantation of cells selected in cultures of chronic myeloid leukemia marrow. Blood 1990;76:2404–10.

534. Brandwein JM, Dube ID, Laraya P, et al. Maintenance of Philadelphia-chromosome–positive progenitors in long-term marrow cultures from patients with advanced chronic myeloid leukemia. Leukemia 1992;6:556–61.

535. Carlo-Stella C, Mangoni L, Piovani G, et al. In vitro marrow purging in chronic myelogenous leukemia: effect of mafosfamide and recombinant granulocyte-macrophage colony-stimulating factor. Bone Marrow Transplant 1991;8:265–73.

536. Rizzoli V, Mangoni L, Piovani G, et al. Mafosfamide purged autografts for chronic myelogenous leukemia [abstract]. Blood 1992;80(Suppl 1):66a.

537. McGlave P, Miller J, Miller W, et al. Autologous marrow transplant therapy for CML using marrow treated ex vivo with human recombinant interferon gamma [abstract]. Blood 1992;80(Suppl 1):537a.

538. Ratajczak MZ, Hijiya N, Catani L, et al. Acute- and chronic-phase chronic myelogenous leukemia colony-forming units are highly sensitive to the growth inhibitory effects of c-myb antisense oligodeoxynucleotides. Blood 1992;79:1956–61.

539. Szczylik C, Skorski T, Nicolaides NC, et al. Selective inhibition of leukemia cell proliferation by BCR-ABL antisense oligodeoxynucleotides. Science 1991;253:562–5.

540. Mahon FX, Belloc F, Barbot C, et al. Chronic myelogenous leukemia: in vitro study with antisense oligomers. Blood 1992;80(Suppl 1):211a.

541. Martiat P, Lewalle P, Taj AS, et al. Retrovirally transduced antisense sequences stably suppress P210BCR/ABL and inhibit the proliferation of BCR/ABL-containing cell lines. Blood 1993;81:502–9.

542. Rowe JM, Ryan D, Dipersio J, et al. Autografting in chronic myelogenous leukemia followed by immunotherapy. Stem Cells 1993;11:34–42.

543. de Fabritiis P, Petti MC, Montefusco E, et al. BCR-ABL antisense oligodeoxynucleotide in vitro purging and autologous bone marrow transplantation for patients with chronic myelogenous leukemia in advanced phase. Blood 1998;91:3156–62.

544. Kantarjian HM, O'Brien SM, Keating M, et al. Results of decitabine therapy in the accelerated and blastic phases of chronic myelogenous leukemia. Leukemia 1997;11:1617–20.

545. Kantarjian HM, O'Brien SM, Estey E, et al. Decitabine studies in chronic and acute myelogenous leukemia. Leukemia 1997;11:S35–6.

546. Buchdunger E, Muller M, et al. A potent protein-tyrosine kinase inhibitor which inhibits PDGF receptor and C-Kit mediated in vitro signal transduction and in vivo tumor growth. Submitted.

547. Heinrich M, Zigler A, Griffith D, et al. Selective pharmacological inhibition of wild type and mutant c-kit receptor tyrosine kinase activity in hematopoietic cells [abstract]. Blood 1999;94:265.

548. Druker BJ, Tamura S, Buchdunger E, et al. Effects of a selective inhibitor of the Abl tyrosine kinase on the growth of Bcr-Abl positive cells. Nat Med 1996; 2:561–6.

549. Druker BJ, Talpaz M, Resta D, et al. Clinical efficacy and safety of an abl specific therapy for chronic myelogenous leukemia [abstract]. Blood 1999;94:1639.

550. Druker BJ, Kantarjian H, Sawyers CL, et al. Activity of an abl specific tyrosine kinase inhibitor in patients with bcr-abl positive acute leukemias including chronic myelogenous leukemia in blast crisis [abstract]. Blood 1999;94:3082.

551. Thiesing JT, Ohno-Jones S, Kolibaba KS, Druker B. Efficacy of an abl tyrosine kinase inhibitor in conjunction with other anti-neoplastic agents against bcr/abl positive cells [abstract]. Blood 1999;94:440.

552. Mahon FX, Deininger MW, Schultheis B, et al. Selection and characterization of BCR-ABL positive cell lines with differential sensitivity to the tyrosine kinase inhibitor STI571: diverse mechanisms of resistance. Blood 2000;96:1070–9.

553. Kantarjian HM, Talpaz M, Kontoyiannis D, et al. Treatment of chronic myelogenous leukemia in accelerated and blastic phases with daunorubicin, high-dose cytarabine, and granulocyte-macrophage colony-stimulating factor. J Clin Oncol 1992;10:398–405.

554. Kouides PA, Rowe JM. A dose intensive regimen of cytosine arabinoside and daunorubicin for chronic myelogenous leukemia in blast crisis. Leukemia 1995;19:763–70.

555. Lipton JH, Messner HA, Curtis JE, et al. Intensive remission induction therapy for chronic myeloid leukemia in blast phase with a goal of post-remission bone marrow transplant—a pilot study. Eur J Haematol 1996;57:42–5.

556. Montefusco E, Petti MC, Alimenta G, et al. Etoposide, intermediate-dose cytarabine and carboplatin (VAC): a combination therapy for the blastic phase of chronic myelogenous leukemia. Ann Oncol 1997;8:175–9.

557. Dann EJ, Anastasi J, Larson RA. High-dose cladribine therapy for chronic myelogenous leukemia in the accelerated or blast phase. J Clin Oncol 1998;16:1498–504.

8

Complications of Treatment

PETER H. WIERNIK, MD

This chapter deals with select toxicities of certain drugs used in the treatment of the leukemias in adults and emphasizes important toxicities of newer agents. Whenever possible, preventive and corrective measures are discussed.

CARDIAC TOXICITY

Anthracyclines

The cardiac toxicity of anthracycline antineoplastic agents became evident almost immediately after these agents were first introduced into clinical trial. The major manifestation of this toxicity is decreased left ventricular ejection fraction and congestive heart failure (Figure 8–1).[1] Heart failure results from impaired left ventricular contractility and, especially in children and young adults, increased afterload secondary to left ventricular wall thinning.[2] Myocardial fibrosis is seen microscopically in affected patients.[3] A number of risk factors for anthracycline-induced cardiac toxicity have been identified. In children, black race and trisomy 21 increase the risk of anthracycline car-

diotoxicity, and female gender is a risk factor for patients of all ages.[2] The cumulative anthracycline dose, rate of administration, mediastinal irradiation, history of heart disease, and electrolyte imbalance, especially hypokalemia and hypomagnesemia, are major risk factors for children and adults.[4] The mechanism of anthracycline cardiac toxicity involves anthracycline-iron complexes that generate highly reactive oxygen species that cause lipid peroxidation in the myocyte membrane, which results in myocyte damage and eventual fibrosis.[5,6]

In an early investigation of clinical anthracycline cardiac toxicity, Steinherz and colleagues[3] studied 201 patients who had survived pediatric malignancies treated a median of 7 years prior to the study. They found abnormal cardiac function on noninvasive cardiac testing in 23 percent of patients. The prevalence of cardiac dysfunction was 38 percent in 56 patients studied 10 years or more after completion of treatment who had received a median anthracycline dose of 495 mg/m^2, and the prevalence of cardiac functional abnormalities was 63 percent in patients who received 500 mg/m^2 or more total dose of anthracycline 10 or more years post-treatment.

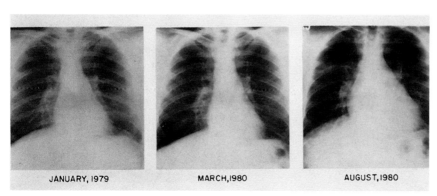

Figure 8–1. Chest radiographs showing progressive cardiomegaly over a 19-month period due to anthracycline cardiac toxicity in a patient with AML who received re-induction therapy for her third relapse in October 1978.

Frank cardiac failure and dysrhythmia were evident in 9 of the entire study group of 201 patients, and an additional 3 patients had suddenly died. The existence of anthracycline-induced late ventricular dysfunction was subsequently confirmed in an extensive literature review by Shan and colleagues[7]

More recently, Kremer and colleagues[8] studied the incidence of early and late anthracycline-induced clinical heart failure in 607 patients who had been treated as children between 1976 and 1996. The mean follow-up time was 6.3 years. The cumulative incidence of clinical heart failure was 2.8 percent, and the mean cumulative dose of anthracycline was only 301 mg/m^2. Patients who had received a higher cumulative anthracycline dose had a higher incidence of congestive heart failure, and the risk of failure increased over time post-treatment (2% after 2 years, 5% after 15 years).

A number of pharmacologic approaches to reducing anthracycline-induced cardiac toxicity have been studied. The bisdioxopiperazine dexrazoxane was shown in randomized trials of patients with breast cancer or pediatric sarcoma to allow for the administration of greater cumulative anthracycline doses while decreasing the risk of an adverse cardiac event from 31 to 14 percent.[1,5] Dexrazoxane administration did not significantly reduce response rates in those trials that involved more than 700 patients. However, not all studies have resulted in confidence that the addition of dexrazoxane to anthracycline-based chemotherapy does not impair response rates. In fact, the largest study of that question did show a significantly lower response rate with dexrazoxane compared with placebo.[5]

Dexrazoxane binds free and bound iron and decreases the formation of anthracycline-iron complexes, which are thought to initiate myocyte damage. It may markedly increase the granulocytopenia associated with anthracycline administration and may make anthracycline dosage reduction necessary, which may compromise treatment efficacy.

Batist and colleagues[9] studied liposome-encapsulated doxorubicin and cyclophosphamide in patients with metastatic breast cancer. Approximately 300 patients were randomized to receive encapsulated or free doxorubicin with the same dose of cyclophosphamide. Clinically significant cardiotoxicity occurred in 6 percent of patients receiving encapsulated doxorubicin and 21 percent of those treated with free anthracycline. Objective response rates, median time to progression, median time to treatment failure, and median survival were virtually identical in the two treatment groups. In addition, leukopenia was reduced in the encapsulated drug group. Similar studies are required for patients with acute leukemia treated with daunorubicin. Idarubicin seems less cardiotoxic than daunorubicin.[10] Therefore, it may be more difficult to demonstrate the efficacy of this or any other approach to the prevention of cardiotoxicity in patients with leukemia treated with that anthracycline.

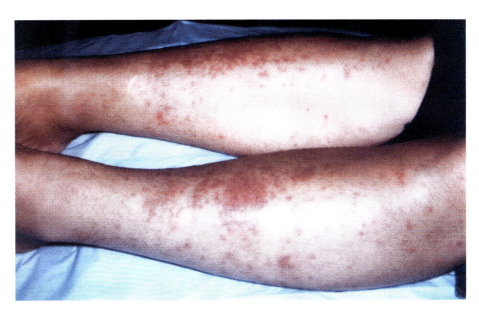

Figure 8–2. Macular erythematous skin reaction to all-*trans* retinoic acid (ATRA) in a patient with acute promyelocytic leukemia. The lesions were dry but not pruritic and were evident on the seventh day of daily treatment. About 10 percent of patients develop a skin rash with ATRA.

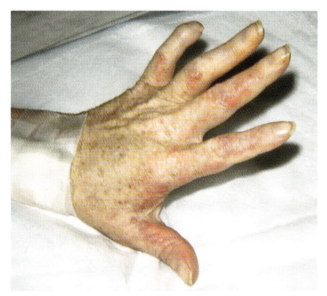

Figure 8–3. Patchy macular erythematous asymptomatic skin reaction to cytarabine. The lesions were confined to the hands and feet, which are typical of cytarabine reactions and occur in 2 to 3 percent of patients during the first exposure

There is a suggestion in the literature that amifostine administration may protect against anthracycline-induced cardiotoxicity.[11] It may be productive to formally follow that lead with a prospective, randomized trial.

Anagrelide

Anagrelide is a new oral agent used primarily in the treatment of essential thrombocytosis and for the control of thrombosis in polycythemia vera. Serious cardiovascular adverse events, including congestive heart failure[12] and cardiac arrhythmias,[13] have been reported with its use. The incidence of these complications is not known, but, although these toxicities appear to be uncommon, they have been reported in virtually all series.[14,15] The mechanism of cardiotoxicity is thought to be the inhibition of phosphodiesterase, which may result in positive inotropic activity and vasodilation.[12,13]

Arsenic Trioxide

Arsenic trioxide has major activity against relapsed and refractory acute promyelocytic leukemia (APL) and is being investigated in other hematologic malignancies. Isolated reports of cardiac toxicity

with this agent have appeared over the last few years.[16,17] Recently, Ohnishi and colleagues[18] used continuous monitoring to prospectively follow electrocardiograms and echocardiograms to determine the cardiac toxicity in 8 patients treated with arsenic trioxide for APL. They reported prolonged QT intervals in all 8 patients studied and serious arrhythmias in 4 of those patients. They recommended that patients receiving arsenic trioxide should be carefully monitored for QT interval prolongation, and, if such prolongation should occur, patients should be monitored for serious arrhythmias.

Unnikrishnan and colleagues[19] reported torsades de pointes, a ventricular tachycardia with QRS complexes of changing amplitude that twist around the isoelectric baseline and are known to occur with arsenic poisoning, in three patients with hematologic malignancies while undergoing treatment with arsenic trioxide. They pointed out that arsenic-induced ventricular arrhythmias are refractory to correction by most techniques, including cardioversion.

Although the incidence of serious arsenic trioxide–induced cardiac toxicity is not known at this time, it seems clear that significant toxicity may occur with commercially available[18] and investigational drugs.[19] Patients should be informed and monitored accordingly.

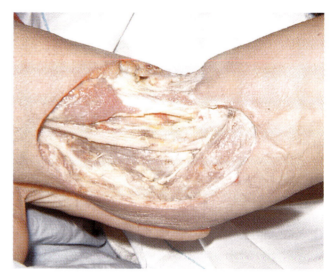

Figure 8–4. Life-threatening soft-tissue necrosis exposing underlying tendons secondary to paravenous extravasation of a vesicant investigational agent. Such agents should only be administered through an intravenous catheter or other access device demonstrated to be functioning well prior to drug administration to prevent such devastating complications.

ALL-*TRANS* RETINOIC ACID SYNDROME

All-*trans* retinoic acid (ATRA) syndrome was first described by Frankel and colleagues as a potentially fatal pulmonary complication of ATRA treatment of patients with APL.[20] They reported that a minority of patients whose white blood cell counts rose after ATRA administration developed an acute pulmonary distress syndrome, which could be fatal. Autopsy revealed engorgement of pulmonary microvasculature with partially differentiated white blood cells. They also presented evidence that the administration of dexamethasone at the first evidence of the syndrome was usually successful in reversing it. Subsequently, De Botton and colleagues[21] reviewed a large series of patients in an effort to learn more about the diagnosis and management of the ATRA syndrome. They analyzed the data from 64 of 413 (15%) patients who developed the syndrome within a median of 7 days after beginning induction treatment. The most common manifestations of the syndrome were respiratory distress (89%), fever (81%), pulmonary infiltrates (81%), weight gain (50%), and pleural effusion (47%). In addition, renal failure occurred in 39% of patients, and pericardial effusion, cardiac failure, and hypotension each occurred in 19% or less of patients. Most of the patients had several of those manifestations of the syndrome, and mechanical ventilation was required by 13 patients. Fourteen percent of patients who developed the ATRA syndrome died (1.2% of all patients treated). All-*trans* retinoic acid syndrome occurred only during induction therapy and was not seen in patients who received ATRA maintenance therapy while in complete remission. When this syndrome was first described, it was thought that it occurred most frequently in patients with an elevated white blood cell count, but no relationship between pretreatment count and incidence of ATRA syndrome was found in the study by De Botton and colleagues.[21] Curiously, dexamethasone was not found to be useful in treating the ATRA syndrome in that study. Another important and surprising finding in that study was that the occurrence of the ATRA syndrome was associated with a significantly lower event-free and overall survival rate compared with the study group as a whole. Therefore, the ATRA syndrome in APL has implications beyond the acute distress that led to its description.

Other data on the effect of the ATRA syndrome on event-free survival have been presented. Ko and colleagues[22] suggested that the ATRA syndrome was a risk factor for extramedullary relapse in APL. They reported such relapses in three of five patients with ATRA syndrome, compared with none of eight patients treated with ATRA who did not develop the ATRA syndrome. These provocative data have not, to date, been confirmed by others. In the intergroup experience reported by Tallman and colleagues,[23] data similar to that of De Botton and colleagues[21] were reported. ATRA also can cause cutaneous eruptions as shown in Figure 8–2.

Che-Pin and colleagues[24] reported a syndrome identical to the ATRA syndrome in a patient with APL treated for relapse with arsenic trioxide. They suggested that any agent that can induce leukocytosis in APL may cause this syndrome. Several authors have suggested that expression of certain adhesion molecules expressed by partially matured leukemic cells may be the unifying factor that leads to pulmonary leukostasis in these syndromes.

TUMOR LYSIS SYNDROME WITH RITUXIMAB

Rituximab is an anti-CD20 monoclonal antibody with activity against low-grade lymphoma and chronic lymphocytic leukemia. Byrd and colleagues[25] reported on five patients who received rituximab at a time when high numbers of tumor cells were circulating and experienced sudden, acute respiratory distress. All had bulky lymphadenopathy and organomegaly and rapid clearance of circulating abnormal lymphoid cells. Mild electrolyte imbalance consistent with tumor lysis syndrome developed as well. All patients survived and were subsequently retreated with rituximab without incident. These observations have been confirmed by others, and it is now recommended that rituximab be administered only to patients whose circulating abnormal lymphocyte count is 20,000/μL or less and in the absence of bulky lymphoid tumor. Winkler and colleagues[26] reported that the phenomenon described after infusion of rituximab to patients

with chronic lymphocytic leukemia (CLL) with a high white blood cell count is due to release of certain cytokines, such as tumor necrosis factor-α and interleukin-6. Their release caused fever, chills, nausea, vomiting, hypotension, and/or dyspnea in some patients. They also noted a rapid, substantial drop in circulating lymphocyte and platelet counts and a major increase in liver enzymes and prolongation of the prothrombin time. They recommended that in patients with CLL and leukocytosis, rituximab therapy should be initiated at a dose of 50 mg/m² on day 1, followed by 150 mg/m² on day 2 and the balance of the usual 375 mg/m² dose on day 3. No adverse reactions were seen with this dose and schedule of administration.

In our center, we use leukapheresis to lower the white blood cell count to normal in patients with CLL and then proceed to full- or higher-dose[27] rituximab therapy without incident.

NEUROTOXICITY OF INTRATHECAL CHEMOTHERAPY

Resar and colleagues[28] reported on two teenagers who developed severe neurotoxicity after intrathecal drug administration for acute leukemia. In one, a rapidly ascending myelopathy and encephalopathy developed within a day of receiving the third daily dose of intrathecal cytarabine alone, which persisted for 10 months until the boy's death. The other patient had resolution of her encephalopathy and seizures after a month. She had received both cytarabine and methotrexate intrathecally. Others have reported focal leukoencephalopathy after intraventricular administration of methotrexate or cytarabine to children and adults.[29] Burch and colleagues[30] demonstrated in rabbits that 67 to 99 percent of the total area of the spinal cord is exposed to intrathecally administered drug about an hour after injection and that high drug levels were measured in the area of the substantia gelatinosa and peripheral white matter, which correspond to the sites of pathologic changes seen in the cord and brain of patients with intrathecal chemotherapy-induced neurotoxicity.[31] Fortunately, neurotoxicity from intrathecal chemotherapy is rare, although we have observed permanent paraplegia in adults from

intrathecal cytarabine properly administered on two occasions. There is no effective treatment for this complication.

NEUROTOXICITY OF INTRAVENOUS CYTARABINE

Although cytarabine frequently causes cutaneous eruptions (Figure 8–3), other more serious complications, such as neurotoxicity, are less well known. Nand and colleagues[32] reported a 23 percent incidence of cerebellar toxicity in adults receiving high-dose cytarabine and found preexisting and progressive hepatic dysfunction to be a major predisposing factor. Damon and colleagues[33] reported neurotoxicity from high-dose cytarabine in 18 percent of 101 patients who received 147 courses of treatment. It was reversible in 76 percent of patients who experienced it. The most significant predisposing factor in their study was renal insufficiency. Neurotoxicity was observed in 62 percent of patients with a serum creatinine level of ≥ 1.5 mg/dL and only 8 percent of patients with normal renal function. Rubin and colleagues[34] confirmed the relationship between hepatic and renal dysfunction and the development of neurotoxicity after high-dose cytarabine and extended the observations of others. They also found age ≥ 40 years to be a risk factor. In their study, patients under the age of 40 years with normal hepatic and renal function had an incidence of neurotoxicity after high-dose cytarabine administration of only 1 percent, compared with 37 percent for patients who had two or more of the three risk factors identified.

Although neurotoxicity from high-dose cytarabine is usually manifested by cerebellar dysfunction and somnolence, optic neuropathy, anosmia, hemiparesis, dysarthria, and coma have each rarely been reported.[35] Courtney and Coffey[36] studied mechanisms of cytarabine neurotoxicity in vitro and found that cytarabine-induced death of differentiating cerebellar neurons is prevented by cycloheximide at concentrations that prevent protein synthesis and that the activity of certain cyclin-dependent kinases may play a major role in cerebellar neuron death. The neurotoxicity of other chemotherapeutic agents has been thoroughly reviewed previously.[37,38]

CYTARABINE CORNEAL TOXICITY

High-dose cytarabine may cause ocular pain, tearing, a sensation of a foreign body in the eye, photophobia, or blurred vision.[39] These symptoms are frequently accompanied by conjunctival hyperemia and fine corneal epithelial opacities. All of these problems, due to cytarabine inhibition of corneal epithelial DNA synthesis, may spontaneously resolve within a week of discontinuing cytarabine administration. However, cataracts may occasionally occur. Lass and colleagues[40] demonstrated that 1 percent prednisolone phosphate eyedrops administered 12 hours before and at the time of each high-dose cytarabine dose could virtually eliminate the corneal toxicity of high-dose cytarabine, and the use of steroid eyedrops for this purpose has become standard. The same group[41] demonstrated similar efficacy for 2-deoxycytidine eyedrops, but that preparation is not generally available.

NEUROPSYCHIATRIC TOXICITY OF INTERFERON

Many patients with chronic myelogenous leukemia (CML) find interferon a difficult treatment, primarily because of its neuropsychiatric toxicity. Some patients experience severe neuropsychiatric problems with this biologic, but the frequency of and risk factors for developing such toxicity have only recently been determined. Hensley and colleagues[42] studied 91 patients with previously untreated CML treated with recombinant interferon-α2b plus low-dose cytarabine for the development of grade 3 to 4 neuropsychiatric toxicity, which they found in 22 patients, or 24 percent of the study group. The toxic effects of the treatment resolved after discontinuation of treatment in all patients but commonly recurred in patients who were re-treated with the same agent. The authors made the very important observation that 63 percent of patients with a pretreatment diagnosis of a neurologic or psychiatric disorder developed grade 3 to 4 neuropsychiatric toxicity from interferon, compared with 14 percent of patients without a prior neuropsychiatric problem. Therefore, a neuropsychiatric history is important in determining whether a patient is a candidate for interferon therapy. The study also demonstrated that patients who discontinue interferon therapy because of serious neuropsychiatric toxicity should not be rechallenged.

Musselman and colleagues[43] recently conducted a study to determine whether paroxetine could prevent depression in patients receiving high-dose interferon. In a double-blind study in patients receiving high-dose interferon-α2b for malignant melanoma, they randomly assigned 20 patients to receive paroxetine and 20 others to receive placebo. Treatment with paroxetine was initiated 2 weeks before starting interferon therapy and continued during the first 3 months of interferon administration. Major depression occurred in 2 of 18 patients in the paroxetine group and 9 of 20 in the placebo group. They concluded that paroxetine can minimize depression related to interferon treatment. It therefore seems prudent to pretreat patients with paroxetine prior to interferon administration and to continue the antidepressant during interferon therapy.

FLUDARABINE TOXICITY

A number of uncommon yet serious toxicities of fludarabine therapy for CLL and low-grade lymphoma have recently come to light. Neurotoxicity with this agent, when given at a high dose, is well documented.[44] However, it is not generally appreciated that serious neurotoxicity may rarely occur with standard doses (0.2% of patients who receive 125 mg/m^2 per course).[45] Visual defects are the most common complaint, but progressive encephalopathy has also been reported. The drug appears to cause progressive demyelination in those patients.[45]

At least two cases of autoimmune thrombocytopenia have been reported after fludarabine administration,[46] but, more commonly, hemolytic anemia has been observed.[47] The anemia may occur with the first or subsequent courses of the drug, and hematocrit declines of 8 to 29 points (median 14) have been reported,[47] and seven patients are known to have died as a result of hemolytic anemia.[47] Rechallenge of patients who developed hemolytic anemia almost always leads to another episode; therefore, rechallenge should not be attempted. We have treated one patient with CLL with standard doses of fludarabine who developed fatal aplastic anemia.

That patient had also developed myasthenia gravis just prior to the diagnosis of CLL, which suggests that an autoimmune phenomenon may have been responsible for the development of aplastic anemia. Such a mechanism is thought to underlie fludarabine-induced hemolytic anemia.[47]

Diffuse interstitial pneumonitis responsive to corticosteroids has been observed at least once after fludarabine administration to a patient with CLL.[48]

CLADRIBINE TOXICITY

Although usually well tolerated as a treatment for hairy cell leukemia and CLL,[49] some of the same uncommon toxicities (and others) observed with fludarabine have been reported with cladribine. Autoimmune hemolytic anemia refractory to corticosteroid treatment may occur early or late[50] during treatment, and pure red cell aplasia in patients with CLL treated with cladribine has been reported as well.[51] Gillis and colleagues[52] found a high prevalence of hypoplastic or aplastic foci in bone marrow biopsies of patients with hairy cell leukemia after treatment with cladribine. They observed such foci in only 13 percent of pretherapy biopsies and in 66 percent of post-therapy biopsies. Most of the patients with hypoplastic biopsies had normal blood counts, but the long-term significance of this finding, if any, is not yet known.

Cladribine has been reported to rarely cause severe, even life-threatening skin reactions in patients with hairy cell leukemia.[53]

AVASCULAR NECROSIS OF BONE

It was recognized more than a decade ago that corticosteroid therapy for graft-versus-host disease increased the risk for avascular necrosis of bone in survivors of bone marrow transplantation.[54] The magnitude of the problem was studied by Enright and colleagues,[55] who reviewed the records of 902 consecutive bone marrow transplant patients and found 28 who had developed avascular necrosis of bone. Only allogeneic transplant patients developed this complication (28 of 642: 0.4% incidence), and autologous transplant patients were not at risk. Symptoms of affected patients began a median of 1 year post-transplantation, and multiple joints were usually involved. Hip and knee involvement was more common than ankle, shoulder, or elbow involvement. Almost all affected patients had received corticosteroid prophylaxis and therapy for graft-versus-host disease, and there was a significant correlation between the total cumulative corticosteroid dose and number of joints involved. Increasing age was also an independent risk factor for avascular necrosis of bone in these patients. Half of the afflicted patients required surgery for joint replacement or repair.

Avascular necrosis of bone has also been observed in adult acute leukemia patients treated with corticosteroid-containing regimens that do not include bone marrow transplantation, at about the same rate.[56]

MISCELLANEOUS TOXICITIES

A number of infrequent complications of leukemia treatment that have been well described appear not to be fully appreciated (Figure 8–4). Physicians acquainted with these problems will better serve patients who experience them.

Anemia develops to a mild or moderate degree after long-term administration of anagrelide in approximately one-quarter of patients.[15] There are no data on the efficacy or lack thereof of recombinant erythropoietin in this situation, but transfusion is rarely required.

Methotrexate, by any route of administration, including intrathecal,[57] may rarely cause a pneumonitis characterized by nonproductive cough, fever, dyspnea, cyanosis, eosinophilia, and bilateral pulmonary infiltrates. Corticosteroid therapy has been helpful to some patients.

Porphyria cutanea tarda (Figures 8–5 to 8–7) may be unmasked in patients with acute myelogenous leukemia (AML) by treatment.[58] Iron overload from blood transfusion, hepatotoxicity from estrogens given to block menstruation, or cytarabine hepatotoxicity may be causally related. Signs and symptoms include dark urine, facial pigmentation, and vesicular or ulcerative lesions of the feet, hands, neck, and face. Hypertrichosis with a peculiar distribution involving the forehead, face, and forearms

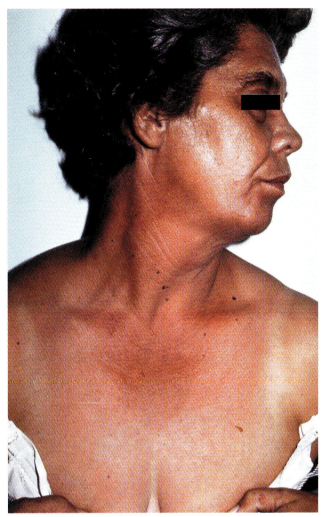

Figure 8–5. Hyperpigmentation of the skin in a woman with AML who developed porphyria cutanea tarda while receiving postremission therapy. She had no history of alcoholism but received multiple courses of estrogens to prevent menstruation during treatment.

may also occur. The mainstay of treatment is phlebotomy to reduce iron stores in the liver.

The anti-CD33 calicheamicin conjugate (gemtuzumab ozogamicin) recently introduced for the

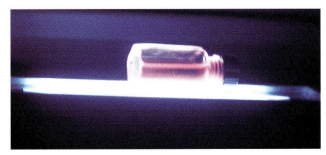

Figure 8–6. The urine of the patient in Figure 8–5 under ultraviolet light fluoresces due to excreted porphyrins.

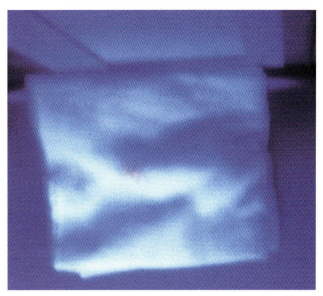

Figure 8–7. Liver biopsy from the patient in Figures 8–5 and 8–6 photographed under ultraviolet light. Porphyrins cause the specimen to fluoresce.

therapy of certain patients with AML is known to be associated with dose-related hepatotoxicity manifested by hepatic enzyme elevation, which is usually clinically insignificant.[59] However, Neumeister and colleagues[60] recently reported hepatic veno-occlusive disease in two patients with relapsed AML after administration of that agent. The patients were heavily pretreated and may have had other risk factors for veno-occlusive disease, but this report requires that caution be observed in treating patients who may be at risk for hepatic veno-occlusive disease with this new agent.

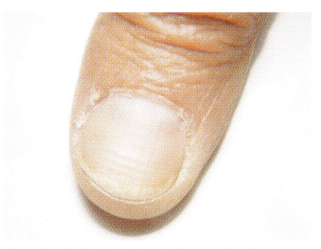

Figure 8–8. Multiple nail horizontal ridges resulting from arrested nail growth with each of three induction therapy courses for AML.

Finally, it is prudent to inform patients that horizontal pigmented banding of the nails (Figure 8–8) may occur with the administration of anthracyclines,[61] cyclophosphamide, and other chemotherapeutic agents[62] and that mitoxantrone administration is likely to result in blue urine.

REFERENCES

1. Hochster H, Wasserheit C, Speyer J. Cardiotoxicity and cardioprotection during chemotherapy. Curr Opin Oncol 1995;7:304–9.
2. Grenier MA, Lipshultz SE. Epidemiology of anthracycline cardiotoxicity in children and adults. Semin Oncol 1998;25:72–85.
3. Steinherz LJ, Steinherz PG, Tan CT, et al. Cardiac toxicity 4 to 20 years after completing anthracycline therapy. JAMA 1991;25:1672–7.
4. Pai VB, Nahata MC. Cardiotoxicity of chemotherapeutic agents: incidence, treatment and prevention. Drug Saf 2000;22:263–302.
5. Wiseman LR, Spencer CM. Dexrazoxane. A review of its use as a cardioprotective agent in patients receiving anthracycline-based chemotherapy. Drugs 1998;56:385–403.
6. Horenstein MS, Vander Heide RS, L'Ecuyer TJ. Molecular basis of anthracycline-induced cardiotoxicity and its prevention. Mol Genet Metab 2000;71:436–44.
7. Shan K, Lincoff AM, Young JB. Anthracycline-induced cardiotoxicity. Ann Intern Med 1996;125:47–58.
8. Kremer LC, van Dalen EC, Offringa M, et al. Anthracycline-induced clinical heart failure in a cohort of 607 children: long-term follow-up study. J Clin Oncol 2001;19:191–6.
9. Batist G, Ramakrishnan G, Rao CS, et al. Reduced cardiotoxicity and preserved antitumor efficacy of liposome-encapsulated doxorubicin and cyclophosphamide compared with conventional doxorubicin and cyclophosphamide in a randomized, multicenter trial of metastatic breast cancer. J Clin Oncol 2001;19:144–54.
10. Anderlini P, Benjamin RS, Wong FC, et al. Idarubicin cardiotoxicity: a retrospective study in acute myeloid leukemia and myelodysplasia. J Clin Oncol 1995; 13:2827–34.
11. Dorr RT, Lagel KE. Anthracycline cardioprotection by amifostine (WR-2721) and its active metabolite (WR-1065) in vitro. Proc Am Soc Clin Oncol 1994;13:435.
12. James CW. Anagrelide-induced cardiomyopathy. Pharmacotherapy 2000;20:1224–7.
13. Pescatore SL, Lindley C. Anagrelide: a novel agent for the treatment of myeloproliferative disorders. Expert Opin Pharmacother 2000;1:537–46.
14. Mills AK, Taylor KM, Wright SJ, et al. Efficacy, safety and tolerability of anagrelide in the treatment of essential thrombocythaemia. Aust N Z J Med 1999; 29:29–35.
15. Storen EC, Tefferi A. Long-term use of anagrelide in young patients with essential thrombocythemia. Blood 2001;97:863–6.
16. Huang SY, Chang CS, Tang JL, et al. Acute and chronic arsenic poisoning associated with treatment of acute promyelocytic leukaemia. Br J Haematol 1998;103:1092–5.
17. Westervelt P, Pollock J, Huang J, et al. Response and toxicity associated with dose escalation of arsenic trioxide in the treatment of resistant acute promyelocytic leukemia. Blood 1997; 90(Suppl 1):249b.
18. Ohnishi K, Yoshida H, Shigeno K, et al. Prolongation of the QT interval and ventricular tachycardia in patients treated with arsenic trioxide for acute promyelocytic leukemia. Ann Intern Med 2000;133:881–5.
19. Unnikrishnan D, Dutcher JP, Varshneya N, et al. Torsades de pointes in 3 patients with leukemia treated with arsenic trioxide. Blood 2001;97:1514–6.
20. Frankel SR, Eardley A, Lauwers G, et al. The "retinoic acid syndrome" in acute promyelocytic leukemia. Ann Intern Med 1992;117:292–6.
21. De Botton S, Dombret H, Sanz M, et al. Incidence, clinical features, and outcome of all trans-retinoic acid syndrome in 413 cases of newly diagnosed acute promyelocytic leukemia. The European APL group. Blood 1998;92:2712–8.
22. Ko BS, Tang JL, Chen YC, et al. Extramedullary relapse after all-trans retinoic acid treatment in acute promyelocytic leukemia—the occurrence of retinoic acid syndrome is a risk factor. Leukemia 1999;13:1406–8.
23. Tallman MS, Andersen JW, Schiffer CA, et al. Clinical description of 44 patients with acute promyelocytic leukemia who developed the retinoic acid syndrome. Blood 2000;95:90–5.
24. Che-Pin L, Huang IY, Lin WY, Sheu YT. Retinoic acid syndrome induced by arsenic trioxide in treating recurrent all-trans retinoic acid resistant acute promyelocytic leukemia. Leuk Lymphoma 2000;38:195–8.
25. Byrd JC, Waselenko JK, Maneatis TJ, et al. Rituximab therapy in hematologic malignancy patients with circulating blood tumor cells: association with increased infusion-related side effects and rapid tumor clearance. J Clin Oncol 1999;17:791–5.
26. Winkler U, Jensen M, Manzke O, et al. Cytokine-release syndrome in patients with B-cell chronic lymphocytic leukemia and high lymphocyte counts after treatment with an anti-CD20 monoclonal antibody (rituximab, IDEC-C2B8). Blood 1999;94:2217–24.
27. O'Brien S, Kantarjian H, Thomas DA, et al. Rituximab dose-escalation trial in chronic lymphocytic leukemia. J Clin Oncol 2001;19:2165–70.

28. Resar LMS, Phillips PC, Kastan MB, et al. Acute neurotoxicity after intrathecal cytosine arabinoside in two adolescents with acute lymphoblastic leukemia of B-cell type. Cancer 1993;71:117–23.

29. Colamaria V, Caraballo R, Borgna-Pignatti C, et al. Transient focal leukoencephalopathy following intraventricular methotrexate and cytarabine. A complication of the Ommaya reservoir: case report and review of the literature. Childs Nerv Syst 1990; 6:231–5.

30. Burch PA, Grossman SA, Reinhard CS. Spinal cord penetration of intrathecally administered cytarabine and methotrexate: a quantitative autoradiographic study. J Natl Cancer Inst 1988;80:1211–6.

31. Honkaniemi J, Kahara V, Dastidar P, et al. Reversible posterior leukoencephalopathy after combination chemotherapy. Neuroradiology 2000;42:895–9.

32. Nand S, Messmore HL Jr, Patel R, et al. Neurotoxicity associated with systemic high-dose cytosine arabinoside. J Clin Oncol 1986;4:571–5.

33. Damon LE, Mass R, Linker CA. The association between high-dose cytarabine neurotoxicity and renal insufficiency. J Clin Oncol 1989;7:1563–8.

34. Rubin EH, Andersen JW, Berg DT, et al. Risk factors for high-dose cytarabine neurotoxicity: an analysis of a Cancer and Leukemia Group B trial in patients with acute myeloid leukemia. J Clin Oncol 1992; 10:948–53.

35. Hoffman DL, Howard JR Jr, Sarma R, Riggs JE. Encephalopathy, myelopathy, optic neuropathy, and anosmia associated with intravenous cytosine arabinoside. Clin Neuropharmacol 1993;16:258–62.

36. Courtney MJ, Coffey ET. The mechanism of Ara-C-induced apoptosis of differentiating cerebellar granule neurons. Eur J Neurosci 1999;11:1073–84.

37. Weiss HD, Walker MD, Wiernik PH. Neurotoxicity of commonly used antineoplastic agents. N Engl J Med 1974;291:75–81, 127–33.

38. Kaplan RS, Wiernik PH. Neurotoxicity of antineoplastic drugs. Semin Oncol 1982;9:103–30.

39. Hopen G, Mondino BJ, Johnson BL, Chervenick PA. Corneal toxicity with systemic cytarabine. Am J Ophthalmol 1981;91:500–4.

40. Lass JH, Lazarus HM, Reed MD, Herzig RH. Topical corticosteroid therapy for corneal toxicity from systemically administered cytarabine. Am J Ophthalmol 1982;94:617–21.

41. Lazarus HM, Hartnett ME, Reed MD, et al. Comparison of the prophylactic effects of 2-deoxycytidine and prednisolone for high-dose intravenous cytarabine-induced keratitis. Am J Ophthalmol 1987;104: 476–80.

42. Hensley ML, Peterson B, Silver RT, et al. Risk factors for severe neuropsychiatric toxicity in patients receiving interferon alfa-2b and low-dose cytara-

bine for chronic myelogenous leukemia: analysis of Cancer and Leukemia Group B 9013. J Clin Oncol 2000;18:1301–8.

43. Musselman DL, Lawson DH, Gumnick JF, et al. Paroxetine for the prevention of depression induced by high-dose interferon alfa. N Engl J Med 2001;344:961–6.

44. Chun HG, Leyland-Jones BR, Caryk SM, Hoth DF. Central nervous system toxicity of fludarabine phosphate. Cancer Treat Rep 1986;70:1225–8.

45. Gonzalez H, Bolgert F, Camporo P, Leblond V. Progressive multifocal leukoencephalitis (PML) in three patients treated with standard-dose fludarabine (FAMP). Hematol Cell Ther 1999;41:183–6.

46. Bay JO, Fouassier M, Beal D, et al. Autoimmune thrombocytopenia after six cycles of fludarabine phosphate in a patient with chronic lymphocytic leukemia. Hematol Cell Ther 1997;39:209–12.

47. Weiss RB, Freiman J, Kweder SL, et al. Hemolytic anemia after fludarabine therapy for chronic lymphocytic leukemia. J Clin Oncol 1998;16:1885–9.

48. Hurst PG, Habib MP, Garewal H, et al. Pulmonary toxicity associated with fludarabine monophosphate. Invest New Drugs 1987;5:207–10.

49. Robak T, Blonski JZ, Kasznicki M, et al. Cladribine with or without prednisone in the treatment of previously treated and untreated B-cell chronic lymphocytic leukaemia—updated results of the multicentre study of 378 patients. Br J Haematol 2000;108:357–68.

50. Tetreault SA, Saven A. Delayed onset of autoimmune hemolytic anemia complicating cladribine therapy for Waldenstrom macroglobulinemia. Leuk Lymphoma 2000;37:125–30.

51. Robak T, Kasznicki M, Blonski JZ, et al. Pure red cell aplasia in patients with chronic lymphocytic leukaemia treated with cladribine. Br J Haematol 2001;112:1083–5.

52. Gillis S, Amir G, Bennett M, Polliack A. Unexpectedly high incidence of hypoplastic/aplastic foci in bone marrow biopsies of hairy cell leukemia patients in remission following 2-chlorodeoxyadenosine therapy. Eur J Haematol 2001;66:7–10.

53. Grey MR, Flanagan NG, Kelsey PR. Severe skin rash in two patients treated with 2-chlorodeoxyadenosine for hairy cell leukaemia at a single institution. Clin Lab Haematol 2000;22:111–3.

54. Atkinson K, Cohen M, Biggs J. Avascular necrosis of the femoral head secondary to corticosteroid therapy for graft-versus-host disease after marrow transplantation: effective therapy with hip arthroplasty. Bone Marrow Transplant 1987; 2:421–6.

55. Enright H, Haake R, Weisdorf D. Avascular necrosis of bone: a common serious complication of allogeneic bone marrow transplantation. Am J Med 1990;89: 733–8.

56. Hui L, Wiernik PH. Avascular necrosis of bone after

adult acute lymphocytic leukemia treatment with methotrexate, vincristine, L-asparaginase, and dexamethasone (MOAD). Am J Hematol 1996;52:184–8.

57. Gutin PH, Green MR, Bleyer WA, et al. Methotrexate pneumonitis induced by intrathecal methotrexate therapy. Cancer 1976;38:1529–34.

58. Dutcher JP, Fisher M, Spivack M, Wiernik PH. Porphyria cutanea tarda in a patient with acute leukemia. Am J Hematol 1986;23:69–75.

59. Sievers EL, Appelbaum FR, Spielberger RT, et al. Selective ablation of acute myeloid leukemia using antibody-targeted chemotherapy: a phase I study of an anti-CD33 calicheamicin immunoconjugate. Blood 1999;93:3678–84.

60. Neumeister P, Eibl M, Zinke-Cerwenka W, et al. Hepatic veno-occlusive disease in two patients with relapsed acute myeloid leukemia treated with anti-CD33 calicheamicin (CMA-676) immunoconjugate. Ann Hematol 2001;80:119–20.

61. Morris D, Aisner J, Wiernik PH. Horizontal pigmented banding of the nails in association with Adriamycin chemotherapy. Cancer Treat Rep 1977;61:499–501.

62. Shetty MR. Case of pigmented banding of the nail caused by bleomycin. Cancer Treat Rep 1977;61:501–2.

9

Extramedullary Manifestations of Adult Leukemia

PETER H. WIERNIK, MD

Granulocytic sarcomas are extramedullary accumulations of leukemic cells that infrequently occur in patients with acute myeloid leukemia (AML), chronic myeloid leukemia (CML), or myelodysplastic syndrome (MDS). They were originally referred to as chloromas because they sometimes have a greenish color due to a high concentration of myeloperoxidase. The green color fades slowly when the tissue is exposed to light. Although the vast majority of granulocytic sarcomas are found in patients with an established diagnosis of a myeloid neoplasm, they sometimes are seen in patients with no other evidence of malignancy.[1,2] In that situation, granulocytic sarcoma is frequently misdiagnosed as non-Hodgkin's lymphoma[2–4] when only routine preparation and staining of biopsied material are performed. The diagnosis of granulocytic sarcoma is greatly facilitated by immunohistochemical studies employing antilysozyme and antimyeloperoxidase antibodies,[4–7] both of which will identify myeloid cells in over 90 percent of cases of granulocytic sarcoma and other myeloid extramedullary leukemic infiltrates. Lymphoma cells will always give negative reactions to those antibodies.[6] Immunohistochemical techniques require minimal tissue, and diagnosis of granulocytic sarcoma by fine-needle aspiration is common.[3,8–10]

Extramedullary accumulation of leukemic cells occurs in acute lymphocytic leukemia (ALL) and chronic lymphocytic leukemia (CLL) also, but virtually always in patients with an established diagnosis of leukemia. This makes the diagnosis of extramedullary leukemia in lymphoid leukemias less difficult than it sometimes is in myeloid leukemias.

Granulocytic sarcoma as the first evidence of relapse after stem cell transplantation with high-dose chemotherapy or total-body radiation therapy is being observed more frequently as patients so treated survive longer. Such relapses have been reported in AML[11–13] and CML,[11,13–15] where the relapse rate with granulocytic sarcoma is in the range of 4 to 5 percent, and in MDS,[17,18] where the rate appears to be lower.

It is not known why some patients with myeloid malignancies develop granulocytic sarcoma or other less prominent extramedullary leukemic infiltrations and others do not. Some studies suggest that neural cell adhesion molecules expressed on the cell surface of certain leukemic cells may play a role in the infiltration of neural structures by leukemic cells. This concept is supported by the observation of a relatively high frequency of extramedullary leukemia, especially of the brain, spinal cord, and orbit, in patients with AML type M4Eo or M2 whose cells often express the neural cell adhesion molecule CD56.[19,20] However, Seymour and colleagues[21] found that CD56 expression was quite common in patients with a variety of AML subtypes and that its expression was not correlated with extramedullary leukemic infiltration. In addition, CD56 expression in ALL is not associated with extramedullary leukemic infiltration.[22] Therefore, it seems unlikely that CD56 expression alone plays a major role in the pathogenesis of extramedullary leukemic infiltration. Despite the fact that a high incidence of extramedullary leukemia characterizes AML FAB M2 with t(8;21), many other cytogenetic abnormalities have been reported in the leukemic cells of patients with granulocytic sarcoma or less clinically evident extramedullary leukemic infiltration, such as complex karyotypes including translocations involving an X chromosome,[23] t(3;4),[24] t(12;13),[25] and t(9;11),[26] to name a few. It must be concluded that, at present, the pathogenesis of extramedullary leukemic infiltration is poorly understood.

There is some confusion in the literature about the influence of extramedullary leukemia on prognosis in AML. In some studies of children, such infiltrates had no prognostic significance,[27,28] but in one study, they actually conferred a good prognosis.[29] Byrd and colleagues[30] reported that adult patients with t(8;21) and extramedullary leukemia had a significantly poorer complete response rate and overall survival compared with adult AML patients with the same FAB type and karyotype but without extramedullary leukemia. Overall survival in another study that included children and adults with M2 and t(8;21) may have been similarly adversely affected by extramedullary leukemia as well.[31]

One of the most important clinical questions concerning patients who present with a granulocytic sarcoma is whether to treat locally with or without systemic chemotherapy. Imrie and colleagues[1] reported that significantly fewer such patients who received chemotherapy at presentation subsequently developed AML significantly less often than those patients who did not receive systemic treatment (41 versus 71%) and that overall survival was also significantly prolonged in patients treated with chemotherapy. On the other hand, Meis and colleagues[2] reported that 25 percent of patients with isolated granulocytic sarcoma who did not receive chemotherapy did not develop AML during a 3.5- to 16-year follow-up period. Therefore, it is uncertain that systemic antileukemia chemotherapy for isolated granulocytic sarcoma prevents the subsequent development of AML.

CUTANEOUS MANIFESTATIONS OF LEUKEMIA

Specific cutaneous manifestations of leukemia are uncommon, but nonspecific lesions such as infections, drug reactions, petechiae, and ecchymoses are obviously quite common. Petechiae represent capillary hemorrhage resulting from thrombocytopenia, and ecchymoses may represent confluent petechial hemorrhage in dependent or traumatized parts of the body or bleeding secondary to clotting factor deficiency. Therefore, the presence of ecchymoses should always raise the question of acute promyelocytic leukemia (APL) (FAB M3) in a newly diagnosed patient with acute leukemia. Other benign skin lesions associated with leukemia include (1) leukocytoclastic vasculitis, which clinically may resemble an allergic vasculitis usually on the extremities and appear as a purpuric, raised annular, or circular rash that may be tender. Histologically, the lesion appears to be a capillary vasculitis associated with a neutrophilic infiltrate.[32] This rare lesion of unknown etiology may be seen in patients with acute or chronic leukemia and usually responds to prednisone. Although this lesion is most commonly seen in patients with active leukemia, it may precede other evidence of acute leukemia by many months.[33] (2) Acute febrile dermatosis, or Sweet's syndrome,[32] is associated with fever and malaise. The skin lesions are pleomorphic and may appear anywhere. Histologically, the lesion is characterized by dense focal infiltration of mature granulocytes into the upper and middle dermis. These lesions of unknown etiology appear rarely during the course of active acute leukemia, myelodysplasia,[34] or CML[35,36] and may require steroids for management.

Of far greater significance than the benign dermatoses discussed above is leukemia cutis, which results from direct infiltration of the skin with leukemic cells. Such lesions are highly variable in appearance. Leukemia cutis may present as multiple small lesions several millimeters in diameter (Figures 9–1 and 9–2), multiple lesions (Figure 9–3), or a single larger lesion (Figure 9–4). Small pinkish or tan papules, nodules, or plaques are perhaps the most common presentations.[37–40] Leukemia cutis has rarely been reported in acute and chronic lymphocytic leukemia but is primarily a complication of AML and CML and of MDS.[32,37–44] The vast majority of patients with leukemia cutis have or will acquire a diagnosis of AML, and approximately 3 percent of AML patients will demonstrate leukemia cutis at some point during the course of their disease.[32,38] Leukemia cutis may precede other evi-

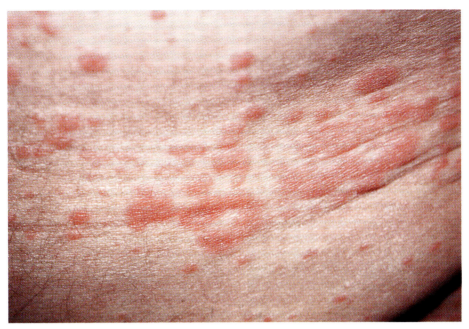

Figure 9–1. Leukemia cutis in an adult with AML M1 in hematologic remission. The lesions are slightly raised and measure 2 to 4 mm in diameter (original magnification ×4).

dence of AML by many months[45,46] or be the first sign of relapse after complete remission.[35,40] Most commonly, it occurs along with other evidence of active disease.

If the diagnosis of leukemia cutis is not entertained, especially in a patient with no other evidence of leukemia, it may be misdiagnosed as lymphoma[47] or anaplastic carcinoma since routine histologic evaluation may reveal only small round cells with nucleoli. In a review of 154 published cases of extramedullary leukemia, 46 percent were initially misdiagnosed.[43] However, with appropriate histo-

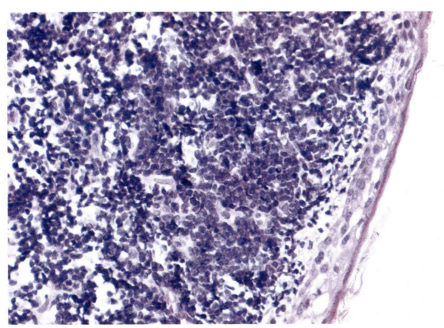

Figure 9–2. Biopsy of a lesion from the patient in Figure 9–1. Leukemic cells infiltrate the dermis and epidermis (hematoxylin and eosin stain; original magnification ×200).

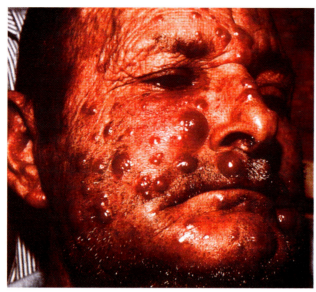

Figure 9–3. Large granulocytic sarcomas of the face in a patient who presented with AML M4Eo. The lesions completely responded to systemic induction therapy.

chemical and immunologic techniques, the true nature of the lesions will be determined. Most helpful in establishing the myeloid nature of the immature cells are monoclonal antibodies to myeloperoxidase, lysozyme, CD43, and CD20.[7,43,48] These agents allow for the exclusion of a diagnosis of lymphoma and the positive identification of the myeloid origin of the infiltrate.

More than 70 percent of patients with leukemia cutis have or develop AML FAB M4 or M5,[38,39,43,49] and there is evidence that expression of T-cell markers such as CD2, CD4, and CD7 by myelomonocytic and monocytic blasts is associated with a high incidence of all types of extramedullary leukemia, including leukemia cutis.[7,50,51] Furthermore, Schiffer and colleagues[49] demonstrated that patients whose blasts demonstrated some degree of maturation in vitro had twice the incidence of extramedullary leukemia compared with those whose blasts did not. They hypothesized that the mechanism of extramedullary leukemia in M4 and M5 most likely involved blast maturation that allowed early egress from the marrow with subsequent tissue invasion, and this has been confirmed by others.[50,51]

Although large (granulocytic sarcoma) and small (leukemia cutis) leukemic cutaneous infiltrates readily respond to systemic chemotherapy and/or local radiotherapy,[38,42,43] relapse is common and is usually

a harbinger of hematologic relapse. There is some evidence, however, that induction chemotherapy for AML given to patients who present with leukemia cutis without other evidence of AML may be curative.

A small number of patients have been reported who have developed leukemia cutis at the site of an indwelling central venous catheter.[52–56] This phenomenon appears to be the result of bleeding into the skin at a time when the blood contains obvious or occult blast cells.

Leukemia cutis may precede other evidence of AML for as long as several years,[57] but the usual interval in such cases is weeks or several months. Leukemia cutis is less common in CML than AML, but it may occur during or prior to blast crisis,[7,58,59] with features identical to those of leukemia cutis in AML, and has been reported at least once in chronic neutrophilic leukemia.[60] Leukemia cutis in CML blast crisis usually demonstrates lymphoblastic infiltration,[59] but sea blue histiocytes may be seen as well.[61]

Extramedullary leukemia in patients with APL, including leukemia cutis, is being recognized with increasing frequency.[62–65] In most cases, the patients had previously received all-*trans* retinoic acid (ATRA) during induction therapy or as postremission therapy, and leukemia cutis developed as a manifestation of relapse.[62,63,65] Leukemia cutis may be much less common in APL patients who have never received ATRA,[62] and when it does occur in

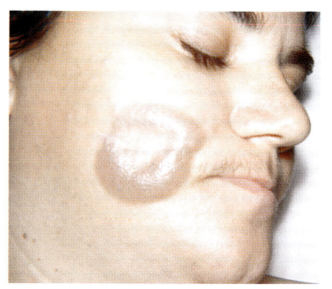

Figure 9–4. Granulocytic sarcoma of the face 1 year prior to the diagnosis of AML M2.

such patients, it may respond to ATRA.[64] Whether ATRA promotes extramedullary disease in patients with APL is currently actively debated. All-*trans* retinoic acid treatment of APL results in remission through differentiation induction, and certain adhesion molecules such as aminopeptidase N may be overexpressed after ATRA therapy. These adhesion molecules may play a role in the pathogenesis of the retinoic acid syndrome and other extramedullary involvement in APL, including leukemia cutis.

A small number of patients who have received allogeneic bone marrow transplantation for AML and CML or myelodysplasia have developed extramedullary leukemia as the first sign of relapse, which, in some cases, has been manifested as leukemia cutis.[66–68]

CENTRAL NERVOUS SYSTEM LEUKEMIA

Epidural Spinal Tumor

Spinal cord compression secondary to epidural granulocytic sarcoma, an uncommon manifestation of leukemia, occurs most frequently in young males[20,69–76] with AML but has also been reported in CML transitioning to blast crisis.[72,77,78] Cord compression from similar masses has also been observed less frequently in ALL[72,79] and at least once in CLL.[72] Leg weakness, back pain, and bladder dysfunction are the most frequent complaints, and paraplegia with or without sphincter dysfunction is the most common sign.[72,76] The thoracic and lumbar cord are most frequently involved,[73,75,76] with the cauda equina involved less frequently.[20,80–82] Paraspinal granulocytic sarcoma has been described as the initial evidence of AML before marrow involvement,[75,80,81] as the first sign of relapse during hematologic remission,[60,73,74] or as occurring concurrently with marrow evidence of AML.[70,71,83]

When patients present with a paraspinal mass and no other evidence of leukemia, an emergency laminectomy is usually necessary for diagnosis and cord decompression. In patients with a known diagnosis of leukemia, a fine-needle aspiration with computed tomographic (CT) assistance may be successful in making the diagnosis. The cerebrospinal fluid usually has an elevated protein concentration but no

pleocytosis. Once the diagnosis is made, local radiation therapy is indicated,[77] whether or not systemic chemotherapy is given for other manifestations of the disease. The completeness of neurologic recovery is inversely related to the interval from onset of neurologic symptoms to initiation of radiation therapy.

The vast majority of patients with AML who develop paraspinal granulocytic sarcoma have FAB M2 bone marrow morphology and a karyotype that includes t(8;21). Interestingly, most such patients have additional karyotypic abnormalities, such as loss of an X or Y chromosome.[20,69–71,83] Although –X or –Y is common in patients with t(8;21), the loss of a sex chromosome appears to be more common in patients with t(8;21), who develop granulocytic sarcoma of the central nervous system (CNS). Furthermore, of all subtypes of AML, granulocytic sarcoma of the CNS is found more frequently in FAB M2 patients with t(8;21). As many as 15 to 25 percent of those patients have developed such granulocytic sarcomas in several series.[20] A possible explanation for the relatively high frequency of CNS granulocytic sarcoma in AML patients with t(8;21) has been proposed by Hurwitz and colleagues,[84] who demonstrated that the neural adhesion molecule CD56 is expressed on the leukemic cells of more than 60 percent of patients with t(8;21) and few others. Others have reported paraspinal granulocytic sarcoma in patients whose marrow blasts demonstrated t(8;21) and expressed CD56.[69,74] Although this possible explanation for CNS granulocytic sarcoma is fascinating, it should be remembered that the second most common leukemia associated with spinal cord involvement is CML[72] and that patients with Philadelphia chromosome-positive AML with spinal epidural granulocytic sarcoma have been reported as well.[72]

Intracranial Granulocytic Sarcoma

Granulocytic sarcomas within the cranium usually arise from the dura[42,85–90] (Figure 9–5), but intracerebral[91–93] and intracerebellar[94–97] lesions have been described. One intracerebellar granulocytic sarcoma was associated with blasts that had a normal karyotype but were CD56+.[97] Headache, seizure, papilledema, and focal weakness are common manifestations.[42,85–90] The cerebrospinal fluid may be nor-

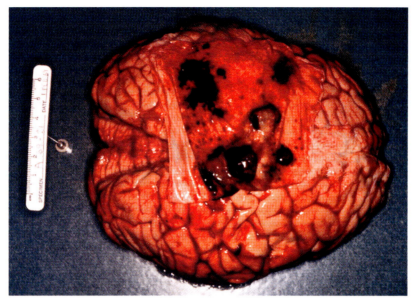

Figure 9–5.   Multiple granulocytic sarcomas of the dura of a patient with AML M1. She initially presented with multiple CNS lesions 11 months prior to the diagnosis of AML. The lesions completely responded to cranial irradiation but recurred at a time of hematologic relapse. The lesions were dark green in color at autopsy but gradually faded over a 48-hour period.

mal,[90] and the tumor or tumors are usually readily seen on CT or magnetic resonance imaging (MRI).[88,90,95,98] The lesions are usually quite sensitive to radiation therapy.[42,87,88,98] Intracranial granulocytic sarcoma most frequently occurs in patients with AML[85–87,91,93,94,98] either as the first sign of AML,[42,85] during hematologic remission,[93,94,98] or concurrently with bone marrow evidence of AML.[86,91] On rare occasions, it may be an isolated finding in patients who never develop other evidence of leukemia.[88,92] Intracranial granulocytic sarcoma has also been reported in patients with polycythemia vera[87] and essential thrombocythemia[89,90] transforming to an acute leukemia.

Orbital and Ocular Granulocytic Sarcoma

Granulocytic sarcoma of the orbit occurs primarily in children, especially those from other than Western industrialized countries, for unknown reasons.[99–101] Its incidence seems to be decreasing in industrialized countries, again for unknown reasons.[99] It rarely occurs in adults (Figures 9–6 and 9–7).[99,102,103] It is usually unilateral but may present bilaterally.[99,104,105] It may precede other evidence of AML,[105,106] occur with bone marrow involve-

ment,[100,101,104,105] or appear during marrow remission.[102,103,105] In most cases in which marrow cytogenetics were evaluated, t(8;21) has been found,[100,104] often in association with –Y.[104] Local radiation therapy may be necessary to save the eye,[102,104] especially if there is retinal hemorrhage (Figure 9–8), but chemotherapy alone may be sufficient if the eye is not severely compromised.[100,101,104]

Choroidal infiltration resulting in retinal detachment (Figure 9–9) has rarely been observed in adults with CML or CLL,[107] and retrobulbar extramedullary hematopoiesis has been reported in myelofibrosis with myeloid metaplasia.[108]

Meningeal Leukemia

In the acute leukemias, several presenting features increase the likelihood of the development of meningeal leukemia sometime during the course of the disease. High white blood cell count and low platelet count at diagnosis are associated with a high incidence of meningeal leukemia. Patients with ALL are more likely than those with AML to develop meningeal leukemia, and in both ALL and AML, there is an inverse relationship between the age of the patient and incidence of meningeal leukemia. In

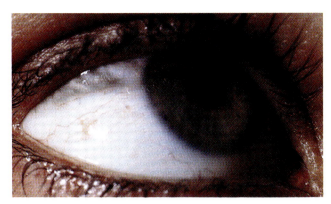

Figure 9–6. Green leukemic infiltrate of the conjunctiva biopsy proven in a patient with AML M1 (original magnification ×4).

patients with AML, the highest incidence of meningeal leukemia (33%) at diagnosis or during hematologic remission appears to be in acute myelomonocytic leukemia patients (FAB M4Eo) with inv(16).[109] In patients with CML, meningeal leukemia is most likely to develop in young patients in blast crisis or late in the chronic phase as the initial manifestation of blast crisis.

Cranial nerve palsies may occur in young patients with ALL, AML, or CML in blast crisis with or without other evidence of meningeal leukemia. If there is no pleocytosis in the cerebrospinal fluid, which frequently is the case, intrathecal therapy is useless, and local irradiation will be required. Cranial nerve palsies are usually unilateral and involve the long cranial nerves (VI, VII) most frequently. Leukemic infiltration of the adventitia of the nerve results in compression of the nerve in long canals of the skull.

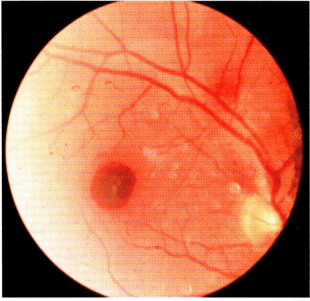

Figure 9–8. Macular hemorrhage in an adult patient with ALL at the time of marrow relapse.

Intracerebral leukostasis occurs in 25 to 50 percent of myeloid leukemia patients with a high peripheral blood blast count (> 200,000/μL) and may lead to sudden death from intracerebral hemorrhage. Blood hyperviscosity leads to sludging of blasts at the venous end of a capillary bed, which results in capillary rupture and hemorrhage. This complication can be completely prevented by

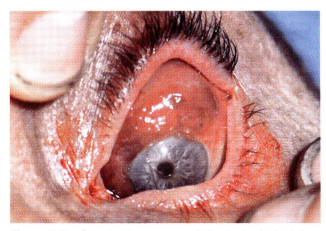

Figure 9–7. Granulocytic sarcoma of the lacrimal gland in a patient with AML M4Eo (original magnification ×4).

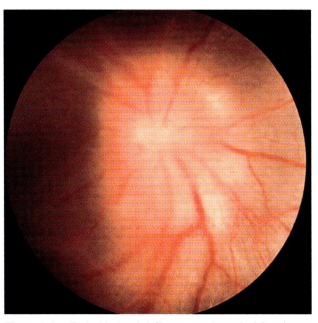

Figure 9–9. Retinal leukemic infiltrates causing retinal detachment in a patient with CLL.

rapidly lowering the circulating blast count with oral hydroxyurea or leukapheresis and by delivering low-dose whole-brain irradiation to eradicate leukemic foci in the brain that may have already been established. Intracerebral leukostasis does not occur in CLL, ALL, or CML in the chronic phase because the leukemic cells in those neoplasms do not increase blood viscosity.

Several theories of the mechanism of meningeal leukemia have been advanced. Petechial hemorrhage in the meninges has been suggested as causative. A more complicated explanation suggests that an expanding mass of leukemic cells erodes skull bones and infiltrates the dura and subsequently infiltrates the adventitia of vessels and nerves that traverse the space between the dura and pia-arachnoid. Once blasts reach the pia-arachnoid, they layer on it, rather than penetrate it. It can be calculated from the average size of a blast cell and the average doubling time of blasts that it would take about 3 months to form a nidus of blasts large enough to interfere with the flow of cerebrospinal fluid between the dura and pia-arachnoid, which would result in a communicating hydrocephalus and cause symptoms related to increased intracranial pressure. The peak incidence of clinically detectable meningeal leukemia is, in fact, 3 to 6 months after bone marrow diagnosis of acute leukemia. Another theory of the pathogenesis of meningeal leukemia is suggested by the work of Bjornson and colleagues,[110] who found that, after transplantation into irradiated hosts, mouse neural stem cells produce a variety of blood cell types, including myeloid and lymphoid cells and early hematopoietic cells. This amazing observation, taken together with the fact that, in some lower animals (sharks), the choroid plexus of the third ventricle is a hematopoietic organ, raises the question as to whether meningeal leukemia can arise de novo within the cranium through dedifferentiation of neural tissue in patients with acute leukemia.

Acute Lymphocytic Leukemia

In a recent review of more than 4,000 patients in the literature, Gokbuget and Hoelzer[111] reported that meningeal leukemia is present at the time of diagno-sis in approximately 6 percent of adult patients with ALL. The incidence is higher in those with T-cell (8%) and B-cell ALL (13%). The incidence is much higher in patients with L3 morphology, compared with those with L1 or L2 morphology.[112] Without meningeal prophylaxis, approximately one-third of adults with ALL will develop meningeal leukemia sometime after the diagnosis of leukemia, usually months after bone marrow remission is obtained. They concluded from their review that prophylaxis with intrathecal therapy alone, intrathecal therapy, and CNS irradiation or high-dose parenteral chemotherapy afforded approximately the same protection from meningeal relapse and that each method was associated with a relapse rate of approximately 15 percent. The relapse rate was lower with high-dose parenteral chemotherapy and intrathecal chemotherapy with or without the addition of CNS irradiation (5–8%). They also noted that the prognosis is extremely poor for adults with ALL and meningeal relapse. Although most such patients had complete resolution of the relapse with intrathecal therapy, CNS relapse was usually followed by marrow relapse, and < 10 percent of patients ultimately survived.

Acute Myeloid Leukemia

In a review of 410 patients with de novo AML treated at one institution, Castagnola and colleagues[113] reported that 2.2 percent developed meningeal leukemia at some point in the course of their disease. Most patients had a complete remission of CNS involvement with intensive treatment consisting of high-dose cytarabine parenterally and intrathecal methotrexate with or without cranial irradiation. Although CNS leukemia is a life-threatening event in AML from which patients rarely ultimately survive, the incidence is too low to advise routine prophylactic meningeal leukemia therapy. It should be remembered that high-dose parenteral cytarabine, which most patients receive during postremission therapy, results in therapeutic cerebrospinal fluid levels and may provide prophylactic meningeal and systemic therapy. This concept is supported by the fact that meningeal leukemia was observed with greater frequency in patients with AML (16%) in the pre–high-dose cytarabine era.[114]

Optic nerve leukemic infiltration has been reported in a patient with APL who had a complete response to ATRA,[115] and infiltration of the pituitary gland was reported to occur in more than 45 percent of 52 adults with acute leukemia of all types. One patient had inappropriate secretion of antidiuretic hormone, but all others had no pituitary dysfunction, and the infiltration was only discovered at autopsy.[116] Peripheral polyneuropathy secondary to leukemic infiltration of somatic and autonomic nerves in a patient with acute monoblastic leukemia in hematologic remission has been documented,[117] and other cases associated with marrow evidence of leukemia have been reported in AML as well.

Chronic Myeloid Leukemia

Meningeal leukemia in CML occurs as the initial event in or during blastic transformation with approximately the same frequency as in AML, and, similarly, the incidence is inversely related to patient age. Schwartz and colleagues[118] found meningeal leukemia in approximately 7 percent of a large series of patients with CML. The major signs were cranial nerve palsies and papilledema, and the cerebrospinal fluid always contained blast cells. All patients were in blastic transformation and all apparently had a myeloid blast crisis, but the authors did not specifically comment on whether the blast crisis was myeloid or lymphoid. Intrathecal methotrexate or cytarabine was as effective in eradicating meningeal infiltration as others have found in AML and ALL. Their seven patients ranged in age from 14 to 48 years, with a median age of 30 years. Since all of their patients were well below the median age of all patients with CML, most physicians have the impression that meningeal leukemia is rare in CML. Autopsy studies have revealed clinically inapparent meningeal leukemia in as many as half of CML patients, however.[118] The highest incidence of meningeal leukemia in patients with CML may be in those with a lymphoid blast crisis.[119,120] The incidence of clinically evident meningeal leukemia in those patients may be as high as 45 percent.[119] On rare occasion, meningeal leukemia in CML may present with unusual manifestations, such as optic nerve involvement.[121]

Chronic Lymphocytic Leukemia

Meningeal leukemia in CLL has been observed, but it is rare. It has been reported in T-cell[122] and B-cell CLL[123,124] and to respond to intrathecal methotrexate alone[123] or in combination with cranial irradiation.[124–126] Most reported patients have been older (age 57–81 years) than acute leukemia or CML patients with meningeal leukemia,[123,124,127] although younger patients with T-cell CLL[122] and CLL evolving into prolymphocytic leukemia[125] have been reported to develop meningeal leukemia.[122]

HEAD AND NECK REGION

Sklansky and colleagues[128] published an early review of otolaryngologic complications of acute leukemia based on a retrospective analysis of 213 patients with AML and 60 with ALL. The vast majority of the patients were adults. The most frequent cause of head and neck pathology in acute leukemia patients was due to infection,[128] and almost 75 percent of patients in that study had hemorrhage in the skin and mucous membranes (Figure 9–10) of the region.[128] Leukemic infiltration of facial skin, maxilla, paranasal sinuses, temporal bone, pharynx, gingiva, and other sites have all been documented in the literature.[128] Granulocytic sarcoma of the head and neck region is uncommon but is reported from time to time, especially from nonindustrialized countries.[129] Granulocytic sarcoma

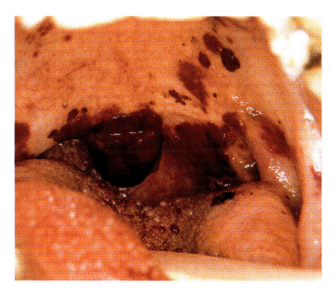

Figure 9–10. Uveal hemorrhage in a thrombocytopenic patient presenting with AML M4Eo.

in patients with CML almost always occurs as a manifestation of blast crisis and frequently results in lymphadenopathy, especially of cervical lymph nodes.[130]

Gingiva

The gingivae are the most common tissues of the head and neck region to be infiltrated with leukemic cells in patients with AML. Gross gingival hypertrophy was noted in 20 percent of patients with AML in one large study and was not observed in patients with ALL (Figure 9–11).[128] However, in other studies, gingival hypertrophy has rarely been observed in patients with ALL and even more rarely in patients with CLL.[131] The incidence was three-fold higher in patients with acute monocytic leukemia (FAB M5) than in patients with other FAB types. Gingival hypertrophy in AML is due to infiltration of leukemic cells into the gingiva, sometimes massive enough to hide most of the teeth. It frequently causes friable and painful gingiva that may ulcerate[132] but usually does not result in significant hemorrhage. Loosening of the teeth may occur in severe cases. Gingival hypertrophy resulting from leukemic infiltration usually responds rapidly to systemic chemotherapy, although, on occasion, local radiotherapy may be employed.[128] Gingival hypertrophy due to phenytoin hypersensitivity is due to dense fibrosis of the gingiva without cellular infiltration. Isolated gingival granulocytic sarcoma without generalized gingival hypertrophy has been reported in APL as a manifestation of relapse after chemother-

apy alone or after ATRA therapy alone or in combination with chemotherapy.[133]

Isolated gingival relapse during complete hematologic remission has been reported in APL (Figure 9–12),[65,134] and intra-alveolar granulocytic sarcoma developing after tooth extraction in a patient with CML has been reported.[135]

Every leukemia patient should be examined by a dentist prior to treatment. Plaque removal will minimize gingivitis, which may worsen during periods of granulocytopenia, and smoldering periapical abscesses can be treated before they result in bacteremia.[136–139]

Larynx

Abundant leukemic infiltration of the larynx causing stridor rarely occurs in AML and CML (Figure 9–13).[128,140,141] Although a significant incidence of laryngeal leukemic infiltration has been noted in autopsy series of acute leukemia patients, such infiltration is only rarely of clinical significance.[140] Laryngeal leukemic infiltration is usually asymmetric[142] and involves the arytenoids and the true and false chords.[128] Chemotherapy is usually sufficient treatment, but cases with significant stridor may require intubation and radiation therapy for rapid resolution.

Mandible

Rare reports of clinically significant leukemic infiltration of the masseteric muscle[143] and mandible[144,145] have appeared, but these problems usually occur in children with AML[145] or ALL[144,146] and only rarely in adults with acute leukemia or as the initial event heralding blast crisis in CML.[147]

Ear

Acute leukemia may rarely present as acute mastoiditis or acute otitis media[148] either as a result of infection or leukemic infiltration, especially in children[149,150] with AML. Leukemic involvement of the temporal bone may result in facial nerve paralysis.[149]

Paparella and colleagues[151] studied the temporal bone and ear at autopsy in 25 patients with leukemia and found leukemic infiltration of the external ear in

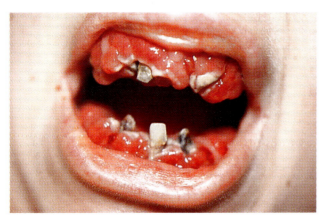

Figure 9–11. Gingival hyperplasia in a patient presenting with AML M5.

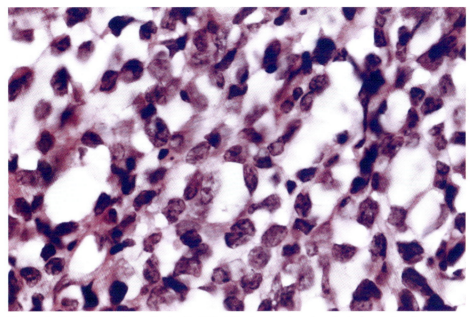

Figure 9–12. Biopsy of a patient with AML M3 who developed a gingival granulocytic sarcoma while in hematologic remission (hematoxylin and eosin stain; original magnification ×900).

1 of 14 patients with AML and 2 of 8 with ALL. The middle ear was infiltrated in 5 of the patients with ALL and in 3 with AML. The inner ear was infiltrated in one patient with ALL, and the VIIIth cranial nerve was infiltrated in 7 patients with AML, 3 with ALL, and in 1 of 3 with CML. Twenty percent of patients with demonstrated leukemic infiltration of ear structures at autopsy had clinical otologic complications, such as sensorineural hearing loss or vertigo. Others have reported similar findings.[128,152,153] Relapse of AML as leukemic infiltration of the external auditory canal has been reported rarely[74,154] and observed by the author in an adult with FAB M2 AML and t(8;21). Some evidence suggests that patients with clinically significant leukemic infiltrations of the head and neck region are more likely to have t(8;21) than other cytogenetic abnormalities.[74,148,149]

THE CHEST

Cardiovascular System

Direct involvement of the heart by acute leukemia was found to be much more common in an autopsy study than suspected clinically. Roberts and colleagues[155] examined the hearts of 420 patients with acute leukemia and found that 69 percent were involved with hemorrhage, leukemic infiltration, or both. Twenty of the patients had had cardiac symptoms such as chest pain or dyspnea terminally. Of the 13 patients who had had chest pain, 9 had pericarditis at autopsy, but in only 2 was the pericarditis a result of leukemic infiltration. Most cases of pericarditis were due to hemorrhage or infection in this series that included both children and adult patients.

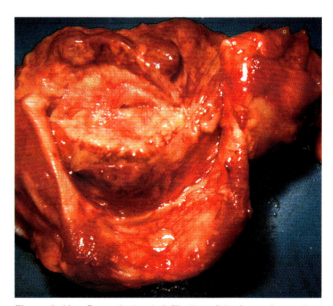

Figure 9–13. Dense leukemic infiltration of the larynx in a patient who presented with AML M5.

Four of the 13 patients who had experienced chest pain had a focus of myocardial necrosis at autopsy due to hemorrhage or infection. Seven of 20 symptomatic patients had dyspnea associated with acute cardiac failure, and 6 of those patients had leukemic infiltration and hemorrhage in the myocardium at autopsy. Therefore, in this large series of acute leukemia patients who died, clinically significant cardiac involvement was quite uncommon despite identification of such involvement in the majority of patients autopsied. Preterminal sudden onset of dyspnea and acute cardiac failure were more likely to be due to direct cardiac involvement with acute leukemia than was chest pain. This point has been emphasized in more recent reports of acute cardiac failure secondary to massive infiltration of the myocardium with leukemic cells. Massive myocardial infiltration has been reported in patients with AML (Figures 9–14, 9–15 and 9–16),[156–159] prolymphocytic leukemia,[160,161] CLL,[162] and CML in chronic phase.[163]

Rare cases of cardiac tamponade secondary to leukemic pericardial infiltration have been observed in adults with ALL,[164,165] AML,[166] and chronic myelomonocytic leukemia,[167,168] and tamponade in a patient with CML secondary to extramedullary hematopoiesis in the pericardium has been reported.[169]

In an extensive review of the electrocardiograms of 480 patients with leukemia,[170] it was determined that most abnormalities resulted from anemia and the age of the patient. However, a number of cases of arrhythmias caused by leukemic infiltration of the conduction system of patients with CML,[171] AML,[172] and prolymphocytic leukemia[173] have been reported, but such conduction defects appear to be quite rare.[157] Other reported rare cardiovascular phenomena directly related to leukemia include infiltration of cardiac valves in AML (Figure 9–17), venous valvular infiltration in a few patients with ALL or CLL,[174] ruptured aortic aneurysm in a patient with AML due to leukemic infiltration of the aneurysm,[175] aortic leukemic infiltration in a patient with CLL (Figure 9–18), myocardial infarction due to leukemic infiltration of the heart of a patient with CML,[163] and endomyocardial fibrosis in CLL (Figure 9–19).

Lungs

Infection is clearly the most common pulmonary complication of acute and chronic leukemia. Minor pulmonary hemorrhage is seen at autopsy in approximately half of acute leukemia patients,[176] and in perhaps 10 percent it is severe and associated with preterminal acute signs and symptoms.[176] The degree

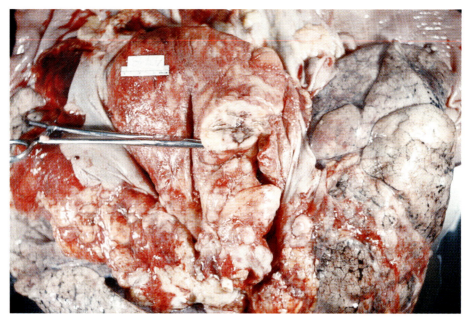

Figure 9–14.   Granulocytic sarcoma of the myocardium in a patient with AML M5 who died with signs and symptoms of myocardial infarction during an attempt to induce a third remission.

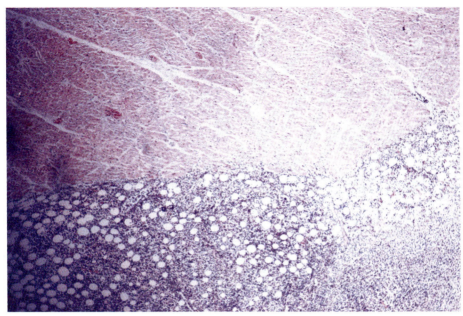

Figure 9–15. Low-power microscopic view of the lesion in Figure 9–14. The lesion does not appear to infiltrate myocardium (hematoxylin and eosin stain; original magnification ×200).

of pulmonary hemorrhage, which is commonly intra-alveolar or intrapleural, usually correlates with the degree of thrombocytopenia,[176] but some evidence suggests that for massive pulmonary hemorrhage to occur in patients with acute leukemia, there has to be not only severe thrombocytopenia but diffuse alveolar and capillary damage as well.[177] It has been proposed that capillary endothelial cell cytoplasmic swelling and bleb formation caused by chemotherapy may set the stage for massive pulmonary hemorrhage in some patients.[177]

Leukemic infiltration of pulmonary parenchyma is usually clinically unimportant and discovered only at autopsy as microscopic lesions.[176,178] Two-thirds or more of acute leukemia patients have such infiltrates, and they are found with equal frequency

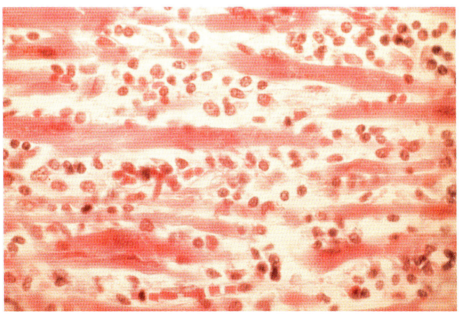

Figure 9–16. High-power view of the lesion in Figures 9–14 and 9–15 showing infiltration between myocardial muscle fibers (hematoxylin and eosin stain; original magnification ×900).

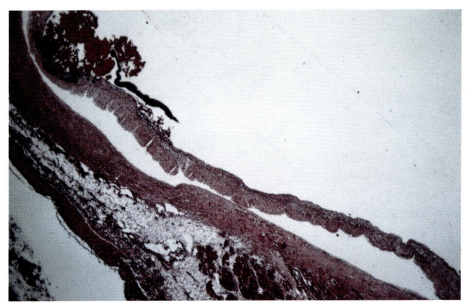

Figure 9–17.   Leukemic infiltration of the mitral valve in a patient with relapsed AML M1 (hematoxylin and eosin stain; original magnification ×200).

in ALL and AML and occasionally in CML patients in blast crisis.[179,180] Such lesions in patients with CLL are quite rare.[179,181] The typical infiltrate is peribronchial or perivascular,[176] and the size and number of such lesions correlate roughly with the circulating blast count. Less than 10 percent of patients with leukemic pulmonary infiltrations have chest radiographic evidence of them. When extensive pulmonary infiltration does result in an abnormal chest radiograph, bilateral diffuse interstitial lung infiltrates are usually seen, and such patients may demonstrate progressive, severe dyspnea.[182] Low-dose whole-lung irradiation may resolve the clinical symptoms and signs within a few days.[182]

Pulmonary leukostasis may occur in patients with acute leukemia or CML in blast crisis who have hyperleukocytosis (Figure 9–20).[183,184] Such patients rapidly develop severe dyspnea and may die within

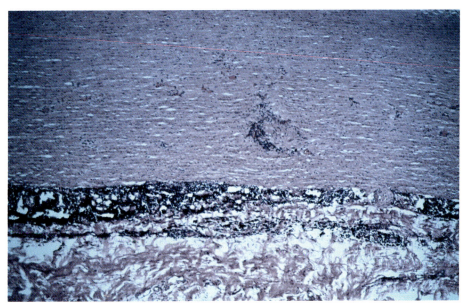

Figure 9–18.   Leukemic infiltration of the aortic intima in a patient with CLL (hematoxylin and eosin stain; original magnification ×200).

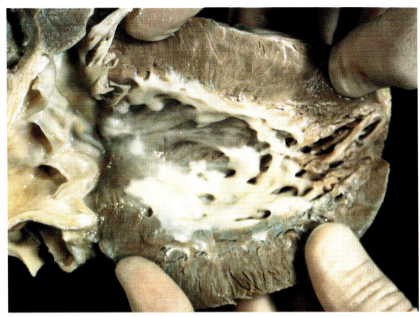

Figure 9–19. Endocardial fibrosis in a patient with CLL.

hours. The pathologic lesion is a rapidly occurring engorgement of pulmonary capillaries and arterioles with blasts.[183,184] The precise mechanism of this complication is unknown, but factors other than hyperleukocytosis must be involved since the syndrome has been occasionally reported in patients with relatively low white blood cell counts and no circulating blasts.[176,185] Patients with pulmonary leukostasis frequently have rapidly developing diffuse alveolar consolidations on chest radiography.[185–187] Whole-lung emergency radiation therapy may be life saving. A similar syndrome may occur after treatment of patients with APL with ATRA (the so-called retinoic acid syndrome). In that situation, vascular engorgement with mature, differentiated granulocytes occurs, and the 10 percent of patients who develop the syn-

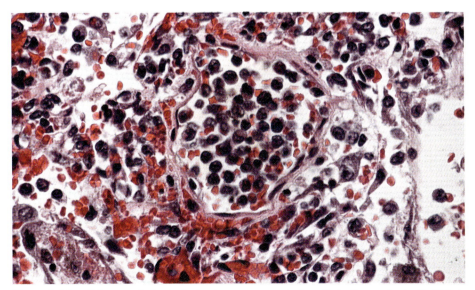

Figure 9–20. Pulmonary leukostasis due to engorgement of capillaries in a patient with CML in blast crisis. The lesions were suspected clinically when the patient developed acute shortness of breath. He responded initially to whole-lung irradiation but died suddenly 6 weeks later when he was severely pancytopenic after systemic chemotherapy (hematoxylin and eosin stain; original magnification ×900).

drome usually respond well to corticosteroids.[188] Treating patients with chemotherapy before giving ATRA may largely prevent the syndrome. In both types of pulmonary leukostasis, an affinity of leukemic cells for pulmonary vascular endothelium may be involved in the mechanism.[185,188]

Endobronchial tumor obstructing a bronchus has been observed in patients with AML.[189,190] Multiple pulmonary nodules associated with cervical lymphadenopathy secondary to granulocytic sarcoma, which was the only evidence of AML, were seen in one elderly patient.[191] A woman with AML who had a T-cell–depleted sibling marrow allograft in remission relapsed 1 year later with an interstitial pneumonitis caused by granulocytic sarcoma. A donor lymphocyte infusion completely resolved the problem.[192]

Extrapulmonary Thoracic Manifestations

Granulocytic sarcoma presenting as a mediastinal mass has on rare occasion been the only manifestation of AML[193–197] or MDS[198] and has also occurred in patients with typical hematologic features of leukemia.[194] Systemic chemotherapy for AML appears to be the treatment of choice rather than local irradiation therapy.[194] Au and colleagues[199] reported three women with mediastinal granulocytic sarcoma and AML whose leukemia had a near tetraploid karyotype, which is usually found only in males. All three patients responded poorly to treatment. Local radiation therapy may be helpful in resolving anterior chest wall granulocytic sarcomas, which may herald systemic relapse of AML.[42,200]

GASTROINTESTINAL TRACT

Esophagus

Although about 7 to 10 percent of autopsied leukemia patients have microscopic infiltration of the esophagus,[201,202] esophageal involvement is rarely of clinical significance. In the largest study to date,[201] only high initial white blood cell count correlated with esophageal involvement. In those patients with clinical evidence of esophageal infiltration, dysphasia was the most common symptom.[201] Acute myelomonocytic leukemia (M4)

appears to be the leukemia most commonly associated with this rare manifestation of AML,[201] but it has been reported in CML also.[202] It should be remembered that infection, especially candidiasis, is by far more commonly the cause of dysphagia in a leukemia patient than is leukemic infiltration of the upper gastrointestinal tract.

Stomach

A unique patient with Philadelphia chromosome-positive ALL was reported by Weisdorf and colleagues,[203] who, while recovering from graft-versus-host disease of the gastrointestinal tract, experienced an exacerbation of symptoms that proved to be due to gastric and duodenal infiltration with lymphoblasts. Chemotherapy induced a complete remission, but the patient relapsed shortly thereafter. Rarely, gastric involvement with leukemia has been observed in patients with CLL, and in almost all reports of gastric infiltration with leukemia, marrow involvement is present as well.[203–205] Granulocytic sarcoma of the stomach has also been rarely reported, even in the absence of other evidence of AML.[206]

Small Bowel

Small bowel infiltration occurs rarely in leukemia patients and primarily in patients with CLL.[207] Increased abdominal girth, diarrhea, and an abnormal upper gastrointestinal radiography series with small bowel follow-through have heralded this complication frequently,[207] and the diagnosis is made by biopsy. Standard therapy for CLL may resolve the problem. Granulocytic sarcoma of the small bowel (Figure 9–21), also exceedingly rare as a clinical problem, may perforate and result in peritonitis[208] or may cause small bowel obstruction.[209–211] Chemotherapy may initially completely resolve the bowel leukemia, but virtually all patients have subsequently relapsed with hematologic evidence of AML.[206,209] At least one patient with small bowel granulocytic sarcoma and AML survived in complete remission after induction chemotherapy.[212] A case of a child with CML who had leukemic infiltration of the ileum that resulted in a protein-losing enteropathy has been reported,[210] but this has apparently not been seen in adults.

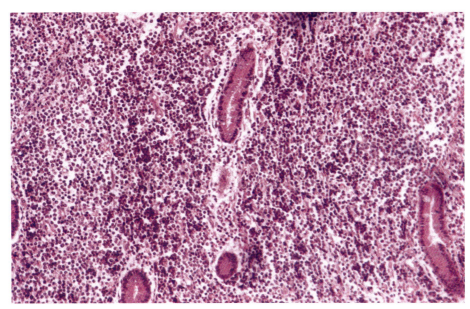

Figure 9–21. Granulocytic sarcoma of the jejunum in a patient without other evidence of AML. Glandular remnants are almost completely obliterated. The patient died of sepsis during induction therapy (hematoxylin and eosin stain; original magnification ×200).

Large Bowel

Granulocytic sarcoma infiltrating adenomatous polyps of the colon has been reported in AML,[213] and granulocytic sarcoma of otherwise normal colonic mucosa has been observed in patients with myelodysplasia.[214,215] Colonoscopic evaluation may suggest Crohn's disease in patients with leukemic infiltration of the large bowel.[215] Such infiltration has also been reported in patients with CLL.[216] Rarely, large bowel granulocytic sarcoma may result in perforation.[217] Abdominal pain and rectal bleeding are apparently the most common signals of large bowel granulocytic sarcoma.[213,215,217] Rectal pain is far more likely to be due to perirectal abscess, especially in patients with AML with a monocytic component, than granulocytic sarcoma.[218] Perirectal abscess may be difficult to diagnose in granulocytopenic leukemia patients due to the absence of signs of inflammation.[218]

Pancreas, Liver, and Gall Bladder

Obstructive jaundice due to granulocytic sarcoma in the head of the pancreas,[219] biliary ductal system,[220] or the gall bladder itself[221] has rarely been encountered, as has pancreatic granulocytic sarcoma without obstruction.[222] Most such patients have had or even-

tually were diagnosed with AML,[219,221] but patients with CML and biliary tract obstruction secondary to granulocytic sarcoma have been also reported.[220] The liver is very frequently infiltrated with leukemia of all types (Figure 9–22), but such involvement is rarely important clinically. Hepatomegaly is uncommon in adults with acute leukemia but may be evident in the end stages of CLL (Figure 9–23) and in the blast phase of CML. Massive leukemic infiltration is common in myelofibrosis with myeloid metaplasia, especially after splenectomy.

FEMALE ORGANS

Oliva and colleagues[223] reported on 11 patients with granulocytic sarcoma of the female genital tract seen at the Massachusetts General Hospital. The ovary was involved in 7 cases, the vagina in 3, and the cervix in 1. In 3 patients, the bone marrow was also involved, but in 2 others, granulocytic sarcoma was the only evidence of AML. In 2 other patients, granulocytic sarcoma occurred after marrow relapse.

Cervix and Vagina

Granulocytic sarcoma of the cervix is a rare manifestation of AML and occurs much less commonly

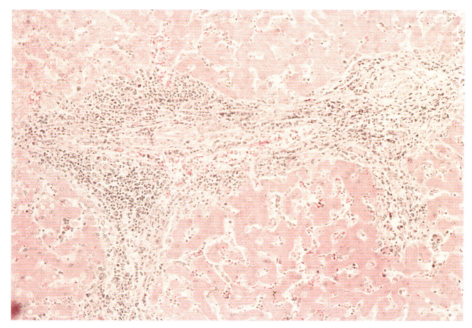

Figure 9–22. Leukemic infiltration of the liver in an adult with ALL (hematoxylin and eosin stain; original magnification ×400).

than ovarian leukemic infiltration.[223] Granulocytic sarcoma of the cervix may occur without other evidence of AML,[224,225] simultaneously with such evidence,[226] or as the first sign of relapse of AML.[227] Patients are usually elderly[224,227,228] or at least middle-aged.[223,226,228,229] Vaginal bleeding is the most common presentation.[223–229] Vaginal extension of a cervical mass is common.[223] Infiltration of the cervix with ALL has not been reported.

Ovary

Leukemic infiltration of the ovary is an uncommon but well-recognized complication of childhood

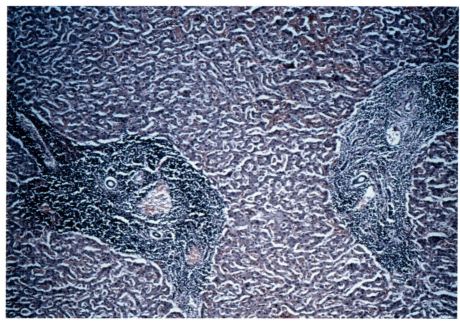

Figure 9–23. Leukemic infiltration of the portal triads of the liver in a patient with CLL. Liver function was mildly abnormal (hematoxylin and eosin stain; original magnification ×400).

ALL.[230] Adult patients with ALL who develop this problem are usually young. Isolated ovarian relapse with ALL may be curable with induction chemotherapy alone.[231,232] Granulocytic sarcoma of the ovary also seems to occur more commonly in children and young women,[233–235] and it may occur unilaterally[233,236] or bilaterally[234] as the only manifestation of relapse of AML,[233] along with other, more conventional evidence of relapse,[237] or in patients at the time of initial diagnosis of AML[234–236] or before other evidence of AML.[238] The most common presentation is an abdominal or pelvic mass or masses, and patients with ovarian granulocytic sarcoma seem to have a worse prognosis than those with ALL involving the ovary.

Other Gynecologic Presentations

A woman with a huge abdominal granulocytic sarcoma and CML was reported, but the origin of the mass was uncertain.[239] Another woman presented with a serous ascitic effusion, and cytologic examination revealed abundant myeloblasts.[240] No focal granulocytic sarcoma was evident, and there was no other evidence of leukemia.

There are four reports of examination of the placenta of leukemia patients who gave birth.[241] In two, there was decidual leukemic infiltration of the placenta, one case had intervillous infiltration, and one had infiltration of the maternal surface. Three of those pregnancies resulted in apparently healthy children, but the placenta with intervillous leukemic infiltration was associated with a partial mole. Three of the patients had acute monocytic leukemia (M5), and the fourth had ALL.

Breast

The female breast may rarely be infiltrated with leukemia unilaterally[242–245] or bilaterally[246–248] when there is no other evidence of leukemia[242,245,246,249,250] at the time of bone marrow diagnosis[244,251] or as the first sign of relapse after complete remission.[252,253] Massive granulocytic sarcoma of the breast has occasionally been reported.[244,248,251,253] In one review, it was estimated that more than one-third of all granulocytic sarcomas diagnosed by fine-needle aspiration occurred in the breast.[247] However, gran-

ulocytic sarcoma of the breast is by far the least common hematopoietic neoplasm of the breast, and it occurs much less commonly than lymphoma of the breast, which is itself quite uncommon.[249] At least one case of breast granulocytic sarcoma in a male has been documented.[252] The vast majority of cases of leukemic infiltration of the breast have been in patients with AML, but granulocytic sarcoma of the breast has also been reported in CML.[247] Leukemic breast masses in patients with ALL are exceedingly rare. The author has observed one case during hematologic remission in a young woman in which local irradiation was curative, and the patient remained in complete remission for decades until she was lost to follow-up.

Some patients who presented with isolated granulocytic sarcoma of the breast treated with systemic chemotherapy developed a bone marrow relapse months later,[246] whereas others have remained disease-free.[245,250] Local radiotherapy may resolve the local problem but does not seem to influence the systemic evolution of the leukemia. The male who relapsed from AML with an isolated breast granulocytic sarcoma had a complete response to allogeneic bone marrow transplantation but subsequently had an isolated second relapse in the same breast and failed to respond to further therapy, which included donor lymphocyte infusion, radiation therapy, and chemotherapy.[252]

GENITOURINARY SYSTEM

Prostate

Flaherty and colleagues[254] were the first to report prostatic obstruction secondary to acute leukemia. They described a 38-year-old man who was admitted with acute urinary retention and found to have acute leukemia. The patient died shortly after admission and at autopsy was found to have a diffusely enlarged prostate heavily infiltrated with monoblasts. The bladder, liver, and peripheral blood were infiltrated as well. Subsequently, others presented patients with CLL infiltration of the prostate.[255–258] Those 10 patients presented with urinary tract obstruction and ranged in age from 55 to 76 years (median, 70 years). All had other evidence of CLL when they presented with urinary tract obstruction. Most of these patients in the older literature were treated with transurethral resection and systemic therapy, to which most responded without return of urinary tract symptoms, but local irradiation therapy may be successful as well.[256–259]

Belis and colleagues[260] reported a 19-year-old man who presented with acute myelomonocytic leukemia and acute urinary retention, which resolved after induction chemotherapy, which resulted in complete remission. During complete remission, the patient again presented with urinary tract obstruction, and a prostatic biopsy again demonstrated leukemic infiltration. He had prompt relief of symptoms after a short course of low-dose irradiation and remained disease-free for at least 9 months following irradiation.

Thalhammer and colleagues[261] described a 68-year-old man who developed a granulocytic sarcoma of the prostate after 9 years of complete remission of AML. The tumor responded to systemic chemotherapy, but the patient developed a bone marrow relapse shortly thereafter.

Prostatic infiltration with leukemia has rarely been reported in patients with myelodysplasia,[262] polycythemia vera,[263] and other myeloproliferative disorders.

Urinary tract obstruction secondary to leukemic infiltration of the prostate is most common in CLL and AML.[261–263] The diagnosis is suspected on digital examination and confirmed by biopsy, and should be entertained in any leukemia patient with an enlarged prostate. Local irradiation is currently considered the treatment of choice to relieve acute obstruction.

Bladder

Bladder involvement with leukemia was reviewed by Givler.[264] He reported 4 patients with acute leukemia, 1 with CML, and 1 with CLL who had mucosal leukemic nodules or bladder mucosal thickening due to gross infiltration. In addition, he found macroscopic bladder infiltrates in approximately one-quarter of 229 patients studied at autopsy, as well as similar infiltrates in approximately 17 percent of patients with CLL and CML, with equal frequency. These lesions were rarely of clinical signifi-

cance. Others reported similar lesions in patients who also had prostatic leukemic infiltration.[256]

Kidney

Unilateral renal granulocytic sarcoma seen on CT scan and MRI was reported as the only manifestation of AML in a patient by Bagg and colleagues.[265] The mass, which diffusely involved the kidney, was diagnosed by open renal biopsy and only partially responded to induction therapy for AML. Others have reported an approximately 70 percent incidence of microscopic leukemic infiltration of the kidney at autopsy in patients with acute leukemia, a similar incidence of such infiltrations in CML, and a much lower frequency in CLL (Figure 9–24).[264]

Testis

Although testicular relapse of acute leukemia is common in children, it is uncommon in adults. Young adults experience testicular relapse much more frequently than do older patients,[266–268] and the problem is observed in ALL[266] (Figure 9–25) with greater frequency than in AML.[267] The most common presentation is painless swelling in one testicle, most commonly the left. However, not uncommonly, both testes will be determined to be involved after wedge biopsy. Most patients have isolated testicular relapse, but patients with concurrent bone marrow or other relapse have been reported.[266,269] Irradiation of both testicles is the treatment of choice and usually resolves the local problem. Rarely, testicular granulocytic sarcoma may be the only manifestation of AML, and local radiation plus systemic chemotherapy may be curative.[268]

Granulocytic sarcoma of the testis has been reported at least once in an elderly patient with MDS.[268]

Penis and Clitoris

Priapism due to leukostasis of leukemic cells in the corpora cavernosa and dorsal vein of the penis is an extremely rare complication of ALL, AML, and CML in adults.[270,271] This extremely painful problem is usually managed conservatively, without shunting.[270] It is only seen in patients with active systemic leukemia. Clitorism has been reported in a child[272] but not in adults.

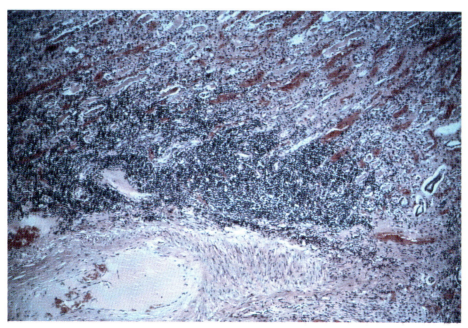

Figure 9–24. Leukemic infiltration of a kidney of the patient in Figure 9–23. Renal function was moderately impaired (hematoxylin and eosin stain; original magnification ×400).

SKELETAL SYSTEM

A generation ago, Thomas and colleagues reviewed autopsies of 85 acute leukemia patients who died at the National Cancer Institute for skeletal manifesta-tions of their disease.[273] They found lesions of the tibia, spine, ribs, and femur to be the most common sources of bone pain in adults. Skeletal pain was one of the initial manifestations of acute leukemia in 5 percent of adults and 25 percent of children. In

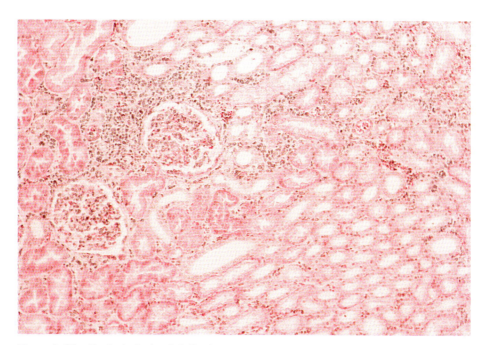

Figure 9–25. Testicular leukemic infiltration in an adult with ALL who presented with an enlarged, painful testicle while in hematologic remission. Radiation therapy resulted in a complete response, but the patient developed meningeal leukemia and bone marrow relapse simultaneously 3 months later (hematoxylin and eosin stain; original magnification ×400).

adults, the most common radiograph lesions directly caused by acute leukemia were osteolytic lesions (Figure 9–26), whereas in children, metaphyseal radiolucent bands, growth arrest lines, and cortical and periosteal lesions were common. The authors did not distinguish between patients with ALL and AML. Others have reported diffuse skeletal muscle infiltration by leukemic cells in patients with acute myelomonocytic leukemia.[274] Chabner and colleagues[275] reported 6 of 205 patients with CML whose initial manifestation of blast crisis was destructive bone lesions. The femur was involved in 2 patients, the humerus in 1, and the ileum in another, and 2 had multiple lesions throughout the skeleton. In another report, a granulocytic sarcoma of the sternum occurred as an early manifestation of CML,[276] and in another case, diffuse osteolytic lesions in a patient with CML in blast crisis were associated with hypercalcemia.[277] Granulocytic sarcoma of the sacrum[278] and scapula[279] as the initial manifestation of AML was reported, and some authors have noted that the most common site of granulocytic sarcoma is bone (Figure 9–27).[7,278] These lesions frequently require local radiation therapy for control of pain. Bone pain as a result of destructive bone lesions in patients with hairy cell

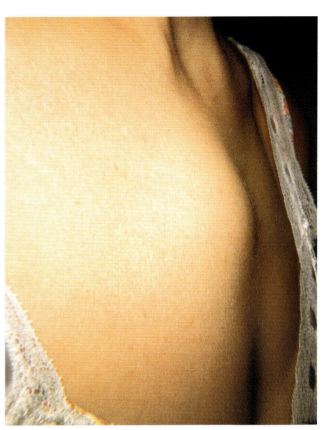

Figure 9–27. Granulocytic sarcoma in a patient with AML M4 arising subperiosteally from a rib at the sternal border. Marrow relapse occurred 2 months later.

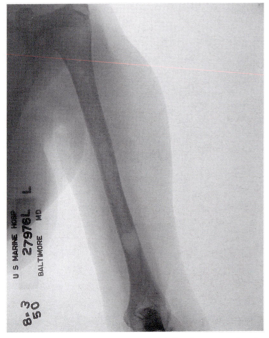

Figure 9–26. Osteolytic lesion of the humerus due to granulocytic sarcoma in a patient presenting with AML M1.

leukemia is uncommon but not rare. The femoral head and neck are frequently involved, and lytic lesions are usually evident on radiography.[280,281] The lesions respond well to local radiation therapy, after which they may not recur.[281] Generalized skeletal involvement with adult T-cell leukemia has been observed,[282] and back pain secondary to leukemic infiltration of lumbar intervertebral discs with partial collapse of vertebrae was observed in a patient with B-CLL.[283] Adults with ALL may present with arthritis[284] due to synovial leukemic infiltration, although this is much more common in children.

REFERENCES

1. Imrie KR, Kovacs MJ, Selby D, et al. Isolated chloroma: the effect of early antileukemic therapy. Ann Intern Med 1995;123:351–3.
2. Meis JM, Butler JJ, Osborne BM, Manning JT. Granulocytic sarcoma in nonleukemic patients. Cancer 1986;58:2697–709.
3. Suh YK, Shin HJ. Fine-needle aspiration biopsy of

granulocytic sarcoma: a clinicopathologic study of 27 cases. Cancer 2000;90:364–72.

4. Menasce LP, Banerjee SS, Beckett E, Harris M. Extramedullary myeloid tumor (granulocytic sarcoma) is often misdiagnosed: a study of 26 cases. Histopathology 1999;34:391–8.

5. Roth MJ, Medeiros LJ, Elenitoba-Johnson K, et al. Extramedullary myeloid tumors. An immunohistochemical study of 29 cases using routinely fixed and processed paraffin-embedded tissue sections. Arch Pathol Lab Med 1995;119:790–8.

6. Hudock J, Chatten J, Miettinen M. Immunohistochemical evaluation of myeloid leukemia infiltrates (granulocytic sarcomas) in formaldehyde-fixed, paraffin-embedded tissue. Am J Clin Pathol 1994;102:55–60.

7. Neiman RS, Barcos M, Berard C, et al. Granulocytic sarcoma: a clinicopathologic study of 61 biopsied cases. Cancer 1981;48:1426–37.

8. Bangerter M, Hildebrand A, Waidmann O, Griesshammer M. Diagnosis of granulocytic sarcoma by fine-needle aspiration cytology. Acta Haematol 2000;103:102–8.

9. Tao J, Wu M, Fuchs A, Wasserman P. Fine-needle aspiration of granulocytic sarcomas: a morphologic and immunophenotypic study of seven cases. Ann Diagn Pathol 2000;4:17–22.

10. Liu K, Mann KP, Garst JL, et al. Diagnosis of posttransplant granulocytic sarcoma by fine-needle aspiration cytology and flow cytometry. Diagn Cytopathol 1999;20:85–9.

11. Koc Y, Miller KB, Schenkein DP, et al. Extramedulary tumors of myeloid blasts in adults as a pattern of relapse following allogeneic bone marrow transplantation. Cancer 1999;85:608–15.

12. Beckassy AN, Hermans J, Gorin NC, Gratwohl A. Granulocytic sarcoma after bone marrow transplantation: a retrospective European multicenter survey. Acute and Chronic Leukemia Working Parties of the European Group for Blood and Marrow Transplantation. Bone Marrow Transplant 1996;17:801–8.

13. Nachbaur D, Duba HC, Feichtinger H, et al. Polychemotherapy combined with G-CSF-mobilized donor buffy coat transfusion for granulocytic sarcoma after allogeneic BMT for AML. Bone Marrow Transplant 1997;19:947–9.

14. Lee JJ, Kim HJ, Kook H, et al. Granulocytic sarcoma as isolated extramedullary relapse after donor lymphocyte infusion in a patient with CML who relapsed after allogeneic bone marrow transplantation: a case report. J Korean Med Sci 1998;13:434–6.

15. Au WY, Chan AC, Lie AK, et al. Isolated extramedullary relapse after allogeneic bone marrow transplantation for chronic myeloid leukemia. Bone Marrow Transplant 1998;22:99–102.

16. De Oliveira JS, Chauffaille ML, Colleoni GW, et al. Granulocytic sarcoma presented as a reactivation of chronic myeloid leukemia after allogeneic bone marrow transplantation. Rev Paul Med 1998;116:1689–91.

17. Szomor A, Passweg JR, Tichelli A, et al. Myeloid leukemia and myelodysplastic syndrome relapsing as granulocytic sarcoma (chloroma) after allogeneic bone marrow transplantation. Ann Hematol 1997;75:239–41.

18. Hancock JC, Prchal JT, Bennett JM, Listinsky CM. Trilineage extramedullary myeloid tumor in myelodysplastic syndrome. Arch Pathol Lab Med 1997;121:520–3.

19. Byrd JC, Weiss RB. Recurrent granulocytic sarcoma. An unusual variation of acute myelogenous leukemia associated with 8;21 chromosomal translocation and blast expression of the neural cell adhesion molecule. Cancer 1994;73:2107–12.

20. Tallman MS, Hakimian D, Shaw JM, et al. Granulocytic sarcoma is associated with the 8;21 translocation in acute myeloid leukemia. J Clin Oncol 1993;11:690–7.

21. Seymour JF, Pierce SA, Kantarjian HM, et al. Investigation of karyotypic, morphologic and clinical features in patients with acute myeloid leukemia blast cells expressing the neural adhesion molecule (CD56). Leukemia 1994;9:823–6.

22. Paietta E, Neuberg D, Richards S, et al. Rare adult acute lymphocytic leukemia with CD56 expression in the ECOG experience shows unexpected phenotypic and genotypic heterogeneity. Am J Hematol 2001;66:189–96.

23. Heimann P, Vamos E, Ferster A, Sariban E. Granulocytic sarcoma showing chromosomal changes other than the t(8;21). Cancer Genet Cytogenet 1994;74:59–61.

24. Myint H, Chacko J, Mould S, et al. Karyotypic evolution in a granulocytic sarcoma developing in a myeloproliferative disorder with a novel (3;4) translocation. Br J Haematol 1995;90:462–4.

25. Adam LR, Angus B, Carey P, Davison EV. Cytogenetic analysis of a granulocytic sarcoma in a patient without systemic leukaemia. J Clin Pathol 1991;44:81–2.

26. Bown NP, Rowe D, Reid MM. Granulocytic sarcoma with the translocation (9;11)(p22;q23): two cases. Cancer Genet Cytogenet 1997;96:115–7.

27. Bischop MM, Revesz T, Bierings M, et al. Extramedullary infiltrates at diagnosis have no prognostic significance in children with acute myeloid leukemia. Leukemia 2001;15:46–9.

28. Felice MS, Zubizarreta PA, Alfaro EM, et al. Good outcome of children with acute myeloid leukemia and t(8;21)(q22;q22), even when associated with granulocytic sarcoma: a report from a single institution in Argentina. Cancer 2000;88:1939–44.

29. Schwyzer R, Sherman GG, Cohn RJ, et al. Granulocytic sarcoma in children with acute myeloblastic leukemia and t(8;21). Med Pediatr Oncol 1998;31:144–9.

30. Byrd JC, Weiss RB, Arthur DC, et al. Extramedullary leukemia adversely affects hematologic complete remission rate and overall survival in patients with t(8;21)(q22;q22): results from Cancer and Leukemia Group B 8461. J Clin Oncol 1997;15:466–475.

31. Rege K, Swansbury GJ, Atra AA, et al. Disease features in acute myeloid leukemia with t(8;21)(q22;q22). Influence of age, secondary karyotype abnormalities, CD19 status, and extramedullary leukemia on survival. Leuk Lymphoma 2000;40:67–77.

32. Dreizen S, McCredie KB, Keating MJ, et al. Leukemia-associated skin infiltrates. Postgrad Med 1989; 85:45–53.

33. Fernandez AM, Abeles M, Wong RL. Recurrent leukocytoclastic vasculitis as the initial manifestation of acute myelomonocytic leukemia. J Rheumatol 1994;21:1972–4.

34. Soppi E, Nousiainen T, Seppa A, Lahtinen R. Acute febrile neutrophilic dermatosis (Sweet's syndrome) in association with myelodysplastic syndromes: a report of three cases and a review of the literature. Br J Haematol 1989;73:43–7.

35. Cohen PR, Kurzrock R. Chronic myelogenous leukemia and Sweet syndrome. Am J Hematol 1989;2:134–7.

36. Hatch ME, Farber SS, Superfon NP, et al. Sweet's syndrome associated with chronic myelogenous leukemia. J Am Osteopath Assoc 1989;89:363–70.

37. Shaikh BS, Frantz E, Lookingbill DP. Histologically proven leukemia cutis carries a poor prognosis in acute nonlymphocytic leukemia. Cutis 1987;39: 57–60.

38. Baer MR, Barcos M, Farrell H, et al. Acute myelogenous leukemia with leukemia cutis. Cancer 1989;63:2192–200.

39. Sepp N, Radaszkiewicz T, Meijer CJLM, et al. Specific skin manifestations in acute leukemia with monocytic differentiation. Cancer 1993;71:124–32.

40. Kaiserling E, Horny H-P, Geerts M-L, et al. Skin involvement in myelogenous leukemia: morphologic and immunophenotypic heterogeneity of skin infiltrates. Mod Pathol 1994;7:771–9.

41. Berger BJ, Gross PR, Daniels RB, et al. Leukemia cutis masquerading as guttate psoriasis. Arch Dermatol 1873;108:416–8.

42. Wiernik PH, Serpick AA. Granulocytic sarcoma (chloroma). Blood 1970;35:361–9.

43. Byrd JC, Edenfield J, Shields DJ, et al. Extramedullary myeloid cell tumors in acute nonlymphocytic leukemia: a clinical review. J Clin Oncol 1995; 13:1800–16.

44. Murakami Y, Nagae S, Matsuishi E, et al. A case of CD56+ cutaneous aleukaemic granulocytic sarcoma with myelodysplastic syndrome. Br J Dermatol 2000;143:587–90.

45. Haubenstock A, Zalusky R, Ghali VS, et al. Isolated leukemia cutis—a case report. Am J Hematol 1987; 24:437–9.

46. Meis JM, Butler JJ, Osborne BM, et al. Granulocytic sarcoma in nonleukemic patients. Cancer 1986; 58:2697–709.

47. Sadahira Y, Sugihara T, Yawata Y, Manabe T. Cutaneous granulocytic sarcoma mimicking immunoblastic large cell lymphoma. Pathol Int 1999;49:347–53.

48. Goldstein NS, Ritter JH, Argenyi ZB, et al. Granulocytic sarcoma. Int J Surg Pathol 1995;2:177–86.

49. Schiffer CA, Sanel FT, Stechmiller BK, Wiernik PH. Functional and morphologic characteristics of the leukemic cells of a patient with acute monocytic leukemia: correlation with clinical features. Blood 1975;46:17–26.

50. Cross AH, Goorha RM, Nuss R, et al. Acute myeloid leukemia with t-lymphoid features: a distinct biologic and clinical entity. Blood 1988;72:579–87.

51. Schwonzen M, Kuehn N, Vetten B, et al. Phenotyping of acute myelomonocytic (AMMOL) and monocytic leukemia (AMOL): association of T-cell-related antigens and skin infiltration in AMMOL. Leuk Res 1989;13:893–8.

52. Amiraian R, Penn TE, Hamann S, et al. Leukemic dermal infiltrates as a complication of central venous catheter placement. Cancer 1988;62:2223–5.

53. Niazi Z, Molt P, Mittelman A, et al. Leukemic dermal infiltrates at permanent indwelling central venous catheter insertion sites. Cancer 1991;68:2281–3.

54. Harakati MS. Cutaneous granulocytic sarcoma at the exit site of Hickman indwelling venous catheter. Int J Hematol 1993;57:39–43.

55. Ariad S, Pizov G, Koretz M. Granulocytic sarcoma of the chest wall at site of Hickman catheter tract. Leuk Lymphoma 1996;23:401–3.

56. Baden TJ, Gammon WR. Leukemia cutis in acute myelomonocytic leukemia. Arch Dermatol 1987; 123:88–90.

57. Frimmer D, Quagliana JM. An unusual case of granulocytic sarcoma (chloroma). J Med Soc N J 1975; 72:137–40.

58. Martinelli G, Vianelli N, De Vivo A, et al. Granulocytic sarcomas: clinical, diagnostic and therapeutic aspects. Leuk Lymphoma 1997;24:349–53.

59. Ansell JE, Bhawan J, Pechet L. Leukemia cutis in blastic transformation of chronic myelocytic leukemia: TdT positive blasts and response to vincristine and prednisone. J Cut Pathol 1980;7:302–9.

60. Willard RJ, Turiansky GW, Genest GP, et al. Leukemia

cutis in a patient with chronic neutrophilic leukemia. J Am Acad Dermatol 2001;44:365–9.

61. Seligman BR, Rosner F, Solomon RB. Chronic myelogenous leukemia. N Y State J Med 1975;75:1271–4.

62. Giralt S, O'Brien S, Weeks E, et al. Leukemia cutis in acute promyelocytic leukemia: report of three cases after treatment with all-trans retinoic acid. Leuk Lymphoma 1994;4:453–6.

63. Weiss MA, Warrell RP Jr. Two cases of extramedullary acute promyelocytic leukemia. Cancer 1994;74:1882–6.

64. Selleri C, Pane F, Notaro R, et al. All-trans-retinoic acid (ATRA) responsive skin relapses of acute promyelocytic leukemia followed by ATRA-induced pseudotumor cerebri. Br J Haematol 1996;92:937–40.

65. Wiernik PH, DeBellis R, Muxi P, et al. Extramedullary acute promyelocytic leukemia. Cancer 1996;78:2510–4.

66. Bekassy AN, Hermans J, Gorin NC, et al. Granulocytic sarcoma after allogeneic bone marrow transplantation: a retrospective European multicenter survey. Bone Marrow Transplant 1996;17:801–8.

67. Prystowsky JH, Johnson BL, Bolwell BJ, et al. Treatment of cutaneous granulocytic sarcoma in a patient with myelodysplasia. Am J Med 1989;86:477–80.

68. Longacre TA, Smoller BR. Leukemia cutis. Am J Clin Pathol 1993;100:276–84.

69. Krishnan K, Ross CW, Adams PT, et al. Neural cell-adhesion molecule (CD 56)-positive, t(8;21) acute myeloid leukemia (AML, M-2) and granulocytic sarcoma. Ann Hematol 1994;69:321–3.

70. Wodzinski MA, Collin R, Winfield DA, et al. Epidural granulocytic sarcoma in acute myeloid leukemia with 8;21 translocation. Cancer 1988;62:1299–300.

71. Aizawa T, Kokubun S, Hatori M, et al. Extradural granulocytic sarcoma of the thoracic spine in acute myelogenous leukemia with 8;21 chromosome translocation. Tohoku J Exp Med 1996;178:431–6.

72. Petursson S, Boggs DR. Spinal cord involvement in leukemia. Cancer 1981;47:346–50.

73. Hildebrand J, Leenaerts L, Nubourgh Y, et al. Epidural spinal cord compression in acute myelogenous leukemia. Arch Neurol 1980;37:319.

74. Byrd JC, Weiss RB. Recurrent granulocytic sarcoma. Cancer 1994;73:2107–12.

75. Lagrange M, Gaspard M-H, Lagrange J-L, et al. Granulocytic sarcoma with meningeal but no bone marrow involvement at presentation. Acta Cytol 1992;36:319–24.

76. Dunnick NR, Heaston DK. Computed tomography of extracranial chloroma. J Comput Assist Tomogr 1982;6:83–5.

77. Muss HB, Moloney WC. Chloroma and other myeloblastic tumors. Blood 1973;42:721–8.

78. Mahendra P, Azer S, Bedlow AJ, et al. Two unusual neurological presentations of granulocytic sarcoma in Philadelphia positive chronic myeloid leukemia. Leuk Lymphoma 1994;15:351–5.

79. Hwang W-L, Gau J-P, Hu H-T, Young J-H. Isolated extramedullary relapse of acute lymphoblastic leukemia presenting as an intraspinal mass. Acta Haematol 1994;91:46–8.

80. Sandhu GS, Ghufoor K, Gonzalez-Garcia J, Elexpuru-Camiruaga JA. Granulocytic sarcoma presenting as cauda equina syndrome. Clin Neurol Neurosurg 1998;100:205–8.

81. Deme S, Deodhare SS, Tucker WS, Bilbao JM. Granulocytic sarcoma of the spine in nonleukemic patients: report of three cases. Neurosurgery 1997;40:1283–7.

82. Mostafavi H, Lennarson PJ, Traynelis VC. Granulocytic sarcoma of the spine. Neurosurgery 2000;46:78–83.

83. Abe R, Umezu H, Uchida T, et al. Myeloblastoma with an 8;21 chromosome translocation in acute myeloblastic leukemia. Cancer 1986;58:1260–4.

84. Hurwitz CA, Raimondi SC, Head D, et al. Distinctive immunophenotypic features of t(8;21)(q22;q22) acute myeloblastic leukemia in children. Blood 1992;80:3182–8.

85. Hurwitz BS, Sutherland JC, Walker MD. Central nervous system chloromas preceding acute leukemia by one year. Neurology 1970;20:771–5.

86. Tripathi BN, Kapoor AK, Chandra M, Agarwal PK. Chloromas with unusual neurological manifestations. J Indian Med Assoc 1974;62:162–3.

87. Roy EP III, Rodgers JS II, Riggs JE. Intracranial granulocytic sarcoma in postpolycythemia myeloid metaplasia. South Med J 1989;82:1564–7.

88. Binder C, Tiemann M, Haase D, et al. Isolated meningeal chloroma (granulocytic sarcoma)—a case report and review of the literature. Ann Hematol 2000;79:459–62.

89. Au WY, Shels TW, Ma SK, et al. Myeloblastoma (chloroma) in leukemia: case 2. Meningeal granulocytic sarcoma (chloroma) in essential thrombocythemia. J Clin Oncol 2000;18:3996–7.

90. Grande M. Central nervous system granulocytic sarcoma in a patient with essential thrombocythemia. Am J Hematol 1996;51:64–7.

91. Vinters HV, Gilbert JJ. Multifocal chloromas of the brain. Surg Neurol 1982;17:47–51.

92. Joselson RA, Beckstead JH, Davis RL. Granulocytic sarcoma of the brain after renal transplantation. J Neuropathol Exp Neurol 1982;41:580–7.

93. Krishnamurthy M, Nusbacher N, Elguezabal A, Seligman BR. Granulocytic sarcoma of the brain. Cancer 1977;39:1542–6.

94. Demaray MJ, Caladonato JP, Parker JC Jr, Rosomoff HL. Intracerebellar chloroma (granulocytic sar-

coma): a neurosurgical complication of acute myelocytic leukemia. Surg Neurol 1976;6:353–6.

95. Parker K, Hardjasudarma M, McClellan R, et al. MR features of an intracerebellar chloroma. AJNR Am J Neuroradiol 1996;17:1592–4.

96. Lorsbach RB, Folkerth RD, Pinkus GS. Relapse of acute myelogenous leukemia as a cerebellar myeloblastoma showing megakaryoblastic differentiation. Mod Pathol 1999;12:1186–91.

97. Hatano Y, Miura I, Horiuchi T, et al. Cerebellar myeloblastoma formation in CD7-positive, neural cell adhesion molecule (CD56)-positive acute myelogenous leukemia (M1). Ann Hematol 1997;75:125–8.

98. Yamamoto K, Hamaguchi H, Nagata K, et al. Isolated recurrence of granulocytic sarcoma of the brain: successful treatment with surgical resection, intrathecal injection, irradiation and prophylactic systemic chemotherapy. Jpn J Clin Oncol 1999;29:214–8.

99. Zimmerman LE, Font RL. Ophthalmologic manifestations of granulocytic sarcoma. Am J Ophthalmol 1975;80:975–90.

100. Tanigawa M, Tsuda Y, Amemiya Y, et al. Orbital tumor in acute myeloid leukemia associated with karyotype 46,XX,t(8;21)(q22;q22): a case report. Ophthalmology 1998;212:202–5.

101. Lakhkar BN, Banovali S, Philip P. Orbital granulocytic sarcoma in acute myelogenous leukemia. Indian J Pediatr 2000;67:234–5.

102. Watkins LM, Remulla HD, Rubin PA. Orbital granulocytic sarcoma in an elderly patient. Am J Ophthalmol 1997;123:854–6.

103. Yaghouti F, Nouri M, Mannor GE. Ocular adnexal granulocytic sarcoma as the first sign of acute myelogenous leukemia relapse. Am J Ophthalmol 1999;127:361–3.

104. Frappaz D, Bertheas MF, Vasselon C, et al. Retroorbital chloroma in children with t(8;21) acute myeloblastic leukemia M2 type. Am J Pediatr Hematol Oncol 1988;10:134–8.

105. Stockl FA, Dolmetsch AM, Saornil MA, et al. Orbital granulocytic sarcoma. Br J Ophthalmol 1997;81:1084–8.

106. Puri P, Grover AK. Granulocytic sarcoma of orbit preceding acute myeloid leukemia: a case report. Eur J Cancer Care 1999;8:113–5.

107. Murphy JA, Pitts JF, Dudgeon J, et al. Retinal detachments due to chronic lymphocytic leukemia. Clin Lab Haematol 1991;13:217–20.

108. Landolf R, Colosimo C Jr, De Candia E, et al. Meningeal hematopoiesis causing exophthalmus and hemiparesis in myelofibrosis: effect of radiotherapy. Cancer 1988;62:2346–9.

109. Glass JP, Van Tassel P, Keating MJ, et al. Central nervous system complications of a newly recognized subtype of leukemia: AMML with a pericentric inversion of chromosome 16. Neurology 1987;37:639–44.

110. Bjornson CRR, Rietze RL, Reynolds BA, et al. Turning brain into blood: a hematopoietic fate adopted by adult neural stem cells in vivo. Science 1999;283:534–7.

111. Gokbuget N, Hoelzer D. Meningeosis leukaemica in adult acute lymphoblastic leukaemia. J Neurooncol 1998;38:167–80.

112. Kantarjian HM, Walters RS, Smith TL, et al. Identification of risk groups for development of central nervous system leukemia in adults with acute lymphocytic leukemia. Blood 1988;72:1784–9.

113. Castagnola C, Nozza A, Corso A, Bernasconi C. The value of combination therapy in adult acute myeloid leukemia with central nervous system involvement. Haematologica 1997;82:577–80.

114. Peterson BA, Brunning RD, Bloomfield CD, et al. Central nervous system involvement in acute nonlymphocytic leukemia. Am J Med 1987;83:464–70.

115. Brown DM, Kimura AE, Ossoinig KC, Weiner GJ. Acute promyelocytic infiltration of the optic nerve treated by oral *trans*-retinoic acid. Ophthalmology 1992;99:1463–7.

116. Masse SR, Wolk RW, Conklin RH. Peripituitary gland involvement in acute leukemia in adults. Arch Pathol 1973;96:141–2.

117. Krendel DA, Albright RE, Graham DG. Infiltrative polyneuropathy due to acute monoblastic leukemia in hematologic remission. Neurology 1987;37:474–7.

118. Schwartz JH, Canellos GP, Young RC, DeVita VT. Meningeal leukemia in blastic phase of chronic granulocytic leukemia. Am J Med 1975;59:819–28.

119. Saikia TK, Dhabkar B, Iyer RS, et al. High incidence of meningeal leukemia in lymphoid blast crisis of chronic myelogenous leukemia. Am J Hematol 1993;43:10–3.

120. Feng C-S. An unusual case of extramedullary blast crisis in chronic myelocytic leukemia. Am J Hematol 1988;29:117–9.

121. Hendrick AM, Rogers JS II, Guliner RJ. Ocular complications following blast transformation in chronic myelogenous leukemia. Am J Hematol 1979;7:389–94.

122. Oshimi K, Akahoshi M, Hagiwara N, et al. A case of T-cell chronic lymphocytic leukemia with an unusual phenotype and central nervous system involvement. Cancer 1985;55:1937–42.

123. Stagg MP, Gumbart CH. Chronic lymphocytic leukemic meningitis as a cause of the syndrome of inappropriate secretion of antidiuretic hormone. Cancer 1987;60:191–2.

124. Cash J, Fehir KM, Pollack MS. Meningeal involvement in early stage chronic lymphocytic leukemia. Cancer 1987;59:798–800.

125. Wang ML, Shih LY, Dunn P, Kuo MC. Meningeal involvement in B-cell chronic lymphocytic leukemia: report of two cases. J Formos Med Assoc 2000;99:775–8.

126. Miller K, Budke H, Orazi A. Leukemic meningitis complicating early stage chronic lymphocytic leukemia. Arch Pathol Lab Med 1997;121:524–7.

127. Diwan RV, Diwan VG, Bellon EM. Brain involvement in chronic lymphocytic leukemia. J Comput Assist Tomogr 1982;6:812–4.

128. Sklansky BD, Jafek BW, Wiernik PH. Otolaryngologic manifestations of acute leukemia. Laryngoscope 1974;84:210–30.

129. Nayak DR, Balakrishnan R, Raj G, et al. Granulocytic sarcoma of the head and neck: a case report. Am J Otolaryngol 2001;22:80–3.

130. Hossain D, Weisberger J, Sreekantaiah C, Seiter K. Biphenotypic (mixed myeloid/T-cell) extramedullary myeloid cell tumor. Leuk Lymphoma 1999;33: 399–402.

131. Presant CA, Safdar SH, Cherrick H. Gingival leukemic infiltration in chronic lymphocytic leukemia. Oral Surg 1973;36:672–4.

132. Tong AC, Lam KY. Granulocytic sarcoma presenting as an ulcerative mucogingival lesion: report of a case and review of the literature. J Oral Maxillofac Surg 2000;58:1055–8.

133. Benekli M, Savas MC, Haznedaroglu C, Dundar AV. Granulocytic sarcoma in acute promyelocytic leukemia. Leuk Lymphoma 1996;22:183–6.

134. Haznedaroglu IC, Ustundag Y, Benekli M, et al. Isolated gingival relapse during complete hematological remission in acute promyelocytic leukemia. Acta Haematol 1995;93:54–5.

135. Thomas CI, Cameselle TJ, Diz DP, et al. Intra-alveolar granulocytic sarcoma developing after tooth extraction. Oral Oncol 2000;36:491–4.

136. McGowan DA. Acute leukaemia and the dental hygienist. Dent Health 1970;9:68–9.

137. Sela MN, Pisanti S. Early diagnosis and treatment of patients with leukemia, a dental problem. J Oral Med 1977;32:46–50.

138. Williford SK, Salisbury PL, Peacock JE, et al. The safety of dental extractions in patients with hematologic malignancies. J Clin Oncol 1989;7:798–802.

139. Segelman AE, Doku HC. Treatment of the oral complications of leukemia. J Oral Surg 1977;35:469–77.

140. Ti M, Villafuerte R, Chase PH, Dosik H. Acute leukemia presenting as laryngeal obstruction. Cancer 1974;34:427–30.

141. Shilling BB, Work WP. Leukemic involvement of larynx. Arch Otolaryngol 1967;85:658–65.

142. Griffiths MV, Choudhry C. Acute leukaemia—an unusual presentation. J Laryngol Otol 1974;88: 683–6.

143. Bassichis B, McClay J, Wiatrak B. Chloroma of masseteric muscle. Int J Pediatr Otorhinolaryngol 2000;53:57–61.

144. Huffman GG. Mandibular involvement in acute lymphocytic leukemia: report of a case. J Oral Surg 1976;34:842–3.

145. Stern MH, Cole WL. Radiographic changes in the mandible associated with leukemic cell infiltration in a case of acute myelogenous leukemia. Oral Med 1973;36:343–7.

146. Sippel HW, Samartano JG. Leukemia manifested as lymphosarcoma of the mandible: report of a case. J Oral Surg 1971;29:363–6.

147. Jacknow G, Frizzera G, Gajl-Peczalska K, et al. Extramedullary presentation of the blast crisis of chronic myelogenous leukaemia. Br J Haematol 1985;61:225–36.

148. Bertrand Y, Lefrere J-J, Leverger G, et al. Acute myeloblastic leukemia presenting as apparent acute otitis media. Am J Hematol 1988;27:136–8.

149. Almadori G, Del Ninno M, Cadoni G, et al. Facial nerve paralysis in acute otomastoiditis as presenting symptom of FAB M2, t8;21 leukemic relapse. Case report and review of the literature. Int J Pediatr Otorhinolaryngol 1996;36:45–52.

150. Wright JLW. Acute leukaemia presenting as acute mastoiditis. J Laryngol Otol 1971;85:1087–91.

151. Paparella MM, Berlinger NT, Oda M, El Fiky F. Otological manifestations of leukemia. Laryngoscope 1973;83:1510–26.

152. Shukla GK, Dayal D, Gupta KR. Otological manifestations of leukaemia. Otolaryngology 1972;44:365–72.

153. La Venuta F, Moore JA. Involvement of the inner ear in acute stem cell leukemia. Ann Otol 1972;81:132–7.

154. Padmore RF, Bedard Y, Chapnik J. Relapse of acute myelogenous leukemia presenting as acute otitis externa. Cancer 1984;53:569–72.

155. Roberts WC, Bodey GP, Wertlake PT. The heart in acute leukemia. Am J Cardiol 1968;21:388–412.

156. Foucar K, Foucar E, Willman C, et al. Nonleukemic granulocytic sarcoma of the heart: a report of a fatal case. Am J Hematol 1987;25:325–32.

157. Wiernik PH, Sutherland JC, Stechmiller BK, Wolff J. Clinically significant cardiac infiltration in acute leukemia, lymphocytic lymphoma, and plasma cell myeloma. Med Pediatr Oncol 1976;2:75–85.

158. Bjorkholm M, Ost A, Biberfeld P. Myocardial rupture with cardiac tamponade as a lethal early manifestation of acute myeloblastic leukemia. Cancer 1982;50:1867–9.

159. Lisker SA, Finkelstein D, Brody JI, et al. Myocardial infarction in acute leukemia. Arch Intern Med 1967;119:532–5.

160. McAdams HP, Schaefer PS, Ghaed VN. Leukemic

infiltrates of the heart: CT findings. J Comput Assist Tomogr 1989;13:525–7.

161. Perry DJ, McCormick D, Vassey S, et al. Right heart obstruction due to intracavitary prolymphocytic leukemia. Am J Med 1986;81:131–4.

162. Appelfeld MM, Milner SD, Vigorito RD, et al. Congestive heart failure and endocardial fibroelastosis caused by chronic lymphocytic leukemia. Cancer 1980;46:1479–84.

163. Bergeron GA, Datnow B. Acute myocardial infarction due to chronic myelogenous leukemia. Chest 1974;65:452–5.

164. Chia BL, Da Costa JL, Ransome GA. Cardiac tamponade due to leukaemic pericardial effusion. Thorax 1973;28:657–9.

165. Armitage JO, Feagler JR. Acute leukemia presenting with pericardial involvement. Nebr Med J 1976; 61:198–201.

166. Rege K, Powles R, Norton J, et al. An unusual presentation of acute myeloid leukaemia with pericardial and pleural effusions due to granulocytic sarcoma. Leuk Lymphoma 1993;11:305–7.

167. Bradford CR, Smith SR, Wallis JP. Pericardial extramedullary haemopoiesis in chronic myelomonocytic leukaemia. J Clin Pathol 1993;46:674–5.

168. Mani S, Duffy TP. Pericardial tamponade in chronic myelomonocytic leukemia. Chest 1994;106:967–70.

169. Shih L-Y, Lin F-C, Kuo T-T. Cutaneous and pericardial extramedullary hematopoiesis with cardiac tamponade in chronic myeloid leukemia. Am J Clin Pathol 1988;89:693–7.

170. Kafkas P, Papaevangelou G, Kanaginis T, et al. Frequency of electrocardio-graphic alterations in patients with leukaemia. Ann Clin Res 1973;5:23–6.

171. Suryaprasad AG, Van Slyck EJ, James TN. The sinus node in chronic granulocytic leukemia. Chest 1972;61:494–6.

172. Hatake K, Saito K, Saga T, et al. A case of acute myelogenous leukemia with advanced atrioventricular block and pericardial effusion caused by leukemic cell infiltration. Jpn J Med 1982;21:115–9.

173. Allen DC, Alderdice JM, Morton P, et al. Pathology of the heart and conduction system in lymphoma and leukaemia. J Clin Pathol 1987;40:746–50.

174. Beckering RE, Titus JL. Leukemic infiltration of valves of thigh veins. Mayo Clin Proc 1969;44:25–7.

175. Shifrin EG, Drenger B, Matzner Y, et al. Ruptured inflammatory abdominal aortic aneurysm due to acute myelomonocytic leukemia. J Cardiovasc Surg 1987;28:32–4.

176. Bodey GP, Powell RD, Hersh EM, et al. Pulmonary complications of acute leukemia. Cancer 1966;19:781–93.

177. Smith LJ, Katzenstein AA. Pathogenesis of massive pulmonary hemorrhage in acute leukemia. Arch Intern Med 1982;142:2149–52.

178. Klatte EC, Yardley J, Smith EB, et al. The pulmonary manifestations and complications of leukemia. AJR Am J Roentgenol 1963;89:598–609.

179. Green RA, Nichols NJ. Pulmonary involvement in leukemia. Am Rev Respir Dis 1959;80:833–44.

180. Vilpo JA, Dryzun B, Klemi P, et al. Extramedullary pleural blast crisis during otherwise chronic phase in chronic granulocytic leukaemia. Eur J Cancer 1980;16:885–91.

181. Doran HM, Sheppard MN, Collins PW, et al. Pathology of the lung in leukaemia and lymphoma: a study of 87 autopsies. Histopathology 1991;18:211–9.

182. Mangal AK, Growe GH. Extensive pulmonary infiltration by leukemic blast cells treated with irradiation. Can Med Assoc J 1983;128:424–6.

183. Lokich JJ, Maloney WC. Fatal pulmonary leukostasis following treatment in acute myelogenous leukemia. Arch Intern Med 1972;130:759–62.

184. Lester TJ, Johnson JW, Cuttner J. Pulmonary leukostasis as the single worst prognostic factor in patients with acute myelocytic leukemia and hyperleukocytosis. Am J Med 1985;79:43–8.

185. Soares FA, Landell GAM, Cardoso MCM. Pulmonary leukostasis without hyperleukocytosis: a clinicopathologic study of 16 cases. Am J Hematol 1992;40:28–32.

186. Van Buchem MA, Wondergem JH, Kool LJS, et al. Pulmonary leukostasis: radiologic-pathologic study. Radiology 1987;165:739–41.

187. Geller SA. Acute leukemia presenting as respiratory distress. Arch Pathol 1971;91:573–6.

188. Frankel SR, Eardley A, Lauwers G, et al. The "retinoic acid syndrome" in acute promyelocytic leukemia. Ann Intern Med 1992;117:292–6.

189. Dugdale DC, Salness TA, Knight L, et al. Endobronchial granulocytic sarcoma causing acute respiratory failure in acute myelogenous leukemia. Am Rev Respir Dis 1987;136:1248–50.

190. Wong KF, Chan JKC, Chan JCW. Acute myeloid leukemia presenting as granulocytic sarcoma of the lung. Am J Hematol 1993;43:77–8.

191. Callahan M, Wall S, Askin F, et al. Granulocytic sarcoma presenting as pulmonary nodules and lymphadenopathy. Cancer 1987;60:1902–4.

192. Kottaridis PD, Ketley N, Peggs K, et al. An unusual case of intrapulmonary granulocytic sarcoma presenting as interstitial pneumonitis following allogeneic bone marrow transplantation for acute myeloid leukemia and responding to donor lymphocyte infusion. Bone Marrow Transplant 1999;24:807–9.

193. Ajarim DSS, Santhosh-Kumar CR, El Saghir NS, et al. Granulocytic sarcoma of the thymus in acute promyelocytic leukaemia. Clin Lab Haematol 1990;12:97–9.

194. Chubachi A, Miura I, Takahashi N, et al. Acute mye-

logenous leukemia associated with a mediastinal tumor. Leuk Lymphoma 1993;12:143–6.

195. McCluggage WG, Boyd HK, Jones FG, et al. Mediastinal granulocytic sarcoma: a report of two cases. Arch Pathol Lab Med 1998;122:545–7.

196. Rosenoff SH, Canellos GP, O'Connell M, Wiernik PH. Mediastinal adenopathy in granulocytic leukemia. Arch Intern Med 1974;134:135–8.

197. Hishima T, Fukayama M, Hayashi Y, et al. Granulocytic sarcoma of the thymus in a nonleukemic patient. Virchows Arch 1999;435:447–51.

198. Ravandi-Kashani F, Cortes J, Giles FJ. Myelodysplasia presenting as granulocytic sarcoma of mediastinum causing superior vena cava syndrome. Leuk Lymphoma 2000;36:631–7.

199. Au WY, Ma SK, Chan AC, et al. Near tetraploidy in three cases of acute myeloid leukemia associated with mediastinal granulocytic sarcoma. Cancer Genet Cytogenet 1998;102:50–3.

200. Wadhwa J, Gujral S, Kumar L, et al. Extramedullary myeloid cell tumor: presentation as anterior chest wall mass during AML relapse. Postgrad Med 1999;75:483–4.

201. Fulp SR, Nestok BR, Pwell BL, et al. Leukemic infiltration of the esophagus. Cancer 1993;71:112–6.

202. Prolla JC, Kirsner JB. The gastrointestinal lesions and complications of the leukemias. Ann Intern Med 1964;61:1084–103.

203. Weisdorf D, Arthur D, Rank J, et al. Gastric recurrence of acute lymphoblastic leukaemia mimicking graft-versus-host disease. Br J Haematol 1989;71:559–64.

204. Cornes GJ, Jones TG. Leukaemic lesions of the gastrointestinal tract. J Clin Pathol 1962;15:305–13.

205. Dewar GJ, Lim CN, Michalyshyn B, Akabutu J. Gastrointestinal complications in patients with acute and chronic leukemia. Can J Surg 1981;29:67–71.

206. Brugo EA, Marshall RB, Riberi AM, Pautasso OE. Preleukemic granulocytic sarcomas of the gastrointestinal tract. Am J Clin Pathol 1977;68:616–21.

207. Wasser AH, Spector JI. Endoscopic evaluation of small-bowel leukemia. Dig Dis 1977;22:1028–32.

208. Takeh H, Farran M, Debaize JP. Granulocytic sarcoma (chloroma) of the small intestine. Acta Chir Belg 1999;99:78–81.

209. Corpechot C, Lemann M, Brocheriou I, et al. Granulocytic sarcoma of the jejunum: a rare cause of small bowel obstruction. Am J Gastroenterol 1998;93:2586–8.

210. Cockington RA. Leukaemic infiltration of the gastrointestinal tract. Med J Aust 1975;1:103–5.

211. Orlandi E, Morra E, Lazzarino M, et al. Multiple granulocytic sarcoma during complete hematologic remission of acute nonlymphoid leukemia. Acta Haematol 1989;81:41–3.

212. Rottenberg GT, Thomas BM. Case report: granulocytic sarcoma of the small bowel—a rare presentation of leukaemia. Clin Radiol 1994;49:501–2.

213. Gorczyca W, Weisberger J, Seiter K. Colonic adenomas with extramedullary myeloid tumor (granulocytic sarcoma). Leuk Lymphoma 1999;34:621–4.

214. Dabbagh V, Broene G, Parapia LA, et al. Granulocytic sarcoma of the rectum: a rare complication of myelodysplasia. J Clin Pathol 1999;52:865–6.

215. Catalano MF, Levin B, Hart RS, et al. Granulocytic sarcoma of the colon. Gastroenterology 1991;100:555–9.

216. Scharschmidt BF. Chronic lymphocytic leukemia presenting as colitis. Dig Dis 1978;23(Suppl):9S–12S.

217. Evans C, Rosenfeld CS, Winkelstein A, et al. Perforation of an unsuspected cecal granulocytic sarcoma during therapy with granulocyte-macrophage colony-stimulating factor. N Engl J Med 1990;322:337–8.

218. Schimpff SC, Wiernik PH, Block JB. Rectal abscesses in cancer patients. Lancet 1972;2:844–7.

219. King DJ, Ewen SW, Sewell HF, Dawson AA. Obstructive jaundice. An unusual presentation of granulocytic sarcoma. Cancer 1987;60:114–7.

220. Fleming DR, Slone SP. CML blast crisis resulting in biliary obstruction following BMT. Bone Marrow Transplant 1997;19:853–4.

221. Matsueda K, Yamamoto H, Doi I. An autopsy case of granulocytic sarcoma of the porta hepatis causing obstructive jaundice. J Gastroenterol 1998;33:428–33.

222. Ravandi-Kashaani F, Estey E, Cortes J, et al. Granulocytic sarcoma of the pancreas: a report of two cases and literature review. Clin Lab Haematol 1999;21:219–24.

223. Oliva E, Ferry JA, Young RH, et al. Granulocytic sarcoma of the female genital tract: a clinicopathologic study of 11 cases. Am J Surg Pathol 1997;21:1156–65.

224. Seo IS, Hull MT, Pak HY. Granulocytic sarcoma of the cervix as a primary manifestation. Cancer 1977;40:3030–7.

225. Kamble R, Kochupillai V, Sharma A, et al. Granulocytic sarcoma of uterine cervix as presentation of acute myeloid leukemia: a case report and review of literature. J Obstet Gynaecol Res 1997;23:261–6.

226. Kapadia SB, Krause JR, Kanbour AI, et al. Granulocytic sarcoma of the uterus. Cancer 1978;41:687–91.

227. Delaflor-Weiss E, Zauber NP, Kintiroglou M, et al. Acute myelogenous leukemia relapsing as granulocytic sarcoma of the cervix. A case report. Acta Cytol 1999;43:1124–30.

228. Harris NL, Scully RE. Malignant lymphoma and granulocytic sarcoma of the uterus and vagina. Cancer 1984;53:2530–45.

229. Friedman HD, Adelson MD, Elder RC, et al. Granulo-cytic sarcoma of the uterine cervix-literature review of granulocytic sarcoma of the female genital tract. Gynecol Oncol 1992;46:128–37.

230. Lane DM, Birdwell RL. Ovarian leukemia detected by pelvic sonography. Cancer 1986;58:2338–42.

231. Heaton DC, Duff GB. Ovarian relapse in a young woman with acute lymphoblastic leukemia. Am J Hematol 1989;30:42–3.

232. Stavem P, Evensen SA, Torkildsen EM, Stenwig J. Ovarian relapse in a young woman with acute lym-phoblastic leukemia. Am J Hematol 1989;32:155.

233. Sreejith G, Gangadharan VP, Elizabath KA, et al. Pri-mary granulocytic sarcoma of the ovary. Am J Clin Oncol 2000;23:239–40.

234. Hinkamp JF, Szanto PB. Chloroma of the ovary. Am J Obstet Gynecol 1959;78:812–6.

235. Osborne BM, Robboy SJ. Lymphomas or leukemia pre-senting as ovarian tumors. Cancer 1983;52:1933–43.

236. Drinkard LC, Waggoner S, Stein RN, et al. Acute myelomonocytic leukemia with abnormal eosinophils presenting as an ovarian mass: a report of two cases and a review of the literature. Gynecol Oncol 1995;56:307–11.

237. Yamamoto K, Akiyama H, Maruyama T, et al. Granulo-cytic sarcoma of the ovary in patients with acute mye-logenous leukemia. Am J Hematol 1991;38:223–5.

238. Jung SE, Chun KA, Park SH, Lee EJ. MR findings in ovarian granulocytic sarcoma. Br J Radiol 1999; 72:301–3.

239. Paydas S, Hazar B, Sahin B, Gonlusen G. Granulocytic sarcoma as the cause of giant abdominal mass: diag-nosis by fine needle aspiration and review of the lit-erature. Leuk Res 2000;24:267–9.

240. Rowlands CG. Cytology of ascitic fluid in a patient with granulocytic sarcoma (extramedullary myeloid tumor). A case report. Acta Cytol 1999;43:227–31.

241. Sheikh SS, Khalifa MA, Marley EF, et al. Acute mono-cytic leukemia (FAB M5) involving the placenta asso-ciated with delivery of a healthy infant: case report and discussion. Int J Gynecol Pathol 1996;15:363–6.

242. Jung SM, Kuo TT, Wu JH, et al. Granulocytic sarcoma presenting as a giant breast tumor in a pregnant woman: a case report. Chang Keng I Hsueh Tsa Chih 1998;21:97–102.

243. Guermazi A, Quoc SN, Socie G, et al. Myeloblastoma (chloroma) in leukemia: case 1. Granulocytic sar-coma (chloroma) of the breast. J Clin Oncol 2000; 18:3993–6.

244. Blackwell B. Acute leukaemia presenting as a lump in the breast. Br J Surg 1963;50:769–71.

245. Eshghabadi M, Shojania AM, Carr I. Isolated granulo-cytic sarcoma: report of a case and review of the lit-erature. J Clin Oncol 1986;4:912–7.

246. Gartenhaus WS, Mir R, Pliskin A, et al. Granulocytic sarcoma of the breast: aleukemic bilateral metachronous presentation and literature review. Med Pediatr Oncol 1985;13:22–9.

247. Ngu IW, Sinclair EC, Greenaway S, Greenberg ML. Unusual presentation of granulocytic sarcoma in the breast: a case report and review of the literature. Diagn Cytopathol 2001;24:53–7.

248. Wiernik PH. Letter to the editor. Cancer 1989;63:1624.

249. Lin Y, Govindan R, Hess JL. Malignant hematopoietic breast tumors. Am J Clin Pathol 1997;107:177–86.

250. Breccia M, Petti MC, Fraternali-Orcioni G, et al. Gran-ulocytic sarcoma with breast and skin presentation: a report of a case successfully treated by local radi-ation and systemic chemotherapy. Acta Haematol 2000;104:34–7.

251. Domanic N, Akman N, Muftuoglu U. Massive breast involvement in acute leukemia. Helvet Paediatr Acta 1972;27:601–5.

252. Au WY, Ma SK, Kwong YL, et al. Acute myeloid leukemia relapsing as gynecomastia. Leuk Lym-phoma 1999;36:191–4.

253. Gralnick HP, Dittmar K. Development of myeloblastoma with massive breast and ovarian involvement during remission in acute leukemia. Cancer 1969;24:746–50.

254. Flaherty SA, Cope HE, Shecket HA. Prostatic obstruc-tion as the presenting symptom of acute monocytic leukemia. J Urol 1940;44:488–97.

255. Johnson MA, Gundersen AH. Infiltration of the prostate gland by chronic lymphatic leukemia. J Urol 1953;69:681–4.

256. Weathers EA, Lahem JE. Leukemic infiltration of the prostate. South Med J 1972;65:417–9.

257. Waddington RT. Leukaemic infiltration of the prostate in a patient with chronic lymphatic leukaemia—a case report. Br J Urol 1973;45:184–6.

258. Butler MR, O'Flynn JD. Prostatic disease in the leukaemic patient—with particular reference to leukaemic infiltration of the prostate—retrospective clinical study. Br J Urol 1973;45:179–83.

259. Fishman A. Taylor WN. Leukemic infiltration of the prostate. J Urol 1963;89:65–72.

260. Belis JA, Lizza EF, Kim JC, et al. Acute leukemic infil-tration of the prostate. Cancer 1983;51:2164–7.

261. Thalhammer F, Gisslinger H, Chott A, et al. Granulo-cytic sarcoma of the prostate as the first manifesta-tion of a late relapse of acute myelogenous leukemia. Ann Hematol 1994;68:97–9.

262. Frame R, Head D, Lee R, et al. Granulocytic sarcoma of the prostate. Cancer 1987;59:142–6.

263. Neiman RS, Barcos M, Berard C, et al. Granulocytic sarcoma: a clinicopathologic study of 61 biopsied cases. Cancer 1981;48:1426–37.

264. Givler RL. Involvement of the bladder in leukemia and lymphoma. J Urol 1971;105:667–70.

265. Bagg MD, Wettlaufer JN, Willadsen DS, et al. Granulocytic sarcoma presenting as a diffuse renal mass before hematological manifestations of acute myelogenous leukemia. J Urol 1994;152:2092–3.

266. Vukelja SJ, Simmson SJ, Knight RD, et al. Testicular relapse in adult acute lymphocytic leukemia: a case report and literature review. Med Pediatr Oncol 1989;17:170–3.

267. Shaffer DW, Burris HA, O'Rourke J. Testicular relapse in adult acute myelogenous leukemia. Cancer 1992;70:1541–4.

268. Ferry JA, Snigley JR, Young RH. Granulocytic sarcoma of the testis: a report of two cases of a neoplasm prone to misinterpretation. Mod Pathol 1997;10:320–5.

269. Pond HS. Priapism as the presenting complaint of myelogenous leukemia. South Med J 1969;62:465–7.

270. Nelson JH, Winter CC. Priapism: evolution of management in 48 patients in a 22-year series. J Urol 1977;117:455–8.

271. Veenhof CHN, Vander Meer J, Goudsmit R. Successfully treated priapism in acute myeloblastic leukemia complicating Hodgkin's disease. Acta Med Scand 1973;194:349–52.

272. Williams DL, Bell BA, Ragat AH. Clitorism at presentation of acute nonlymphocytic leukemia. J Pediatr 1985;107:754–5.

273. Thomas LB, Forkner CE, Frei E III, et al. The skeletal lesions of acute leukemia. Cancer 1963;14:608–21.

274. Taverna C, Vogt P, Pestalozzi BC. Uncommon sites of presentation of hematologic malignancies. Case 2: diffuse muscle infiltration by granulocytic sarcoma seven years after acute myelomonocytic leukemia. J Clin Oncol 1999;17:1642–3.

275. Chabner BA, Haskell CM, Canellos GP. Destructive bone lesions in chronic granulocytic leukemia. Medicine 1969;48:401–10.

276. Blot E, Miquel J, Heron F, et al. Sternum tumor revealing a chronic myeloid leukaemia. Br J Rheumatol 1998;37:1353–4.

277. Tricot G, Boogaerts MA, Broeckaert-Van Orshoven A, et al. Hypercalcemia and diffuse osteolytic lesions in the acute phase of chronic myelogenous leukemia. Cancer 1983;52:841–5.

278. Novick SL, Nicol TL, Fishman EK. Granulocytic sarcoma (chloroma) of the sacrum: initial manifestation of leukemia. Skeletal Radiol 1998;27:112–4.

279. Karnak I, Ciftci AO, Senocak ME, Gogus S. Granulocytic sarcoma of the scapula: an unusual presentation of acute myeloblastic leukemia. J Pediatr Surg 1997;32:121–2.

280. Herold CJ, Wittich GR, Schwarzinger I, et al. Skeletal involvement in hairy cell leukemia. Skeletal Radiol 1988;17:171–5.

281. Lembersky BC, Ratain MJ, Golomb HM. Skeletal complications in hairy cell leukemia: diagnosis and therapy. J Clin Oncol 1988;6:1280–4.

282. Tani A, Nakabeppu Y, Kobayashi M, et al. Numerous sites of increased uptake shown on bone scintigraphy in a case of adult T-cell leukemia. Ann Nucl Med 1997;11:321–3.

283. Jiya TU, Van Royen BJ, Sugihara S, et al. Lumbar intervertebral disc involvement in chronic lymphocytic leukemia. A case report. Spine 1998;23:1895–9.

284. Usalan C, Ozarslan E, Zengin N, et al. Acute lymphoblastic leukaemia presenting with arthritis in an adult patient. Postgrad Med J 1999;75:425–7.

10

Supportive Care

JANICE P. DUTCHER, MD

Supportive care in adult leukemias is a major component of the management of patients with these diseases. Supportive care includes the provision of cellular transfusions for thrombocytopenia, anemia or granulocytopenia, plasma or plasma fraction transfusions for certain blood protein deficiencies, and the management of infectious complications of the diseases and/or their treatments. In addition, removal of certain blood components by apheresis is occasionally necessary. In the acute leukemias, both myeloid (AML) and lymphoid (ALL), clinical problems at diagnosis are often based on the absence of normal cellular components of the blood, which results in bleeding or infection. In chronic myelocytic leukemia (CML), supportive care is less necessary until there is a transformation into the acute blastic phase; at that time, supportive care management is similar to that of the acute leukemias. In chronic lymphocytic leukemias (CLLs), the diseases demonstrate a slow process of proliferation of the abnormal clone, with concomitant loss of the normal lymphoid populations and therefore progressive immunosuppression, as well as usually less dramatic myelosuppression. Thus, infection management is the major component of support in these disorders. In myelodysplasia, which often transforms into acute leukemia, initial support may include hematopoietic growth factors, which may substitute for transfusion in the early phases.

TRANSFUSION SUPPORTIVE CARE

Platelet Transfusion Therapy

Platelet transfusion support is perhaps the most significant component of transfusion therapy in the management of acute leukemias and in patients undergoing bone marrow transplantation.[1] In addition to the marrow impairment caused by the disease process, all successful chemotherapeutic regimens for these diseases are intensely myelosuppressive and therefore initiate a prolonged period of thrombocytopenia until marrow recovery occurs. Platelet transfusion delays the onset and reduces the extent of bleeding in severely thrombocytopenic patients.[2-4] Platelet transfusion support during standard induction therapy in the acute leukemias may be required for anywhere from 2 to 6 weeks, and transfusions may be required every 2 to 3 days (Figure 10–1).[5]

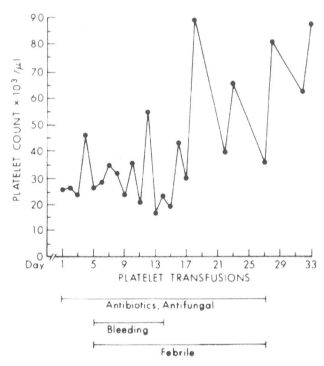

Figure 10–1. The increased frequency of platelet transfusions required during severe illness, with fever and neutropenia, is demonstrated. The frequency diminishes as the marrow and sepsis improves.

Guidelines

In general, for patients with acute leukemia undergoing induction therapy, prophylactic platelet transfusions are recommended to attempt to reduce the incidence of bleeding during this intensive treatment period.[6–13] It is well documented that many concurrent medical problems that arise during induction therapy add to the risk of bleeding and therefore warrant a prophylactic approach.[14,15] These include the mucositis and esophagitis that is induced by chemotherapy, concurrent infections (whether bacterial or yeast) (Figures 10–2 and 10–3), fever, occult infection, certain medications such as some antibiotics, and, occasionally, coagulopathy (Figure 10–4).[14–17] The current platelet count threshold that is used for transfusion in acutely ill patients undergoing active treatment is between 10,000 and 20,000/μL.[12,13,18] In other settings, such as chronic hematologic disorders, with chronically low platelet counts but without medical complications, platelet transfusion is usually only indicated if bleeding occurs. The blood bank community is concerned over excessive use of platelet transfusion for a number of reasons, including cost and exposure to multiple donors with the attendant increased risk of tranfusion-transmitted diseases. Therefore, knowledge and judgment regarding the clinical setting predisposing to bleeding should guide the use of prophylactic platelet transfusions.[1]

Once bleeding develops in a patient with leukemia and thrombocytopenia, frequent, even daily, platelet

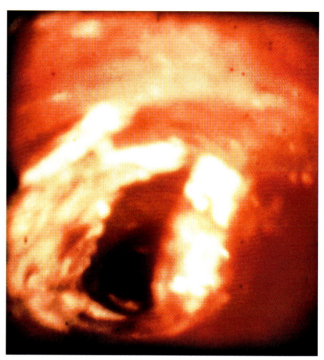

Figure 10–3.   *Candida* esophagitis.

transfusion therapy may be necessary to control bleeding. An attempt should be made to increase the platelet count to approximately 50,000/μL, which will often resolve hemorrhage due to mucositis or uterine bleeding. Prevention of uterine bleeding should be attempted prior to induction chemotherapy in premenopausal women with the prophylactic administration of progesterone, which should be continued until the platelet count normalizes when hematologic remission is attained. It is always much more difficult to stop bleeding than to prevent its occurrence. Should uterine bleeding commence despite the prophylactic administration of progesterone, then combination hormonal therapy with estrogen and progesterone should be administered.

Prophylactic platelet transfusions are also administered in advance of necessary invasive procedures required for management of patients with acute leukemia.[19,20] Examples are the surgical placement of central venous access devices, dental procedures, prior to lumbar puncture, or, rarely, surgical management of infections such as drainage of paranasal sinuses, extraction of infected teeth prior to chemotherapy, or emergency major surgery. Maintenance of the platelet count ≥ 50,000/μL before, during, and after such a procedure will generally prevent

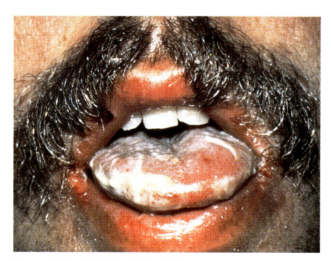

Figure 10–2.   Oral thrush (*Candida*).

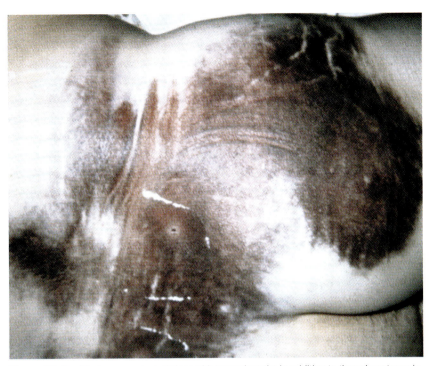

Figure 10–4. Ecchymoses in a patient with coagulopathy in addition to thrombocytopenia.

serious bleeding complications. Once healing has occurred, the platelet count threshold can be reduced to the usual range for prophylactic transfusion.

Evaluation of Response to Platelet Transfusion

Assessing the response to platelet transfusion is usually done by measuring the post-transfusion platelet count, in addition to observing the cessation of active bleeding. The post-transfusion platelet count increment reflects both the size of the patient (body surface area) and the number of platelets transfused. The corrected count increment (CCI), determined 10 to 60 minutes post-transfusion, is used to standardize results among patients and is calculated as the observed increment (count/µL) × body surface area (m²) divided by the number of platelets transfused × 10[11] (Figure 10–5).[21,22] A CCI of 10,000 to 20,000/µL is considered evidence of a successful transfusion. This measure can also provide an indication of the cause of platelet refractoriness (ie, rapid use of platelets owing to clinical causes versus alloimmunization, implying immune-mediated destruction).[17,21–23] With rapid use, there should still be an acceptable CCI at 1 hour, whereas with alloimmunization, there may be no increment as early as

10 minutes following transfusion and never at 1-hour post-transfusion.

Platelet Products

Platelet products for transfusion are currently obtained by two different procedures. The first is called pooled random donor platelets, in which the platelets that have been separated from single units of donated red blood cells are pooled into a transfusion pack that contains 6 to 8 units (each required to contain no less than 0.55 × 10[11] platelets) for adults.[24] These platelets are stored as individual units until requested for transfusion and then are pooled in the blood bank. The second method, apheresis, provides platelets from an individual donor who undergoes a procedure in which a machine mechanically separates platelets from his or her whole blood, during continuous centrifugation and flow, which sepa-

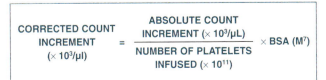

Figure 10–5. Calculation of corrected platelet count increment.

rates the blood into layers and allows collection of the desired layer and return to the donor of the platelet-poor blood (Figure 10–6).[25–27] Such a procedure can be done using dedicated donors identified for an individual patient, or through volunteer donors, who may undergo high-yield plateletpheresis, which may yield sufficient platelets for two transfusions. Analysis of apheresis products is continuing with respect to cost, efficacy, and donor factors.[28] Mechanical apheresis yields a leukodepleted product during the procedure, whereas pooled platelets must undergo bedside filtration if a leukodepleted product is required (Figure 10–7).[29–31]

The advantages of pooled platelets are the potentially greater availability and lower cost. The disadvantage is the exposure to a greater number of donors, one per unit of platelets. The advantages of apheresis platelets are the reduced donor exposure and the ease of leukodepletion. The disadvantages are the cost and longer donor time necessary.

Nevertheless, as platelet use has increased, more blood centers have emphasized apheresis donors since they can repeat their donations much more frequently (monthly, weekly, twice weekly) than if they had donated a unit of blood to provide a unit of random donor platelets (8 weeks).[32] Routine plateletpheresis donation by volunteer donors generally requires a 4-week interval between donations. With these techniques, there is never extreme platelet depletion of donors to reduce the donor platelet count below a safe limit. In fact, in the setting of directed donors, such as human leukocyte antigen (HLA)-matched donors, plateletpheresis can be performed as frequently as twice weekly as long as the donor platelet count is maintained at greater than 150,000/μL and there is medical approval for the donor's participation.[32] The goal of providing HLA-matched platelets is to use sufficient donors to alleviate donor stress and schedule each donor no more often than once per week.

Additionally, cancer centers with apheresis capability use the approach of prescreening dedicated donors for individual patients, who are then readily available when platelets are needed; thus, platelets may be administered as soon as the donation is completed. Repeat screening tests are drawn at the time of collection to maintain current screening data, but results are not required for release of the blood product if the prescreening is within 10 days of donation.[32] In contrast, all donor products from blood centers undergo screening at the time of collection; thus, the product cannot be released until screening results are available, which may require 48 hours. Once the product is released, it must be transported to the requesting hospital, where it is either stored or used. Thus, these transfusion products may be halfway through their shelf-life, prior to transfusion. Thus, the cancer center approach, with prescreened

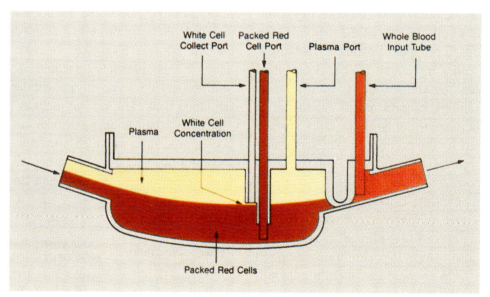

Figure 10–6. Plateletpheresis: diagram of the separation belt of the continuous-flow apheresis machine, with ports accessing each layer of blood cells.

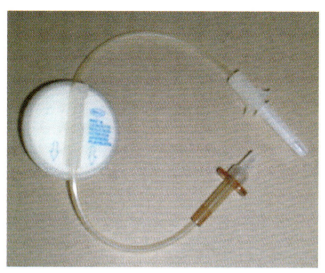

Figure 10–7. Bedside platelet filter to produce leukocyte-poor platelets.

donors providing fresh apheresis platelets, may reduce the numbers of platelets used because their in vivo survival may be greater.

Development of Refractoriness

As stated previously, the evaluation of outcome of platelet transfusion is by means of the post-transfusion count increment.[21,22] The factors that impact on successful transfusion response may be clinical, immunologic, or logistical. The clinical factors that reduce survival of platelet transfusions include fever, sepsis, splenomegaly, active bleeding or oozing from mucositis, coagulopathy, and medications.[14,17,23] A patient with some of these clinical complications may have a very low platelet count on a daily basis and thus require frequent transfusions but, in fact, may not have antibodies that destroy platelets. Such a patient may have a low daily platelet count, but an early CCI (10 minutes or even 1 hour post-transfusion) will demonstrate responsiveness. Logistical factors related to the platelet product that may reduce transfusion viability include storage time, as stated above. A more controversial issue related to transfusion outcome is the effect of ABO compatibility. Older studies demonstrated the adsorption of ABH antigens on the surface of platelets, but the impact on transfusion outcome was debated.[33,34] More recent studies have again suggested that ABO antigens can be adherent

to platelet membranes. In a paired study comparing ABO-compatible with ABO-mismatched random donor platelets, there was decreased platelet transfusion survival with the mismatched transfusions.[35] It appears that there is a different level of expression of ABH antigens in different normal donors, and this may explain the disparate results.[36] However, there are clearly situations where availability dictates the need for ABO-mismatched platelets, and these can be administered safely when absolutely necessary.

Alloimmunization

Finally, immunologic factors impact on the outcome of platelet transfusions. Following exposure to blood products, individuals can develop antibodies that lead to immune-mediated refractoriness to platelet transfusions, or alloimmunization. The majority of the antibodies impacting on platelet transfusion are directed against histocompatibility antigens (HLAs) present on lymphocytes, which are adsorbed onto the surface of platelets.[37,38] The genes for HLAs are present on chromosome 6 (Figure 10–8), and matching of HLA-A and HLA-B, serologic antigens, is used for providing HLA-matched platelet transfusions. Rarely are antibodies directed to platelet-specific antigens in the setting of multiple transfusions since these antigens are almost universally present on platelets. Alloimmunization can predate the development of transfusion needs in the setting of acute leukemia; for example, in women who have been pregnant, there is a greater

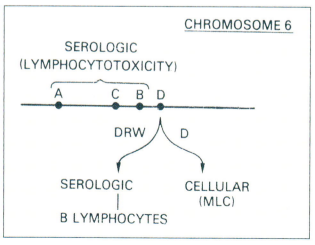

Figure 10–8. Chromosome 6: showing sites of genes for the human leukocyte antigens.

risk, owing to transplacental exposure to paternal antigens, as well as in patients who have had previous red blood cell transfusions. The presence of lymphocytotoxic antibodies against HLAs can be assayed but is rarely done in the setting of transfusion management owing to the expense and laborious nature of the methodology. Occasionally, blood centers will run a panel against high-frequency antigens, but this does not rule out alloimmunization to less common antigens.[39] Suspicion of alloimmunization can be inferred from the outcome of early post-transfusion platelet counts in that even the 10-minute post-transfusion CCI will not demonstrate an adequate increment if the cause of refractoriness is immunologically mediated.[21,22] Alloimmunization reflects a combination of the presence of alloantibodies and refractoriness to random donor transfusions.

Management of transfusion support for those who are alloimmunized uses the support of HLA-matched apheresis platelet donors. This requires the availability of a pool of HLA-typed donors who can be called on to donate in the case of allorefractory patients.[40,41] Usually, the match includes only HLA-A and HLA-B loci (see Figure 10–8), and varying degrees of match occur. Obviously, fully matched donors are preferred, but if only partial matches are available, then the least

degree of mismatch is used (Figure 10–9). It is very important to assess early post-transfusion CCI for all HLA-matched transfusions to assess which donors are actually providing a beneficial transfusion. A single key mismatch can totally obviate the benefit of an HLA-"matched" transfusion. There are cross-reactive HLA antigens that, even when mismatched, do not impact on transfusion outcome; in particular, HLA-B12, HLA-B44, and HLA-B45 are considered to be interchangeable for the purpose of platelet transfusion (see Figure 10–9).[42–44]

In addition to HLA typing for defining potential donors for alloimmunized patients, another technique is platelet crossmatching, although this is not widely available. Moroff and colleagues have used this approach and have demonstrated the ability to define compatible donors, comparable to that of HLA typing.[45]

Attempts have been made to reverse alloimmunization-induced refractoriness, in particular through the use of gamma-globulin infusions, administered immediately prior to platelet transfusion, to block the reticuloendothelial system of the spleen. This has been largely unsuccessful in alloimmunization, despite its success in autoimmune thrombocytopenia.[46–48] However, Kickler and colleagues have demonstrated

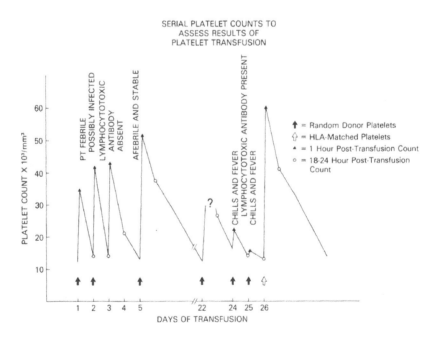

Figure 10–9. Response to human leukocyte antigen-matched platelets with donors who are good and poor matches, as demonstrated by the corrected count increments.

partial success when this approach was used in patients who had become refractory to previously useful HLA-matched donors. In about half of the cases, response was regained with the use of pre-infusion of gamma globulin.[49]

Alloimmunization is not universal in patients undergoing treatment for acute leukemia, despite frequent exposure to blood products containing antigenic stimuli. This has been hypothesized to be due to a somewhat suppressed state of immunity associated with leukemia. However, a phenomenon is noted among recipients of multiple red blood cell transfusions in which not all exposed individuals develop antibodies to blood products. Therefore, this variable development of alloimmunization to platelets may be more patient specific rather than disease specific. In two large studies, the incidence of alloimmunization was evaluated, one in patients with leukemia[50] and one in patients with other malignant diseases.[51] The rate of alloimmunization was approximately 30 percent in each, which is somewhat less than in the general population exposed to red cell antigens, perhaps arguing for a component of immune suppression from the disease or its treatment.

Of interest in both studies was the finding that there was no dose-response relationship between the number of platelet transfusions (all pooled random donor transfusions) administered and the risk of alloimmunization, even among those who had previously been exposed by transfusion or pregnancy (Figure 10–10).[50,51] This is in the context of a baseline requirement for therapeutic platelet transfusion; thus, there was no lowest number that would prevent alloimmunization.[50,51] Of interest also was that there were a substantial number of patients who received a large number of platelets and yet never became alloimmunized.[50,51] Additionally, a small number of immunosuppressed patients have been observed to "lose" their lymphocytotoxic antibodies during subsequent treatment cycles and to resume responsiveness to random donor platelets later (Table 10–1).[50,52,53] Nevertheless, alloimmunization remains a significant supportive care problem in the management of transfusions during treatment of acute leukemia.

Therefore, recent platelet transfusion research has focused on new methods to prevent the development of alloimmunization. Several approaches have focused on the lymphocytes that are often a component of the platelet product and that provide antigens for HLA alloimmunization. Lymphocytes carry both class II and class I HLA antigens and thus can evoke an alloresponse. Studies of lymphocyte-depleted transfusion products suggest that this approach can reduce the frequency of alloimmunization. The recently published Trial to Reduce Alloimmunization to Platelets (TRAP) showed that a number of methods are successful in this regard.[54] Lymphocytes can be removed by filtration, usually at the bedside, using

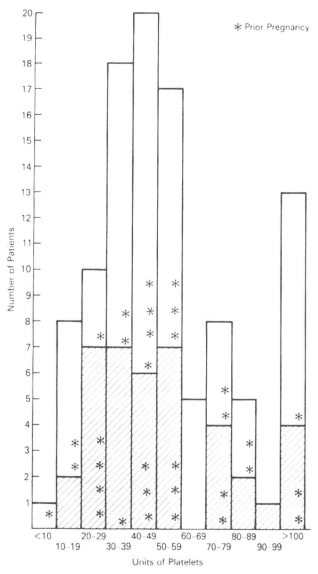

Figure 10–10. A graph demonstrating the number of platelets administered during induction treatment for acute myeloid leukemia. Those patients hatchmarked became alloimmunized during induction therapy. There is no dose-response relationship between the number of platelets given and the development of alloimmunization. Those with asterisks have been previously pregnant.

Table 10–1. LOSS OF ALLOIMMUNIZATION IN AML PATIENTS ALLOIMMUNIZED AND REQUIRING HLA-MATCHED PLATELETS DURING INDUCTION THERAPY

Study	Number Alloimmunized in 1st and 2nd Courses
Dutcher et al.[50]	Induction therapy: 48 patients alloimmunized; all required HLA-matched platelets Maintenance/consolidation therapy: 8 (17%) no longer alloimmunized responsive to random donor platelets
Murphy et al.[53]	Induction therapy: 37 patients alloimmunized; all required HLA-matched platelets Second course of treatment: 16 (43%) no longer required HLA-matched transfusions

prepackaged, polyester, leukoadherent filters, and this provides sufficient leukoreduction (reduction of greater than three logs to $< 10^7$ leukocytes) to reduce alloimmunization (see Figure 10–7).[29,30,55–59] This approach can be used for platelet transfusions provided by pooling individual platelet units. Additionally, the current apheresis protocols using modern equipment (COBE Spectra [Turbo], Lakewood, CO; Fresenius, Redmond, WA; Baxter-Fenwal, Deerfield, IL) provide sufficient leukodepletion (also reduction of greater than three logs to $< 10^7$ leukocytes) to prevent alloimmunization (Figure 10–11).[60] Finally, the third approach used in the TRAP study was to administer ultraviolet B irradiation to the lymphocytes in the platelet product and thus inactivate them and render them incapable of generating an alloresponse.[54,61–63] All of these approaches were found to be equally efficacious in the TRAP study, and all significantly reduced the incidence of alloimmunization.[54] In this study, the development of lymphocytotoxic antibodies occurred in 45 percent of the control patients who received random donor platelets and in 17 to 21 percent of the other treatment groups. Similarly, alloimmunization, in addition to refractoriness to random donor platelets, occurred in 13 percent of the controls and in 3 to 4 percent of the patients who received processed platelets.[54] The rate of refractoriness associated with the presence of lymphocytotoxic antibodies in the control group was considerably lower than that observed in previously published reports.[54]

The other apparent benefit achieved by providing leukodepleted blood products in the setting of acute leukemia and marrow transplantation is the reduction in the risk of transmission of cytomegalovirus (CMV).[59,64–68] Several studies demonstrated the effectiveness of this approach, which is especially helpful if CMV-negative donors are not available.

Platelet Transfusion Reactions and Complications

Reactions to platelet transfusions occur, with an incidence of 5 to 30 percent of transfusions, usually during or shortly after the transfusion is administered. The most common type of reaction is a febrile, non-hemolytic reaction thought to be due to leukocyte antibodies reacting to leukocytes in the product. With the current widespread use of leukocyte-depleted products, this type of reaction is becoming less common. However, stored platelets, if not prefiltered, may contain residual cytokines that have been released during the storage process. These, too, can cause febrile reactions[69–71] that are obviously not pre-

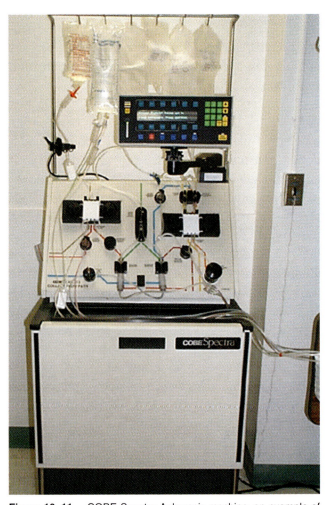

Figure 10–11. COBE Spectra Apheresis machine: an example of a continuous-flow machine.

vented by pretransfusion bedside filtration. Additionally, allergic reactions may occur with platelet transfusions and are thought to be related to substances in the plasma of the product. These often present with urticaria, which can be quite extensive. In one study, however, the presence of elevated levels of interleukin-6 in the platelet product was associated with what appeared to be an allergic reaction.[70] Thus, urticarial reactions may result from multiple causes.

Leukocytes in blood products are also associated with the development of graft-versus-host disease (GVHD) when administered to severely immunocompromised hosts, such as in patients undergoing stem cell transplantation who have been pretreated with intensive chemotherapy. This is a syndrome in which the immunocompetent lymphocytes in the transfusion product attack the organs and tissues of the immunocompromised recipient. The clinical syndrome can be quite severe, and in the stem cell transplantation setting it is mediated by lymphocytes in the stem cell graft itself. In this setting, all blood products undergo gamma irradiation prior to transfusion to inactivate the immune cells in the product and to reduce a contribution from transfusions to the anticipated stem cell–induced graft-versus-host syndrome. Transfusion-associated GVHD is a rare phenomenon in nontransplant recipients. However, transfusion-associated GVHD has been observed in transfusions of fresh whole blood from haplotype-identical donors to immunocompetent recipients,[72–75] and this has created a concern regarding directed family donations. The latter is a common practice in the management of transfusion support of patients with acute leukemia, for example. Thus, donations of red cells or platelets from family members are irradiated prior to transfusion as a precaution. In view of the leukodepletion that is accomplished by modern apheresis systems and the results of the TRAP study, which demonstrated sufficient leukodepletion to reduce alloimmunization,[54,76] it is possible that there are insufficient lymphocytes in apheresis products to engender transfusion-associated GVHD in routine supportive care. However, it is the current policy to irradiate blood products from family members provided specifically for a given patient.

Another potential complication of platelet transfusion is the risk of infection. Platelets obtained from single units of blood are often stored from 2 to 4 days after they are drawn, prior to pooling for transfusion. This storage is at room temperature. Thus, if there had been initial bacterial contamination during the drawing of the unit, there is the opportunity for proliferation of organisms during the storage process. This has been observed, but it is uncommon. [77]

In summary, platelet transfusions are a major and extremely important component of the supportive care of patients with acute leukemia undergoing intensive treatment. The product is generally safe and effective, and with the current expertise available in HLA matching, even refractory patients can be supported for the time necessary to achieve remission. It is rare now to have a hemorrhagic death in a patient with acute leukemia, whereas this was commonplace prior to the advent of apheresis-derived and matched donor platelets. Platelet transfusions have been life-saving to innumerable patients who are currently alive and perhaps cured of their leukemia. They are well worth the effort and expense.

Platelet Cryopreservation

Cryopreservation of autologous platelets for future use in patients who are likely to undergo subsequent treatment is an available but underused technology (Figure 10–12).[78–80] Although the technique is labor intensive and requires several sessions of apheresis on the part of the patient to collect sufficient platelets to support another course of chemotherapy, this technology has been particularly useful in alloimmunized patients who require HLA-matched platelets. Autologous platelet collection and cryopreservation allow these patients to serve as their own matched donor. Cryopreservation methods require the use of the cryopreservative dimethyl sulfoxide,[81,82] and processing is similar to that used for stem cell preservation. Autologous plasma for reinfusion must also be stored. Recoveries after thawing are between 50 and 70 percent of the equivalent fresh platelets, and efficacy is documented in clinical reports.[78,79,83] Alloimmunized patients have been maintained solely with their own cryopreserved platelets throughout courses of postremission treatment (Figure 10–13).[78,79,83]

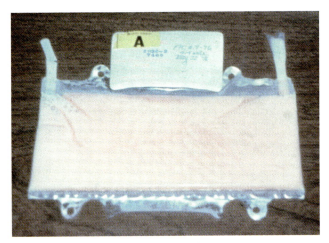

Figure 10–12. Autologous frozen platelets.

Disseminated Intravascular Coagulation

One specific subtype of acute leukemia, promyelocytic leukemia, is associated with the development of a coagulopathy characterized as disseminated intravascular coagulation (DIC). The clinical features of this leukemia include hypergranulated blast cells whose granules contain procoagulants (Figure 10–14). The release of these substances occurs as the disease develops and can be exacerbated by cytotoxic chemotherapy. Additionally, the patients usually manifest thrombocytopenia, prolongation of the prothrombin time, activated partial thromboplastin time, and thrombin time. There is also an increase in fibrin degradation products and hypofibrinogenemia.[84–86] However, controversy remains as to whether the primary process is thrombosis or fibrinolysis, and the malignant promyelocyte could trigger either or both processes. Patients often present with hemorrhage, from probable sites like the gums, uterus, and gastrointestinal tract, or even with an acute intracranial hemorrhage. Ecchymotic bleeding is commonplace when there is a coagulopathy associated with thrombocytopenia (Figure 10–15).

The management of the coagulopathy is with maximal supportive care. Heparin has been recommended as a strategy to inhibit the coagulation cascade and has been successful in several studies.[85,87] This is a low-dose regimen of 250 U/kg per 24 hours and can be adjusted to maintain the fibrinogen level at above 100 mg/dL. As the leukemia resolves, control of the coagulopathy improves. Additional support with platelet transfusions and fresh frozen plasma, containing clotting factors, is also often necessary but, of course, fuels the consumption.[85,87–89] Platelet transfusion is given to maintain a count greater than 20,000/µL in patients who are not bleeding and at 50,000/µL in patients who are bleeding. Fresh frozen plasma is administered to patients with significant prolongation of clotting parameters if there is also bleeding.

Recently, the use of all-*trans* retinoic acid (ATRA) as an antileukemic agent in promyelocytic leukemia appears to improve the coagulopathy long before the leukemia is completely controlled. In the largest study, from France using ATRA, the coagulopathy resolved in 4 ± 3 days compared with 7 ± 4

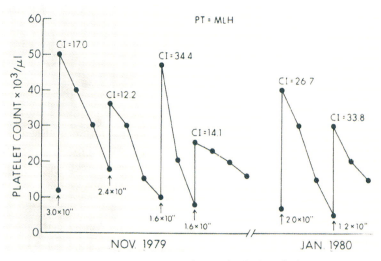

Figure 10–13. Example of response to frozen platelet transfusions.

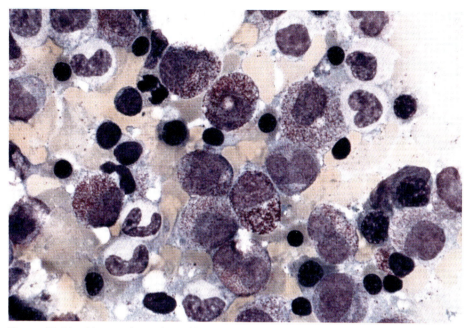

Figure 10–14. Marrow of a patient with acute promyelocytic leukemia, demonstrating the hyper-granulated blasts that contain the procoagulant that triggers disseminated intravascular coagulation.

days among a group of 47 patients treated with chemotherapy alone.[90] This is being studied further in ongoing clinical trials.

Red Blood Cell Transfusions

Patients with hematologic malignancies have reduced marrow capacity for the production of normal blood cells due to their disease and its treatment. Patients with acute leukemia usually require a minimum of 4 weeks of intensive supportive care, which includes the frequent transfusion of red blood cells, often two to three times per week. These patients often have mild or even moderate bleeding episodes from gastrointestinal mucositis, vaginal bleeding, and other sites and thus have both decreased production and blood loss. Patients with CLL may develop severe anemia as a late manifestation of the disease but rarely require red cell transfusions during the early course of the disease. However, hemolytic anemia is a rare immune manifestation of this disease that may occur at any time in its course and may evoke a crisis, the treatment of which is treating the CLL. Initially, this usually requires corticosteroids. Patients with myelodysplasia may present with anemia, which may require transfusions of red blood cells or, in some cases, may be supported

by injections of recombinant erythropoietin. Patients with CML rarely demonstrate anemia in the chronic phase of their disease, but as they progress to the acute phase of the disease, anemia becomes a component of the process, similar to acute leukemia.

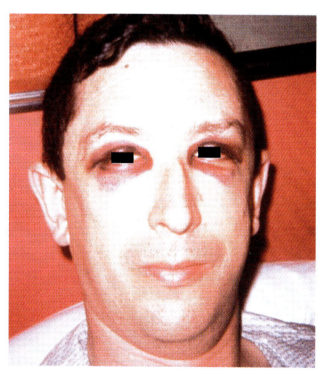

Figure 10–15. Example of ecchymotic bleeding associated with acute promyelocytic leukemia.

Red Cell Products

The usual red blood cell products are red cell concentrates prepared from one unit of donor whole blood, following removal of most of the plasma.[32] In transfusion to patients with hematologic malignancies or during stem cell transplantation, leukocyte-depleted products are usually used to reduce alloimmunization and the risk of infection from CMV. Leukocyte-depleted red blood cells are also indicated for patients who have a history of febrile, nonhemolytic transfusion reactions. Leukodepletion of red cells is achieved by use of filters, either through processing of units at the blood center or using prepackaged, polyester, leukoadherent filters at the bedside (Figure 10–16). Several such filters have been fully evaluated and are readily available.[91–93]

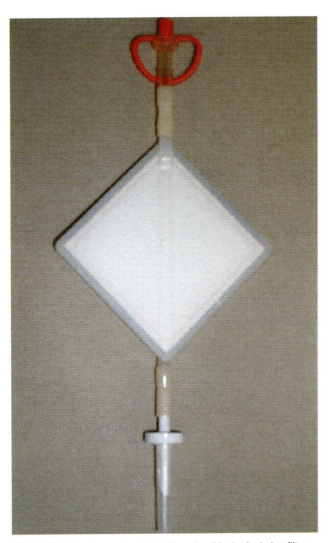

Figure 10–16.   Example of bedside red cell leukodepletion filter.

Gamma-irradiated red blood cells are used to prevent transfusion-associated GVHD, and all cellular products given to patients undergoing stem cell transplantation are irradiated. In addition, gamma irradiation of all cellular products is recommended for other severely immunocompromised patients (ie, severely immunocompromised cancer patients and patients who receive transfusions from relatives).[94,95] Known cases of transfusion-associated GVHD, emanating from the transfusion itself to nonimmunocompromised recipients, have occurred in cases where whole blood was donated by a haplotype-identical relative and administered fresh.[72–75] Such transfusions may induce a fulminant graft-versus-host syndrome that may be fatal.[74] In general, in the setting of support of hematologic malignancy patients, it is highly exceptional to administer fresh whole blood, and, in fact, rarely, if ever, are red blood cells given that are from related donors. Related donors are used for platelets, as discussed above, and irradiation of any product from a relative is recommended.[94,95]

The hematocrit at which red blood cells are administered varies with the clinical situation. Whereas many patients with chronic anemia may do very well with a chronically low hemoglobin level, in patients with other medical problems, particularly cardiac, maintenance of a higher hemoglobin may be indicated. The current recommendation for the perioperative hemoglobin threshold in patients not critically ill is 8 g/dL,[96] after a study showed no adverse effect on short- or long-term survival based on hemoglobin level. However, patients who are seriously ill should be maintained at a higher level, closer to 10 g/dL. Patients with acute leukemia undergoing induction therapy may also be chronically bleeding and therefore may need a higher transfusion threshold hemoglobin to avoid a catastrophic fall in hemoglobin from exacerbated bleeding. Thus, the clinical setting will dictate the transfusion threshold. It is also apparent that red cell transfusions are given more frequently in the setting of acute leukemia than even standards suggest for patients with nonproducing marrows.[97,98] This may be related to chronic bleeding and to the use of red cells with longer storage times prior to transfusion.

Patients with CLL develop progressive marrow infiltration, which usually will manifest as anemia.

These patients may also develop autoimmune hemolytic anemia as a component of their disease or its treatment. Between 10 and 20 percent of patients with this disease develop red cell autoantibodies during the course of their disease.[99] Fludarabine, used to treat CLL, has also been associated with the development of severe autoimmune hemolytic anemia.[100] This may reflect further disruption of T-cell function and subsets, leading to autoimmune manifestations. Clinical signs of hemolysis include the sudden onset of severe anemia, jaundice, and elevated lactate dehydrogenase and bilirubin. Laboratory evaluation will reveal red cell antibodies by the direct antiglobulin test. The indirect antiglobulin test may reveal a panagglutinin as well.

Erythropoietin, mentioned earlier, is a hormone that stimulates red cell production under normal circumstances. Its effectiveness in patients with primary marrow dysfunction is limited. It is not generally used in the treatment of acute leukemia because of lack of effect. However, there are patients with myelodysplasia who do respond to erythropoietin and become transfusion independent with its use.[101,102] It may also have a beneficial effect in some patients with CLL.

Red cell transfusions in patients with CML are rarely necessary in the chronic phase of the disease. Anemia may become a manifestation of the transition from chronic to acute leukemia, and then the transfusion approach is similar to that used in managing acute leukemia. The transformation phase of the disease, with increasing splenomegaly, may produce anemia as an initial indication of the onset of blast crisis.

Transfusion Reactions

The most common type of reaction to red blood cell transfusions is a febrile, nonhemolytic reaction, leading to fever during or at completion of the transfusion. Such reactions are believed to be related to leukoagglutinins (antibodies against donor leukocytes).[103–105] In patients undergoing treatment of acute leukemia, the majority of the products administered are leukodepleted, which minimizes the risk of leukoagglutinin reactions. Febrile reactions in the setting of leukodepleted products are believed to be due to cytokines remaining in the product during storage.[69] Allergic reactions can occur, primarily due to recipient reaction to protein factors in the plasma, and this is usually mild and manifested as urticaria. Severe allergic reactions are rare, but if bronchospasm or hypotension develops, emergency intervention is required with epinephrine and steroids. The best documented cause of such a reaction is in immunoglobulin (Ig)A-deficient recipients, who react to IgA in the transfused plasma. Such patients, when identified, require donors who are IgA deficient or washed red blood cells.[94]

The most serious type of reaction to red blood cells is an acute hemolytic reaction, which reflects antigen-antibody interaction. Fortunately, these are rare but occur with transfusion of ABO-incompatible blood and may be fatal. Clinical symptoms are fever, chills, nausea, and lower back pain. There can be severe hypotension and free hemoglobin in the urine and scrum. Supportive care requires aggressive hydration, diuretics to protect renal function, and blood pressure support as needed (Table 10–2). Disseminated intravascular coagulation can develop, and abnormal clotting parameters may be the first indication of such a transfusion reaction.[94,106] In at least 50 percent of such reactions, the cause is not in the typing laboratory but an error in administering the wrong unit to the patient.[107,108]

It is rare for bacteria to grow during the storage of red blood cells. However, there are reports of bacterial contamination in red cells stored at 4°C by organisms who live well at this temperature and whose growth is enhanced by the presence of iron, in particular, *Yersinia enterocolitica*.[94,106,109]

Transfusion-Transmitted Diseases

Any cellular blood product may transmit organisms that are harbored in the plasma or in the cells or

Table 10–2. HEMOLYTIC TRANSFUSION REACTION	
Features	**Components**
Clinical	Fever, chills, nausea, low back pain, hypotension
Laboratory	Free hemoglobin in serum and urine, elevated lactate dehydrogenase, renal insufficiency, abnormal clotting factors, elevated complement, release of bradykinin and catecholamines
Treatment	Hydration, diuretics, vasopressors, dialysis

through serologic viremias or bacteremias. In particular, viruses have caused concern because they are difficult to detect and because of the latency of the infection and the manifestations of the disease (Table 10–3). Of greatest concern is human immunodeficiency virus (HIV). To decrease the risk of transfusion-transmitted HIV disease, donor screening currently involves a detailed history, the ability to self-defer, and multiple antibody screening tests, including by enzyme-linked immunosorbent assay and Western blot, and testing for the p24 antigen of the virus. This multiplicity of testing provides a strong basis for safety of blood products. In the screening of more than 6 million donations, only 2 positive blood donors were identified (both were negative for antibodies to HIV but were positive for the p24 antigen).[110]

In addition, transmission of hepatitis B and C is strongly associated with blood product administration. Other hepatitis viruses (A and G) are less of a risk. In the 1970s, reduced use of paid blood donors and the development of better screening tests for hepatitis B surface antigen led to a reduction in transfusion-transmitted hepatitis B.[111] However, non-A and non-B hepatitis were still of concern. In fact, the careful assessment of HIV-related risk factors among donors led also to a reduction in transfusion-associated non-A and non-B hepatitis, along with the use of other surrogate markers such as elevated liver function tests to defer donors.[112] Now, hepatitis C has been identified as the major component of non-A and non-B hepatitis, and testing for antibodies to hepatitis C is accurate, providing another serologic test for donor deferral. Thus, the current risk of transfusion-associated transmission of hepatitis C is

greatly reduced.[113] The importance of this infection is its chronicity from transfusions administered 10 or more years ago, leading to chronic liver disease, cirrhosis, and hepatocellular carcinoma.

Cytomegalovirus remains latent in tissues and is believed to be sequestered in white blood cells. Cytomegalovirus causes clinical disease in severely immunocompromised patients and is of particular concern in patients undergoing stem cell transplantation. Cytomegalovirus pneumonia accounts for as much as 40 percent of post-transplant pneumonitis and is frequently fatal. The clinical manifestations may reflect a primary new infection, which is the most severe situation, or reactivation of the virus that the recipient carries. Patients undergoing stem cell transplantation or treatment for acute leukemia who carry no antibody for CMV should receive CMV-negative blood products. Leukodepletion of blood products has become an alternative when CMV-negative products are not available and appear to be sufficiently leukodepleted to prevent primary infection.[64–68]

Other viruses associated with transfusion are human T-cell leukemia virus types I and II (HTLV-I and II), and testing is routinely done for these organisms. Epstein-Barr virus is another leukocyte-associated virus that can be transmitted, and testing for this has recently been added to the required donor profile.[106]

The risk of transfusion-transmitted diseases is another argument for single donor platelets and for a reduced hemoglobin transfusion threshold. The frequency of current screening procedures detecting HIV ranges from 1 in 200,000 to 1 in 2,000,000 U,[103] whereas the frequency of hepatitis B ranges from 1 in 30,000 to 1 in 250,000 U, and the frequency of hepatitis C ranges from 1 in 30,000 to 1 in 150,000 U.[113]

Blood components remain an important and necessary component of support for patients with hematologic malignancies. Safety remains the greatest transfusion concern and is the greatest area of research in transfusion medicine.[106,114]

Granulocyte Transfusion

The potential value of granulocyte transfusion therapy in infection control in neutropenic patients has been recognized for more than 50 years.[115,116] Initial

Table 10–3. TRANSFUSION-TRANSMITTED VIRUSES AND FREQUENCY[106]

Virus	Estimated Frequency (per unit)
Human immunodeficiency virus	1/200,000–1/2,000,000
Hepatitis B	1/30,000–1/250,000
Hepatitis C	1/30,000–1/150,000
Hepatitis A	1/1,000,000
Human T-cell leukemia virus types I and II	1/250,000–1/2,000,000
Parvovirus B19	1/10,000

Adapted from Goodnough et al.[106]

studies took advantage of the high white blood cell counts of patients with CML, and transfusions from such patients to neutropenic, septic patients both increased the circulating white blood cell count and also were demonstrated to migrate to sites of infection.[117,118] Clinical outcome was also improved with resolution of infections.[117–120] A dose of 1 to 4×10^{10} CML granulocytes led to reduction of fever, and higher doses led to circulating granulocytes and resolution of infections.[121,122] A persistence of granulocytes in the circulation and the observation of earlier circulating precursors were also noted, providing a progressive maturation of infection-fighting cells from the single transfusion (Figure 10–17).[119]

However, the lack of availability of such donors made this source of granulocytes impractical, and with the development of apheresis technology in the 1970s, attempts were made to use normal donors for granulocyte transfusions. In the 1970s, there were a number of randomized trials to evaluate granulocyte transfusions in severely ill, neutropenic patients,[123–130] several of which supported the use of granulocytes in conjunction with antibiotic therapy in patients with documented infection.[124,128] Additionally, granulocytes appeared to be beneficial in those patients who had prolonged granulocytopenia and conferred a survival advantage to them.[125,129] Therefore, the overall recommendations for granulocyte transfusions have been for patients with documented bacterial or fungal

infections who fail broad-spectrum antibiotics and whose marrow recovery is not imminent. The major concern of granulocyte transfusions from normal donors, despite premedication with corticosteroids, has been the relatively small yield of cells available for transfusion. As stated above, the dose of transfused cells was directly related to the success of the transfusions in eradicating fever and infection.

Over the past 20 years, improved, more potent broad-spectrum antibiotics, the earlier empiric use of antibiotics in febrile, neutropenic patients, and the use of hematopoietic growth factors to hasten marrow recovery have markedly reduced the use of granulocyte transfusions. All of these measures appear to shorten the duration of febrile neutropenia. Nevertheless, infection remains the major cause of death among leukemia and marrow transplantation patients, and more effective means of managing infection are needed.

The indications for granulocyte transfusions include treatment of both gram-negative and gram-positive sepsis in neutropenic patients who do not appear to be responding to appropriate antibiotics (Table 10–4 and Figure 10–18). Animal studies initially documented the effectiveness of granulocytes in experimental gram-negative bacterial sepsis.[131–133] The major source of uncontrolled infection is fungal infection, which is particularly resistant to antibiotic therapy without the added benefit of granulocytes.

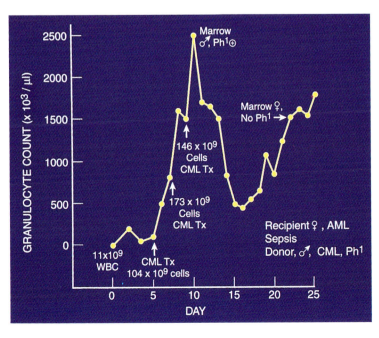

Figure 10–17. Response of a septic neutropenic female patient with acute myeloid leukemia (AML) to multiple granulocyte transfusions from a male patient with chronic myelocytic leukemia (CML). The elevated white blood cell count with CML granulocytes corrected the infection. As the patient with AML approached remission, the CML granulocytes disappeared.

Granulocyte recovery remains critical to survival from fungal infections. Animal data demonstrated the benefit of granulocyte transfusions in dogs infected with *Candida albicans*.[134,135] Fungal infection continues to be an indication for granulocyte transfusion if the patient is not responding to appropriate antibiotics and in the setting of marrow aplasia (Figures 10–2, 10–3, 10–19, 10–20, 10–21).[136]

Recently, attempts to enhance granulocyte donation yield have capitalized on the development of recombinant hematopoietic growth factors. Several studies have now been reported in which donors are premedicated with the combination of corticosteroids and granulocyte colony-stimulating factor (G-CSF), producing a markedly enhanced yield of granulocytes, in the range of 4 to 8×10^{10} cells per transfusion.[137–141] This higher yield results in elevations of peripheral granulocyte counts and appears to be beneficial in eradicating fungal infections.[142–144]

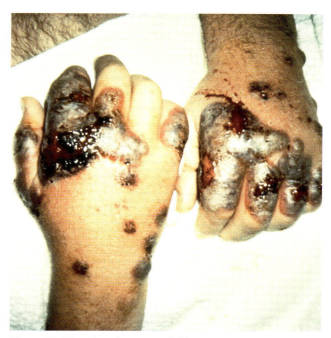

Figure 10–18. *Pseudomonas* cellulitis.

Evaluation of Granulocyte Transfusions

Evaluation of effectiveness, in the usual sense in transfusion therapy, has been difficult because there usually is very little count increment, if any, after granulocyte transfusions. Early studies used indium-111 labeling to evaluate granulocyte migration and demonstrated rapid accumulation of labelled granulocytes at the site of infection[145] (Figure 10–22). Rapid localization of transfused granulocytes to the infectious site may be one reason that circulating granulocyte count increments are difficult to obtain. However, in comparing studies with large doses of CML-derived cells with those using normal donors,[118,119] there is clearly a dose effect, and it is expected that larger doses of granulocytes currently available with donor stimulation will yield better clinical results. With the use of growth factor premedica-

tion of donors and the subsequent larger granulocyte yields, white blood cell count increments in the recipient are now frequently noted.[137,139,140] Thus, an effective course of daily granulocyte transfusions for a minimum of 4 and as many as 7 to 10 days should produce a sustained elevation of granulocytes in the recipient's peripheral blood. The ultimate sign of effectiveness, of course, is eradication of the infection, and this is being re-investigated in current clinical trials.[136,143,144]

Finally, a practical tool in assessing the localization of granulocytes that have circulated in the blood

Table 10–4. CRITERIA FOR EARLY GRANULOCYTE TRANSFUSION

In the setting of expected prolonged granulocytopenia,
  Progressive infection on presumed correct antibiotics
  Antibiotic-resistant organisms
  Fungal infection
  Infection in life-threatening site
  Pneumonia
  Elderly, debilitated patients

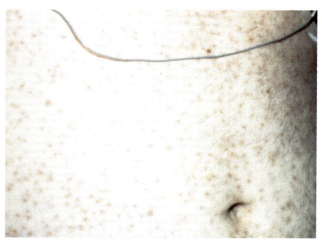

Figure 10–19. *Candida* septicemia with cutaneous lesions.

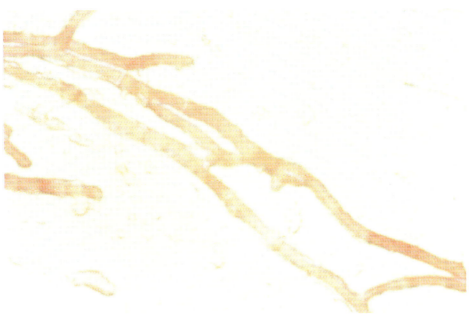

Figure 10–20. *Aspergilllus* hyphae in a pulmonary biopsy specimen.

that is returning to favor is the measurement of oral cavity granulocytes.[115,144,146] The number of granulocytes in the oral cavity is proportional to the number circulating in the peripheral blood. Therefore, following a transfusion, quantification of oral granulocytes suggests the effectiveness of transfused cells to migrate to a source of inflammation and thus potentially to the site of infection.[115,144,146]

Granulocyte Collection

Granulocytes are almost exclusively collected by apheresis techniques and have been for the past 20 years, with continued technologic improvements.[147,148] Hydroxyethyl starch is used in the procedure to help separate granulocytes from red blood cells that have similar density.[149] However, yield is

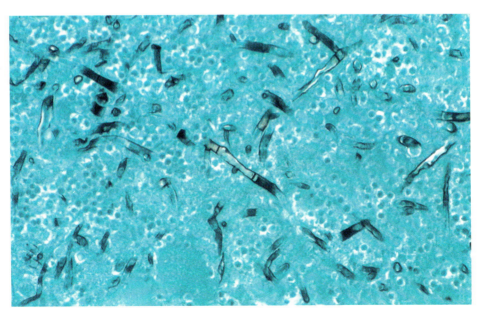

Figure 10–21. Silver stain of lung tissue demonstrating the hyphae of *Aspergillus* infection (original magnification ×50).

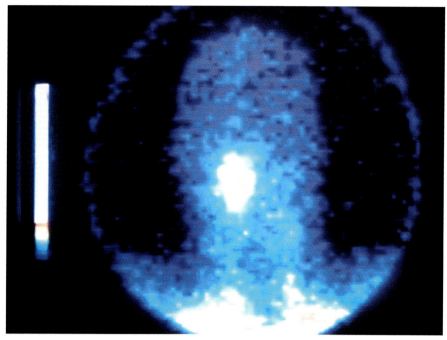

Figure 10–22. Rapid (30-minute) localization of granulocytes to the site of infection. A 30-minute indium-111–labeled granulocyte scan shows uptake in the sinus of a patient with sinusitis. Yellow/red reflects intensive radioactive tracer uptake.

directly dependent on donor premedication to enhance circulating granulocyte count. The initial approach to this has been with corticosteroids, which induce demargination of granulocytes into the peripheral bloodstream.[150,151] However, it is now apparent that the optimum premedication technique, in terms of numbers of granulocytes obtained, involves both corticosteroids and hematopoietic growth factors (Table 10–5).[115,137–144,152,153] Although most major cancer centers have their own apheresis facility to provide such specialized transfusion products and rely heavily on family donors, Price and colleagues have demonstrated that this can be done with the use of community donors, who accept the need for premedication and tolerate it very well.[144] Donor issues include the need to medicate normal volunteers with medications that are known to produce reactions in a small percentage of individuals, and this is not without concern in the blood banking community. Nevertheless, the incidence of reactions is less than 5 percent. Donors dedicated to a specific patient may undergo granulocyte collection on multiple occasions and

Table 10–5. PREMEDICATION SCHEMA FOR GRANULOCYTE DONORS	
Example	**Premedication Regimans**
Original regimen[150]	Dexamethasone, 8 mg orally, night before Dexamethasone, 10 mg IV day of collection Yield: $5–15 \times 10^9$
New approaches[115,144,152,153]	G-CSF 3–6 mg/kg/d subcutaneous injection starting 24 hours prior to collection and continuing for 9–14 d, during granulocyte collection Yield: 41.6×10^9/d
	G-CSF 300 µg/kg as a single dose, 12–16 hours before starting collection Yield: 44×10^9, processing 5–7 L of blood
	Dexamethasone, 8 mg orally, and G-CSF, single dose, 600 µg subcutaneously, both 16 hours before collection Yield: $81.9 \pm 2.3 \times 10^9$
	G-CSF 2, 5, 7.5, or 10 µg/kg subcutaneously, daily × 5 days, starting collection on day 2 Yield: $20–60 \times 10^9$, depending on dose

therefore may receive multiple doses of G-CSF. These donors are more likely to develop marrow expansion side effects, such as bone pain. Multiple dosing can produce sustained granulocyte elevations, and several daily collections of granulocytes can be obtained with outstanding yields (greater than 4×10^{10}).[152] To date, there is no evidence of adverse effects from serial granulocyte collections from the same donor. Nonspecific volunteer donors can still provide a substantial yield after premedication with steroids and growth factor, usually given 12 hours prior to donation.

Several laboratories have tested the function of granulocytes produced using donor premedication, and these cells demonstrate normal chemotaxis and phagocytosis and perhaps enhanced enzymatic activity, such as chemiluminescence and superoxide formation.[138,142,153,154] Other studies have demonstrated that cytotoxicity and production of hydrogen peroxide for bacterial killing are functioning normally in these collected cells.[154–156] Recipients also receive additional hematopoietic growth factor to sustain the transfused cells and to stimulate their own marrow recovery, and this may enhance the function of transfused granulocytes as well.

Granulocyte Storage

Granulocytes should be transfused as soon as they are collected because storage causes rapid deterioration of granulocyte function. There is a 30 to 50 percent decline in chemotaxis after 24 hours of cold storage and at least 30 percent with room temperature storage according to earlier studies.[157–160] There is also a reduction in the percentage of cells able to circulate after prolonged storage (24 hours).[161] Although function appears to be reasonably preserved with 8 hours of room temperature storage,[162] it is recommended that granulocytes be transfused as soon as possible after collection. Administration is usually 1 hour per 2×10^{10} cells, so there is storage time in the hanging bag that must also be taken into consideration.

Histocompatibility Issues in Granulocyte Transfusions

Febrile reactions and pulmonary infiltrates were commonly associated with granulocyte transfusions in the past.[163] However, not all of these reactions are immunologic. Nevertheless, histocompatibility factors are important in granulocyte transfusion therapy. Granulocytes must be ABO compatible, essentially because of the red blood cells, which contaminate granulocyte transfusions. Although previously thought to be present, more recent work has determined that ABO antigens are not present in the granulocyte cell membrane.[164] Therefore, if complete or near-complete removal of red blood cells could be accomplished, perhaps ABO matching would not be a requirement for granulocyte transfusion.[164] Granulocytes have both HLAs and neutrophil-specific antigens (the latter are not linked to HLA) on their surface. In the past, it was not possible to use transfusion count increments to demonstrate limitations in effectiveness caused by histocompatibility factors because the count increments were not measurable. Studies using indium-111–labelled granulocytes were able to evaluate the success of migration of granulocytes to infectious sites in patients receiving histoincompatible granulocytes.[165–167] Studies of granulocyte agglutinating antibodies and lymphocytotoxic antibodies demonstrated the failure of incompatible granulocytes to localize to sites of infection[165,166] and sequestration of histoincompatible granulocytes in the pulmonary capillary bed[167] (Figure 10–23). The latter may explain some of the pulmonary transfusion reactions observed with unmatched granulocyte transfusions in early studies. Although there was added information from the use of granulocyte agglutination assays, this is not practical in the blood bank setting. Thererfore, patients who demonstrate anti-HLA antibodies are unlikely to benefit from unmatched granulocytes. McCullough and colleagues have recommended serial screening of the patient's sera against a panel of cells periodically to determine if the subject is becoming immunized.[115] Others use anti-HLA antibody assays. If antibodies develop, HLA-matched donors will be necessary, if available.

Transfusion Reactions

Febrile reactions due to granulocytes are quite common and are likely multifactorial. Possible components of such reactions are cytokines released during

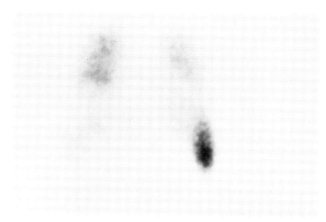

Figure 10–23. Pulmonary and splenic uptake on an indium-111–labeled granulocyte scan in an alloimmunized patient given random granulocytes: 30-minute scan.

granulocyte storage and transport, localization to sites of ongoing inflammation, and aggregates. Patients with pre-exiting pneumonia may manifest localization to the infection as acute respiratory distress and fever. Granulocyte transfusions should be administered slowly, over at least 1 to 2 hours, and in cases of large numbers of cells at a rate approximating 2×10^{10} cells per hour. Although in the past there was concern regarding interactions of amphotericin B with concurrent granulocyte transfusions (perhaps an interaction with the cell membrane), there is no statistically significant increased risk of reactions with concurrent administration, and, in fact, such reactions occur with either modality alone. Nevertheless, because reactions with either are common, the two modalities should not be administered together but rather serially, to define the cause of any difficulties that may arise.[168–170]

Complications of Granulocyte Transfusions

In addition to transfusion reactions, another possible complication of granulocyte transfusions is the transmission of disease. The most common concern is that of CMV transmission. This virus lives in granulocytes and therefore is easily transmitted. Development of a de novo CMV infection in a CMV-negative recipient is a major complication of bone marrow transplantation, and current practice in leukemia management and transplantation is to screen donors and recipients for CMV status. If the recipient is CMV positive, there is no benefit from restricting

CMV-positive products. However, if the recipient is CMV negative, every attempt should be made to do so. Current practice is to use either CMV-negative products as available or leukocyte filters that remove three logs of leukocytes. Obviously, the filters are not appropriate when the goal is to transfuse granulocytes. Therefore, if granulocytes are needed, CMV-negative donors must be used if at all possible.

Graft-versus-host disease is a known complication of products with transfusion of viable lymphocytes to severely immunodeficient recipients. There have been reports of GVHD following granulocyte transfusions from normal donors, but this is exceedingly rare.[171–174] Nevertheless, this can be a fatal complication, and care must be taken in selecting donors and in irradiating related donors. Routine irradiation of all granulocyte transfusions is not recommended, however.

In summary, granulocyte transfusion therapy is returning as a therapeutic modality using the same criteria for indications (ie, severe neutropenia in a patient with an unresponsive bacterial or fungal infection who is likely to remain profoundly granulocytopenic for at least another week). The promise of the new approach to granulocyte collection and donor premedication with growth factors is that severe infections can be eradicated and survival enhanced, thus allowing such patients to regenerate their own or transplanted marrow.

HEMATOPOIETIC GROWTH FACTORS IN PATIENTS WITH LEUKEMIAS

Treatment of acute leukemia induces profound neutropenia with the attendant risk of onset of serious infection. In this setting, due to the intensity of the treatment and the marrow status of the disease itself, the use of hematopoietic colony-stimulating factors (CSFs) will not eliminate severe neutropenia. However, there is the possibility that CSFs will shorten the duration of neutropenia, which could impact on the incidence or seriousness of new infections.

A summary of evidence-based studies was presented in the American Society of Clinical Oncology Guidelines updated for the year 2000 for the use of CSFs.[175] The results of several placebo-controlled, randomized studies using G-CSF or granulocyte-macrophage CSF (GM-CSF) administered after induction chemotherapy in patients with AML were evaluated.[176–184] Most, but not all, trials evaluated growth factors in older patients primarily. The overall conclusions were quite consistent and demonstrated a reduction in time to granulocyte recovery to 500 neutrophils/mm³ by 2 to 6 days. There was no positive or negative impact on remission rate[177–184] or on survival[176,178–184] in the vast majority of these studies, and the variant results in single studies were explained by issues related to each study's design or conduct. Durations of hospital stay and antibiotic use were shortened significantly in most of these studies. Therefore, the year 2000 recommendations state that there may be a cost-benefit improvement with the use of CSFs following induction chemotherapy in patients with AML by shortening hospital stay and a modest reduction in the incidence of serious infections. This benefit is observed primarily in patients older than age 54 years. Perhaps the greater benefit was observed with the use of CSFs following consolidation therapy of patients with AML treated after achieving remission. In contrast, there is no evidence that "priming" leukemia patients with CSFs before starting antileukemia treatment is of benefit, and this approach is not recommended.[175]

With respect to myelodysplasia, although administration of CSFs can raise the neutrophil count in neutropenic patients, chronic administration is not recommended.[175] Colony-stimulating factors should be used as supportive care for the management of infections only.[185,186]

The year 2000 guidelines also include an evaluation of CSF use in studies of patients with ALL.[175] Studies were more heterogeneous, and some gave CSFs concurrently with chemotherapy and some following completion of chemotherapy, at differing timepoints. The summary, however, is similar to that of CSF use in AML, with a reduction in duration of profound neutropenia by approximately 1 week but no impact on disease-free or overall survival.[187–192] Most benefit was noted in older adults, with a reduction in hospital days and use of antibiotics.[187–192] In studies in children, there was a similar reduction in the duration of neutropenia.[188,193] Therefore, CSFs are considered cost effective in patients undergoing induction therapy for ALL, particularly in adults.[175]

INFECTION MANAGEMENT IN ACUTE LEUKEMIA

Infection is a major complication in patients with acute leukemia because of the nature of the disease and its treatment, which both render the patient neutropenic. Without the defenses of granulocytes, and with chemotherapy inducing damage to mucosal barriers, the stage is set for infection. In addition, the advent of the use of central venous catheters has led to an increase in infection due to skin organisms by providing a portal of entry.

Because such patients are so profoundly neutropenic, it takes a minimal bacterial dose to cause a febrile episode, usually a bacteremia.[131–133] However, it is rare to obtain a positive culture from the blood during a fever spike, again because the bacterial load able to cause infection in neutropenic patients is so small. Early studies in dogs showed that two logs less bacteria could lead to sepsis in neutropenic hosts, compared with animals with adequate defenses.[131–133] Thus, in humans, the concept of empiric antibiotics for fever, and even with subsequent negative cultures, has been life saving in protecting neutropenic patients from potent but low doses of bacteria. Small fevers can represent bacteremias and produce serious consequences (Figure 10–24).

Additionally, most of the organisms that cause serious bacterial and fungal infections in neutropenic patients are of low virulence and are derived from the normal body flora.[194] Experience has taught that coverage must be broad in neutropenic patients and not be narrowed to cover a single identified or suspected organism.

The usual pattern of infection during the induction treatment of acute leukemia is the development of fever several days after the onset of profound neutropenia, less than 500 white cells per microliter, and more likely at less than 100 white cells per microliter. When there is a fever spike of more than 100.4°F and after cultures of blood, urine, and any visible lesions, patients are empirically placed on broad-spectrum antibiotics. The most common organisms to cause the first infections in this setting are still gram-negative bacilli, although they are less commonly isolated in cultures than previously (see Figure 10–18). Nevertheless, initial antibiotic cover-

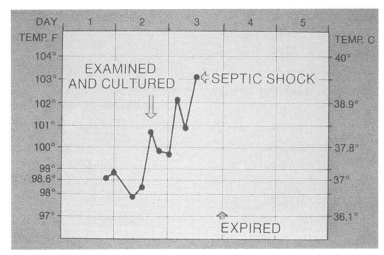

Figure 10–24.   Fever curve not treated with antibiotics, thought to be a transfusion reaction, ending in septic shock.

age must be capable of combating these bacteria because they have the capacity to induce endotoxic shock. The most common gram-negative organism in most institutions is *Escherichia coli* and the second most common is *Klebsiella* sp. *Pseudomonas aeruginosa* has long been the most serious gram-negative infection, but, fortunately, in most institutions, it has decreased in frequency, although it has

not disappeared (see Figure 10–18). Each hospital has its characteristic flora, which should be known to the infection control team.

There are three antibiotic schemes that have gained prominence in the approach to this initial fever[195] (Figure 10–25). The most commonly used is the combination of an antipseudomonal beta-lactam and an aminoglycoside agent. The addition of van-

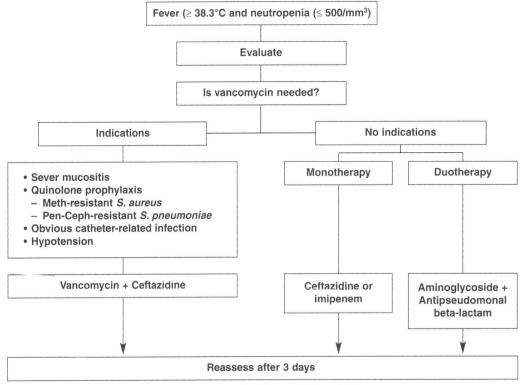

Figure 10–25.   Algorithm for empiric antibiotics at initial fever: initial antibiotic regimens.

comycin to the initial combination has been used by some or may be given earlier. A single agent such as ceftazidime or imipenem has been successful in many cases, but in at least 50 percent of patients, an aminoglycoside must subsequently be added due to persistent fever.[196,197] If fever continues after 3 days, the patient must be reassessed and recultured to identify other causes of fever (Figure 10–26). Antibiotic coverage may also have to be reassessed. When there is recurrence of fever after several days of broad-spectrum antibiotics, the possibility of antibiotic-induced fever must be considered. If there is evidence of new infection, antibiotics may need to be changed (see Figure 10–26). However, if there is no other obvious source and the patient appears well, yet there is a spiking fever pattern, it is occasionally necessary to stop all antibiotics and reculture. The fever may resolve with cessation of antibiotics. If this approach is being tested, the patient must be watched very carefully for signs of progressive infection. However, antibiotic-induced fever is not uncommon, and the patient may defervesce with this approach.

However, if with this new fever, the patient appears ill, then an additional infectious source must be evaluated and covered with antibiotics. The patient must again be cultured, and in this era of venous access devices, the second infection is likely to be due to a gram-positive organism, admitted to the body through the exit site of the catheter (see Figure 10–26). This is most likely to be a skin organism, either *Staphylococcus aureus* or *S. epidermidis*.[198–201] Coagulase-negative *Staphylococcus (epidermidis)* is the most common blood culture isolate. Other less common skin organisms include gram-negative bacilli, which may colonize the skin in sick patients. This fever spike is treated empirically with vancomycin to cover *Staphylococcus* sp while the cultures are pending. Although it is considered acceptable to add the gram-positive coverage with the initial fever spike, most infectious disease experts recommend against this and suggest waiting for the next temperature spike (see Figure 10–26).[202–204] This recommendation is for three reasons: (1) unless there is a history of access line infections, this is very unlikely to be a source of infection early on in the course; (2) the goal is to limit exposure to antistaphylococcal antibiotics to avoid development of antibiotic resistance; and (3) there is some coverage provided by initial broad-spectrum antibiotics. There is great concern regarding the development of resistant gram-positive organisms, and this is becoming a major issue in centers that use a great deal of vancomycin. Currently, the recommendation is to administer no more than 3 to 4 days of vancomycin if cultures do not grow gram-positive organisms. If, in fact, there is a gram-positive coccus identified, then all three antibiotics are usually continued. Attempts to reduce antibiotic exposure can be made, but more than 50 percent of patients will need antibiotics restarted.

Randomized studies in which temporary central lines have been impregnated with antiseptic coatings to prevent infection have yielded promising results in the critical care or general hospital setting in

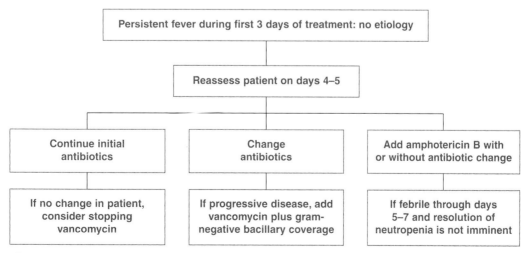

Figure 10–26. Algorithm for management of second fever spike in neutropenic patients.

terms of reduction in line colonization and in bacteremias.[205,206] However, in a recent report of a randomized study of benzalkonium chloride-impregnated temporary central venous catheters used in neutropenic cancer patients, the majority of whom had acute leukemia, there was no difference in the incidence of catheter colonization or in the frequency of bacteremias.[207] These patients were at high risk for infection, and in this study, the antiseptic was not sufficient to prevent infection.

These initial fevers are often without bacterial confirmation, and the episode resolves quickly and the patient becomes afebrile quickly. However, serious complications may develop if the antibiotics are not initiated rapidly, within a few hours of the fever spike. Nurses in oncology units, highly experienced in the management of these patients, usually have instructions to immediately culture and begin empiric antibiotics, and this has saved many patients who have otherwise life-threatening infections.

In patients who require additional time for marrow recovery or a second course of induction therapy, the risk of additional infectious episodes is very high. These are likely to be caused by either additional, resistant bacterial organisms or fungal organisms. If, after the initial antibiotic therapy, fever either persists or returns, and if fever persists after a change in antibacterial antibiotics, then empiric antifungal therapy should be added.

In most hospital settings, if there is no ongoing construction, the initial fungal infection is most likely to be *Candida* sp, part of the normal flora and likely to grow out after broad-spectrum antibiotic therapy. In most cases, systemic or mucocutaneous candidiasis can be treated with fluconazole. The exception are *Candida tropicalis* and *krusei,* which require amphotericin B. Candidal infections develop in the setting of prolonged neutropenia and prolonged treatment with broad-spectrum antibiotics (Figure 10–27).

Recent evaluations point to an increasing incidence of hepatosplenic candidiasis (see Figure 10–27).[208] This entity classically arises as the patient is recovering from severe neutropenia, and as the white blood cell count recovers, elevated liver function tests and new fever are noted. Prolonged neutropenia has always been a factor in the development of this infection, but additional factors contributing

to the increase in incidence are more intensive treatment regimens and a statistically significant association with the use of high-dose cytosine arabinoside as both induction and consolidation therapy.[208,209] This regimen facilitates the development of disseminated candidiasis even in patients treated at a time when their blood counts are normalized, just prior to consolidation therapy (Wiernik PH, personal communication, 2000) (see Figure 10–27). The usual diagnostic tests for hepatosplenic candidiasis include ultrasound and computed tomographic (CT) scans. This may be followed by CT-guided biopsy. A recent article suggested that magnetic resonance imaging may be useful in the diagnosis and monitoring of response in this entity and may obviate the need for invasive diagnostic measures.[210]

The use of prophylactic fluconazole remains controversial in the leukemia treatment setting, although it is routinely used in transplantation centers. A decrease in infectious episodes has been documented,[211] but there is an additional risk of selection of resistant organisms, such as *C. krusei*, particularly in patients who do not immediately achieve remission and require additional therapy.[212,213] Others report an increased association of *Torulopsis glabrata* infections with the use of fluconazole prophylaxis in the setting of bone marrow transplantation.[214]

The other major fungal pathogen in acute leukemia is *Aspergillus* sp. This fungus is associated with pulmonary infections, which, again, are most likely after prolonged neutropenia (see Figures

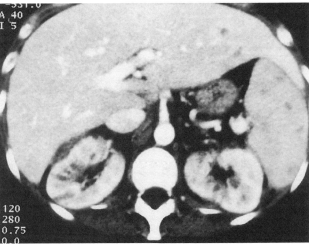

Figure 10–27. Hepatosplenic candidiasis with multiple small abscesses in the liver, spleen, and kidneys.

10–20 and 10–21). Environmental factors contribute to its development, and if there is construction, or if the patient develops a new pulmonary infiltrate, there must be concern about *Aspergillus* sp, which requires amphotericin B therapy.[194]

New antifungal agents are under investigation, directed at targets such as the cell wall, as well as more potent or more bioavailable triazoles. Clinical trials are ongoing. One agent to recently reach the clinic is itraconazole, a new triazole, with a broader antifungal spectrum than fluconazole.[215] Both oral and intravenous formulations are now available. With this agent, the efficacy is directly related to the serum level achieved, and this is dependent on bioavailability.[216] Itraconazole has a broader spectrum and has antifungal activity against *Aspergillus* sp and against fluconazole-resistant yeasts in animal studies. Its exact positioning in the human treatment setting is still being defined, but it has been relatively successful in the prophylactic setting.[217] A combination of intravenous administration followed by oral administration has led to successful treatment of invasive aspergillosis.[218]

Other peculiar fungi may be isolated in the setting of prolonged neutropenia, and these rely on the microbiology laboratory for specific identification. While waiting for final identification, the standard approach remains empiric. If fever persists with the use of fluconazole, then a change is made to amphotericin B. If fever persists when the liposomal preparations are used, then standard amphotericin B is needed. There continues to be better tissue penetration with the standard preparation of amphotericin B.

In the setting of persistent fever, the possible causes are antibiotic fever or persistent serious infection. If, after antibiotic adjustment occurs, the patient remains profoundly neutropenic and febrile, granulocyte transfusions are then indicated. In general, if the white blood cell count recovers, almost all patients survive these infectious episodes. However, in patients who do not achieve remission or have very prolonged granulocytopenia, there is significant risk of mortality from infection.

In patients with acute leukemia who continue to have a central venous catheter, the management and the decision to remove the catheter because of persistent infection have been outlined in the infectious disease literature. The decision to remove the catheter is determined by the severity of the infection, whether there are persistently positive cultures, and whether there is a tunnel infection in the skin and not simply bacteremias. In patients who have recovered their white blood cell count and are clinically well, it is often possible to clear the catheter of infection. However, if episodes of bacteremia persist, the catheter must be removed. Similarly, in neutropenic patients, if they are persistently febrile and ill and the catheter is the source, then it must be removed.

As stated above, the majority of febrile episodes in patients with leukemia are a result of host flora traversing disrupted mucosal or skin barriers. It is quite uncommon for these patients to develop more "standard" infections, such as isolated urinary tract infections or meningitis. Of course, in the setting of bacteremias, any site may become infected.

INFECTIOUS COMPLICATIONS IN PATIENTS WITH LYMPHOCYTIC LEUKEMIAS AND DISORDERS

In general, the infections associated with B-cell diseases, in particular, CLL and myeloma, are related to impairments of humoral immunity, whereas the infections associated with T-cell disorders, such as cutaneous T-cell lymphoma/leukemia and HTLV-I–associated T-cell leukemia, are related to impairments of cellular immunity and neutropenia. In this section, because of the frequency of the disease, the focus is on the infectious complications of CLL, which is almost always a B-cell disorder. However, the spectrum of infections that occurs in this disease has changed with more aggressive treatment; therefore, a discussion of infections common to both B- and T-cell disorders is necessary.

Chronic lymphocytic leukemia is characterized by progressive immunodeficiency. Initially, patients maintain their ability to combat infections, but as time progresses, and with therapy that is also immunosuppressive, these patients are at risk for bacterial, viral, and opportunistic infections. This risk develops from the combination of immunologic deficits inherent in the disease itself, with poor B-cell function and progressive loss of neutrophils, which predisposes these patients to bacterial infections and infections of mucosal surfaces due to loss of normal immunoglobulins.[219] In addition, more recently entering the spectrum of infections are those resulting from the additional T-cell deficits induced by agents used to treat CLL, such as fludarabine and 2-chlorodeoxyadenosine.[219] Patients are also often treated with corticosteroids as part of therapy, and this can also predispose to infectious complications.

The initial manifestation of the immunocompromised state in patients with this disease is often the development of herpes zoster, a reactivation of *Varicellavirus* (Figure 10–28). Additionally, even early in the course of the disease, there is increased susceptibility to upper respiratory infections and bacterial pneumonia as a result of inherently low immunoglobulins and defects in opsonization. Defects in mucosal immunoglobulins may predispose to some of these infections.[219]

In patients who are treated with the new nucleoside analogues, considerable T-cell depletion occurs, in addition to the preexisting B-cell deficit; therefore, a variety of opportunistic infections have been reported.[219–222] These include *Listeria monocytogenes, Pneumocystis carinii*, mycobacteria, and opportunistic fungal and viral infections. These organisms are also prevalent in infections in patients with chronic T-cell lymphomas.

Odd types of infections that have been reported in patients with CLL include painful red nodules in the skin, which were caused by gram-negative bacterial infections,[223,224] and cryptococcosis,[225] both in patients who had and not had nucleoside analogues. Viral infections may also be more severe in patients

with CLL having been recently treated with nucleoside analogues, and reports include severe respiratory syncytial virus pulmonary infection[226] and Richter's syndrome associated with the presence of Epstein-Barr virus.[227,228]

Recently, the agent CAMPATH-1 has been approved for use in CLL. This is a monoclonal antibody directed toward CD52, which is expressed on most indolent lymphoid disorders. This agent is highly immunosuppressive and is also associated with a wide number of opportunistic infections.[229]

The T-cell–derived indolent lymphomas, with or without a leukemic phase, are associated with the infections described above that are related to T-cell defects but rarely those associated with humoral immunity. In addition, patients with cutaneous lymphoma/leukemia (ie, mycosis fungoides and Sézary syndrome) are susceptible to *Staphylococcus* sp infections because of the extensive skin involvement with tumor. The clinical differences between these types of infections are usually readily apparent.

Management of patients with CLL requires close attention to early symptoms of infection complications and early empiric treatment. Serious complications in these patients can be reduced by early intervention. Such patients should be adequately advised of the need to contact medical staff early when symptoms arise. These patients, when complaining of upper respiratory infection symptoms, should be evaluated in the event that this represents early pneumonia. Additional attention to possible opportunistic infections must be sought in patients treated with the newer agents since these are often more subtle in symptoms but are potentially very serious.

As a result of the observation of hypogammaglobulinemia in patients with CLL, studies of replacement gamma globulin have been conducted. In one large, placebo-controlled, multicenter trial, gamma globulin was administered at a dose of 400 mg/kg every 3 weeks. There were significantly fewer minor or moderate bacterial infections among those receiving gamma globulin.[230] However, there was no decrease in major or life-threatening infections or in viral or fungal infections among those who did or did not receive gamma globulin. A subsequent analysis was unable to determine an improvement in quality or length of life as a result of reducing minor infections, nor was rou-

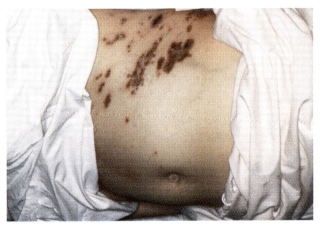

Figure 10–28. Herpes zoster in a dermatomal pattern.

tine gamma globulin administration considered cost effective.[231,232] Similar randomized studies using lower doses of gamma globulin also showed that its use reduced febrile episodes but did not reduce the incidence of serious infections.[233–235] In part, the limited benefit derived from prophylactic gamma globulin administration may reflect the absence of IgM or IgA in the infusion product.[219] Therefore, routine prophylactic gamma globulin infusions are not recommended in patients with CLL. There may be special clinical circumstances where such infusions may seem appropriate, but this must be individualized.

Finally, fever does occur in patients with CML, but in the chronic phase, this is unlikely to represent an opportunistic infection since the granulocytes of these patients are functional and they are not immunocompromised. Fever in the chronic phase should be evaluated for routine, bacterial infections, or it may be the result of initiation of interferon therapy. However, persistent fever in a patient in the chronic phase of CML must be evaluated as a possible indicator of transition to the accelerated or blastic phase of CML. Fever in a patient with blastic crisis of CML should be evaluated as disease related or related to the development of neutropenia, in which case the rules related to empiric antibiotics are used, as in AML.

In summary, infection complications are a major part of the morbidity of leukemias. Careful attention to subtle signs and symptoms of infection are a major part of management of patients with acute leukemia. In the chronic leukemias, particularly during treatment, a high level of suspicion is needed to identify infections due to both expected and unexpected organisms.

LEUKOPHERESIS IN THE SUPPORTIVE CARE OF LEUKEMIA PATIENTS

Patients with acute leukemia may present with an extremely high blast count, > 100,000/μL. This presentation is associated with a high risk of early death due to hemorrhagic complications of leukostasis of blasts in the capillary bed of the brain or to respiratory failure from the same process in the capillary bed of the lungs.[236–241] Extreme leukocytosis is most dangerous in the myeloid leukemias, AML, or blast crisis of CML. It is extremely uncommon for this clinical syndrome to occur in chronic-phase CML because of the greater deformability of the more mature cells.[242] Similarly, it is uncommon in ALL, even with a high blast count, due to the deformability of these blast cells, and it is almost never observed in patients with CLL.[242]

When patients are symptomatic with a very high blast count, rapid reduction of the blast cell count is necessary to prevent acute complications. Numerous reports document the practical usefulness of intensive leukapheresis to produce a rapid reduction in blast counts, with improvement in symptoms.[243–247] To maintain this acute reduction in counts, either concomitant hydroxyurea is given or definitive induction chemotherapy is begun. However, the benefit of chemotherapy may take several days to reduce the white blood cell count, and several apheresis procedures may be necessary. Those patients with the most rapidly rising counts may be the most difficult to control simply because of the technical limitations of the procedure, and chemotherapy must be initiated as quickly as it is safe to do so, given the likelihood of metabolic abnormalities occurring in this setting as well.[248]

Leukapheresis has been used in the management of patients with advanced CLL, often after more standard approaches have failed.[249–252] These older reports demonstrate control of blood counts, reduction of organomegaly, and control of hemolytic anemia but no immunologic reconstitution.[249–252] More recent experience has again demonstrated the ability to control hemolytic anemia by controlling the white blood cell count and obviating the need for chronic corticosteroid administration (Dutcher JP, personal communication, 1990), and in occasional patients who are chemotherapy naive, there has been a reversal in cytopenias.[253] Another approach that is being explored is the role of pretherapy leukapheresis in patients with CLL to allow safer administration of the new agent, rituximab, which requires a lower white blood cell count for administration.[254]

In summary, aggressive supportive care for patients with leukemia related to blood product support and infection prevention and management remains a critical component for the successful outcome of treatment of these diseases. Hematologists and oncologists caring for these patients must be knowledgeable in the supportive care aspects and the chemotherapy required for treatment. Additionally, transfusion medicine and infectious disease physicians with particular interest in the management of pancytopenic patients provide expertise in this very specialized area of clinical medicine. Nevertheless, the treating oncologist must remain current in all aspects, including supportive care, when caring for patients with adult leukemias.

REFERENCES

1. McCullough J. Current issues with platelet transfusion in patients with cancer. Semin Hematol 2000;37:2–10.

2. Han T, Stutzman L, Cohen E, et al. Effect of platelet transfusion on hemorrhage in patients with acute leukemia. An autopsy study. Cancer 1966;19:1937–42.

3. Higby DJ, Cohen E, Holland JF, Sinks L. The prophylactic treatment of thrombocytopenic leukemic patients with platelets: a double blind study. Transfusion 1974;14:440–6.

4. Murphy S, Litwin S, Herring LM, et al. Indications for platelet transfusion in children with acute leukemia. Am J Hematol 1982;12:347–56.

5. Hanson SR, Slichter SJ. Platelet kinetics in patients with bone marrow hypoplasia: evidence for a fixed platelet requirement. Blood 1985;66:1105–9.

6. Duke WW. Relationship of blood platelets to hemorrhagic disease: description of a method to determine bleeding time and coagulation time and report of cases of hemorrhagic disease relieved by transfusion. JAMA 1910;55:1185–92.

7. Gaydos LA, Freireich EJ, Mantel N. The quantitative relation between platelet count and hemorrhage in patients with acute leukemia. N Engl J Med 1962;266:905–9.

8. Patten E. Controversies in transfusion medicine: prophylactic platelet transfusion revisited after 25 years. Con Transfusion 1992;32:381–5.

9. Baer MR, Bloomfield CD. Controversies in transfusion medicine: prophylactic platelet transfusion therapy. Pro Transfusion 1992;32:377–80.

10. Schiffer CA. Prophylactic platelet transfusion. Transfusion 1992;32:295–8. [editorial]

11. Aderka D, Praff G, Santo M, et al. Bleeding due to thrombocytopenia in acute leukemia and reevaluation of the prophylactic platelet transfusion policy. Am J Med Sci 1986;291:147–51.

12. NIH Consensus Conference. Platelet transfusion therapy. JAMA 1987;257:1777–80.

13. Slichter SJ. Platelet transfusion therapy. Hematol Oncol Clin North Am 1991;4:291–7.

14. Bishop JF, McGrath K, Wolf WW, et al. Clinical factors influencing the efficacy of pooled platelet tranfusions. Blood 1988;71:383–7.

15. Gralnick HR, Bagley J, Abrell E. Heparin treatment for the hemorrhagic diathesis of acute progranulocytic leukemia. Am J Med 1971;52:167–74.

16. Daly PA, Schiffer CA, Wiernik PH. Acute progranulocytic leukemia—clinical management of 15 patients. Am J Hematol 1980;8:347–59.

17. Bishop JF, Matthews JP, McGrath K, et al. Factors influencing 20-hour increments after platelet transfusion. Transfusion 1991;31:392–6.

18. Beutler E. Platelet transfusions: the 20,000/μl trigger. Blood 1993;81:1411–3.

19. Bishop JF, Schiffer CA, Aisner J, et al. Surgery in acute leukemia: a review of 167 operations in thrombocytopenic patients. Am J Hematol 1987;26:147–55.

20. Williford SK, Salisbury PL III, Peacock JE Jr, et al. The safety of dental extractions in patients with hematologic malignancies. J Clin Oncol 1989;7:798–802.

21. Daly PA, Schiffer CA, Aisner J, Wiernik PH. Platelet transfusion therapy. One hour post-transfusion increments are valuable in predicting the need for HLA-matched preparations. JAMA 1980;243:435–8.

22. O'Connell B, Lee EJ, Schiffer CA. The value of 10-minute posttransfusion platelet counts. Transfusion 1988;28:66–7.

23. Bishop JF, Matthews JP, Yuen K, et al. The definition of refractoriness to platelet transfusions. Transfus Med 1991;2:35–41.

24. Mourad N. A simple method for obtaining platelet concentrates free of aggregates. Transfusion 1968;8:48.

25. Simon TL. The collection of platelets by apheresis procedures. Transfus Med Rev 1994;8:132–45.

26. Hester J, Ventura G, Boucher T. Platelet concentrate collection in a dual stage channel using computer generated algorithms for collection and prediction of yield. Plasma Ther Transfus Technol 1987;8:377–85.

27. Maresh S, Randels MJ, Strauss RG, et al. Comparison of plateletpheresis with a standard and an improved collection device. Transfusion 1993;33:835–7.

28. Goodnough LT, Kuter D, McCullough J, Brecher ME. Apheresis platelets: emerging issues related to donor platelet count, apheresis platelet yield, and platelet transfusion dose. J Clin Apheresis 1998;13:114–9.

29. Sniecinski I, St. Jean J, Nowicki B. Preparation of leukocyte-poor platelets by filtration. J Clin Apheresis 1989;5:7–11.

30. Kickler TS, Bell W, Ness PM, et al. Depletion of white cells from platelet concentrates with a new adsorption filter. Transfusion 1989;29:411–4.

31. Miyamoto M, Sasakawa S, Ishikawa Y, et al. Leukocyte-poor platelet concentrates at the bedside by filtration through Sepacell-PL. Vox Sang 1989;57:164–7.

32. Standards for blood banks and transfusion services.

19th Ed. Bethesda, MD: AABB Press; 1999. p. 10, 26, 51–2.

33. Aster RH. Effect of anticoagulant and ABO incompatibility on recovery of transfused human platelets. Blood 1965;26:732–43.

34. Kelton JG, Hamid C, Aker S, Blajchman MA. The amount of blood group A substance on platelets is proportional to the amount in the plasma. Blood 1982;59:980–5.

35. Lee EJ, Schiffer CA. ABO compatibility can influence the results of platelet transfusion: results of a randomized trial. Transfusion 1989;29:384–9.

36. Curtis BR, Edwards JT, Hessner MJ, et al. Blood group A and B antigens are strongly expressed on platelets of some individuals. Blood 2000;96:1574–81.

37. Hogge DE, Dutcher JP, Aisner J, Schiffer CA. Lymphocytotoxic antibody is a predictor of response to random donor platelet transfusion. Am J Hematol 1983;14:363–9.

38. Yankee RA, Grumet FC, Rogentine GN. Platelet transfusion therapy. The selection of compatible platelet donors for refractory patients by lymphocyte HLA typing. N Engl J Med 1969;281:1208–12.

39. Mittal KK, Terasaki PI. Serologic cross-reactivity in the HLA system. Tissue Antigens 1974;4:146–52.

40. Chow MP, Yung HY, Hu JL, et al. Platelet crossmatching with lymphocytotoxicity test: an effective method in alloimmunized Chinese patients. Transfusion 1991;31:595–9.

41. Schiffer CA, Keller C, Dutcher JP, et al. Potential HLA matched platelet donor availability for alloimmunized patients. Transfusion 1983;23:286–9.

42. Aster RH, Szatkowski N, Liebert M. Expression of HLA-B12, HLA-B8, W4 and W6 on platelets. Transplant Proc 1977;9:1695–6.

43. Liebert M, Aster RH. Expression of HLA-B12 on platelets, on lymphocytes and in serum. A quantitative study. Tissue Antigens 1977;9:199–208.

44. Schiffer CA, O'Connell B, Lee EJ. Platelet transfusion therapy for alloimmunized patients: selective mismatching for HLA-B12, an antigen with variable expression on platelets. Blood 1989;74:1172–6.

45. Moroff G, Garratty G, Heal J, et al. Selection of platelets for refractory patients by HLA matching and prospective crossmatching. Transfusion 1992;32:633–40.

46. Fehr J, Hofmann V, Kappeler U. Transient reversal of thrombocytopenia in idiopathic thrombocytopenic purpura by high-dose intravenous gamma globulin. N Engl J Med 1982;305:1254–8.

47. Schiffer CA, Hogge DE, Aisner J, et al. High dose intravenous gamma globulin in alloimmunized platelet transfusion recipients. Blood 1984;64:937–40.

48. Lee EJ, Norris D, Schiffer CA. Intravenous immune globulin for patients alloimmunized to random donor platelet transfusion. Transfusion 1987;27:245–7.

49. Kickler TS, Braine HG, Piantadosi S, et al. A randomized, placebo-controlled trial of intravenous gamma globulin in alloimmunized thrombocytopenic patients. Blood 1990;75:313–6.

50. Dutcher JP, Schiffer CA, Aisner J, et al. Long-term follow-up of patients with leukemia receiving platelet transfusions: identification of a large group of patients who do not become alloimmunized. Blood 1981;58:1007–11.

51. Holohan TV, Terasaki PI, Deisseroth AB. Suppression of transfusion-related alloimmunization in intensively treated cancer patients. Blood 1981;58:122–8.

52. Lee EJ, Schiffer CA. Serial measurement of lymphocytotoxic antibody and response to nonmatched platelet transfusions in alloimmunized patients. Blood 1987;70:1727–9.

53. Murphy MF, Metcalfe P, Ord J, et al. Disappearance of HLA and platelet-specific antibodies in acute leukaemia patients alloimmunized by multiple transfusions. Br J Haematol 1987;67:255–60.

54. The Trial to Reduce Alloimmunization to Platelets Study Group. Leukocyte reduction and ultraviolet B irradiation of platelets to prevent alloimmunization and refractoriness to platelet transfusions. N Engl J Med 1997;337:1861–9.

55. Freedman JJ, Blajchman MA, McCombie N. Canadian Red Cross Society symposium on leukodepletion: report of proceedings. Transfus Med Rev 1994;8:1–14.

56. Heddle NM. The efficacy of leukodepletion to improve platelet transfusion response: a critical appraisal of clinical studies. Transfus Med Rev 1994;8:15–28.

57. Oksanen K, Kekomaki R, Ruutu T, et al. Prevention of alloimmunization in patients with acute leukemia by use of white cell-reduced blood components—a randomized trial. Transfusion 1991;31:588–94.

58. van Marwijk Kooy M, van Prooijen HC, Moes M, et al. Use of leukocyte-depleted platelet concentrates for the prevention of refractoriness and primary HLA alloimmunization: a prospective, randomized trial. Blood 1991;77:201–5.

59. Lane TA, Anderson KC, Goodnough LT, et al. Leukocyte reduction in blood component therapy. Ann Intern Med 1992;117:151–62.

60. Burgstaler EA, Pineda AA, Bryant SC. Prospective comparison of plateletpheresis using four apheresis systems on the same donors. J Clin Apheresis 1999;14:163–70.

61. Slichter SJ, Deeg HJ, Kennedy MS. Prevention of platelet alloimmunization in dogs with systemic cyclosporine and by UV-irradiation or cyclosporine loading of donor platelets. Blood 1987;69:414–8.

62. Kahn RA, Duffy BF, Rodey GG. Ultraviolet irradiation of platelet concentrates abrogates lymphocyte activation without affecting platelet function in vitro. Transfusion 1985;25:547–50.

63. Deeg HJ, Aprile J, Storb R, et al. Functional dendritic cells are required for transfusion-induced sensitization in canine marrow graft recipients. Blood 1988;71:1138–40.

64. Bowden RA, Sayers M, Flournoy N, et al. Cytomegalovirus immune globulin and seronegative blood products to prevent primary cytomegalovirus infection after marrow transplantation. N Engl J Med 1986;314:1006–10.

65. Gilbert GL, Hayes K, Hudson IL, et al. Prevention of transfusion-acquired cytomegalovirus infection in infants by blood filtration to remove leucocytes. Lancet 1989;1:1228–31.

66. deGraan-Hentzen YCE, Gratama JW, Mudde GC, et al. Prevention of primary cytomegalovirus infection in patients with hematologic malignancies by intensive white cell depletion of blood products. Transfusion 1989;29:757–60.

67. Bowden RA, Slichter SJ, Sayers MH, et al. Use of leukocyte-depleted platelets and cytomegalovirus seronegative red blood cells for prevention of primary cytomegalovirus infection after marrow transplant. Blood 1991;78:246–50.

68. Bowden RA, Slichter SJ, Sayers M, et al. A comparison of filtered leukocyte-reduced and cytomegalovirus (CMV) seronegative blood products for the prevention of transfusion-associated CMV infection after marrow transplant. Blood 1995;86:3598–603.

69. Heddle NM, Klama L, Singer J, et al. The role of the plasma from platelet concentrates in transfusion reactions. N Engl J Med 1994;331:625–8.

70. Muylle L, Wouters E, Peetermans ME. Febrile reactions to platelet transfusion: the effect of increased interleukin 6 levels in concentrates prepared by the platelet-rich plasma method. Transfusion 1996;36:886–90.

71. Goodnough LT, Riddell J, Lazarus H, et al. Prevalence of platelet transfusion reaction before and after implementation of leukocyte-depleted platelet concentrates by filtration. Vox Sang 1993;65:103–7.

72. Linden JV, Pisciotto PT. Transfusion-associated graft-versus-host disease and blood irradiation. Transfus Med Rev 1992;6:116–23.

73. Kanter MH. Transfusion-associated graft-versus-host disease: do transfusions from second-degree relatives pose a greater risk than those from first-degree relatives? Transfusion 1992;32:323–7.

74. Petz LD, Calhoun L, Yam P, et al. Transfusion-associated graft-versus-host disease in immunocompetent patients: report of a fatal case associated with transfusion of blood from a second-degree relative, and a survey of predisposing factors. Transfusion 1993;33:742–50.

75. McMilin KD, Johnson RL. HLA homozygosity and the risk of related-donor transfusion-associated graft-versus-host disease. Transfus Med Rev 1993;7:37–41.

76. Heddle NM, Blajchman MA. The leukodepletion of cellular blood products in the prevention of HLA-alloimmunization and refractoriness to allogeneic platelet transfusion. Blood 1995;85:603–6.

77. Chiu EKW, Yuen KY, Lie AKW, et al. A prospective study of symptomatic bacteremia following platelet transfusion and of its management. Transfusion 1994;34:950–4.

78. Schiffer CA, Aisner J, Wiernik PH. Frozen autologous platelet transfusion for patients with leukemia. N Engl J Med 1978;299:7–12.

79. Dutcher JP, Spivack M, Mohandas K, Wiernik PH. A clinical program of platelet cryopreservation. In: Proceedings of the 8th International Meeting of Society of Haematology. Warsaw, September 8–13, 1985.

80. Herve P, Otron G, Droule C, et al. Human platelets frozen with glycerol in liquid nitrogen: biological and clinical aspects. Transfusion 1981;21:384–90.

81. Kim BK, Baldini MG. Biochemistry, function and hemostatic effectiveness of frozen human platelets. Proc Soc Exp Biol Med 1974;145:830.

82. Valeri CR, Feingold H, Marchionni LL. A simple method for freezing human platelets using 6 percent dimethylsulfoxide and storage at –80°C. Blood 1974;43:131–6.

83. Daly PA, Schiffer CA, Aisner J, Wiernik PH. Successful transfusion of platelets cryopreserved for more than 3 years. Blood 1979;54:1023–7.

84. Rand JJ, Maloney WD, Sise HS. Coagulation defects in acute promyelocytic leukemia. Arch Intern Med 1969;123:39–44.

85. Gralnick HR, Sultan C. Acute promyelocytic leukemia: haemorrhagic manifestations and morphologic criteria. Br J Haematol 1979;7:373–9.

86. Groopman J, Ellman C. Acute promyelocytic leukemia. Am J Hematol 1979;7:395–401.

87. Daly PA, Schiffer CA, Wiernik PH. Acute promyelocytic leukemia—clinical management of 15 patients. Am J Hematol 1980;8:347–59.

88. Goldberg MA, Ginsburg D, Mayer RJ, et al. Is heparin administration necessary during induction chemotherapy for patients with acute promyelocytic leukemia? Blood 1987;69:187–94.

89. Feldman EJ, Arlin ZA, Ahmed T, et al. Acute promyelocytic leukemia: a 5-year experience with new antileukemic agents and a new approach to preventing fatal hemorrhage. Acta Haematol 1989;82:117–21.

90. Fenaux P, Le Deley MC, Castaigne S, et al. Effect of all trans-retinoic acid in newly diagnosed acute promyelocytic leukemia. Results of a multicenter randomized trial. Blood 1993;82:3241–9.

91. Bock M, Wagner M, Knuppel W, et al. Preparation of

white cell-depleted blood: comparison of two bedside filter systems. Transfusion 1990;30:26–9.
92. Koerner K, Sahlmen P, Zimmermann B, Kubanek B. Preparation of leukocyte-poor red cell concentrates: comparison of five different filters. Vox Sang 1991;60:61–2.
93. Lane TA. Leukocyte reduction of cellular blood components: effectiveness, benefits, quality control, and costs. Arch Pathol Lab Med 1994;118:392–404.
94. King KE, Ness PM. Red cell transfusions in patients with hematologic malignancies. In: Wiernik PH, Canellos GP, Dutcher JP, Kyle RA, editors. Neoplastic diseases of the blood. 3rd Ed. New York: Churchill-Livingstone; 1996. p. 1077–88.
95. Brubaker DB. Transfusion-associated graft-versus-host disease. In: Anderson KC, Ness PM, editors. Scientific basis for transfusion medicine: implications for clinical practice. Philadelphia: WB Saunders; 1994. p. 544–60.
96. Office of Medical Application of Research, National Institutes of Health Consensus conference: perioperative red cell transfusion. JAMA 1988;260:2700–4.
97. American College of Physicians. Practice strategies for elective red blood cell transfusion. Ann Intern Med 1992;116:403–6.
98. Expert Working Group. Guidelines for red blood cell and plasma transfusion for adults and children. Can Med Assoc J 1997;156(Suppl 11):S1–24.
99. Sthoeger ZM, Sthoeger D, Shtalrid M, et al. Mechanism of autoimmune hemolytic anemia in chronic lymphocytic leukemia. Am J Hematol 1993;43:259–64.
100. Tosti S, Caruso R, D'Adamo F, et al. Severe autoimmune hemolytic anemia in chronic lymphocytic leukemia responsive to fludarabine-based treatment. Ann Hematol 1992;65:238–9.
101. Cazzola M, Ponchia L, Beguin Y, et al. Subcutaneous erythropoietin for treatment of refractory anemia in hematologic disorders. Results of a phase I/II clinical trial. Blood 1992;79:29–37.
102. Ludwig H, Fritz E, Leitgeb C, et al. Erythropoietin treatment for chronic anemia of selected hematologic malignancies and solid tumors. Ann Oncol 1993;4:161–7.
103. Payne R. The association of febrile transfusion reactions with leuko-agglutinins. Vox Sang 1957;2:233–6.
104. Brittingham RE, Chaplin H. Febrile transfusion reactions caused by sensitivity to donor leukocytes and platelets. JAMA 1957;165:819–23.
105. Perkins HA, Payne R, Ferguson J, Wood M. Nonhemolytic febrile transfusion reactions: quantitative effects of blood components with emphasis on isoantigenic incompatibility of leukocytes. Vox Sang 1966;11:578–600.
106. Goodnough LT, Brecher ME, Kanter MH, AuBuchon JP. Transfusion medicine, part I. Blood transfusion. N Engl J Med 1999;340:438–47.
107. Linden JV, Paul B, Dressler KP. A report of 104 transfusion errors in New York State. Transfusion 1992;32:601–6.
108. Linden JV, Tourault MA, Scribner CL. Decrease in frequency of transfusion fatalities. Transfusion 1997; 37:243–4.
109. Red blood cell transfusion contaminated with *Yersinia enterocolitica*—United States, 1991–1996, and initiation of a national study to detect bacteria-associated transfusion reactions. MMWR Morb Mortal Wkly Rep 1997;46:553–5.
110. Pau CP, Hu DJ, Spruill C, et al. Surveillance for human immunodeficiency virus type I group O infections in the United States. Transfusion 1996;36:398–400.
111. Domen RE. Paid-versus-volunteer blood donation in the United States: a historical review. Transfus Med Rev 1995;9:53–9.
112. Aach RD, Szmuness W, Mosley JW, et al. Serum alanine aminotransferase of donors in relation to the risk of non-A, non-B hepatitis in recipients: the Transfusion-Transmitted Viruses Study. N Engl J Med 1981;304:989–94.
113. Schreiber GB, Busch MP, Kleinman SH, Korelitz JJ. The risk of transfusion-transmitted viral infections. N Engl J Med 1996;334:1685–90.
114. AuBuchon JP, Birkmeyer JD, Busch MP. Safety of the blood supply in the United States: opportunities and controversies. Ann Intern Med 1997;127:904–9.
115. McCullough J. Granulocyte transfusion. In: Petz LD, Swisher SN, Kleinman S, et al., editors. Clinical practice of transfusion medicine. New York: Churchill-Livingstone; 1996. p. 413–22.
116. Dutcher JP. Platelet and granulocyte transfusion. In: Wiernik PH, Canellos GP, Dutcher JP, Kyle RA. editors. Neoplastic diseases of the blood. 3rd Ed. New York: Churchill-Livingstone, 1996. p. 1089–109.
117. Freireich EJ, Levin RH, Whang J, et al. The function and fate of transfused leukocytes from donors with chronic myelocytic leukemia in leukopenic recipients. Ann N Y Acad Sci 1965;113:1081–9.
118. Morse EE, Freireich EJ, Carbone PP, et al. The transfusion of leukocytes from donors with chronic myelocytic leukemia to patients with leukopenia. Transfusion 1966;6:183–8.
119. Schiffer CA, Aisner J, Dutcher JP, Wiernik PH. Sustained post-transfusion granulocyte count increments following transfusion of leukocytes obtained from donors with chronic myelogenous leukemia. Am J Hematol 1983;15:65–74.
120. Eyre HJ, Goldstein IM, Perry S, Graw RG Jr. Leukocyte transfusions: function of transfused granulocytes from donors with chronic myelocytic leukemia. Blood 1970;36:432–42.
121. Schwarzenberg L, Mathe G, Amiel JL, et al. A study of factors determining the usefulness and complica-

tions of leukocyte transfusions. Am J Med 1967; 43:206–13.

122. Schwarzenberg L, Mathe G, DeGrouchy J, et al. White blood cell transfusions. Isr Med J 1965;1:925–56.

123. Graw RG Jr, Herzig G, Perry S, Henderson ES. Normal granulocyte transfusion therapy. Treatment of septicemia due to gram-negative bacteria. N Engl J Med 1972;287:367–71.

124. Higby DJ, Yates JW, Henderson ES, Holland JF. Filtration leukapheresis for granulocyte transfusion therapy—clinical laboratory studies. N Engl J Med 1975;1292:761–6.

125. Alavi JB, Root RK, Djerrasi I, et al. A randomized clinical trial of granulocyte transfusions for infection in acute leukemia. N Engl J Med 1977;296:706–11.

126. Vogler WR, Winton EF. A controlled study of the efficacy of granulocyte transfusions in patients with neutropenia. Am J Med 1977;63:548–55.

127. Fortuny IE, Bloomfield CD, Hadlock DC, et al. Granulocyte transfusions: a controlled study in patients with acute nonlymphocytic leukemia. Transfusion 1975;15:548–58.

128. Winston DJ, Ho WG, Gale RP. Therapeutic granulocyte transfusions for documented infections. Ann Intern Med 1982;97:509–15.

129. Herzig GP, Graw RG Jr. Granulocyte transfusions for bacterial infections. In: Brown EB, editor. Progress in hematology. Vol. 9. Orlando, FL: Grune & Stratton; 1975. p. 209–25.

130. Herzig RH, Herzig GP, Graw RG Jr, et al. Successful granulocyte transfusion therapy for gram-negative septicemia. A prospective randomized controlled study. N Engl J Med 1977;296:701–5.

131. Epstein RB, Waxman FJ, Bennett BT, Andersen BR. *Pseudomonas* septicemia in neutropenic dogs. I. Treatment with granulocyte transfusions. Transfusion 1974;14:51–7.

132. Appelbaum FR, Bowles CA, Makuch RW, Deisseroth AB. Granulocyte transfusion therapy of experimental *Pseudomonas* septicemia: study of cell dose and collection technique. Blood 1978;52:323–31.

133. Epstein RB, Chow HS. An analysis of quantitative relationships of granulocyte transfusion therapy in canines. Transfusion 1981;21:360–2.

134. Ruthe RC, Andersen BR, Cunningham BL, Epstein RB. Efficacy of granulocyte transfusions in the control of systemic candidiasis in leukopenic host. Blood 1978;52:493–8.

135. Chow HS, Sarpel SC, Epstein RB. Experimental candidiasis in neutropenic dogs: tissue burden of infection and granulocyte transfusion effects. Blood 1982;59:328–33.

136. Bhatia S, McCullough J, Perry EH, et al. Granulocyte transfusion: efficacy in treating fungal infections in neutropenic patients following bone marrow transplantation. Transfusion 1994;34:226–32.

137. Price TH. Granulocyte colony-stimulating factor-mobilized granulocyte concentrate transfusion. Curr Opin Hematol 1998;5:381–95.

138. Dale DC, Liles WC, Llewellyn C, et al. Neutrophil transfusions: kinetics and function of neutrophils mobilized with granulocyte-colony-stimulating factor and dexamethasone. Transfusion 1998;38:713–21.

139. Dale DC, Liles WC. Return to granulocyte transfusion. Curr Opin Pediatr 2000;12:18–22.

140. Price TH. The current prospects for neutrophil transfusions for the treatment of granulocytopenic infected patients. Transfus Med Rev 2000;14:2–11.

141. Schiffer CA. Granulocyte transfusion therapy. Curr Opin Hematol 1999;6:3–7.

142. Gaviria JM, van Burik JA, Dale DC, et al. Modulation of neutrophil-mediated activity against the pseudo-hyphal form of *Candida albicans* by granulocyte colony-stimulating factor administered in vivo. J Infect Dis 1999;179:1301–4.

143. Peters C, Minkov M, Matthes-Martin S, et al. Leucocyte transfusions from rhG-CSF or prednisolone stimulated donors for treatment of severe infections in immunocompromised neutropenic patients. Br J Haematol 1999;106:689–96.

144. Price TH, Bowden RA, Boeckh M, et al. Phase I/II trial of neutrophil transfusion from donors stimulated with G-CSF and dexamethasone for treatment of patients with infections in hematopoietic stem cell transplantation. Blood 2000;95:3302–9.

145. Dutcher JP, Schiffer CA, Johnson GS. Rapid migration of [111]indium-labeled granulocytes to sites of infection. N Engl J Med 1981;304:586–9.

146. Arnold R, Pflieger H, Dietrich M, Heimpel H. The clinical efficacy of granulocyte transfusions: studies on the oral cavity. Blut 1977;35:405–14.

147. Hester JP, Kellogg RM, Mulzet AP, et al. Principles of blood separation and component extraction in a disposable continuous-flow single-stage channel. Blood 1979;54:254–68.

148. Wagner B, Moore R, Grima K, Dutcher JP. Granulocytopheresis efficiency: comparison of COBE 2997 to the COBE Spectra automated granulocyte protocol. J Clin Apheresis 1991;6:186. [abstract]

149. Huestis DW, White RF, Price MJ, Inman M. Use of hydroxyethyl starch to improve granulocyte collection in the Latham blood processor. Transfusion 1975;15:559–64.

150. Winton EF, Vogler WR. Development of a practical oral dexamethasone premedication schedule leading to improved granulocyte yields with the continuous flow centrifugal blood cell separator. Blood 1978;52:249–53.

151. Glasser L, Huestis DW, Jones JF. Functional capabilities of steroid-recruited neutrophils harvested for clinical transfusion. N Engl J Med 1977;297:1033–6.

152. Bensinger WI, Price TH, Dale DC, et al. The effects of daily recombinant human granulocyte colony-stimulating factor administration on normal granulocyte donors undergoing leukapheresis. Blood 1993;81:1883–8.

153. Caspar CB, Seger RA, Burger J, Gmur J. Effective stimulation of donors for granulocyte transfusions with recombinant methionyl granulocyte colony-stimulating factor. Blood 1993;81:2866–71.

154. Khwaja A, Carver JE, Linch DC. Interactions of granulocyte-macrophage colony-stimulating factor (CSF), and tumor necrosis factor α in the priming of the neutrophil respiratory burst. Blood 1992;79:745–53.

155. Ohsaka A, Kitagawa S, Sakamoto S, et al. In vivo activation of human neutrophil functions by administration of recombinant human granulocyte colony-stimulating factor in patients with malignant lymphoma. Blood 1989;74:2743–8.

156. Lindemann A, Herrmann F, Oster W, et al. Hematologic effects of recombinant granulocyte colony-stimulating factor in patients with malignancy. Blood 1989;74:2644–51.

157. Glasser L. Functional considerations of granulocyte concentrates used for clinical transfusions. Transfusion 1979,19.1–6.

158. Glasser L. Effect of storage on normal neutrophils collected by discontinuous-flow centrifugation leukapheresis. Blood 1977;50:1145–50.

159. McCullough J. Liquid preservation of granulocytes. Transfusion 1980;20:129–37.

160. Glasser L, Fiederlein RL, Huestis DW. Granulocyte concentrates: glucose concentration and glucose utilization during storage at 22°C. Transfusion 1985;25:68–9.

161. Price TH, Dale DC. Blood kinetics and in vivo chemotaxis of transfused neutrophils: effect of collection method, donor corticosteroid treatment, and short term storage. Blood 1979;54:977–86.

162. Christensen RD, Bradley PP, Rothstein G. The leukocyte left shift in clinical and experimental neonatal sepsis. J Pediatr 1981;98:101–5.

163. Strauss RG, Connett JE, Gale RP, et al. A controlled trial of prophylactic granulocyte transfusions during initial induction chemotherapy for acute myeloid leukemia. N Engl J Med 1981;305:597–603.

164. McCullough J, Clay ME, Loken MK, Hurd JJ. Effect of ABO incompatibility on fate in vivo of [111]indium granulocytes. Transfusion 1988;28:358–61.

165. McCullough J, Clay M, Hurd D, et al. Effect of leukocyte antibodies and HLA matching on the intravascular recovery, survival and tissue localization of 111-indium granulocytes. Blood 1986;67:522–8.

166. Dutcher JP, Schiffer CA, Johnston GS, et al. Alloimmunization prevents the migration of transfused [111]indium-labeled granulocytes to sites of infection. Blood 1983;62:354–60.

167. Dutcher JP, Riggs C, Fox JJ, et al. The effect of histocompatibility factors on pulmonary retention of indium-111-labeled granulocytes. Am J Hematol 1990;33:238–43.

168. Wright DG, Robichaud KJ, Pizzo PA, Deisseroth AB. Lethal pulmonary reactions associated with the combined use of amphotericin B and leukocyte transfusions. N Engl J Med 1981;304:1185–90.

169. Dana BW, Durie BGM, White RF, Huestis DW. Concomitant administration of granulocyte transfusions and amphotericin B in neutropenic patients: absence of significant pulmonary toxicity. Blood 1981;47:90–4.

170. Dutcher JP, Kendall J, Papenberg D, et al. Granulocyte transfusion therapy and amphotericin B: adverse reactions? Am J Hematol 1989;31:102–8.

171. Ford JM, Lucey JJ, Cullen MH, Tobias JS. Fatal graft-versus-host disease following transfusion of granulocytes from normal donors. Lancet 1976;2:1167–71.

172. Rosen RC, Huestis DW, Corrigan JJ. Acute leukemia and granulocyte transfusion: fatal graft-versus-host reaction following transfusion of cells obtained from normal donors. J Pediatr 1978;93:268–73.

173. Betzhold JB, Hong R. Fatal graft-versus-host disease after a small leukocyte transfusion in a patient with lymphoma and varicella. Pediatrics 1978;62:63–8.

174. Weiden PL, Zuckerman N, Hansen JA, et al. Fatal graft-versus-host disease in a patient with lymphoblastic leukemia after normal granulocyte transfusion. Blood 1981;57:328–32.

175. Ozer H, Armitage JO, Bennett CL, et al. 2000 update of recommendations of the use of hematopoietic colony-stimulating factors: evidence based, clinical practice guidelines. J Clin Oncol 2000;18:3558–85.

176. Dombret H, Chastang C, Fenaux P, et al. A controlled study of recombinant human granulocyte colony-stimulating factor in elderly patients after treatment for acute myeloid leukemia. AML Cooperative Study Group. N Engl J Med 1995;332:1678–83.

177. Rowe JM, Andersen JW, Mazza JJ, et al. A randomized placebo-controlled phase III study of granulocyte-macrophage colony-stimulating factor in adult patients (> 55 to 70 years of age) with acute myelogenous leukemia: a study of the Eastern Cooperative Oncology Group (E1490). Blood 1995;86:457–62.

178. Stone RM, Berg DT, George SL, et al. Granulocyte-macrophage colony-stimulating factor after initial chemotherapy for elderly patients with primary acute myelogenous leukemia: Cancer and Leukemia Group B. N Engl J Med 1995;332:1671–7.

179. Heil G, Hoelzer D, Sanz MA, et al. The International Acute Myeloid Leukemia Study Group: a randomized, double-blind, placebo controlled, phase III study of filgrastim in remission induction and consolidation therapy for adults with de novo acute myeloid leukemia. Blood 1997;90:4710–8.

180. Godwin JE, Kopecky KJ, Head DR, et al. A double-blind placebo-controlled trial of granulocyte colony-stimulating factor in elderly patients with previously untreated acute myeloid leukemia: a Southwest Oncology Group study (9031). Blood 1998;91:3607–15.

181. Lowenberg B, Boogaerts MA, Daenen SMGJ, et al. Value of different modalities of granulocyte-macrophage colony-stimulating factor applied during or after induction therapy of acute myeloid leukemia. J Clin Oncol 1997;15:3496–506.

182. Lowenberg B, Suciu S, Archimbaud E, et al. Use of recombinant GM-CSF during and after remission induction chemotherapy in patients aged 61 years and older with acute myeloid leukemia: final report of AML-111, a phase III randomized study of the Leukemia Cooperative Group of European Organisation of the Research and Treatment of Cancer and the Dutch-Belgian Hemato-Oncology Cooperative Group. Blood 1997;90:2952–61.

183. Zittoun R, Suciu S, Archimbaud E, et al. Granulocyte-macrophage colony-stimulating factor associated with induction treatment of acute myelogenous leukemia: a randomized trial by the European Organization for Research and Treatment of Cancer Leukemia Cooperative Group. J Clin Oncol 1996;14:2150–9.

184. Witz F, Sadoun A, Perrin M-C, et al. A placebo-controlled study of recombinant human granulocyte-macrophage colony-stimulating factor administered during and after induction treatment of de novo acute myelogenous leukemia in elderly patients. Blood 1998;91:2722–30.

185. Vadhan-Raj S, Keating M, LeMaistre A, et al. Effects of human granulocyte-macrophage colony-stimulating factor in patients with myelodysplastic syndromes. N Engl J Med 1987;317:1545–52.

186. Negrin RS, Nagler A, Kobayashi Y, et al. Maintenance treatment of patients with myelodysplastic syndromes using recombinant human granulocyte colony stimulating factor. Blood 1990;78:36–43.

187. Larson RA, Dodge RK, Linker CA, et al. A randomized controlled trial of filgrastim during remission induction and consolidation for adults with acute lymphoblastic leukemia. Blood 1998;92:1556–64.

188. Pui C, Boyett JM, Hughes WT, et al. Human granulocyte colony-stimulating factor after induction chemotherapy in children with acute lymphoblastic leukcmia. N Engl J Med 1997;336:1781–7.

189. Ottmann OG, Hoelzer D, Gracien E, et al. Concomitant granulocyte colony-stimulating factor and induction chemoradiotherapy in adult acute lymphoblastic leukemia: a randomized phase III trial. Blood 1995;86:444–50.

190. Welte K, Reiter A, Mempel K, et al. A randomized phase III study of the efficacy of granulocyte colony-stimulating factor in children with high-risk acute lymphoblastic leukemia. Blood 1996;87:3143–50.

191. Geissler K, Koller E, Hubmann E, et al. Granulocyte colony-stimulating factor as an adjunct to induction chemotherapy for adult acute lymphoblastic leukemia: a randomized phase III study. Blood 1997;90:590–6.

192. Scherrer R, Geissler K, Kyrle PA, et al. Granulocyte colony-stimulating factor (G-CSF) as an adjunct to induction chemotherapy of adult acute lymphoblastic leukemia (ALL). Ann Hematol 1993;66:283–9.

193. Laver J, Amylon M, Desai S, et al. Effects of r-metHuG-CSF in an intensive treatment for T-cell leukemia and advanced stage lymphoblastic lymphoma of childhood. A Pediatric Oncology Group pilot study. J Clin Oncol 1998;16:522–6.

194. Hughes WT. Treatment of established bacterial and fungal infections in patients with hematologic malignancy. In: Wiernik PH, Canellos GP, Dutcher JP, Kyle RA, editors. Neoplastic diseases of the blood. 3rd Ed. New York: Churchill-Livingstone; 1996. p. 1027–40.

195. Infectious Disease Society of America: Guidelines for use of antimicrobial agents in neutropenic patients with unexplained fever: a statement by the Infectious Diseases Society of America. J Infect Dis 1990;161:381–6.

196. Wade JC, Standiford HC, Drusano GL, et al. Potential of imipenem as single agent empiric antibiotic therapy for febrile neutropenic patients with cancer. Am J Med 1985;78:62–72.

197. Pizzo PA, Hathorn JW, Hiemenz J, et al. A randomized trial comparing ceftazidime alone with combination antibiotic therapy in patients with fever and neutropenia. N Engl J Med 1986;315:552–8.

198. Patrick CC. Coagulase-negative staphylococci: pathogens with increasing clinical significance. J Pediatr 1990;116:497–507.

199. Wade JC, Schimpff SC, Newman KA, et al. *Staphylococcus epidermidis*: an increasing cause of infection in patients with granulocytopenia. Ann Rev Intern Med 1982;97:503–8.

200. Maki DG. Infections caused by intravascular devices used for infusion therapy: pathogenesis, prevention, and management. In Bistro AI, Waldvogel FA, editors. Infections associated with indwelling medical devices. 2nd Ed. Washington, DC: ASM Press, 1994. p. 155–205.

201. Tenney JH, Moody MR, Newman KA, et al. Adherent microorganisms on lumenal surfaces of long-term intravenous catheters. Importance of *Staphylococcus epidermidis* in patients with cancer. Arch Intern Med 1986;146:1949–54.

202. Greene JN, Linch DA, Miller CB. Current treatments

230. Cooperative Group for the Study of Immunoglobulin in Chronic Lymphocytic Leukemia. Intravenous immunoglobulin for the prevention of infection in chronic lymphocytic leukemia. N Engl J Med 1988;319:902–7.

231. Weeks JC, Tierney MR, Weinstein MC. Cost effectiveness of prophylactic intravenous immune globulin in chronic lymphocytic leukemia. N Engl J Med 1991;325:81–6.

232. Stiehm ER. New uses of intravenous immune globulin. N Engl J Med 1991;325:123–5.

233. Dicato M, Chapel H, Gamm H, et al. Use of intravenous immunoglobulin in chronic lymphocytic leukemia. A brief review. Cancer 1991;68:1437–9.

234. Gamm H, Huber H, Chapel H, et al. Intravenous immune globulin in chronic lymphocytic leukemia. Clin Exp Immunol 1994;97 (Suppl 1):17–20.

235. Jurlander J, Hartmann GC, Hansen MM. Treatment of hypogammaglobulinaemia in chronic lymphocytic leukemia by low-dose intravenous gammaglobulin. Eur J Haematol 1994;53:114–8.

236. Wiernik PH, Serpick AA. Factors affecting remission and survival in adult acute non-lymphocytic leukemia. Medicine 1970;49:505–13.

237. McKee LC, Collins RD. Intravascular leukocyte thrombi and aggregates as a cause of morbidity and mortality in leukemia. Medicine 1974;53:463–78.

238. Fritz RD, Forkner CE, Freireich EJ, et al. The association of fatal intracranial hemorrhage and "blastic crisis" in patients with acute leukemia. N Engl J Med 1959;261:59–64.

239. Green RA, Nichols NJ, King EJ. Alveolar-capillary block due to leukemic infiltration of the lung. Am Rev Respir Dis 1959;80:895–901.

240. Resnick ME, Berkowitz RD, Rodman T. Diffuse interstitial leukemic infiltration of the lungs producing the alveolar-capillary block syndrome. Am J Med 1961;31:149–53.

241. Lester TJ, Johnson JW, Cuttner J. Pulmonary leukostasis as the single worst prognostic factor in patients with acute myelocytic leukemia and hyperleukocytosis. Am J Med 1975;79:43–8.

242. Lichtman MA, Rowe JM. Hyperleukocytic leukemias: rheological, clinical and therapeutic considerations. Blood 1982;60:279–84.

243. Vernant JP, Brun B, Mannoni P, Dreyfus B. Respiratory distress of hyperleukocytic granulocytic leukemias. Cancer 1979;44:264–71.

244. Bloom R, Taviera DA, Silva AM, Bracey A. Reversible respiratory failure due to intravascular leukostasis in chronic myelogenous leukemia. Am J Med 1979;67:679–84.

245. Eisenstaedt RS, Berkman EM. Rapid cytoreduction in acute leukemia: management of cerebral leukostasis by cell pheresis. Transfusion 1978;18:113–9.

246. Lane TA. Continuous-flow leukapheresis for rapid cytoreduction in leukemia. Transfusion 1980;20:455–61.

247. Meyer RJ, Cuttner J, Truog P, et al. Therapeutic leukopheresis of acute myelomonocytic leukemia in pregnancy. Med Pediatr Oncol 1978;4:77–82.

248. Schiffer CA. Therapeutic cytapheresis and plasma exchange. In: Wiernik PH, Canellos GP, Dutcher JP, Kyle RA, editors. Neoplastic diseases of the blood. 3rd ed. New York: Churchill-Livingstone; 1996. p. 1065–76.

249. Fortuny IE, Hadlock DC, Kennedy BJ, et al. The role of continuous flow centrifuge leucapheresis in the management of chronic lymphocytic leukaemia. Br J Haematol 1976;32:609–15.

250. Curtis JE, Hersh EM, Freireich EJ. Leukapheresis therapy of chronic lymphocytic leukemia. Blood 1972;39:163–75.

251. Goldfinger D, Capostagno V, Lowe C, et al. Use of long-term leukapheresis in the treatment of chronic lymphocytic leukemia. Transfusion 1980;20:450–4.

252. Cooper IA, Ding JD, Adams PB, et al. Intensive leukapheresis in the management of cytopenias in patients with chronic lymphocytic leukaemia and lymphocytic lymphoma. Am J Hematol 1979;6:387–98.

253. Mackower D, Venkatraj U, Dutcher JP, Wiernik PH. Occurrence of myeloma in a chronic lymphocytic leukemia patient after response to differentiation therapy with interleukin-4. Leuk Lymphoma 1996;23:617–9.

254. Talusan R, Dutcher JP, Wiernik PH. The use of large volume leukapheresis followed by full-dose rituximab in chronic lymphocytic leukemia. A case report. J Clin Apheresis 2001. [In press]

Index

Page numbers followed by f indicate figure. Pages numbers followed by t indicate table.

for infection in neutropenic patients with hematologic malignancy. Oncology 2000;14(Suppl 6):31–4.

203. Hughes W, Armstrong D, Bodey G, et al. 1997 guidelines for the use of antimicrobial agents in neutropenic patients with unexplained fever. Clin Infect Dis 1997;25:551–73.

204. DePauw BE, Raemaekers JMM, Schattenberg T, et al. Empirical and subsequent use of antibacterial agents in the febrile neutropenic patient. J Intern Med 1997;242:69–77.

205. Maki DG, Stolz SM, Wheeler S, Mermel LA. Prevention of central venous catheter-related bloodstream infection by use of an antiseptic-impregnated catheter. Ann Intern Med 1997;127:257–66.

206. Raad I, Darouiche R, Dupuis J, et al. Central venous catheters coated with minocycline and rifampin for the prevention of catheter-related colonization and bloodstream infections: a randomized double-blind trial. Ann Intern Med 1997;127:267–74.

207. Jaeger K, Osthaus JK, Heine J, et al. Efficacy of a benzalkonium chloride-impregnated central venous catheter to prevent catheter-associated infection in cancer patients. Chemotherapy 2001;47:50–5.

208. Winston DW, Hathorn JW, Schuster MG, et al. A multicenter, randomized trial of fluconazole versus amphotericin B for empiric antifungal therapy of febrile neutropenic patients with cancer. Am J Med 2000;108:282–9.

209. Sallah S. Hepatosplenic candidiasis in patients with acute leukemia: increasingly encountered complication. Anticancer Res 1999;19:757–60.

210. Woolley I, Curtis D, Szer J, et al. High dose cytosine arabinoside is a major risk factor for the development of hepatosplenic candidiasis in patients with leukemia. Leuk Lymphoma 1997;27:469–74.

211. Sallah S, Semelka R, Kelekis N, et al. Diagnosis and monitoring response to treatment of hepatosplenic candidiasis in patients with acute leukemia using magnetic resonance imaging. Acta Haematol 1998;100:77–81.

212. Rotstein C, Bow EJ, Laverdiere M, et al. Randomized placebo-controlled trial of fluconazole prophylaxis for neutropenic cancer patients: benefit based on purpose and intensity of cytotoxic therapy. The Canadian Fluconazole Prophylaxis Study Group. Clin Infect Dis 1999;28:331–40.

213. Wingard JR, Merz WG, Rinaldi MG, et al. Increase in *Candida krusei* infection among patients with bone marrow transplantation and neutropenia treated prophylactically with fluconazole. N Engl J Med 1991;325:1274–7.

214. Wingard JR, Merz WG, Rinaldi MG, et al. Association of *Torulopsis glabrata* infections with fluconazole prophylaxis in neutropenic bone marrow transplant patients. Antimicrob Agents Chemother 1993;37:1847–9.

215. Bradford CR, Prentice AG, Warnock DW, Copplestone JA. Comparison of the multiple dose pharmacokinetics of two formulations of itraconazole during remission induction for acute myeloblastic leukemia. J Antimicrob Chemother 1997;41:233–5.

216. Boogaerts MA, Verboef GE, Zachee P, et al. Antifungal prophylaxis with itraconazole in prolonged neutropenia: correlation with plasma levels. Mycoses 1989;32:103–8.

217. Glasmacher A, Molitor E, Hahn C, et al. Antifungal prophylaxis with itraconazole in neutropenic patients with acute leukaemia. Leukemia 1998;12:1338–43.

218. Caillot D, Bassaris H, Seifert WF, et al. Efficacy, safety, and pharmacokinetics of intravenous (IV) followed by oral intraconzole (ITR) in patients with invasive pulmonary aspergillosis. In: Proceedings of the 39th Interscience Conference on Antimicrobial Agents and Chemotherapy, London, 1999;39:574a. [abstract]

219. Morrison VA. The infectious complications of chronic lymphocytic leukemia. Semin Oncol 1998;25:98–106.

220. Anaissie EJ, Kontoyiannis DP, O'Brien S, et al. Infections in patients with chronic lymphocytic leukemia treated with fludarabine. Ann Intern Med 1998;129:559–66.

221. Tsiodras S, Samonis G, Keating MJ, Kontoyiannis DP. Infection and immunity in chronic lymphocytic leukemia. Mayo Clin Proc 2000;75:1039–54.

222. Morra E, Nosari A, Montillo M. Infectious complications in chronic lymphocytic leukaemia. Hematol Cell Ther 1999;41:145–51.

223. Nieves DS, James WD. Painful red nodules of the legs: a manifestation of chronic infection with gram-negative organisms. J Am Acad Dermatol 1999;41:319–21.

224. Watanakunakorn C. Multiple painful indurated erythematous nodular skin lesions associated with *Pseudomonas aeruginosa* septicemia. Clin Infect Dis 1998;27:662–3.

225. Melzer M, Colbridge M, Keenan F, et al. Cryptococcosis: an unusual opportunistic infection complicating B cell lymphoproliferative disorders. J Infect 1998;36:220–2.

226. Eftekhari P, Lassoued K, Oksenhendler E, et al. Severe respiratory syncytial virus pulmonary infection in a patient treated with fludarabine for chronic lymphocytic leukemia. Ann Hematol 1998;76:225–6.

227. Ansell SM, Li CY, Lloyd RV, Phyliky RL. Epstein-Barr virus infection in Richter's transformation. Am J Hematol 1999;60:99–104.

228. Lazzarino M, Orlandi E, Baldanti F, et al. The immunosuppression and potential for EBV reactivation of fludarabine combined with cyclophosphamide and dexamethasone in patients with lymphoproliferative disorders. Br J Haematol 1999;107:877–82.

229. Flynn IM, Byrd JC. Campath-1H monoclonal antibody therapy. Curr Opin Oncol 2000;12:574–81.